Obesity and Metabolic Surgery

Obesity and Metabolic Surgery

Editor: Ivan Robinson

FOSTER ACADEMICS

www.fosteracademics.com

www.fosteracademics.com

FOSTER ACADEMICS

Cataloging-in-Publication Data

Obesity and metabolic surgery / edited by Ivan Robinson.
p. cm.
Includes bibliographical references and index.
ISBN 978-1-64646-552-1
1. Obesity--Surgery. 2. Metabolism--Disorders--Surgery. 3. Surgery. I. Robinson, Ivan.
RD540 .O24 2023
61743--dc23

Foster Academics,
118-35 Queens Blvd., Suite 400,
Forest Hills, NY 11375, USA

ISBN 978-1-64646-552-1 (Hardback)

Contents

Preface IX

Chapter 1 **Do Bariatric Surgeries Enhance Brown/Beige Adipose Tissue Thermogenesis?** 1
Mohammed K. Hankir and Florian Seyfried

Chapter 2 **Obesity Surgery and Cancer: What Are the Unanswered Questions?** 12
Lidia Castagneto-Gissey, James Casella-Mariolo, Giovanni Casella and Geltrude Mingrone

Chapter 3 **Metabolic Surgery to Treat Obesity in Diabetic Kidney Disease, Chronic Kidney Disease and End-Stage Kidney Disease: What Are the Unanswered Questions?** 24
William P. Martin, James White, Francisco J. López-Hernández, Neil G. Docherty and Carel W. le Roux

Chapter 4 **Glucocorticoid Metabolism in Obesity and Following Weight Loss** 47
Elina Akalestou, Laurent Genser and Guy A. Rutter

Chapter 5 **Eligibility and Awareness Regarding Metabolic Surgery in Patients with Type 2 Diabetes Mellitus in the Real-World Clinical Setting: Estimate of Possible Diabetes Remission** 56
Chrysi Koliaki, Evangelia Tzeravini, Eleftheria Papachristoforou, Ioanna Severi, Elina El Deik, Melina Karaolia, Marina Noutsou, Anastasia Thanopoulou, Aikaterini Kountouri, Konstantinos Balampanis, Vaia Lambadiari, Nicholas Tentolouris and Alexander Kokkinos

Chapter 6 **Plasma N-Acetylaspartate is Related to Age, Obesity and Glucose Metabolism: Effects of Antidiabetic Treatment and Bariatric Surgery** 64
Giuseppe Daniele, Beatrice Campi, Alessandro Saba, Simone Codini, Annamaria Ciccarone, Laura Giusti, Stefano Del Prato, Russel L. Esterline and Ele Ferrannini

Chapter 7 **The Clinical Obesity Maintenance Model: A Theoretical Framework for Bariatric Psychology** 72
Jayanthi Raman, Dean Spirou, Lisbeth Jahren and Trine Tetlie Eik-Nes

Chapter 8 **Bariatric Surgery and Type 1 Diabetes: Unanswered Questions** 80
Emmanouil Korakas, Aikaterini Kountouri, Athanasios Raptis, Alexander Kokkinos and Vaia Lambadiari

Chapter 9 **Male Obesity Associated Gonadal Dysfunction and the Role of Bariatric Surgery** 92
Sana Sultan, Ameet G. Patel, Shamsi El-Hassani, Benjamin Whitelaw, Bianca M. Leca, Royce P. Vincent, Carel W. le Roux, Francesco Rubino, Simon J. B. Aywlin and Georgios K. Dimitriadis

Chapter 10 **The Impact of Post-Bariatric Abdominoplasty on Secondary Weight Regain after Roux-en-Y Gastric Bypass** 102
Jorunn Sandvik, Torstein Hole, Christian Klöckner, Bård Kulseng and Arne Wibe

Chapter 11 **Comparison of Short and Long-Term Outcomes of Metabolic and Bariatric Surgery in Adolescents and Adults** 110
Fatima Cody Stanford, Tasnim Mushannen, Priscilla Cortez, Karen J. Campoverde Reyes, Hang Lee, Denise W. Gee, Janey S. Pratt, Paul A. Boepple, Miriam A. Bredella, Madhusmita Misra and Vibha Singhal

Chapter 12 **The Effect of Metabolic Surgery on the Complications of Diabetes: What Are the Unanswered Questions?** 118
Karl J. Neff and Carel W. Le Roux

Chapter 13 **Bariatric Surgery Modulates Urinary Levels of MicroRNAs Involved in the Regulation of Renal Function** 127
Abdullah Alkandari, Hutan Ashrafian, Thozhukat Sathyapalan, Ara Darzi, Elaine Holmes, Thanos Athanasiou, Stephen L. Atkin and Nigel J. Gooderham

Chapter 14 **Metabolic and Endocrine Consequences of Bariatric Surgery** 137
Isabel Cornejo-Pareja, Mercedes Clemente-Postigo and Francisco J. Tinahones

Chapter 15 **Obesity-Related Epigenetic Changes after Bariatric Surgery** 162
Andrea G. Izquierdo and Ana B. Crujeiras

Chapter 16 **Diabetic and Elder Patients Experience Superior Cardiovascular Benefits after Gastric Bypass Induced Weight Loss** 174
Pedro R. Pereira, Marta Guimarães, Tiago Morais, Sofia S. Pereira, Mário Nora and Mariana P. Monteiro

Chapter 17 **Mechanisms Underlying Type 2 Diabetes Remission after Metabolic Surgery** 182
Belén Pérez-Pevida, Javier Escalada, Alexander D. Miras and Gema Frühbeck

Chapter 18 **Diabetic Ketoacidosis Post Bariatric Surgery** 191
Ivania M. Rizo and Caroline M. Apovian

Chapter 19 **Obesity, Male Reproductive Function and Bariatric Surgery** 195
Angelo Di Vincenzo, Luca Busetto, Roberto Vettor and Marco Rossato

Chapter 20 **Short-Term Changes in Mental, Physical, and Social Factors after Metabolic Bariatric Surgery in Adolescents** 204
Ariela Goldenshluger, Tamar Maor, Renana Via-Kagan, Orly Zelekha and Yftach Gepner

Chapter 21 **Altered Glucose Metabolism and Glucose Transporters in Systemic Organs after Bariatric Surgery** 211
Ju Hun Oh, Chan Woo Kang, Eun Kyung Wang, Jung Ho Nam, Soohyun Lee, Kyeong Hye Park, Eun Jig Lee, Arthur Cho and Cheol Ryong Ku

Chapter 22 **Metabolite Changes after Metabolic Surgery - Associations to Parameters Reflecting Glucose Homeostasis and Lipid Levels** 220
Sofie Ahlin, Consuelo Cefalo, Isabel Bondia-Pons, Kajetan Trošt, Esmeralda Capristo, Luca Marini, Montserrat Romero, Antonio Zorzano, Amalia Gastaldelli, Geltrude Mingrone and John J Nolan

Chapter 23 **Metabolic Surgery on Patients with Polycystic Ovary Syndrome** **229**
Wenwen Yue, Xin Huang, Wenjing Zhang, Shumin Li, Xu Liu, Yian Zhao, Jiaxin Shu, Teng Liu, Weihua Li and Shaozhuang Liu

Permissions

List of Contributors

Index

Preface

Obesity is a term used to describe a condition wherein a person's body has an excessive percentage of fat. Metabolic surgery is an effective and long-term treatment for managing the cases of morbid obesity. It leads to significant weight loss and helps improve, resolve or prevent a variety of related diseases such as hypertension, type-2 diabetes, sleep apnea, heart disease and some types of cancers. Metabolic surgery is highly effective in achieving significant and durable weight loss at a low perioperative risk when proper patient selection and long-term follow-up are ensured. It is also a potentially effective treatment option for type-2 diabetes patients who are obese. Metabolic surgery, also called bariatric surgery, involves making surgical changes in the organs of the digestive system in order to improve the health of the patient. Common surgical processes involved in metabolic surgery include sleeve gastrectomy, gastric bypass, bilio-pancreatic diversion, gastric band and duodenal switch. Within days to weeks after metabolic surgery, diabetes condition of the patient begins to improve. However, weight loss happens gradually. This book presents researches and studies performed by experts across the globe with respect to obesity and metabolic surgery. Those in search of information to further their knowledge will be greatly assisted by this book.

After months of intensive research and writing, this book is the end result of all who devoted their time and efforts in the initiation and progress of this book. It will surely be a source of reference in enhancing the required knowledge of the new developments in the area. During the course of developing this book, certain measures such as accuracy, authenticity and research focused analytical studies were given preference in order to produce a comprehensive book in the area of study.

This book would not have been possible without the efforts of the authors and the publisher. I extend my sincere thanks to them. Secondly, I express my gratitude to my family and well-wishers. And most importantly, I thank my students for constantly expressing their willingness and curiosity in enhancing their knowledge in the field, which encourages me to take up further research projects for the advancement of the area.

Editor

1

Do Bariatric Surgeries Enhance Brown/ Beige Adipose Tissue Thermogenesis?

Mohammed K. Hankir[1*] *and Florian Seyfried*[2]

[1] *Department of Experimental Surgery, University Hospital Wuerzburg, Wuerzburg, Germany,* [2] *Department of General, Visceral, Vascular and Pediatric Surgery, University Hospital Wuerzburg, Wuerzburg, Germany*

Correspondence:
Mohammed K. Hankir
hankir_m@ukw.de

Bariatric surgeries induce marked and durable weight loss in individuals with morbid obesity through powerful effects on both food intake and energy expenditure. While alterations in gut-brain communication are increasingly implicated in the improved eating behavior following bariatric surgeries, less is known about the mechanistic basis for energy expenditure changes. Brown adipose tissue (BAT) and beige adipose tissue (BeAT) have emerged as major regulators of whole-body energy metabolism in humans as well as in rodents due to their ability to convert the chemical energy in circulating glucose and fatty acids into heat. In this Review, we critically discuss the steadily growing evidence from preclinical and clinical studies suggesting that Roux-en-Y gastric bypass (RYGB) and vertical sleeve gastrectomy (VSG), the two most commonly performed bariatric surgeries, enhance BAT/BeAT thermogenesis. We address the documented mechanisms, highlight study limitations and finish by outlining unanswered questions in the subject. Further understanding how and to what extent bariatric surgeries enhance BAT/BeAT thermogenesis may not only aid in the development of improved obesity pharmacotherapies that safely and optimally target both sides of the energy balance equation, but also in the development of novel hyperglycemia and/or hyperlipidemia pharmacotherapies.

Keywords: Roux-en-Y gastric bypass, vertical sleeve gastrectomy, brown adipose tissue, beige adipose tissue, thermogenesis, obesity, uncoupling protein 1, molecular and thermal imaging

INTRODUCTION

The growing obesity pandemic is thought to primarily stem from the increased intake of processed, caloric-dense foods coupled with an overall less active way of life (1). Despite the major health complications, heightened mortality risk, and significant socioeconomic burden associated with obesity (2–4), currently available treatments are of generally limited efficacy with the exception of bariatric surgeries (5). Roux-en-Y gastric bypass (RYGB) and vertical sleeve gastrectomy (VSG) are the two most commonly opted for procedures in the clinic (6), and sustainably induce marked weight loss associated with a host of other health benefits (7, 8). However, these procedures are last-resort measures due to their irreversible nature, expense and potential for complications (9). It is therefore a pressing medical need to develop safer, noninvasive alternatives to bariatric surgeries with wider applicability, which will invariably require a deeper understanding of their mechanistic underpinnings.

Because of the way they alter gastrointestinal anatomy, RYGB and VSG were first mistakenly (and still commonly) assumed to physically limit energy intake solely through the malabsorption and/or volumetric restriction of ingested food (10). It is now clear; however, that RYGB and VSG both lower defended body fat mass through complex effects on physiology (11, 12). This, to a large extent in humans, engenders marked and lasting reductions in food intake driven by alterations in gut-brain communication (13, 14). On the other hand, numerous clinical studies indicate that RYGB and VSG paradoxically decrease resting energy expenditure within the first year after surgery (15), although when normalized to body weight or fat-free mass, this converts to an increase which scales with the weight loss that they achieve (16–18). Adding further to the uncertainty, the situation in preclinical models appears to be quite the opposite, since food intake suppression by both RYGB and VSG are transient (19), while for the former procedure, total energy expenditure increases when expressed in absolute terms (20–22), or when normalized to body weight (23–25). These considerations and caveats aside, RYGB has reproducibly been shown to enhance diet-induced thermogenesis across species (17, 18, 23, 26, 27). Furthermore, while only established so far in rodents (25, 28), both RYGB and VSG likely at least limit the decrease in total energy expenditure that usually accompanies weight loss in humans too (29), possibly playing a decisive role in the successful long-term maintenance of a negative energy balance post-operatively. Indeed, weight regain in patients 2 years following RYGB has been attributed to its diminished effects on energy expenditure (30).

Incentivized by the rediscovery of functional brown adipose tissue (BAT) by 18F-Flurodeoxyglucose positron emission tomography-computed tomography (^{18}F-FDG PET-CT) imaging in adult humans (31–37), surgical scientists wasted little time in addressing whether enhanced BAT thermogenesis may be responsible for the influences on total energy expenditure produced by RYGB and VSG described above. Similarly, the increased realization that energy-storing white adipose tissue (WAT) can adopt BAT-like characteristics by transforming into beige adipose tissue (BeAT) [also referred to as WAT "browning" (38)], has kindled interest in how RYGB and VSG may affect BeAT thermogenesis as well. In this Review, we will first provide a brief background to BAT and BeAT. We will then discuss, in chronological order, the steadily growing number of preclinical and clinical studies on the effects of RYGB and VSG on BAT and BeAT with particular emphasis on their methodology, limitations, mechanistic insights, and implications. We will finally highlight outstanding questions and present future perspectives.

BAT AND BeAT

Because of the high energy demands and circulating nutrient uptake by BAT, ^{18}F-FDG PET-CT imaging reveals the main classical depot in rodents and adult humans to be located in the interscapular region and the supraclavicular region, respectively (39). Physiologically, BAT is activated by sympathetic nerves when ambient temperatures drop to below thermoneutrality (referred to as temperature-induced thermogenesis) and during feeding (referred to as diet-induced thermogenesis) as part of physiological defense mechanisms in place to protect against hypothermia and weight gain, respectively (40, 41). Both these forms of adaptive thermogenesis absolutely depend on mitochondrial uncoupling protein 1 (UCP1) (42–45), a symporter embedded in the inner mitochondrial membrane that exothermically dissipates the proton gradient generated between the intermembrane space and the mitochondrial matrix by oxidative phosphorylation (46). Brown adipocytes are in fact optimized to generate heat in this way because of their high mitochondrial and UCP1 content as well as their multilocular morphology, which allows free fatty acids released by adrenergic-mediated lipolysis to efficiently activate UCP1 (47).

The anti-obesity potential of BAT was realized early on when its pharmacologic activation by selective beta 3 adrenergic receptor agonists protected leptin-deficient *ob/ob* mice and leptin receptor deficient *fa/fa* rats as well as wild-type rats on a high-fat diet from weight gain (48, 49). Furthermore, the sufficiency of BAT activation/expansion in protecting *ob/ob* mice and wild-type mice on a high-fat diet from weight gain has also been established (50). However, while acutely activating BAT with the selective beta 3 adrenergic agonist mirabegron or cold exposure markedly increases energy expenditure in healthy humans (37, 51), chronically activating/expanding BAT through daily mirabegron treatment, cold exposure or capsinoid treatment does not sufficiently cause weight loss *per se* (51, 52), although mirabegron treatment does markedly improve various aspects of glyceamic control (52). These findings suggest that in the clinical setting, recruiting BAT thermogenesis may better serve as an adjunct to promote and/or maintain weight loss and/or to exert other metabolic benefits (51, 52).

The term BeAT was coined to reflect its intermediate nature between WAT and BAT (38). BeAT forms when cells similar in size and morphology (multilocular and mitochondria-rich) and function (highly nutrient-consuming and thermogenic) to brown adipocytes arise in various WAT depots, most readily in subcutaneous WAT (such as the inguinal depot in rodents or the abdominal depot in humans), but also in visceral WAT [such as the gonadal depot in rodents and the omentum in humans (38)]. Evidence suggests that this can occur either through trans-differentiation of existing white adipocytes (53–57), or commitment of dedicated precursor cells (53, 58–60). As for BAT thermogenesis, BeAT thermogenesis is physiologically triggered in response to cold exposure and feeding through sympathetic nerve activation (61, 62).

Despite total BeAT depots quantitatively contributing $\sim$ 60% less than BAT to temperature-induced thermogenesis due to lower UCP1 protein content (63), chronic activation of inguinal or gonadal BeAT thermogenesis by a variety of pharmacologic and genetic manipulations are sufficient to cause weight loss or protect from weight gain in mice on a high-fat diet (64–66). However, as for BAT thermogenesis (52), chronic activation of abdominal subcutaneous BeAT thermogenesis by mirabegron treatment in prediabetic, obese humans does not lead to significant weight loss, but it does markedly improve glycaemic control (67).

RYGB AND BAT/BeAT THERMOGENESIS

An effective obesity treatment would in principle ideally target both sides of the energy balance equation. Indeed, evidence from preclinical studies suggests that in addition to suppressing food intake, liraglutide, which is a stable analog of the gut hormone glucagon-like peptide 1 (GLP-1) and 1 out of 5 currently approved obesity pharmacotherapies by the FDA (68), increases energy expenditure through stimulatory effects on BAT and BeAT thermogenesis (69, 70). However, this does not appear to be the case in diabetic patients (71), which may in part explain why liraglutide achieves relatively modest weight loss compared to bariatric surgeries in the clinic (5–10 vs. 20–30% within the first year, respectively) (72, 73).

In the first study attempting to address whether bariatric surgeries enhance BAT thermogenesis, Hankir et al. (74) performed small-animal ^{18}F-FDG PET-CT imaging on high-fat diet-induced obese RYGB-operated and sham-operated male Wistar rats following acute treatment with a selective beta-3 adrenergic receptor agonist. Unexpectedly, they found that BAT ^{18}F-FDG uptake was similar between surgical groups, as was BAT *Ucp1* mRNA expression determined by Northern Blot analysis following the same thermogenic stimulus (74). These findings provided early evidence against the outright enhancement of BAT thermogenesis by RYGB, although ^{18}F-FDG PET-CT imaging has more recently been shown not to reliably reflect UCP1 thermogenic function in BAT (75, 76). Moreover, no measurements were made of energy expenditure by indirect calorimetry or heat production in this particular study, precluding any definitive conclusions about the effects of RYGB on BAT thermogenesis (74).

In a subsequent more rigorous study using the same RYGB model as Hankir et al. (74) applied to high-fat diet-induced obese male Wistar rats, Abegg et al. (77) performed indirect calorimetry as well as core-body and BAT temperature measurements by radiotelemetry. Here, the authors also cleverly varied the ambient housing temperature from mild cold stress (22°C), typically used in most rodent studies, to thermoneutrality (32°C), with the expectation that any increase in oxygen consumption from enhanced temperature-induced BAT thermogenesis in RYGB-operated rats at 22°C would be abrogated at 32°C (77). In addition to an obese sham-operated group, they also incorporated a body weight-matched (BWM) sham-operated control group to assess the specific weight loss-independent effects of RYGB. Unexpectedly, but in line with the earlier findings of Hankir et al. (74), there were no differences in energy expenditure between obese sham-operated and RYGB-operated groups or BAT/core-body temperatures regardless of the ambient housing temperature. However, RYGB clearly prevented the marked drop in these measures that was found for the BWM sham-operated control group (77). These findings suggest that while RYGB may not enhance temperature-induced thermogenesis *per se*, it does prevent the marked decrease that typically occurs with weight loss. These findings are also in line with comparable indirect calorimetry experiments performed on high-fat diet-induced obese mice in which RYGB similarly prevented the decrease in energy expenditure that occurs in BWM sham-operated mice—both under mild cold stress conditions and thermoneutrality (25). Interestingly, RYGB-operated mice had almost a third higher energy expenditure compared to BWM sham-operated mice during the onset of the dark period when they normally eat, further suggesting that RYGB enhances diet-induced thermogenesis (25). One way this could be achieved is through enhanced post-prandial release of the BAT-stimulating gut hormone secretin (78). Indeed, RYGB has recently been shown to markedly enhance post-prandial release of secretin in obese patients at both 1 week and 3 months post-operatively (79), although how this influences BAT thermogenesis remains to be formally assessed.

Due to the lack of a clear stimulatory effect of RYGB on BAT function in the study of Hankir et al. (74), two independent studies published at about the same time then addressed the effects of RYGB on BeAT formation (80, 81). Again using high-fat diet-induced obese RYGB-operated and sham-operated male Wistar rats as well as a BWM sham-operated control group, Hankir et al. (80) measured the mRNA expression by RT-qPCR of various genes that are essential for the thermogenic program in adipocytes including those that encode the mitochondrial proteins UCP1 and Cidea (82), the nuclear receptor co-activator and regulator of mitochondrial biogenesis peroxisome proliferator associated receptor gamma co-activator-1 alpha (PGC1-alpha) (83) and PRD1-BF1-RIZ1 homologous domain containing 16 (Prdm16) (84), as well as BeAT-specific markers such as V-erbA-related protein (Ear2) and transmembrane protein 26 (Tmem26) (85) in inguinal WAT and gonadal WAT. This analysis somewhat disappointingly revealed that there were no differences between any of the groups studied (80), although administering a beta 3 adrenergic agonist may have unmasked BeAT formation (38). Notably, RYGB at least partially prevented the decrease in BAT *Ucp1* mRNA expression that was found in the BWM sham-operated group compared to the obese sham-operated group (80). However, it should stressed that *Ucp1* mRNA levels do not provide a reliable indicator of UCP1 thermogenic function (86, 87), and no oxygen consumption or heat production measurements were made in this particular study - again precluding any definitive conclusions.

In the other study assessing BeAT formation by RYGB, Neinast et al. (81) employed high-fat diet-induced obese female C57BL/6 mice, which is highly relevant since a vast majority of bariatric surgeries in the clinic are performed on women. It was unexpectedly found that RYGB-operated mice had increased *Ucp1* mRNA expression determined by RT-qPCR and UCP1 protein expression determined by representative immunohistochemistry in gonadal WAT as opposed to in inguinal WAT, compared to obese sham-operated and BWM sham-operated mice (81). Additionally, in line with the lack of a stimulatory effect of RYGB on BAT thermogenic markers in male rats described above, RYGB had no effect on BAT *Ucp1* mRNA and UCP1 protein expressions. In order to gain insight into the mechanisms behind increased gonadal BeAT formation after RYGB, the authors next turned their attention to natriuretic peptides and their receptors, which have established roles in stimulating BeAT thermogenesis (88). They found using RT-qPCR an increase in gonadal WAT mRNA expression of B-natriuretic peptide (*Nppb*) and natriuretic peptide receptor 2 (*Npr2*) in RYGB-operated mice compared to both obese and BWM sham-operated mice in association with an increase in mRNA expression of the beta-3 adrenergic receptor (*Adrb3*). Together, these data suggest that RYGB increases B-natriuretic peptide synthesis in gonadal WAT to cell-autonomously enhance natriuretic peptide receptor 2 signaling in association with increased sympathetic tone, thereby enhancing BeAT formation in a weight-loss independent manner (81). However, it should be kept in mind that the findings from this particular study were only observational in nature and no energy expenditure or heat production measurements were made. Future studies are required employing indirect calorimetry on mice lacking either B-natriuretic peptide or natriuretic peptide receptor 2 to establish if RYGB does indeed enhance BeAT thermogenesis through the aforementioned mechanism.

The enhanced BeAT formation by RYGB would receive further support in subsequent observational mouse studies. He et al. (89) demonstrated using RT-qPCR that *Ucp1* and *Prdm16* as well as thermogenic *Ucp3* (90) mRNA expressions are higher in both the subcutaneous WAT and gonadal WAT of RYGB-operated diet-induced obese male mice compared to obese sham-operated mice. Further, in a comprehensive tissue-wide translational study, Ben-Zvi et al. (91) demonstrated using RNA-sequencing that *Ucp1* and *Cidea* mRNA expressions are higher in the inguinal WAT of RYGB-operated high-fat diet-induced obese male C57BL/6 mice compared to BWM sham-operated mice, as was UCP1 protein expression determined by representative immunohistochemistry. Importantly, this was complemented with indirect calorimetry measurements which confirmed higher energy expenditure in RYGB-operated mice compared to BWM sham-operated mice (91). While the underlying causal mechanisms for enhanced BeAT thermogenesis after RYGB compared to chronic caloric restriction-induced weight loss were not established in this particular study, mRNA expression of the anti-inflammatory cytokine interleukin-33 (*Il33*) was markedly increased in the inguinal WAT of RYGB-operated mice (91). This is relevant since systemically administered IL-33 can potently induce iWAT browning through a complex localized immune cell response involving type 2 innate lymphoid cell-derived IL-13 and eosinophil-derived IL-4 converging on IL-4 receptors on beige adipocyte precursors to induce their differentiation (92). Furthermore, growth hormone receptor expression was markedly reduced for RYGB-operated mice compared to BWM sham-operated mice throughout different tissues (91), which in the hypothalamus has the remarkable effect of sufficiently preventing the drop in BAT thermogenesis that usually accompanies chronic caloric-restriction induced weight loss (93).

The findings discussed so far collectively suggest that RYGB enhances BeAT thermogenesis but not BAT thermogenesis. However, this has been challenged in the most recent study on the subject by Chen et al. (94). The authors performed small-animal 18F-FDG PET-CT imaging on high-fat diet-induced obese RYGB-operated and obese sham-operated male C57BL/6 mice following acute treatment with insulin. They found that BAT ^{18}F-FDG uptake on this occasion was increased by RYGB, but this simply means that BAT insulin sensitivity, as opposed to its thermogenic function, is enhanced (94). Nevertheless, RYGB increased BAT *Ucp1* and *Prdm16* mRNA expressions determined by RT-qPCR in association with increased energy expenditure determined by indirect calorimetry (94).

As informative as preclinical studies are, the ultimate goal is to understand if RYGB enhances BAT/BeAT thermogenesis in humans. Unfortunately, the number of clinical studies addressing this question is limited, likely due to the difficulties associated with obtaining ethical approval and recruiting patients. In an important early clinical study by Rachid et al. (95) addressing whether RYGB enhances BAT metabolic function, 12 obese, non-diabetic patients underwent 18F-FDG PET-CT imaging following acute cold exposure at baseline and 8 months post-operatively. To further establish whether RYGB enhances BAT thermogenic markers, supraclavicular biopsies were also collected at these time-points for gene expression analysis by RT-qPCR. It was found that while cold-induced supraclavicular BAT 18F-FDG uptake was unchanged by RYGB, *UCP1* mRNA expression increased (95) although how this would affect energy expenditure or heat production was not established. These findings are nevertheless in line with those of Piquer-Garcia et al. (96), who showed using infrared thermal imaging in 15 obese patients (9 with type 2 diabetes) that acute temperature-induced thermogenesis is not changed at 6 months after RYGB.

Concerning BeAT formation by RYGB, the tissue-wide RNA-sequencing translational study described above by Ben-Zvi et al. (91) revealed no effect on abdominal subcutaneous *UCP1* mRNA expression or any other standard thermogenic marker, although this was at a very early 1 month time-point post-operatively. Interestingly, in a study performed on 23 obese women by de Oliviera et al. (97) at baseline and the later 6 month time-point after RYGB, abdominal subcutaneous *UCP2* mRNA and perilipin 1 (PLIN1) mRNA expressions determined by RT-qPCR independently positively predicted weight loss. However, this did not correlate with the weight-adjusted increase in energy expenditure caused by RYGB (97). These preliminary findings nevertheless suggest that in humans, RYGB may increase BeAT thermogenesis through a UCP1-independent mechanism involving PLIN1-mediated fatty acid transfer from lipid droplets to UCP2. Under conditions of oxidative stress, potentially due to extensive remodeling of adipose tissue following RYGB, these liberated fatty acids could be rapidly oxidized to lipid hydroperoxides which activate UCP2-mediated proton transport and heat production (98).

VSG AND BAT/BeAT THERMOGENESIS

Unlike RYGB, VSG does not involve gastrointestinal reconfiguration so it can reasonably be assumed to have a different effect on BAT/BeAT thermogenesis. Indeed, while there is considerable overlap in terms of the physiological changes after both procedures (99), there are some noticeable differences such as their effects on the gut microbiota (100–105) which have reported roles in positively regulating BAT/BeAT thermogenesis (106–109). In the first study addressing whether VSG enhances BAT thermogenesis, Baraboi et al. (110) performed a comprehensive set of experiments on high-fat diet-induced obese VSG-operated and sham-operated as well as BWM sham-operated male Wistar rats including small-animal ^{18}F-Fluoro-6-thiaheptadecanoic acid (^{18}F-FTHA) and ^{11}C-acetate PET-CT imaging, which measure fatty acid utilization and mitochondrial beta oxidation, respectively, in conjunction with indirect calorimetry measurements (110). Similar to RYGB in rats described by Abegg et al. (77), VSG did not increase total energy expenditure, but it did prevent the drop that occurred in BWM sham-operated rats compared to obese sham-operated rats (110). Additionally, similar to RYGB in rats described by Hankir et al. (80), VSG prevented the drop in BAT *Ucp1* mRNA expression determined by RT-qPCR that occurred in BWM sham-operated rats compared to obese sham-operated rats (110). Interestingly, VSG increased both BAT ^{18}F-FTHA and ^{11}C-acetate uptake, indicating increased brown adipocyte fatty acid utilization and beta-oxidation, respectively, compared to both obese sham-operated and BWM sham-operated rats (110). These findings suggest that while VSG may enhance BAT thermogenesis, it is only sufficient to prevent the decrease in total energy expenditure that usually accompanies caloric restriction-induced weight loss rather than enhancing it overall. This is nevertheless consistent with a subsequent study by Moncada et al. (111) on high-fat diet-induced obese VSG-operated and obese sham-operated as well as pair-fed (PF) sham-operated male Wistar rats that underwent core-body temperature measurements. It was found that VSG increased core-body temperature compared to obese sham-operated rats in association with increased BAT UCP1 protein levels determined by Western Blot (111). Interestingly, the increase in these measures for VSG-operated rats compared to PF sham-operated rats was only noticeable in those not characterized as obesity-prone, suggesting that there is a genetic component to the effectiveness of VSG in enhancing BAT thermogenesis (111).

Having established that VSG consistently enhances BAT thermogenesis in rats, efforts were then made to elucidate the underlying mechanisms. Because plasma bile acids are known to be markedly increased by VSG (112), and agonists of the bile acid receptor TGR5 promote BAT thermogenesis in rodents and humans (113, 114), their role in enhanced BAT thermogenesis after VSG was tested in male high-fat diet-induced obese mice (115). First, it was shown that TGR5 knockout mice regained weight after VSG, unlike wild-type mice, and that this was despite similar food intake between genotypes (115). Accordingly, TGR5 knockout mice did not exhibit the increase in energy expenditure determined by indirect calorimetry after VSG that occurs in wild-type mice (115). In line with these findings, the increase in BAT *Ucp1, Ucp3,* and *Pgc1alpha* mRNA expressions determined by RT-qPCR caused by VSG in wild-type mice was not seen in TGR5 knockout mice (115). These results strongly suggest that the increase in circulating bile acids caused by VSG leads to TGR5-mediated enhancement in BAT thermogenesis thereby contributing to a negative whole-body energy balance (115). However, this conclusion would be more strongly supported by performing VSG on mice lacking TGR5 specifically in BAT.

To evaluate if VSG enhances BeAT formation and assess in detail the underlying mechanisms, Liu et al. (116) employed streptozotocin-induced diabetic VSG-operated, obese sham-operated and FR sham-operated male Sprague Dawley rats. It was found that VSG increased *Ucp1* and *Pgc1alpha* mRNA expressions determined by RT-qPCR as well as UCP1 and PGC-1alpha protein levels determined by both Western Blot and representative immunohistochemistry in inguinal WAT (116). This was associated with a strong (20-fold) increase in sirtuin 1 (*Sirt1*) and adiponectin (*Adipoq*) mRNA expressions and an increase in Sirt1 and adiponectin protein levels in inguinal WAT. Mechanistic experiments in cultured 3T3-L1 cells, a mouse white adipocyte cell line, then revealed that forced overexpression of adiponectin increased Sirtuin 1, UCP1, and PGC-1alpha protein levels. In turn, forced overexpression of Sirt1 increased AMPK activation determined by phosphorylated threonine 172 immunoblotting. Because AMPK can increase the expression of PGC-1alpha and UCP1 in BeAT (117), its causal role in BeAT formation after VSG was tested (115). Strikingly, chronic (1 month) weekly administration of the AMPK inhibitor compound C prevented the increase in *Ucp1* and *Pgc1alpha* mRNA expressions as well as UCP1 and PGC1-alpha protein levels in inguinal WAT caused by VSG (115). Taken together, these impressive results suggest that VSG first increases adiponectin expression and release from WAT, which in turn cell-autonomously increases SIRT1 and AMPK activities to drive BeAT formation (116). It is unfortunate however that no measurements of energy expenditure were made by indirect calorimetry in this particular study. Moreover, it is unclear how inhibition of BeAT formation by compound C may have affected body weight or any other metabolic parameter in VSG-operated animals.

In a recent study by Harris et al. (118) aimed at elucidating the weight loss-independent mechanisms behind improved glycaemic control following VSG, interesting effects on adipose tissue metabolic function and gene expression pertinent to thermogenesis were made. Non-obese C57Bl/6 male mice maintained on a normal chow diet first underwent VSG or sham surgeries. Two weeks later, they were orally administered ^{18}F-FDG and its tissue distribution after 1 h was quantified *ex vivo*. Remarkably, this revealed that VSG significantly increased ^{18}F-FDG uptake in iWAT and eWAT compared to sham surgery despite similar body weights and energy expenditure determined by indirect calorimetry between groups. Additionally, VSG-operated mice exhibited improved oral glucose tolerance and increased systemic carbohydrate metabolism (118). Since ^{18}F-FDG uptake by iWAT is increased by beta 3 adrenergic receptor agonist-induced and cold-induced browning (39), these findings provide further functional evidence of iWAT browning after VSG and novel evidence of eWAT browning and suggest that this contributes to improved glycaemic control but not to energy expenditure changes post-operatively. Interestingly, eWAT browning by VSG may be independent of sympathetic nervous system function, since neither chronic pharmacologic beta 3 adrenergic receptor activation nor cold exposure increases eWAT ^{18}F-FDG uptake (39). The authors further went on to show through RNA-sequencing that VSG reduces eWAT mRNA levels of suppressor of zeste 12 protein homolog (*Suz12*) which forms part of the polycomb repressor complex 2 (PRC2) (119). This could potentially contribute to reduced methyltransferase activity of PRC2, leading to reduced lysine 27 trimethylation of histone H3 at the *Ucp1* and *Pgc1alpha* promoters, thereby disinhibiting their transcription (119). It would be interesting in future studies to perform similar experiments as those of Harris et al. (118) on mice at later timepoints after VSG to assess its long-term effects on whole-body energy and glucose balance in relation to brown and beige adipose tissue thermogenesis.

Lastly, to ascertain the effects of bariatric surgery (8 RYGB and 15 VSG) on BAT function in humans, Dadson et al. (120) performed ^{18}F-FTHA PET-CT imaging on 23 obese patients (10 with type 2 diabetes) at baseline and 6 months post-operatively. It was found that bariatric surgery increased supraclavicular BAT ^{18}F-FTHA uptake to the level of lean controls. Notably, BAT triglyceride content was reduced by bariatric surgery as revealed by CT, which is a proxy of enhanced BAT thermogenesis (121). While this did not correlate with post-operative changes in energy expenditure determined by indirect calorimetry, it positively correlated with post-operative improvements in insulin sensitivity (120). The findings again suggest that while VSG may enhance BAT thermogenesis, this does not increase energy expenditure overall but may contribute to improved glycaemic control. The enhanced BAT thermogenesis by VSG would receive direct support in a subsequent study by Picquer-Garcia et al. (96). They demonstrated using infrared thermal imaging on 15 obese patients (5 with type 2 diabetes) that VSG significantly increased acute temperature-induced thermogenesis at the 6 month post-operative time-point.

Concerning the effects of VSG on BeAT formation, Jahansouz et al. (122) collected abdominal subcutaneous adipose tissue samples from 20 obese patients at baseline and 1 week post-operatively (122). Surprisingly, UCP1 protein levels determined by Western Blot were reduced by VSG. In contrast, *UCP2* mRNA,

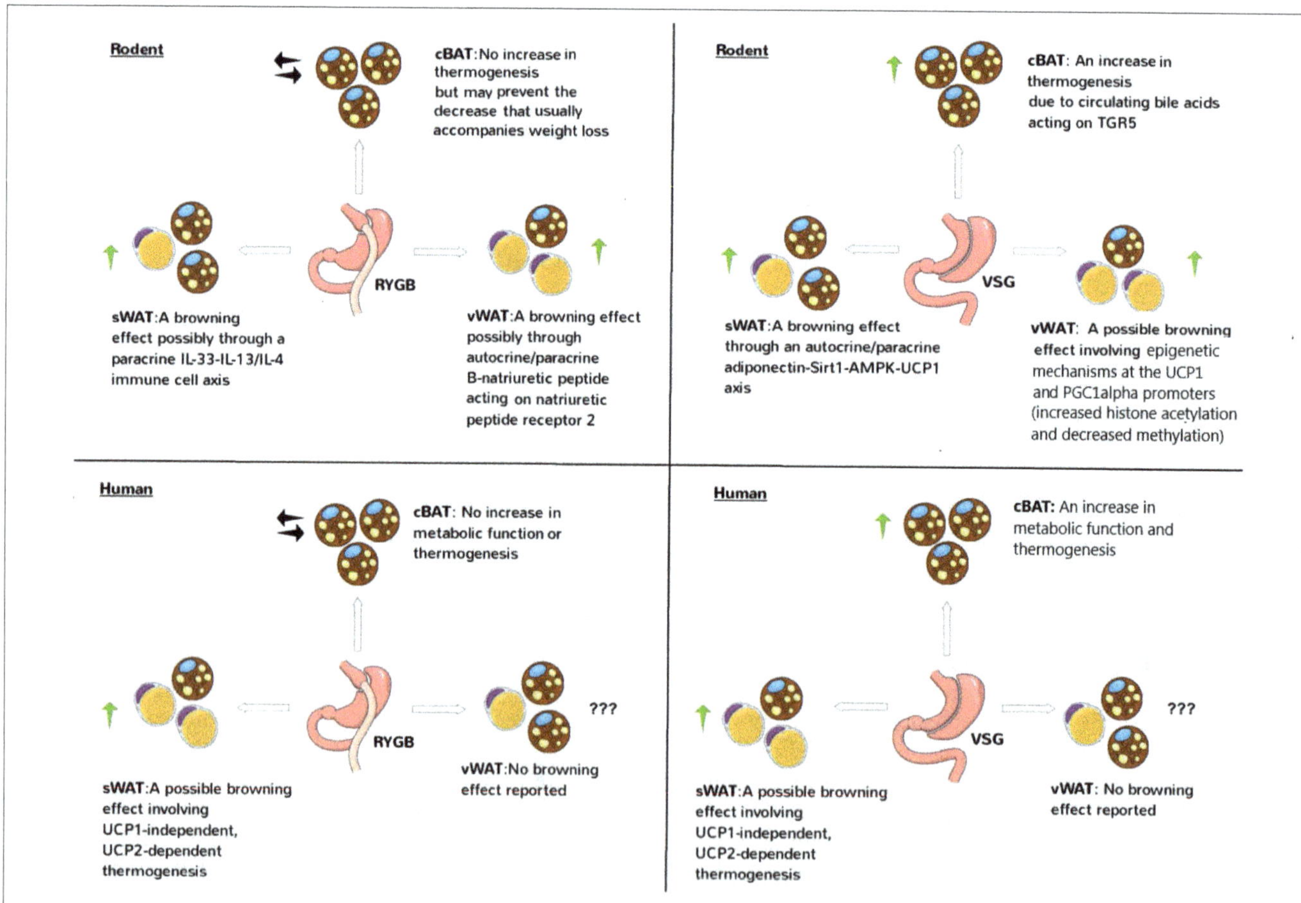

FIGURE 1 | Effects of RYGB and VSG on brown and beige adipose tissue thermogenesis in rodents and humans. The studies discussed in this Review generally show a stimulatory effect of RYGB and VSG on brown and/or beige adipose tissue thermogenesis involving canonical, UCP1-dependent or non-canonical, UCP1-independent mechanisms. cBAT refers to classical BAT which is the interscapular depot in rodents and supraclavicular depot in humans. sWAT refers to subcutaneous WAT which is the inguinal depot in rodents and abdominal depot in humans. vWAT refers to visceral WAT which is the epigonadal depot in rodents and omental depot in humans. Note how sWAT in rodents and vWAT in humans have more browning potential, respectively.

and *PLIN2* mRNA expressions in abdominal subcutaneous adipose tissue determined by RT-qPCR were increased by VSG which associated with a 15-fold higher beta-oxidation rate *ex vivo* (122). These findings are in line with those of Tarabra et al. (123) who collected abdominal subcutaneous adipose tissue from 4 to 9 obese girls at baseline and 10 months after VSG. It was found that VSG markedly increased PLIN1 protein levels determined by Western Blot with no changes in *UCP1* mRNA levels determined by RT-qPCR. However, VSG increased mRNA expression of *PGC1alpha, CIDEA, TBX1, and ADIPOQ.* Interestingly, they found that omental adipose tissue had greater *UCP1, PGC1alpha,* and *CIDEA* mRNA expressions determined by RT-qPCR and UCP1 protein expression revealed by representative immunohistochemistry than abdominal subcutaneous adipose tissue at baseline in these patients, which may have further increased following VSG. Together, the findings of Jahansouz et al. (122) and Tarabra et al. (123) intriguingly suggest that as for RYGB in humans described earlier (97), VSG may enhance (abdominal subcutaneous) BeAT thermogenesis through a UCP1-independent, PLIN1/2- and UCP2-dependent mechanism under conditions of oxidative stress.

CONCLUSIONS AND FUTURE STUDIES

The rodent and human studies discussed in this Review together suggest that RYGB mainly enhances BeAT thermogenesis while VSG mainly enhances BAT thermogenesis (**Figure 1**). Interestingly, in the rodent studies in which BAT/BeAT were not clearly recruited by RYGB (74, 77, 80), animals were post-operatively maintained on a low-fat diet unlike the high-fat diet used in other studies (81, 89, 91, 94). This suggests that high-fat diets are key determinants of BAT/BeAT thermogenesis post-operatively.

Apart for bile acids in the case for VSG, it is unclear which peripheral signals are causally required for enhanced BAT/BeAT thermogenesis after bariatric surgeries which could differ according to procedure. A role for GLP-1 and the co-released gut hormone peptide tyrosine tyrosine (PYY), the augmented post-prandrial levels of which are a hallmark of both RYGB and VSG (99), is at least unlikely for RYGB. This is because systemic and central administration of the GLP-1 receptor antagonist exendin-9 was shown not to influence total energy expenditure in RYGB-operated rats (124, 125) and mice with combined deficiency in the GLP-1 receptor and Y2 receptor remain fully protected by RYGB from the decrease in energy expenditure that usually accompanies caloric-restriction-induced weight loss (126). Postoperative shifts in the intestinal microbiota could also potentially be responsible, especially considering that their depletion by antibiotics prevents some of the metabolic benefits of VSG in diet-induced obese mice through effects on inguinal WAT (127). Moreover, the causal role of BAT/BeAT thermogenesis in weight loss after bariatric surgeries is still unclear. One way to formally address this issue is to perform VSG and RYGB on UCP1-deficient mice. In the event that these mice respond normally to bariatric surgeries, then a role for BAT/BeAT thermogenesis in causing weight loss post-operatively should not be fully discounted as UCP1-independent modes of thermogenesis are increasingly being described in BAT/BeAT (128). Indeed, a UCP1-independent form of thermogenesis involving AMPK in inguinal WAT has recently been shown (129), which may operate after VSG in particular (116).

The fact that increases in energy expenditure and BAT/BeAT thermogenesis seem to be weaker or even absent in humans compared to rodents and especially mice after RYGB and VSG (19), serves only to emphasize that animal models of bariatric surgeries can provide novel mechanisms for how to promote marked and lasting weight loss. Furthermore, a direct comparison between the effects of dieting-induced weight loss with RYGB and VSG on energy expenditure and BAT/BeAT thermogenesis still needs to be performed in humans, which may translate what has already been shown in rodents. Finally, it is possible that BAT/BeAT thermogenesis may play important roles beyond the body weight loss induced by bariatric surgeries, such as in improving glycaemic control and lipid homeostasis (52, 67, 130, 131).

AUTHOR CONTRIBUTIONS

MH wrote the manuscript and produced the figure. FS contributed to the manuscript.

REFERENCES

1. Swinburn BA, Sacks G, Hall KD, McPherson K, Finegood DT, Moodie ML, Gortmaker SL. The global obesity pandemic: shaped by global drivers and local environments. *Lancet.* (2011) 378:804–14. doi: 10.1016/S0140-6736(11)60813-1
2. Global BMI Mortality Collaboration, Di Angelantonio E, Bhupathiraju S, Wormser D, Gao P, Kaptoge S, et al. Body-mass index and all-cause mortality: individual-participant-data meta-analysis of 239 prospective studies in four continents. *Lancet.* (2016) 388:776–86. doi: 10.1016/S0140-6736(16)30175-1
3. Afshin A, Forouzanfar MH, Reitsma MB, Sur P, Estep K, Lee A, et al. Health effects of overweight and obesity in 195 countries over 25 Years. *N Engl J Med.* (2017) 377:13–27. doi: 10.1056/NEJMoa1614362
4. Kent S, Green J, Reeves G, Beral V, Gray A, Jebb SA, et al. Hospital costs in relation to body-mass index in 1.1 million women in England: a prospective cohort study. *Lancet Public Health.* (2017) 2:e214–22. doi: 10.1016/S2468-2667(17)30062-2
5. Bray GA, Fruhbeck G, Ryan DH, Wilding JP. Management of obesity. *Lancet.* (2016) 387:1947–56. doi: 10.1016/S0140-6736(16)00271-3
6. Welbourn R, Hollyman M, Kinsman R, Dixon J, Liem R, Ottosson J, et al. Bariatric surgery worldwide: baseline demographic description and one-year outcomes from the fourth IFSO global registry report 2018. *Obes Surg.* (2019) 29:782–95. doi: 10.1007/s11695-018-3593-1
7. Schauer PR, Bhatt DL, Kashyap SR. Bariatric surgery or intensive medical therapy for diabetes after 5 years. *N Engl J Med.* (2017) 376:1995–7. doi: 10.1056/NEJMoa1600869
8. Reges O, Greenland P, Dicker D, Leibowitz M, Hoshen M, Gofer I, et al. Association of bariatric surgery using laparoscopic banding, Roux-en-Y Gastric Bypass, or Laparoscopic sleeve gastrectomy vs usual care

obesity management with all-cause mortality. *JAMA.* (2018) 319:279–90. doi: 10.1001/jama.2017.20513

9. Lewis KH, Arterburn DE, Callaway K, Zhang F, Argetsinger S, Wallace J, et al. Risk of operative and nonoperative interventions up to 4 years after Roux-en-Y gastric bypass vs vertical sleeve gastrectomy in a Nationwide US commercial insurance claims database. *JAMA Netw Open.* (2019) 2:e1917603. doi: 10.1001/jamanetworkopen.2019.17603
10. Stefater MA, Wilson-Perez HE, Chambers AP, Sandoval DA, Seeley RJ. All bariatric surgeries are not created equal: insights from mechanistic comparisons. *Endocr Rev.* (2012) 33:595–622. doi: 10.1210/er.2011-1044
11. Evers SS, Sandoval DA, Seeley RJ. The physiology and molecular underpinnings of the effects of bariatric surgery on obesity and diabetes. *Annu Rev Physiol.* (2017) 79:313–34. doi: 10.1146/annurev-physiol-022516-034423
12. Hao Z, Mumphrey MB, Morrison CD, Munzberg H, Ye J, Berthoud HR. Does gastric bypass surgery change body weight set point? *Int J Obes Suppl.* (2016) 6:S37–43. doi: 10.1038/ijosup.2016.9
13. Hankir MK, Seyfried F, Miras AD, Cowley MA. Brain feeding circuits after Roux-en-Y gastric bypass. *Trends Endocrinol Metab.* (2018) 29:218–37. doi: 10.1016/j.tem.2018.01.009
14. Zakeri R, Batterham RL. Potential mechanisms underlying the effect of bariatric surgery on eating behaviour. *Curr Opin Endocrinol Diabetes Obes.* (2018) 25:3–11. doi: 10.1097/MED.0000000000000379
15. Lamarca F, Melendez-Araujo MS, de Toledo IP, Dutra ES, de Carvalho KMB. Relative energy expenditure decreases during the first year after bariatric surgery: a systematic review and meta-analysis. *Obes Surg.* (2019) 29:2648–59. doi: 10.1007/s11695-019-03934-0
16. Li K, Zheng L, Guo J, Shi W, Zhao F, Yang C, et al. Increased resting energy expenditure/body weight and decreased respiratory quotient correlate with satisfactory weight loss after sleeve gastrectomy: a 6-month follow-up. *Obes Surg.* (2020) 30:1410–6 doi: 10.1007/s11695-019-04308-2
17. Faria SL, Faria OP, Cardeal Mde A, Ito MK, Buffington C. Diet-induced thermogenesis and respiratory quotient after Roux-en-Y gastric bypass surgery: a prospective study. *Surg Obes Relat Dis.* (2014) 10:138–43. doi: 10.1016/j.soard.2013.09.020
18. Faria SL, Faria OP, Cardeal Mde A, de Gouvea HR, Buffington C. Diet-induced thermogenesis and respiratory quotient after Roux-en-Y gastric bypass. *Surg Obes Relat Dis.* (2012) 8:797–802. doi: 10.1016/j.soard.2012.06.008
19. Lutz TA, Bueter M. The use of rat and mouse models in bariatric surgery experiments. *Front Nutr.* (2016) 3:25. doi: 10.3389/fnut.2016.00025
20. Zechner JF, Mirshahi UL, Satapati S, Berglund ED, Rossi J, Scott MM, et al. Weight-independent effects of roux-en-Y gastric bypass on glucose homeostasis via melanocortin-4 receptors in mice and humans. *Gastroenterology.* (2013) 144:580–90.e7. doi: 10.1053/j.gastro.2012.11.022
21. Mokadem M, Zechner JF, Margolskee RF, Drucker DJ, Aguirre V. Effects of Roux-en-Y gastric bypass on energy and glucose homeostasis are preserved in two mouse models of functional glucagon-like peptide-1 deficiency. *Mol Metab.* (2014) 3:191–201. doi: 10.1016/j.molmet.2013.11.010
22. Nestoridi E, Kvas S, Kucharczyk J, Stylopoulos N. Resting energy expenditure and energetic cost of feeding are augmented after Roux-en-Y gastric bypass in obese mice. *Endocrinology.* (2012) 153:2234–44. doi: 10.1210/en.2011-2041
23. Bueter M, Lowenstein C, Olbers T, Wang M, Cluny NL, Bloom SR, et al. Gastric bypass increases energy expenditure in rats. *Gastroenterology.* (2010) 138:1845–53. doi: 10.1053/j.gastro.2009.11.012
24. Stylopoulos N, Hoppin AG, Kaplan LM. Roux-en-Y gastric bypass enhances energy expenditure and extends lifespan in diet-induced obese rats. *Obesity.* (2009) 17:1839–47. doi: 10.1038/oby.2009.207
25. Hao Z, Mumphrey MB, Townsend RL, Morrison CD, Munzberg H, Ye J, et al. Body composition, food intake, and energy expenditure in a murine model of Roux-en-Y gastric bypass surgery. *Obes Surg.* (2016) 26:2173–82. doi: 10.1007/s11695-016-2062-y
26. Wilms B, Ernst B, Schmid SM, Thurnheer M, Schultes B. Enhanced thermic effect of food after Roux-en-Y gastric bypass surgery. *J Clin Endocrinol Metab.* (2013) 98:3776–84. doi: 10.1210/jc.2013-1087
27. Werling M, Olbers T, Fandriks L, Bueter M, Lonroth H, Stenlof K, et al. Increased postprandial energy expenditure may explain superior long term weight loss after Roux-en-Y gastric bypass compared to vertical banded gastroplasty. *PLoS ONE.* (2013) 8:e60280. doi: 10.1371/journal.pone.0060280
28. Stefater MA, Perez-Tilve D, Chambers AP, Wilson-Perez HE, Sandoval DA, Berger J, et al. Sleeve gastrectomy induces loss of weight and fat mass in obese rats, but does not affect leptin sensitivity. *Gastroenterology.* (2010) 138:2426–36.e1–3. doi: 10.1053/j.gastro.2010.02.059
29. Leibel RL, Rosenbaum M, Hirsch J. Changes in energy expenditure resulting from altered body weight. *N Engl J Med.* (1995) 332:621–8. doi: 10.1056/NEJM199503093321001
30. Faria SL, Kelly E, Faria OP. Energy expenditure and weight regain in patients submitted to Roux-en-Y gastric bypass. *Obes Surg.* (2009) 19:856–9. doi: 10.1007/s11695-009-9842-6
31. Cypess AM, Lehman S, Williams G, Tal I, Rodman D, Goldfine AB, et al. Identification and importance of brown adipose tissue in adult humans. *N Engl J Med.* (2009) 360:1509–17. doi: 10.1056/NEJMoa0810780
32. Virtanen KA, Lidell ME, Orava J, Heglind M, Westergren R, Niemi T, et al. Functional brown adipose tissue in healthy adults. *N Engl J Med.* (2009) 360:1518–25. doi: 10.1056/NEJMoa0808949
33. van Marken Lichtenbelt WD, Vanhommerig JW, Smulders NM, Drossaerts JM, Kemerink GJ, Bouvy ND, et al. Cold-activated brown adipose tissue in healthy men. *N Engl J Med.* (2009) 360:1500–8. doi: 10.1056/NEJMoa0808718
34. Cohade C, Osman M, Pannu HK, Wahl RL. Uptake in supraclavicular area fat ("USA-Fat"): description on 18F-FDG PET/CT. *J Nucl Med.* (2003) 44:170–6.
35. Yeung HW, Grewal RK, Gonen M, Schoder H, Larson SM. Patterns of (18)F-FDG uptake in adipose tissue and muscle: a potential source of false-positives for PET. *J Nucl Med.* (2003) 44:1789–96.
36. Hany TF, Gharehpapagh E, Kamel EM, Buck A, Himms-Hagen J, von Schulthess GK. Brown adipose tissue: a factor to consider in symmetrical tracer uptake in the neck and upper chest region. *Eur J Nucl Med Mol Imaging.* (2002) 29:1393–8. doi: 10.1007/s00259-002-0902-6
37. Cypess AM, Weiner LS, Roberts-Toler C, Franquet Elia E, Kessler SH, Kahn PA, et al. Activation of human brown adipose tissue by a beta3-adrenergic receptor agonist. *Cell Metab.* (2015) 21:33–8. doi: 10.1016/j.cmet.2014.12.009
38. Harms M, Seale P. Brown and beige fat: development, function and therapeutic potential. *Nat Med.* (2013) 19:1252–63. doi: 10.1038/nm.3361
39. Zhang F, Hao G, Shao M, Nham K, An Y, Wang Q, et al. An adipose tissue atlas: an image-guided identification of human-like BAT and beige depots in rodents. *Cell Metab.* (2018) 27:252–62.e3. doi: 10.1016/j.cmet.2017.12.004
40. Nedergaard J, Cannon B. Brown adipose tissue as a heat-producing thermoeffector. *Handb Clin Neurol.* (2018) 156:137–52. doi: 10.1016/B978-0-444-63912-7.00009-6
41. Fischer AW, Schlein C, Cannon B, Heeren J, Nedergaard J. Intact innervation is essential for diet-induced recruitment of brown adipose tissue. *Am J Physiol Endocrinol Metab.* (2019) 316:E487–503. doi: 10.1152/ajpendo.00443.2018
42. Enerback S, Jacobsson A, Simpson EM, Guerra C, Yamashita H, Harper ME, et al. Mice lacking mitochondrial uncoupling protein are cold-sensitive but not obese. *Nature.* (1997) 387:90–4. doi: 10.1038/387090a0
43. Feldmann HM, Golozoubova V, Cannon B, Nedergaard J. UCP1 ablation induces obesity and abolishes diet-induced thermogenesis in mice exempt from thermal stress by living at thermoneutrality. *Cell Metab.* (2009) 9:203–9. doi: 10.1016/j.cmet.2008.12.014
44. von Essen G, Lindsund E, Cannon B, Nedergaard J. Adaptive facultative diet-induced thermogenesis in wild-type but not in UCP1-ablated mice. *Am J Physiol Endocrinol Metab.* (2017) 313:E515–27. doi: 10.1152/ajpendo.00097.2017
45. Golozoubova V, Hohtola E, Matthias A, Jacobsson A, Cannon B, Nedergaard J. Only UCP1 can mediate adaptive nonshivering thermogenesis in the cold. *FASEB J.* (2001) 15:2048–50. doi: 10.1096/fj.00-0536fje
46. Fedorenko A, Lishko PV, Kirichok Y. Mechanism of fatty-acid-dependent UCP1 uncoupling in brown fat mitochondria. *Cell.* (2012) 151:400–13. doi: 10.1016/j.cell.2012.09.010
47. Hankir MK. Loading and firing the brown adipocyte. *Adipocyte.* (2018) 7:4–11. doi: 10.1080/21623945.2017.1405879
48. Himms-Hagen J, Cui J, Danforth E Jr, Taatjes DJ, Lang SS, Waters BL, et al. Effect of CL-316,243, a thermogenic beta 3-agonist, on energy balance and

brown and white adipose tissues in rats. *Am J Physiol.* (1994) 266:R1371–82. doi: 10.1152/ajpregu.1994.266.4.R1371
49. Arch JR, Ainsworth AT, Ellis RD, Piercy V, Thody VE, Thurlby PL, et al. Treatment of obesity with thermogenic beta-adrenoceptor agonists: studies on BRL 26830A in rodents. *Int J Obes.* (1984) 1(Suppl. 8):1–11.
50. Pan D, Mao C, Quattrochi B, Friedline RH, Zhu LJ, Jung DY, et al. MicroRNA-378 controls classical brown fat expansion to counteract obesity. *Nat Commun.* (2014) 5:4725. doi: 10.1038/ncomms5725
51. Yoneshiro T, Aita S, Matsushita M, Kayahara T, Kameya T, Kawai Y, et al. Recruited brown adipose tissue as an antiobesity agent in humans. *J Clin Invest.* (2013) 123:3404–8. doi: 10.1172/JCI67803
52. O'Mara AE, Johnson JW, Linderman JD, Brychta RJ, McGehee S, Fletcher LA, et al. Chronic mirabegron treatment increases human brown fat, HDL cholesterol, and insulin sensitivity. *J Clin Invest.* (2020). doi: 10.1172/JCI131126. [Epub ahead of print].
53. Jiang Y, Berry DC, Graff JM. Distinct cellular and molecular mechanisms for β3 adrenergic receptor-induced beige adipocyte formation. *Elife.* (2017) 6:e30329. doi: 10.7554/eLife.30329
54. Himms-Hagen J, Melnyk A, Zingaretti MC, Ceresi E, Barbatelli G, Cinti S. Multilocular fat cells in WAT of CL-316243-treated rats derive directly from white adipocytes. *Am J Physiol Cell Physiol.* (2000) 279:C670–81. doi: 10.1152/ajpcell.2000.279.3.C670
55. Vitali A, Murano I, Zingaretti MC, Frontini A, Ricquier D, Cinti S. The adipose organ of obesity-prone C57BL/6J mice is composed of mixed white and brown adipocytes. *J Lipid Res.* (2012) 53:619–29. doi: 10.1194/jlr.M018846
56. Rosenwald M, Perdikari A, Rulicke T, Wolfrum C. Bi-directional interconversion of brite and white adipocytes. *Nat Cell Biol.* (2013) 15:659–67. doi: 10.1038/ncb2740
57. Barbatelli G, Murano I, Madsen L, Hao Q, Jimenez M, Kristiansen K, et al. The emergence of cold-induced brown adipocytes in mouse white fat depots is determined predominantly by white to brown adipocyte transdifferentiation. *Am J Physiol Endocrinol Metab.* (2010) 298:E1244–53. doi: 10.1152/ajpendo.00600.2009
58. Berry DC, Jiang Y, Graff JM. Mouse strains to study cold-inducible beige progenitors and beige adipocyte formation and function. *Nat Commun.* (2016) 7:10184. doi: 10.1038/ncomms10184
59. Wang QA, Tao C, Gupta RK, Scherer PE. Tracking adipogenesis during white adipose tissue development, expansion and regeneration. *Nat Med.* (2013) 19:1338–44. doi: 10.1038/nm.3324
60. Long JZ, Svensson KJ, Tsai L, Zeng X, Roh HC, Kong X, et al. A smooth muscle-like origin for beige adipocytes. *Cell Metab.* (2014) 19:810–20. doi: 10.1016/j.cmet.2014.03.025
61. Dodd GT, Andrews ZB, Simonds SE, Michael NJ, DeVeer M, Bruning JC, et al. A hypothalamic phosphatase switch coordinates energy expenditure with feeding. *Cell Metab.* (2017) 26:375–93.e7. doi: 10.1016/j.cmet.2017.08.001
62. Jiang H, Ding X, Cao Y, Wang H, Zeng W. Dense Intra-adipose sympathetic arborizations are essential for Cold-Induced Beiging of mouse white adipose tissue. *Cell Metab.* (2017) 26:686–92.e3. doi: 10.1016/j.cmet.2017.08.016
63. Shabalina IG, Petrovic N, de Jong JM, Kalinovich AV, Cannon B, Nedergaard J. UCP1 in brite/beige adipose tissue mitochondria is functionally thermogenic. *Cell Rep.* (2013) 5:1196–203. doi: 10.1016/j.celrep.2013.10.044
64. Hankir MK, Kranz M, Gnad T, Weiner J, Wagner S, Deuther-Conrad W, et al. A novel thermoregulatory role for PDE10A in mouse and human adipocytes. *EMBO Mol Med.* (2016) 8:796–812. doi: 10.15252/emmm.2015 06085
65. Seale P, Conroe HM, Estall J, Kajimura S, Frontini A, Ishibashi J, et al. Prdm16 determines the thermogenic program of subcutaneous white adipose tissue in mice. *J Clin Invest.* (2011) 121:96–105. doi: 10.1172/JCI44271
66. Yu J, Lv Y, Wang F, Kong X, Di W, Liu J, et al. MiR-27b-3p inhibition enhances browning of epididymal fat in high-fat diet induced obese mice. *Front Endocrinol.* (2019) 10:38. doi: 10.3389/fendo.2019.00038
67. Finlin BS, Memetimin H, Zhu B, Confides AL, Vekaria HJ, El Khouli RH, et al. The beta3-adrenergic receptor agonist mirabegron improves glucose homeostasis in obese humans. *J Clin Invest.* (2020). doi: 10.1172/JCI134892. [Epub ahead of print].
68. May M, Schindler C, Engeli S. Modern pharmacological treatment of obese patients. *Ther Adv Endocrinol Metab.* (2020) 11:2042018819897527. doi: 10.1177/2042018819897527
69. Zhou J, Poudel A, Chandramani-Shivalingappa P, Xu B, Welchko R, Li L. Liraglutide induces beige fat development and promotes mitochondrial function in diet induced obesity mice partially through AMPK-SIRT-1-PGC1-alpha cell signaling pathway. *Endocrine.* (2019) 64:271–83. doi: 10.1007/s12020-018-1826-7
70. Zhu E, Yang Y, Zhang J, Li Y, Li C, Chen L, et al. Liraglutide suppresses obesity and induces brown fat-like phenotype via Soluble Guanylyl Cyclase mediated pathway *in vivo* and *in vitro*. *Oncotarget.* (2016) 7:81077–89. doi: 10.18632/oncotarget.13189
71. van Eyk HJ, Paiman EHM, Bizino MB, IJzermans SL, Kleiburg F, Boers TGW, et al. Liraglutide decreases energy expenditure and does not affect the fat fraction of supraclavicular brown adipose tissue in patients with type 2 diabetes. *Nutr Metab Cardiovasc Dis.* (2019) 30:616–24. doi: 10.1016/j.numecd.2019.12.005
72. Astrup A, Rossner S, Van Gaal L, Rissanen A, Niskanen L, Al Hakim M, et al. Effects of liraglutide in the treatment of obesity: a randomised, double-blind, placebo-controlled study. *Lancet.* (2009) 374:1606–16. doi: 10.1016/S0140-6736(09)61375-1
73. Arterburn DE, Johnson E, Coleman KJ, Herrinton LJ, Courcoulas AP, Fisher D, et al. Weight outcomes of sleeve gastrectomy and gastric bypass compared to nonsurgical treatment. *Ann Surg.* (2020). doi: 10.1097/SLA.0000000000003826. [Epub ahead of print].
74. Hankir M, Bueter M, Gsell W, Seyfried F, Khalil M, Smith KL, et al. Increased energy expenditure in gastric bypass rats is not caused by activated brown adipose tissue. *Obes Facts.* (2012) 5:349–58. doi: 10.1159/000339742
75. Hankir MK, Kranz M, Keipert S, Weiner J, Andreasen SG, Kern M, et al. Dissociation between brown adipose tissue (18)F-FDG uptake and thermogenesis in uncoupling protein 1-deficient mice. *J Nucl Med.* (2017) 58:1100–3. doi: 10.2967/jnumed.116.186460
76. Olsen JM, Csikasz RI, Dehvari N, Lu L, Sandstrom A, Oberg AI, et al. β3-Adrenergically induced glucose uptake in brown adipose tissue is independent of UCP1 presence or activity: Mediation through the mTOR pathway. *Mol Metab.* (2017) 6:611–9. doi: 10.1016/j.molmet.2017.02.006
77. Abegg K, Corteville C, Bueter M, Lutz TA. Alterations in energy expenditure in Roux-en-Y gastric bypass rats persist at thermoneutrality. *Int J Obes.* (2016) 40:1215–21. doi: 10.1038/ijo.2016.55
78. Li Y, Schnabl K, Gabler SM, Willershauser M, Reber J, Karlas A, et al. Secretin-activated brown fat mediates prandial thermogenesis to induce satiation. *Cell.* (2018) 175:1561–74.e12. doi: 10.1016/j.cell.2018.10.016
79. Modvig IM, Andersen DB, Grunddal KV, Kuhre RE, Martinussen C, Christiansen CB, et al. Secretin release after Roux-en-Y gastric bypass reveals a population of glucose-sensitive S cells in distal small intestine. *Int J Obes.* (2020). doi: 10.1038/s41366-020-0541-7. [Epub ahead of print].
80. Hankir MK, Bronisch F, Hintschich C, Krugel U, Seyfried F, Fenske WK. Differential effects of Roux-en-Y gastric bypass surgery on brown and beige adipose tissue thermogenesis. *Metabolism.* (2015) 64:1240–9. doi: 10.1016/j.metabol.2015.06.010
81. Neinast MD, Frank AP, Zechner JF, Li Q, Vishvanath L, Palmer BF, et al. Activation of natriuretic peptides and the sympathetic nervous system following Roux-en-Y gastric bypass is associated with gonadal adipose tissues browning. *Mol Metab.* (2015) 4:427–36. doi: 10.1016/j.molmet.2015.02.006
82. Zhou Z, Yon Toh S, Chen Z, Guo K, Ng CP, Ponniah S, et al. Cidea-deficient mice have lean phenotype and are resistant to obesity. *Nat Genet.* (2003) 35:49–56. doi: 10.1038/ng1225
83. Puigserver P, Wu Z, Park CW, Graves R, Wright M, Spiegelman BM. A cold-inducible coactivator of nuclear receptors linked to adaptive thermogenesis. *Cell.* (1998) 92:829–39. doi: 10.1016/S0092-8674(00)81410-5
84. Seale P, Kajimura S, Yang W, Chin S, Rohas LM, Uldry M, et al. Transcriptional control of brown fat determination by PRDM16. *Cell Metab.* (2007) 6:38–54. doi: 10.1016/j.cmet.2007.06.001
85. Wu J, Bostrom P, Sparks LM, Ye L, Choi JH, Giang AH, et al. Beige adipocytes are a distinct type of thermogenic fat cell in mouse and human. *Cell.* (2012) 150:366–76. doi: 10.1016/j.cell.2012.05.016
86. Bertholet AM, Kazak L, Chouchani ET, Bogaczynska MG, Paranjpe I, Wainwright GL, et al. Mitochondrial patch clamp of beige adipocytes

reveals UCP1-positive and UCP1-negative cells both exhibiting futile creatine cycling. *Cell Metab.* (2017) 25:811–22.e4. doi: 10.1016/j.cmet.2017.03.002

87. Nedergaard J, Cannon B. UCP1 mRNA does not produce heat. *Biochim Biophys Acta.* (2013) 1831:943–9. doi: 10.1016/j.bbalip.2013.01.009
88. Bordicchia M, Liu D, Amri EZ, Ailhaud G, Dessi-Fulgheri P, Zhang C, et al. Cardiac natriuretic peptides act via p38 MAPK to induce the brown fat thermogenic program in mouse and human adipocytes. *J Clin Invest.* (2012) 122:1022–36. doi: 10.1172/JCI59701
89. He R, Yin Y, Li Y, Li Z, Zhao J, Zhang W. Esophagus-duodenum gastric bypass surgery improves glucose and lipid metabolism in mice. *EBioMedicine.* (2018) 28:241–50. doi: 10.1016/j.ebiom.2018.01.032
90. Gong DW, He Y, Karas M, Reitman M. Uncoupling protein-3 is a mediator of thermogenesis regulated by thyroid hormone, beta3-adrenergic agonists, and leptin. *J Biol Chem.* (1997) 272:24129–32. doi: 10.1074/jbc.272.39.24129
91. Ben-Zvi D, Meoli L, Abidi WM, Nestoridi E, Panciotti C, Castillo E, et al. Time-dependent molecular responses differ between gastric bypass and dieting but are conserved across species. *Cell Metab.* (2018) 28:310–23.e6. doi: 10.1016/j.cmet.2018.06.004
92. Lee MW, Odegaard JI, Mukundan L, Qiu Y, Molofsky AB, Nussbaum JC, et al. Activated type 2 innate lymphoid cells regulate beige fat biogenesis. *Cell.* (2015) 160:74–87. doi: 10.1016/j.cell.2014.12.011
93. Furigo IC, P.Teixeira DS, de Souza GO, Couto GCL, Romero GG, Perello M, et al. Growth hormone regulates neuroendocrine responses to weight loss via AgRP neurons. *Nat Commun.* (2019) 10:662. doi: 10.1038/s41467-019-08607-1
94. Chen Y, Yang J, Nie X, Song Z, Gu Y. Effects of bariatric surgery on change of brown adipocyte tissue and energy metabolism in obese mice. *Obes Surg.* (2018) 28:820–30. doi: 10.1007/s11695-017-2899-8
95. Rachid B, van de Sande-Lee S, Rodovalho S, Folli F, Beltramini GC, Morari J, et al. Distinct regulation of hypothalamic and brown/beige adipose tissue activities in human obesity. *Int J Obes.* (2015) 39:1515–22. doi: 10.1038/ijo.2015.94
96. Piquer-Garcia I, Cereijo R, Corral-Perez J, Pellitero S, Martinez E, Taxeras SD, et al. Use of infrared thermography to estimate brown fat activation after a cooling protocol in patients with severe obesity that underwent bariatric surgery. *Obes Surg.* (2020). doi: 10.1007/s11695-020-04502-7. [Epub ahead of print].
97. de Oliveira BAP, de Souza Pinhel MA, Nicoletti CF, de Oliveira CC, Quinhoneiro DCG, Noronha NY, et al. UCP2 and PLIN1 expression affects the resting metabolic rate and weight loss on obese patients. *Obes Surg.* (2017) 27:343–8. doi: 10.1007/s11695-016-2275-0
98. Diano S, Horvath TL. Mitochondrial uncoupling protein 2 (UCP2) in glucose and lipid metabolism. *Trends Mol Med.* (2012) 18:52–8. doi: 10.1016/j.molmed.2011.08.003
99. Kim KS, Sandoval DA. Endocrine function after bariatric surgery. *Compr Physiol.* (2017) 7:783–98. doi: 10.1002/cphy.c160019
100. Chen G, Zhuang J, Cui Q, Jiang S, Tao W, Chen W, et al. Two bariatric surgical procedures differentially alter the intestinal microbiota in obesity patients. *Obes Surg.* (2020). doi: 10.1007/s11695-020-04494-4. [Epub ahead of print].
101. Duboc H, Nguyen CC, Cavin JB, Ribeiro-Parenti L, Jarry AC, Rainteau D, et al. Roux-en-Y Gastric-Bypass and sleeve gastrectomy induces specific shifts of the gut microbiota without altering the metabolism of bile acids in the intestinal lumen. *Int J Obes.* (2019) 43:428–31. doi: 10.1038/s41366-018-0015-3
102. Murphy R, Tsai P, Jullig M, Liu A, Plank L, Booth M. Differential changes in gut microbiota after gastric bypass and sleeve gastrectomy bariatric surgery vary according to diabetes remission. *Obes Surg.* (2017) 27:917–25. doi: 10.1007/s11695-016-2399-2
103. Sanchez-Alcoholado L, Gutierrez-Repiso C, Gomez-Perez AM, Garcia-Fuentes E, Tinahones FJ, Moreno-Indias I. Gut microbiota adaptation after weight loss by Roux-en-Y gastric bypass or sleeve gastrectomy bariatric surgeries. *Surg Obes Relat Dis.* (2019) 15:1888–95. doi: 10.1016/j.soard.2019.08.551
104. Shao Y, Ding R, Xu B, Hua R, Shen Q, He K, et al. Alterations of gut microbiota after Roux-en-Y gastric bypass and sleeve gastrectomy in sprague-dawley rats. *Obes Surg.* (2017) 27:295–302. doi: 10.1007/s11695-016-2297-7
105. Arble DM, Evers SS, Bozadjieva N, Frikke-Schmidt H, Myronovych A, Lewis A, et al. Metabolic comparison of one-anastomosis gastric bypass, single-anastomosis duodenal-switch, Roux-en-Y gastric bypass, and vertical sleeve gastrectomy in rat. *Surg Obes Relat Dis.* (2018) 14:1857–67. doi: 10.1016/j.soard.2018.08.019
106. Li B, Li L, Li M, Lam SM, Wang G, Wu Y, et al. Microbiota depletion impairs thermogenesis of brown adipose tissue and browning of white adipose tissue. *Cell Rep.* (2019) 26:2720–37.e5. doi: 10.1016/j.celrep.2019.02.015
107. Worthmann A, John C, Ruhlemann MC, Baguhl M, Heinsen FA, Schaltenberg N, et al. Cold-induced conversion of cholesterol to bile acids in mice shapes the gut microbiome and promotes adaptive thermogenesis. *Nat Med.* (2017) 23:839–49. doi: 10.1038/nm.4357
108. Zietak M, Kovatcheva-Datchary P, Markiewicz LH, Stahlman M, Kozak LP, Backhed F. Altered microbiota contributes to reduced diet-induced obesity upon cold exposure. *Cell. Metab.* (2016) 23:1216–23. doi: 10.1016/j.cmet.2016.05.001
109. Chevalier C, Stojanovic O, Colin DJ, Suarez-Zamorano N, Tarallo V, Veyrat-Durebex C, et al. Gut microbiota orchestrates energy homeostasis during cold. *Cell.* (2015) 163:1360–74. doi: 10.1016/j.cell.2015.11.004
110. Baraboi ED, Li W, Labbe SM, Roy MC, Samson P, Hould FS, et al. Metabolic changes induced by the biliopancreatic diversion in diet-induced obesity in male rats: the contributions of sleeve gastrectomy and duodenal switch. *Endocrinology.* (2015) 156:1316–29. doi: 10.1210/en.2014-1785
111. Moncada R, Becerril S, Rodriguez A, Mendez-Gimenez L, Ramirez B, Catalan V, et al. Sleeve gastrectomy reduces body weight and improves metabolic profile also in obesity-prone rats. *Obes Surg.* (2016) 26:1537–48. doi: 10.1007/s11695-015-1915-0
112. Myronovych A, Kirby M, Ryan KK, Zhang W, Jha P, Setchell KD, et al. Vertical sleeve gastrectomy reduces hepatic steatosis while increasing serum bile acids in a weight-loss-independent manner. *Obesity.* (2014) 22:390–400. doi: 10.1002/oby.20548
113. Watanabe M, Houten SM, Mataki C, Christoffolete MA, Kim BW, Sato H, et al. Bile acids induce energy expenditure by promoting intracellular thyroid hormone activation. *Nature.* (2006) 439:484–9. doi: 10.1038/nature04330
114. Broeders EP, Nascimento EB, Havekes B, Brans B, Roumans KH, Tailleux A, et al. The bile acid chenodeoxycholic acid increases human brown adipose tissue activity. *Cell Metab.* (2015) 22:418–26. doi: 10.1016/j.cmet.2015.07.002
115. Ding L, Sousa KM, Jin L, Dong B, Kim BW, Ramirez R, et al. Vertical sleeve gastrectomy activates GPBAR-1/TGR5 to sustain weight loss, improve fatty liver, and remit insulin resistance in mice. *Hepatology.* (2016) 64:760–73. doi: 10.1002/hep.28689
116. Liu L, Zhang T, Hu J, Ma R, He B, Wang M, et al. Adiponectin/SIRT1 axis induces white adipose browning after vertical sleeve gastrectomy of obese rats with type 2 diabetes. *Obes Surg.* (2019) 30:1392–403. doi: 10.1007/s11695-019-04295-4
117. Shan T, Liang X, Bi P, Kuang S. Myostatin knockout drives browning of white adipose tissue through activating the AMPK-PGC1alpha-Fndc5 pathway in muscle. *FASEB J.* (2013) 27:1981–9. doi: 10.1096/fj.12-225755
118. Harris DA, Mina A, Cabarkapa D, Heshmati K, Subramaniam R, Banks AS, et al. Sleeve gastrectomy enhances glucose utilization and remodels adipose tissue independent of weight loss. *Am J Physiol Endocrinol Metab.* (2020). doi: 10.1152/ajpendo.00441.2019. [Epub ahead of print].
119. Li F, Wu R, Cui X, Zha L, Yu L, Shi H, et al. Histone deacetylase 1 (HDAC1) negatively regulates thermogenic program in brown adipocytes via coordinated regulation of histone H3 Lysine 27 (H3K27) deacetylation and methylation. *J Biol Chem.* (2016) 291:4523–36. doi: 10.1074/jbc.M115.677930
120. Dadson P, Hannukainen JC, Din MU, Lahesmaa M, Kalliokoski KK, Iozzo P, et al. Brown adipose tissue lipid metabolism in morbid obesity: effect of bariatric surgery-induced weight loss. *Diabetes Obes Metab.* (2018) 20:1280–8. doi: 10.1111/dom.13233
121. Baba S, Jacene HA, Engles JM, Honda H, Wahl RL. CT Hounsfield units of brown adipose tissue increase with activation: preclinical and clinical studies. *J Nucl Med.* (2010) 51:246–50. doi: 10.2967/jnumed.109.068775
122. Jahansouz C, Xu H, Hertzel AV, Kizy S, Steen KA, Foncea R, et al. Partitioning of adipose lipid metabolism by altered expression and function

of PPAR isoforms after bariatric surgery. *Int J Obes.* (2018) 42:139–46. doi: 10.1038/ijo.2017.197

123. Tarabra E, Nouws J, Vash-Margita A, Nadzam GS, Goldberg-Gell R, Van Name M, et al. The omentum of obese girls harbors small adipocytes and browning transcripts. *JCI Insight.* (2020) 5:135448. doi: 10.1172/jci.insight.135448
124. Abegg K, Schiesser M, Lutz TA, Bueter M. Acute peripheral GLP-1 receptor agonism or antagonism does not alter energy expenditure in rats after Roux-en-Y gastric bypass. *Physiol Behav.* (2013) 121:70–8. doi: 10.1016/j.physbeh.2013.03.027
125. Ye J, Hao Z, Mumphrey MB, Townsend RL, Patterson LM, Stylopoulos N, et al. GLP-1 receptor signaling is not required for reduced body weight after RYGB in rodents. *Am J Physiol Regul Integr Comp Physiol.* (2014) 306:R352–62. doi: 10.1152/ajpregu.00491.2013
126. Boland BB, Mumphrey MB, Hao Z, Townsend RL, Gill B, Oldham S, et al. Combined loss of GLP-1R and Y2R does not alter progression of high-fat diet-induced obesity or response to RYGB surgery in mice. *Mol Metab.* (2019) 25:64–72. doi: 10.1016/j.molmet.2019.05.004
127. Jahansouz C, Staley C, Kizy S, Xu H, Hertzel AV, Coryell J, et al. Antibiotic-induced disruption of intestinal microbiota contributes to failure of vertical sleeve gastrectomy. *Ann Surg.* (2019) 269:1092–100. doi: 10.1097/SLA.0000000000002729
128. Chang SH, Song NJ, Choi JH, Yun UJ, Park KW. Mechanisms underlying UCP1 dependent and independent adipocyte thermogenesis. *Obes Rev.* (2019) 20:241–51. doi: 10.1111/obr.12796
129. Pollard AE, Martins L, Muckett PJ, Khadayate S, Bornot A, Clausen M, et al. AMPK activation protects against diet induced obesity through Ucp1-independent thermogenesis in subcutaneous white adipose tissue. *Nat Metab.* (2019) 1:340–9. doi: 10.1038/s42255-019-0036-9
130. Chondronikola M, Volpi E, Borsheim E, Porter C, Annamalai P, Enerback S, et al. Brown adipose tissue improves whole-body glucose homeostasis and insulin sensitivity in humans. *Diabetes.* (2014) 63:4089–99. doi: 10.2337/db14-0746
131. Chondronikola M, Volpi E, Borsheim E, Porter C, Saraf MK, Annamalai P, et al. Brown adipose tissue activation is linked to distinct systemic effects on lipid metabolism in humans. *Cell Metab.* (2016) 23:1200–6. doi: 10.1016/j.cmet.2016.04.029

2

Obesity Surgery and Cancer: What Are the Unanswered Questions?

Lidia Castagneto-Gissey [1], James Casella-Mariolo [1], Giovanni Casella [1] and Geltrude Mingrone [2,3,4]*

[1] Department of Surgical Sciences, Sapienza University of Rome, Rome, Italy, [2] Division of Diabetes & Nutritional Sciences, Fondazione Policlinico Universitario A. Gemelli IRCCS, Rome, Italy, [3] Division of Diabetes & Nutritional Sciences, Università Cattolica del Sacro Cuore Rome, Rome, Italy, [4] Division of Diabetes & Nutritional Sciences, Faculty of Life Sciences & Medicine, King's College London, London, United Kingdom

***Correspondence:**
Lidia Castagneto-Gissey
lidia.castagnetogissey@uniroma1.it

Obesity has become a global epidemic with a soaring economic encumbrance due to its related morbidity and mortality. Amongst obesity-related conditions, cancer is indeed the most redoubtable. Bariatric surgery has been proven to be the most effective treatment for obesity and its associated metabolic and cardiovascular disorders. However, the understanding of whether and how bariatric surgery determines a reduction in cancer risk is limited. Obesity-related malignancies primarily include colorectal and hormone-sensitive (endometrium, breast, prostate) cancers. Additionally, esophago-gastric tumors are growing to be recognized as a new category mainly associated with post-bariatric surgery outcomes. In fact, certain types of surgical procedures have been described to induce the development and subsequent progression of pre-cancerous esophageal and gastric lesions. This emerging category is of great concern and further research is required to possibly prevent such risks. Published data has generated conflicting results. In fact, while overall cancer risk reduction was reported particularly in women, some authors showed no improvement or even increased cancer incidence. Although various studies have reported beneficial effects of surgery on risk of specific cancer development, fundamental insights into the pathogenesis of obesity-related cancer are indispensable to fully elucidate its mechanisms.

Keywords: bariatric surgery, cancer incidence, mortality, hormone-sensitive cancer, gastroesophageal cancer

INTRODUCTION

The incessant rise of obesity and overweight have configured a state of global epidemic, affecting 1.9 billion and 650 million adults worldwide by 2016, respectively (1). Overall mortality is increased by obesity and its related conditions (2). Amongst these, cancer is indeed the most redoubtable. High body mass index (BMI), namely BMI > 40 kg/m^2, has clearly been linked to a greater risk of both common a rare malignancy incidence and mortality rates (3, 4).

Obesity-related neoplasms primarily include colorectal and hormone-sensitive (endometrium, postmenopausal breast, prostate) cancers. Bariatric/metabolic surgery (BMS) has been extensively acknowledged to be the most efficacious treatment option for the cure of severe obesity and the number of procedures performed is exponentially growing globally (5–7) (**Figure 1**). Overall mortality has also been demonstrated to be decreased after BMS (8). On the contrary, it is uncertain whether BMS has any influence over cancer-related mortality.

It is certainly the remission of obesity that has been postulated to be at the basis of cancer incidence reduction or prevention (3, 9–11). Mechanisms involved in obesity-related cancer genesis are multiple and not completely elucidated. Some of these have been suggested to occur through a depauperation of adipose tissue, which causes in parallel a drop in estrogen circulating levels, thereby altering the risk of hormone-sensitive cancers, especially in postmenopausal women (12, 13). Insulin resistance, which is known to often co-exist with obesity, might also have a role in augmented estrogen levels through interaction in insulin signaling pathways, possibly causing exogenous estrogen synthesis (14). Furthermore, several weight loss independent modalities have been proposed to be involved in post-bariatric surgery cancer risk decrease (15) and include lowering of systemic inflammation and inflammatory markers, changes in gastrointestinal hormones, alteration of gastrointestinal anatomy which in turn produces alteration of gut microbiota, fat, glucose and bile metabolism (16).

Available data has generated differing results; while overall cancer risk reduction was reported particularly in women, some authors showed no improvement or even increased cancer incidence.

Herein, we analyze the link between obesity and cancer, reported influence of BMS on outcomes in terms of obesity-associated cancer incidence and mortality and possible mechanisms involved in its genesis.

OBESITY AND OVERALL CANCER RISK

There is a well-established association between the risk of developing several types of cancers and the presence of an increased BMI (i.e., $\geq$ 25 kg/m^2) (3). With an ever-growing obesity and overweight prevalence worldwide, it would be sensible to also expect a concomitant rise in cancer incidence.

Approximately 481,000 or 3.6% of all newly diagnosed cancers worldwide in adults aged 30 years or more were considered to be presumably caused by an increased BMI, in 2012. In turn, 13% of all cancers correlated to obesity could be attributable to a raised BMI in the adult population (17, 18). A projected rise of cancer risk development ranging 3-10% was associated to every unit increase in BMI (3). Another projection by the Global Burden of Disease group estimated a 3.9% of all cancer deaths to be linked to excess BMI (19). However, it is likely that these reckonings might be inaccurate due to several possible confounding factors or modifiers such as additional effects of smoking or replacement hormonal therapy. Additionally, most computations do not take into account the latency time, of ~10 years, which elapses between the rise in BMI and the development of a malignancy.

Abbreviations: BMI, Body Mass Index; BMS, Bariatric/Metabolic Surgery; NK, Natural Killer; Treg, Regulatory T Cells; IGF-1, Insulin-Like Growth Factor 1; VAT, Visceral Adipose Tissue; SAT, Subcutaneous Adipose Tissue; HIF-1-α, Hypoxia-Inducible Factor 1 Alpha; COX-2, Cycloxygenase 2; PGE2, Prostaglandin E2; SHBG, Sex-Hormone Binding Globulin; NAFLD, Non-Alcoholic Fatty Liver Disease; NASH, Non-Alcoholic Steatohepatitis; HCC, Hepatocellular Carcinoma; SOS, Swedish Obese Subjects; SIR, Standardized Incidence Ratio; GERD, Gastroesophageal Reflux Disease; VBG, Vertical Banded Gastroplasty; AGB, Adjustable Gastric Banding; SG, Sleeve Gastrectomy; RYGB, Roux-en-Y Gastric Bypass; OAGB, One Anastomosis Gastric Bypass; IFSO, International Federation for the Surgery of Obesity and Metabolic Disorders.

A recent population-based registry study analyzing the incidence of cancer in Nigeria amongst subjects affected by obesity and overweight, found an estimated 1.4%, similarly to other developing countries. Interestingly, when comparing such incidence with other developed countries such as United States, United Kingdom and Australia, this was substantially lower. In fact, the incident cancers attributable to obesity and overweight were 6.0% in the United States, 5.5% in United Kingdom, and 3.4% in Australia, due to a higher prevalence of overweight and obesity in the aforementioned countries (20). Distinctively, North America showed the greatest obesity-related cancer incidence with an ~23% or 111,000 cases, while the Sub-Saharan Africa had the lowest rates of 1.5% or 7,300 cases (17). Hence, it is evident how obesity and overweight rates go hand in hand with cancer risk and that profound variations exist in its incidence according to the countries' level of development.

Excess BMI significantly influences cancer risk according to difference in gender. In fact, while it was estimated to affect 1.9% or 136,000 males in 2012, the risk was more than doubled in females (i.e., 5.4% or 345,000 cases). Furthermore, cancer sites vary greatly amongst genders. Breast (33.1% of all obesity/overweight-related cancers) and uterus (31.1%) were the most represented malignancies in females followed by colorectal (10.4%), gallbladder (9.3%), renal (8.7%), pancreatic (3.4%), and esophageal (1.2%) cancer. On the other hand, the most common obesity/overweight-related cancer in males were colorectal neoplasms (54%) accompanied by renal (24.8%), pancreatic (10.9%), and esophageal (10.2%) cancer (17, 18). Thus, excess BMI-related cancer risk was found to be substantially greater in women compared to men, regardless of the geographical location (**Figure 2**).

OBESITY-RELATED CANCER AND SYSTEMIC INFLAMMATION

Obesity is characterized by a state of low-grade systemic inflammation. This chronic generalized inflammatory condition contributes to the development of metabolic morbidities distinctive of obesity, in addition to possibly mediating cancer genesis (21). Chronic inflammation has been demonstrated to be at the basis of tumor promotion and growth. In fact, inflammatory cells and its mediators have been shown to be present in tumoral tissue and are able to induce cell proliferation and migration, also contributing to neoangiogenesis (22).

Obesity per se is not directly considered to be a cancer risk predictor. In contrast, it is indeed the coexistence of a chronic low-grade systemic inflammation, which is thought to be fundamental in promoting cancer. Confirming this observation, is the fact that "metabolically healthy" obese subjects are characteristically not affected by metabolic dysfunction which is in turn caused by chronic inflammation. In "metabolically unhealthy" obese individuals, instead, an inflammatory status is responsible for the onset of metabolic dysregulation, increased cardiovascular risk and obesity-related cancers (21).

Adipose tissue is growing to be considered as the vastest endocrine organ of the human body, secreting numerous

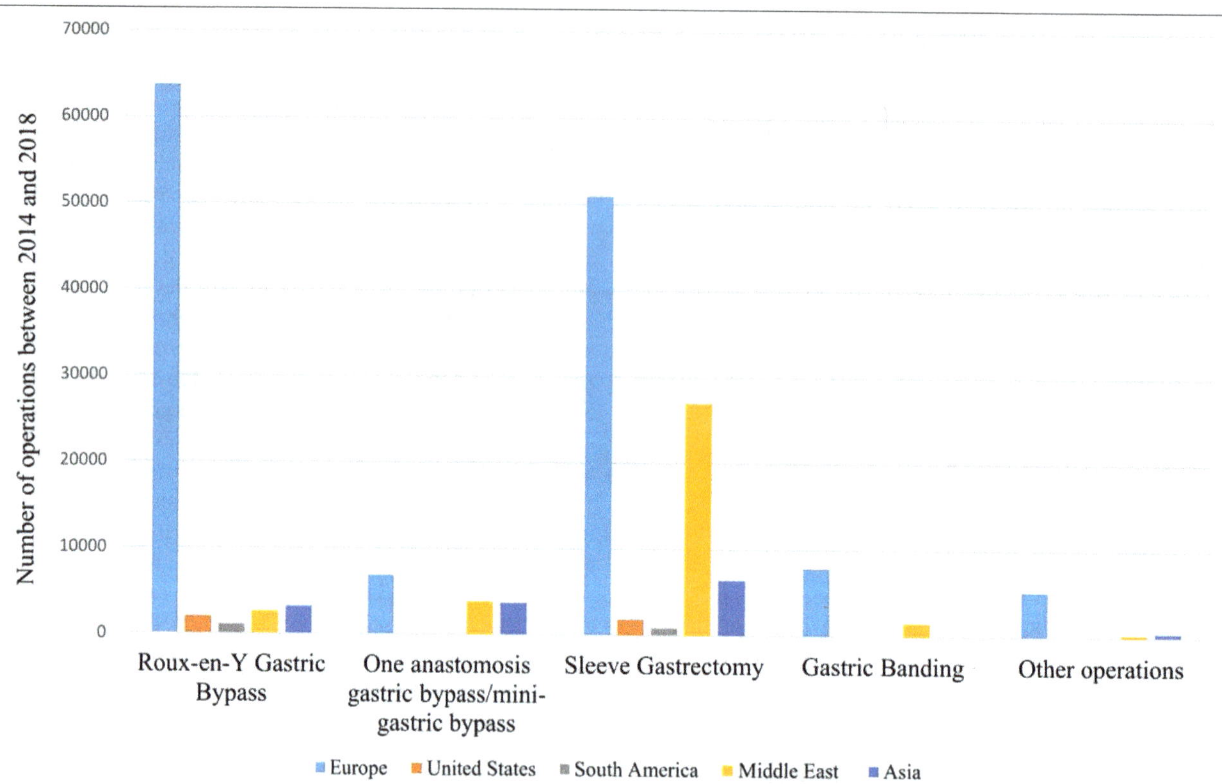

	Roux-en-Y Gastric Bypass	One anastomosis gastric bypass/mini-gastric bypass	Sleeve Gastrectomy	Gastric Banding	Other operations	TOTAL
Europe	63715	6901	50885	7915	5203	134619
United States	2017	7	1858	40	1	3923
South America	1087	46	849	2	9	1993
Middle East	2585	3851	26983	1561	316	35296
Asia	3235	3711	6440	16	486	13888

FIGURE 1 | Bariatric/metabolic operations performed worldwide by region between 2014 and 2018 This figure is original and based on data from Welbourn et al. [7].

cytokines, adypokines and chemokines. Imbalance between caloric intake and expenditure leads to excessive fat deposition and adipose depot expansion. This adipose depot overgrowth causes tissue dysfunction and alteration of its histology due to increased apoptosis, macrophage recruitment and release of several pro-inflammatory molecules, typical of adipose inflammation. Consequently, this contributes to peripheral insulin resistance, hyperglycemia, dyslipidemia, all of which are involved in inducing oxidative stress, cancer development and sustainment (23).

It is important to note how not all types of inflammatory processes are linked to cancer. In actual fact, a distinctive feature of acute inflammation is the presence of natural killer (NK) and CD8+ T cells at the interested site, also involved in tumor immunity. On the contrary, chronic inflammatory sites are lacking these types of cell populations (24). This tissue is instead characterized by a reduction of anti-inflammatory T_H2 and regulatory T cells (Treg) with an increase in the population of T_H1 and CD8+ T cells, in addition to a shift of the M2:M1 macrophage ratio (25). It is this very same type of chronic inflammation of the adipose tissue, which is involved in metabolic dysfunction, cardiovascular risk and carcinogenesis.

A balance between anti-inflammatory and pro-inflammatory factors and immune system cells is present in healthy lean adipose tissue and is capable of maintaining its normal storage capacity, endocrine and whole-body metabolic function. Alteration of this fine equilibrium is responsible of adipocyte hypertrophy, mitochondrial dysregulation, endoplasmic reticulum and oxidative stress, ultimately leading to the release of pro-inflammatory factors and finally cellular apoptosis. This configures a state of adipose inflammation. Adipose tissue ability to store energy and to perform its normal endocrine

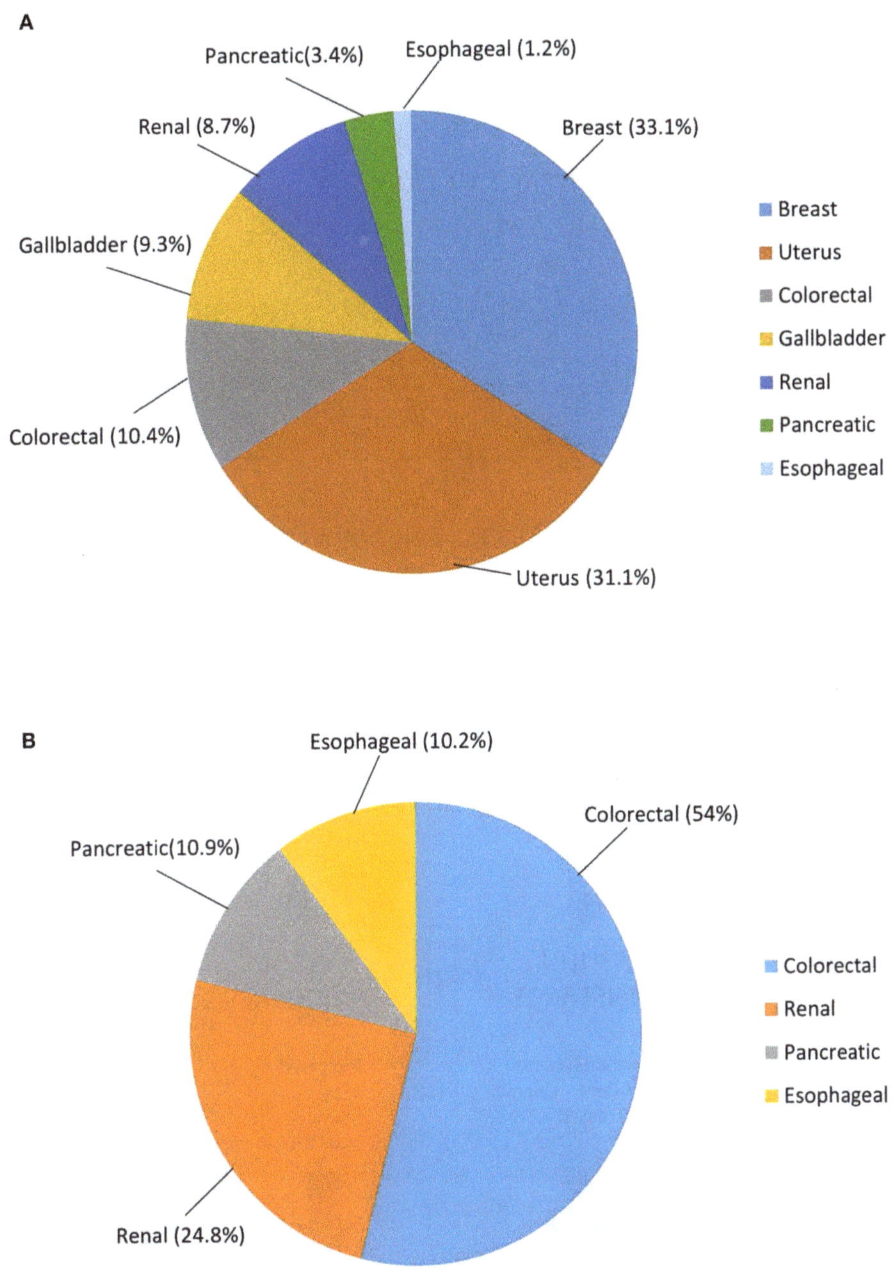

FIGURE 2 | Cancer risk worldwide attributable to overweight and obesity, according to gender. **(A)** Females; **(B)** Males. Data are expressed in %. This figure is original and based on data from Arnold et al. [16].

functions is deeply hampered in obese subjects. In regular conditions, stromal cells are responsible of suppressing tumor growth. Adipose inflammation and the altered adipokine and cytokine secretion can modify this microenvironment and also promote tumor growth, progression and tumor cell migration. Additionally, this inflammatory state causes insulin resistance which translates into a state of hyperglycemia, hyperinsulinemia, increased circulating insulin-like growth factor 1 (IGF-1) which have also been recognized to be involved in carcinogenesis (25) (**Figure 3**).

Local inflammation seems to also play a substantial role especially in breast cancer development. White adipose tissue inflammation in the breast causes histological alterations and release of NFκB, which leads to augmented aromatase activity and estrogen-androgen ratio in the breast tissue. Local and systemic raised estrogen levels are ideal for tumor formation and progression (21).

Epigenetic variations in DNA over time have also been proposed among chief determinants linking obesity and cancer. Several environmental factors, including nutrition, physical

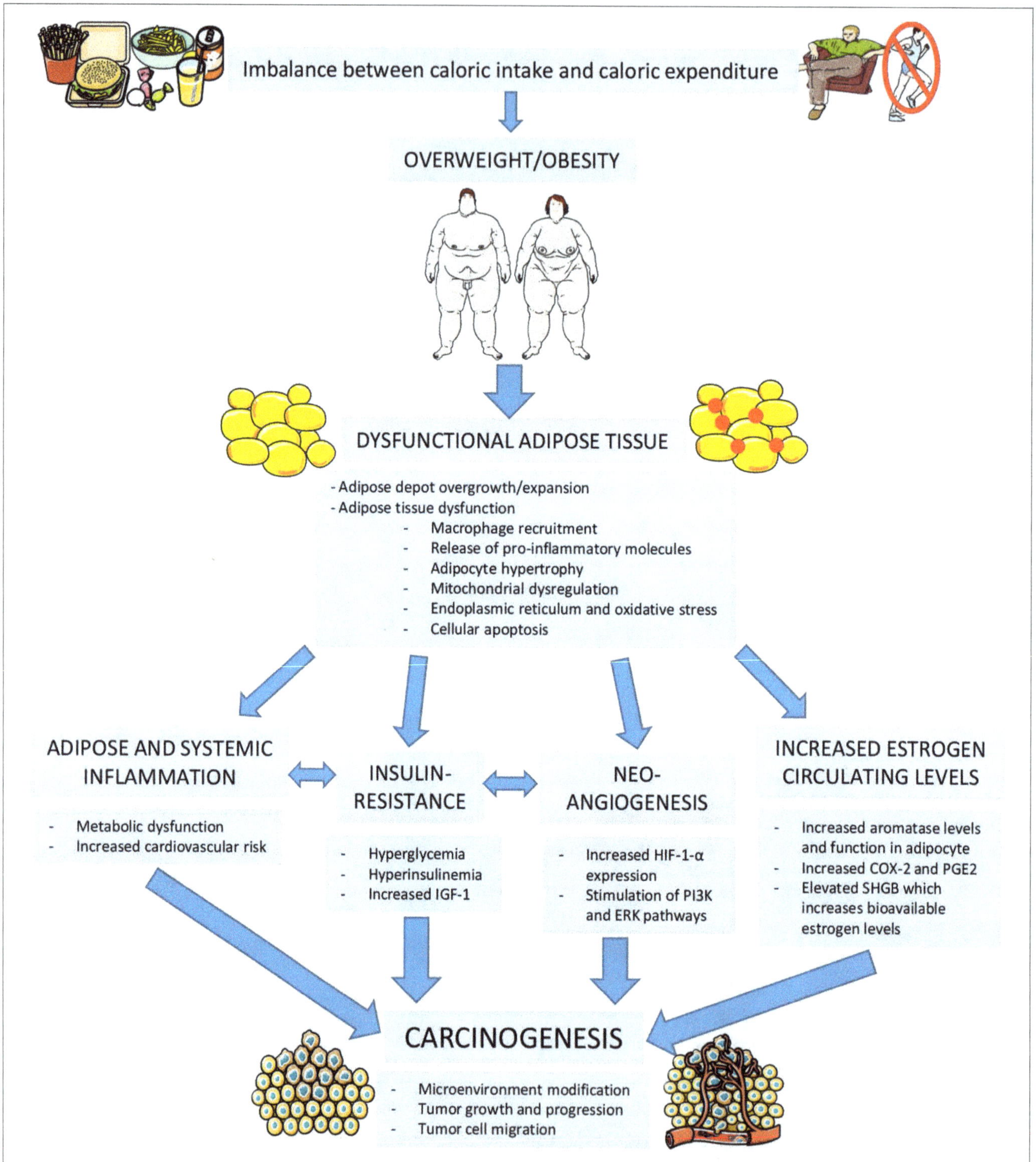

FIGURE 3 | Mechanisms linking obesity to carcinogenesis. IGF-1, Insulin-Like Growth Factor 1; HIF-1-α, Hypoxia-Inducible Factor 1 Alpha; PI3K, Phosphoinositide 3-kinase; ERK, extracellular signal-regulated kinase; COX-2, Cycloxygenase 2; PGE2, Prostaglandin E2; SHBG, Sex-Hormone Binding Globulin. (The figure was created using Servier Medical Art).

exercise and lifestyle, may be involved in such mechanisms, via the activation of inflammatory processes (26). Recent investigations in animal models have shown how diet-induced obesity can decrease DNA methylation and downregulate expression of certain genes, promoting breast cancer with a worsened prognosis. Preventive measures and strategies targeting epigenetic changes are starting to be developed in order to disrupt this linkage (27).

OBESITY-RELATED CANCER AND INSULIN RESISTANCE

Central obesity measured by waist circumference has been found to be a direct predictor of cancer risk. In other words, it is visceral fat rather than peripheral adipose tissue which is correlated with this very risk (28, 29). To this regard, visceral adipose tissue (VAT) has increased lipolytic and lipogenic action additionally to its greater pro-inflammatory factors secretion, compared to subcutaneous adipose tissue (SAT). Metabolic dysfunction and cardiovascular risk are both associated with greater VAT depots (29).

Excess body weight contributes to inducing a state of insulin resistance, characterized by augmented hepatic gluconeogenesis, reduced peripheral glucose uptake and hyperinsulinemia. Prolonged hyperinsulinemia may lead to increased IGF-1 secretion (30). *In vitro* studies have demonstrated the fundamental role of IGF-1 and insulin itself in stimulating tumoral cell growth. Similarly, epidemiological investigations have shown a direct correlation between increased insulin and IGF-1 circulating levels and the development of certain types of malignancies (i.e., pancreatic, liver, colorectal, breast, and endometrium). Furthermore, IGF-1 is capable of promoting tumoral development and sustainment, also stimulating hypoxia-inducible factor 1 alpha (HIF-1-α) release that is associated with specific tumor migration and metastasis and may inhibit certain tumor suppressor genes such as p53. Insulin, on the other hand, also has a role in tumor progression and metastasis through stimulation of different intracellular pathways comprising PI3K and ERK (31, 32) (**Figure 3**).

Mounting evidence has additionally shown that cancer prognosis is affected by insulin and IGF-1 circulating levels, independently of cancer risk. Specifically, a state of hyperinsulinemia is associated with worst cancer prognosis and outcomes. In consideration of the ever-growing obesity global epidemic, insulin resistance and hyperinsulinemia, closely interrelated with obesity, are receiving increasing attention and new experimental antineoplastic drugs—targeting IGF-1 and/or insulin signaling pathways—are being employed in clinical trials (31).

OBESITY-RELATED CANCER AND CIRCULATING ESTROGEN LEVELS

There is a rise in estrone, free and bound estradiol levels in parallel to a rise in BMI (33). The main source of aromatase in the human body resides in preadipocytes, adipocytes, and mesenchymal stem cells found in the adipose tissue. This enzyme is responsible for transforming androgens to estrogens. Levels and function of aromatase increase proportionally to adiposity and aging, with adipose tissue becoming the main secretion site in postmenopausal women. Furthermore, chronic adipose inflammation produces an increased cycloxygenase-2 (COX-2) expression and prostaglandin E_2 (PGE_2) secretion which combines with the already high levels of local pro-inflammatory cytokines; this scenario is capable of inducing aromatase expression and augmented estrogen production, configuring an optimal microenvironment for carcinogenesis. Eicosanoids have also shown to generate tumor cell migration, neoangiogenisis and cell growth, due to its anti-apoptotic and pro-mitotic pathways (34).

Sex-hormone binding globulin (SHBG) levels are also profoundly affected by the amount of adipose tissue as they decrease when adiposity rises. A reduction in SHBG concentration causes a greater portion of estrogen to be bioactive and readily available (35).

Hence, obesity is responsible of increasing estradiol production in adipose tissue and elevating the fraction of biologically active estrogen by influencing SHBG synthesis by the liver (34). The augmented concentration of total serum estrogens and low SHGB levels have been demonstrated to have a causal relationship with postmenopausal breast and endometrial cancer risk development (**Figure 3**).

OBESITY-RELATED CANCER AND GUT MICROBIOTA

Over the past decade, a large body of literature has been dedicated to investigating the role of gut microbiota in the physiopathological mechanisms involved in metabolic regulation in the ambit of cardio-metabolic disorders. Gut microbiota is mostly present in the ileum and colon and is involved in the host defensive action from pathogens, growth and development of the digestive tract, immune response, balance of energy homeostasis, and digestion of nutrients. Its composition is greatly influenced by genetic background, diet, exercise and antibiotics. Obesity and type 2 diabetes mellitus in humans have been linked to alteration in gut microbiota composition. In turn, through energy harvesting of dietary nutrients, gut microbiota can indirectly affect insulin signaling and systemic low-grade inflammation (36). A direct relationship between gut microbiota and gastrointestinal cancers has been shown to occur by way of systemic inflammation and immune response regulation. The gut barrier dysfunction was proven to activate several different pathways, able to promote the development of certain gastrointestinal cancers, including colorectal, hepatocellular and pancreatic cancers (37). BMS induces changes in gut microbiota, which is involved in weight loss, fat deposition normalization, indirectly contributing to cancer risk reduction (36).

OBESITY-RELATED CANCER AND NON-ALCOHOLIC FATTY LIVER DISEASE

Non-alcoholic fatty liver disease (NAFLD) includes a clinical continuum of hepatopathies that range from simple steatosis to non-alcoholic steatohepatitis (NASH) and possibly evolving to liver fibrosis, cirrhosis and hepatocellular carcinoma (HCC). As a result of the ever-rising incidence of overweight, obesity and type 2 diabetes mellitus worldwide, NAFLD has become the most commonly diagnosed liver condition in industrialized countries. Approximately 25% of subjects with NASH develop progressive fibrosis and subsequent cirrhosis (38). Several authors have demonstrated how NAFLD has presently become the main risk factor for the development of HCC, compared to previously recognized predisposing causes such as hepatitis B and C infection (39).

BMS is recommended in those patients affected by morbid obesity in which pharmacotherapy and lifestyle modifications have failed. However, no randomized controlled trials (RCTs) comparing BMS with standard of care have been published until now. A prospective study including 109 subjects demonstrated histological resolution of NASH 1 year after RYGB, bilio-intestinal bypass or gastric banding in 85% of the cases (40). The same authors (41) showed in 381 subjects undergoing liver biopsy during BMS, mainly RYGB, that the percentage of subjects with NASH declined from 27.4 to 14.2% at 5 years, even though, fibrosis somewhat worsened.

A recent meta-analysis (42) including 3093 liver biopsies demonstrated resolution of steatosis in 66%, inflammation in 50%, ballooning in 76%, and fibrosis in 40% of the cases. However, in 12% of subjects fibrosis worsened if present at the baseline or appeared if absent.

The reduction of NAFLD or NASH prevalence in subjects operated of BMS should translate in a future reduction in the incidence of HCC.

EFFECTS OF BARIATRIC/METABOLIC SURGERY ON OBESITY-RELATED CANCER

Bariatric/metabolic surgery seems to have protective effects with regards to cancer development and prognosis. However, this anticarcinogenic action has been shown to be multifactorial and may include weight-dependent and independent mechanisms. Interestingly, several studies have shown a lack of correlation between the entity of weight loss after BMS and the decrease in cancer incidence (15, 43). This is to further confirm how BMS exercises its effects not solely through excess weight loss, but is rather likely to be mediated by various mechanisms. These might include substantial reduction in pro-inflammatory molecule secretion, alteration of gut microbiota, changes in glucose and fat metabolism, improvement of insulin sensitivity, modification of gastrointestinal peptides (15, 21, 24, 31, 32).

Some authors found beneficial effects of BMS in terms of reduction of cancer incidence and mortality in females, especially in the postmenopausal subgroup; the same benefit was not proven in males (43, 44). Such positive outcomes in females are likely to be associated with a substantial decrease in estrogen production and bioavailability, translating in a decline of hormone-sensitive breast and endometrial cancers after BMS (15).

A 2-cohort observational study by Christou et al. comparing patients who received BMS to a control group who did not undergo surgery, demonstrated in parallel with an excess weight loss of 67.1%, a 76% overall reduction of hospital visits for all types of cancers in the post-bariatric group (2.0 and 8.45%, respectively). Moreover, relative risk of breast cancer incidence in the study group had an additional 82% reduction (45). Similarly, Adams et al. conducted a retrospective analysis assessing the effects of BMS (specifically, gastric bypass) compared to non-surgical obese patients, on cancer incidence and mortality over a 24-year period. Significantly lower cancer frequency was found in the surgical group compared to non-operated controls, with cancer-specific mortality decreased by 46% in the former group. Although cancer incidence declined only for obesity-related malignancies (i.e., esophagus, colorectal, pancreas, postmenopausal breast, uterus, kidney, liver, gallbladder), mortality dropped for all cancer types (45, 46).

McCawley et al. further investigated the influence of BMS in female obese subjects in a retrospective study compared to a non-surgical control group. Both groups were found to be younger in age at diagnosis in comparison to the general non-obese population. Furthermore, the non-operated control group had a higher incidence of cancer rates compared to operated subjects (5.8 vs. 3.6%, respectively). Most commonly diagnosed malignancies in both groups were breast, endometrial, cervix and colorectal cancers (47).

The Swedish Obese Subjects (SOS) study was the first prospective controlled intervention trial to evaluate the impact of BMS on cancer rates and outcomes after a mean 10.9-year follow up period. Authors concluded that surgical patients had substantially lower cancer prevalence, however, this was confirmed in women but not the same was found in operated men (43).

A systematic review and meta-analysis involving six observational studies comparing outcomes in terms of cancer risk and mortality in surgical vs. non-surgical obese subjects concluded that BMS is capable of reducing overall cancer incidence and related mortality. Nevertheless, after stratifying patients by gender, beneficial effects of surgery were seen in women but not confirmed in post-bariatric surgical men (48).

To further investigate the observation that substantial weight loss might prevent the risk of developing endometrial hyperplasia and type 1 endometrial cancer, Argenta et al. performed a prospective, blinded, non-interventional pilot study on 45 premenopausal morbidly obese women candidate to BMS. Authors found endometrial pathology (simple or complex endometrial hyperplasia) in 6.8% of the study group at baseline and observed a complete regression of the endometrial lesions in all patients 12–18 months postoperatively. In this group of patients a significant risk reduction of endometrial malignancies was recorded but not abolished (49). Clinical trials are currently underway to establish whether bariatric surgery coupled with hormonal therapy is an effective treatment for endometrial cancer/atypical hyperplasia in obese women of childbearing age who wish to maintain their fertility and might help to unravel possible molecular mechanisms causing endometrial cancer reduction after BMS.

A Swedish nationwide population-based cohort study on 13,123 subjects, by Ostlund et al. analyzed the effect of BMS on long-term obesity-related cancer (breast, prostate, colorectal, endometrial, and kidney) risk and mortality over a 26-year period, calculated by a standardized incidence ratio (SIR). In contrast to the aforementioned studies, Ostlund et al. failed to show a protective effect of surgery on oncologic outcomes in the long term after BMS. Specifically, authors found no reduction of SIRs after BMS over time for all obesity-related cancers, except for colorectal cancer, which had an increased SIR in the long-term for post-bariatric subjects (50).

Colorectal cancer has been shown to be closely associated with obesity, increasing alongside the rise in BMI. It has been suggested that for every increase of 5 kg/m^2 in BMI, colorectal cancer risk increases by 24% in males and 9% in females (3). A recent systematic review and meta-analysis by Afshar et al., analyzing the effects of BMS solely on colorectal cancer incidence, demonstrated a significantly diminished risk, by an estimated 27% in obese operated patients compared to controls (49, 51). However, data in literature regarding this specific risk is inconsistent. Several authors have highlighted the protective effects of BMS on overall cancer risk (3, 36, 45). However, the majority of studies did not demonstrate adequate statistical power nor sufficient length of follow up, which is needed especially for colorectal malignancies, which do have indeed a long decennary carcinogenetic process.

Similarly to findings by Ostlund et al. (50), Derogar et al. (52) highlighted the rise in SIRs for colorectal cancer in the post-bariatric surgical group composed of 15,095 patients, which increased concurrently with time after surgery, compared to the non-operated group (62,016 subjects) who's SIRs continued to be stable also in the long term. Interestingly, authors did not find any difference in SIRs for colorectal cancer in-between the different surgical procedures analyzed in the study (i.e., VBG, AGB, and RYGB). The grounds for such increase is unclear, but the same authors also demonstrated in a previous study how patients who underwent RYGB developed rectal mucosal hyperproliferation persisting at least 3 years postoperatively. Furthermore, a raised mucosal expression of the pro-tumorigenic cytokine macrophage migration inhibitory factor was found (53). It has been hypothesized that colorectal cancer development might increase as a consequence of the malabsorptive effects caused by certain bariatric procedures, where RYGB is the most studied one. The altered intestinal absorption and the surgical bowel rearrangement might lead to the increased mucosal bile salt exposure and modification of gut microbiota. Additionally, the modified dietary intake after surgery, principally composed of proteins and low in carbohydrates, can contribute to the production of harmful metabolites in the colonic tract with possible cytotoxic effects on the mucosa and playing a role in the complex interaction with gut microbiota and bile salts (54, 55).

Existing evidence derives largely from observational retrospective studies, which might represent a selection bias and may influence the reliability of results. Nevertheless, the vast majority of studies available in literature undeniably highlight the positive impact of BMS on specific cancer incidence, prognosis and mortality. This may occur through several pathways that are correlated to weight loss but also involve multiple mechanisms that go beyond mere weight reduction and that seem to be also associated to metabolic modifications that occur after surgery.

BARIATRIC/METABOLIC SURGERY AND NEW ONSET OF GASTROESOPHAGEAL CANCER

Overweight and obesity have been linked to a raised risk of esophageal and gastric cancer development and this has been shown to increase along with rising BMI (56). This correlation (particularly present for malignancies of the distal esophagus and cardia) has been attributed to the higher coexistence in this population of gastroesophageal reflux disease (GERD), hiatal hernia and subsequent erosive esophagitis of variable degrees which may seldom evolve to Barrett's esophagus (57, 58). Helicobacter pylori infection concurrently plays a role in cancer development, especially for gastric malignancies and is in fact classified as a type 1 carcinogen (59). Additionally, hormonal effects generated by dysregulation of insulin and IGF-1 secretion, generally altered in obese subjects, may be implicated in this carcinogenic process (30, 31).

By surgically inducing weight loss, BMS could presumably reduce some risk factors implicated in gastroesophageal tumorigenesis. However, scarce and contrasting evidence has been reported in literature to this regard.

Bariatric procedures encompassing a restriction of the gastric outlet, such as vertical banded gastroplasty (VBG), adjustable gastric banding (AGB), and sleeve gastrectomy (SG), are characterized by certain pathophysiologic modifications possibly involved in gastroesophageal malignancy development. These might comprise alimentary bolus stasis and impaction in the esophagus or gastric pouch due to the presence of a narrowed outlet, local inflammation adjacent to the gastric band location, alteration of gastroesophageal intraluminal pressures and motility with consequent appearance of differing types of gastroesophageal reflux.

The protracted stasis of food content in the distal esophagus or gastric reservoir might expose the mucosa to the harmful effects of exogenous carcinogens (60, 61). Furthermore, certain studies have investigated the local alterations arising in correspondence to the gastric band or mesh (i.e., VBG, ABG). The presence of a foreign body in fact, causes the formation of adhesions, scar retraction, erosion, ulceration, local blood flow reduction and mucosal changes leading to metaplasia that in rare cases may evolve to dysplasia and adenocarcinoma (62–64).

The role of chronic GERD has been proven to have a fundamental role in the genesis of gastroesophageal malignancies. Due to this, extensive research has been dedicated to further understand the effects of BMS on GERD. Specifically, SG was the bariatric procedure which raised the greatest concerns in consideration of its exponentially rising popularity. The effects of SG on GERD are rather conflicting (65). However, several studies have demonstrated that SG substantially causes de novo or a worsening of preexisting GERD, development of erosive esophagitis and hiatal hernia as evaluated by the use of endoscopy (66, 67). Interestingly, no correlation was found between the presence of GERD symptoms and endoscopic findings; indeed authors demonstrated how the vast majority of patients often were asymptomatic for pyrosis, reflux or regurgitation (68). Furthermore, a peculiarity of SG is that the composition of refluxate undergoes profound modifications after surgery and is characterized by the greater presence of bile (66, 67). Our previously published data on endoscopy before and after SG actually confirmed the consensual increase of bile stagnation into the esophagus, which strongly correlated with the degree of erosive esophagitis and Barrett's metaplasia (66). Earlier investigations suggest that biliary or mixed types of gastroesophageal reflux are responsible for esophageal mucosal injury contributing to the development of Barrett's esophagus (69). Several studies actually reported a significantly elevated number of Barrett's esophagus after SG (66, 67, 70), reaching a prevalence as high as 18.8% 5 years after this bariatric operation (70). Barrett's esophagus is considered to be a precancerous lesion and some authors have suggested that this histological alteration might evolve to dysplasia even more rapidly after SG (66, 69). Esophageal adenocarcinoma is in fact the most common malignancy emerging after SG and this might occur on previous metaplasia. However, to this regard, reported cases in literature are sporadic and do not allow to make definitive conclusions on the actual prevalence of such malignancies (70).

After bypass surgery, namely, Roux-en-Y gastric bypass (RYGB), the second most commonly performed bariatric operation, several authors have described tumors arising mainly from the gastric remnant. The excluded stomach might be a site of carcinogenesis due to the accumulation of pancreatic and biliary content at this level that has been shown to generate in experimental studies the progression to intestinal metaplasia and adenocarcinoma (71). Helicobacter Pylori infection has been clearly linked to gastric cancer and some studies have shown how this infection may persist in the gastric remnant after RYGB despite eradication (72). This further supports the importance of its treatment and eradication prior to RYGB (73).

One anastomosis gastric bypass (OAGB) has gained popularity over the past five years and was recently accepted as a standard bariatric procedure by the International Federation for the Surgery of Obesity and Metabolic Disorders (IFSO). This procedure has been hypothesized to potentially cause the development of gastric cancer, owing to its peculiar bypass reconstruction. Previous studies have clearly shown the appearance of gastric adenocarcinoma at the level of the gastro-jejunostomy after Billroth II reconstruction (74, 75). Considering the fact that in OAGB a similar loop reconstruction is performed, it could presumably be linked to a similar carcinogenetic risk to that seen after Billroth II (76). Furthermore, biliary reflux in the distal esophagus is a major concern as this has been shown to be associated with increased incidence of metaplasia, dysplasia, and finally esophageal adenocarcinoma (69). Nevertheless, data in literature is widely lacking due to the relatively recent nature of this procedure.

Preoperative endoscopic screening is of paramount importance in order to rule out possible intraluminal pathological alterations, including erosive esophagitis, hiatal hernia, Barrett's esophagus, malignant tumors, etc. This evaluation is also necessary to properly assess patients who are often asymptomatic for GERD, might have the aforementioned conditions and might go unnoticed if a preoperative endoscopy is not performed. A proper and complete examination, in fact, can contribute to the correct patient selection and submission to the best bariatric operation in that specific case, also contributing to the reduction of postoperative complications.

The reported cases of esophagogastric cancers after BMS are sporadic and insufficient, not allowing to reliably draw a relationship between such types of malignancies and each bariatric surgical procedure. Additionally, epidemiological studies do not show a greater incidence of esophageal and gastric cancers in post-bariatric subjects compared to the general population (77). Nevertheless, higher-level evidence is necessary to fully understand and eventually confirm or deny any intercorrelation. Endoscopic surveillance after all types of bariatric operations seems to be of paramount importance for early detection of esophagogastric malignancies.

OBESITY SURGERY AND CANCER: WHAT ARE THE UNANSWERED QUESTIONS?

Which Types of Cancers Benefit More From BMS?

BMS appears to have protective effects on cancer development. This anticarcinogenic action is multifactorial and includes weight-dependent and independent mechanisms. There is a lack of correlation between the entity of weight loss after BMS and the decrease in cancer incidence. This is to confirm how BMS exercises its effects not solely through weight loss, but is rather likely to be mediated by various mechanisms (15).

The beneficial effects of BMS in terms of reduction of cancer incidence and mortality has especially been shown in females, specifically in the postmenopausal group (12, 13). Such positive outcomes in females are likely to be associated with a substantial decrease in estrogen production and bioavailability, translating in a decline of hormone-sensitive breast and endometrial cancers after BMS (34).

Why Does BMS Benefit More Women Than Men?

It is certainly the remission of obesity that has been postulated to be at the basis of cancer incidence reduction or prevention. Mechanisms involved in obesity-related cancer genesis are multiple and not completely elucidated. Some of these have been suggested to occur through a depauperation of adipose tissue, which causes in parallel a drop in estrogen circulating levels, thereby altering the risk of hormone-sensitive cancers, especially in postmenopausal women (12–15). Insulin resistance, which is known to often co-exist with obesity, might also have a role in augmented estrogen levels through interaction in insulin signaling pathways, possibly causing exogenous estrogen synthesis. Furthermore, several weight loss independent modalities have been proposed to be involved in post-bariatric surgery cancer risk decrease and include lowering of systemic inflammation, changes in gastrointestinal hormones, alteration of gastrointestinal anatomy which in turn produces alteration of gut microbiota, fat, glucose, and bile metabolism. Hence, hormonal levels are at the basis of the improved cancer risk especially in postmenopausal women (34, 35). However, several mechanisms involved in this phenomenon are still waiting to be clarified.

Does Only Cancer Risk Improve or Is Also Prognosis Affected After BMS?

BMS not only affects cancer incidence but has also been shown to profoundly influence cancer prognosis. This may occur through several pathways that are in part correlated to weight loss but also involve multiple mechanisms that go beyond mere weight reduction and that seem to be associated to metabolic modifications occurring after surgery. In fact, evidence suggests that cancer prognosis is affected by insulin and IGF-1 circulating levels, independently of cancer risk. Specifically, a state of hyperinsulinemia is associated with worst cancer prognosis and outcomes. In consideration of the ever-growing prevalence of obesity and insulin resistance, an increasing interest to the development of new experimental antineoplastic drugs—targeting IGF-1 and/or insulin signaling pathways—are being employed in clinical trials (14, 32).

Which Operation Should Be Recommended for Each Specific Type of Cancer?

No evidence is available at present regarding the beneficial effects of different bariatric procedures on specific cancer types. In consideration of this, the various surgical bariatric procedures available should be advised by the bariatric surgeon based on the preoperative work-up and available institutional and international guidelines (78).

Does GERD Contraindicate Specific Bariatric Procedures?

Currently, GERD, regardless of its severity, is not considered as an absolute contraindication to any specific bariatric procedure. However, several bariatric surgeons may oftentimes advice the patient to undergo operations such as RYGB, which is most effective in leading to GERD resolution, as opposed to "refluxigenic" procedures such as SG (78, 79). In fact, SG is controversially associated with an increase or worsening of GERD and the appearance of hiatal hernia and erosive esophagitis. The role of chronic GERD has been proven to have a fundamental role in the genesis of gastroesophageal malignancies. It is for this very reason that SG is often not recommended in patients who have pre-existing GERD. Several studies actually reported a significantly elevated number of Barrett's esophagus after SG. Barrett's esophagus is indeed a precancerous lesion and some authors have suggested that this histological alteration might evolve to dysplasia even more rapidly after this operation (66, 67). Esophageal adenocarcinoma is in actual fact the most common malignancy emerging after SG and postoperative endoscopic surveillance is fundamental for early diagnosis in this group of patients (69, 70, 77).

CONCLUSIONS

Available data has shown that obesity is indeed associated with an increased cancer risk and BMS is capable, through several diverse pathways, to generate a significant reduction in overall cancer prevalence and mortality. However, awareness should be raised with regards to the possibility of increasing the incidence of gastroesophageal cancers after BMS and the necessity of postoperative endoscopic surveillance. Further understanding of involved mechanisms in the development or reduction of such neoplasms in this specific type of patients is required in order to possibly formulate public health strategies in such setting.

AUTHOR CONTRIBUTIONS

All authors listed have made a substantial, direct and intellectual contribution to the work, and approved it for publication.

REFERENCES

1. World Health Organization (WHO). *World Health Statistics, Fact Sheet Obesity and Overweight*. (2020). Available online at: https://www.who.int/news-room/fact-sheets/detail/obesity-and-overweight.
2. Pischon T, Boeing H, Hoffmann K, Bergmann M, Schulze MB, Overvad K, et al. General and abdominal adiposity and risk of death in Europe. *N Engl J Med.* (2008) 359:2105–20. doi: 10.1056/NEJMoa0801891
3. Renehan AG, Tyson M, Egger M, Heller RF, Zwahlen M. Body-mass index and incidence of cancer: a systematic review and meta-analysis of prospective observational studies. *Lancet.* (2008) 371:569–78. doi: 10.1016/S0140-6736(08)60269-X
4. Calle EE, Rodriguez C, Walker-Thurmond K, Thun MJ. Overweight, obesity, mortality from cancer in a prospectively studied cohort of U.S. adults. *N Engl J Med.* (2003) 348:1625–38. doi: 10.1056/NEJMoa021423
5. Colquitt JL, Pickett K, Loveman E, Frampton GK. Surgery for weight loss in adults. *Cochrane Database Syst Rev.* (2014) 8:CD003641. doi: 10.1002/14651858.CD003641.pub4
6. Buchwald H, Avidor Y, Braunwald E, Jensen MD, Pories W, Fahrbach K, et al. Bariatric surgery: a systematic review and meta-analysis. *JAMA.* (2004) 292:1724–37. doi: 10.1001/jama.292.14.1724
7. Welbourn R, Hollyman M, Kinsman R, Dixon J, Liem R, Ottosson J, et al. Bariatric surgery worldwide: baseline demographic description and one-year outcomes from the fourth IFSO global registry report (2018). *Obes Surg.* (2019) 29:782–95. doi: 10.1007/s11695-018-3593-1
8. Cardoso L, Rodrigues D, Gomes L, Carrilho F. Short- and long-term mortality after bariatric surgery: A systematic review and meta-analysis. *Diabetes Obes Metab.* (2017) 19:1223–32. doi: 10.1111/dom.12922
9. Anveden Å, Taube M, Peltonen M, Jacobson P, Andersson-Assarsson JC, Sjöholm K, et al. Long-term incidence of female-specific cancer after bariatric surgery or usual care in the Swedish Obese Subjects Study. *Gynecol Oncol.* (2017) 145:224–9. doi: 10.1016/j.ygyno.2017.02.036
10. Schauer DP, Feigelson HS, Koebnick C, Caan B, Weinmann S, Leonard AC et al. Bariatric surgery and the risk of cancer in a large multisite cohort. *Ann Surg.* (2019) 269:95–101. doi: 10.1097/SLA.0000000000002525
11. Mackenzie H, Markar SR, Askari A, Faiz O, Hull M, Purkayastha S, et al. Obesity surgery and risk of cancer. *Br J Surg.* (2018) 105:1650–7. doi: 10.1002/bjs.10914
12. de Waard F, Poortman J, de Pedro-Alvarez Ferrero M, Baanders-van Halewijn EA. Weight reduction and oestrogen excretion in obese post-menopausal women. *Maturitas.* (1982) 4:155–62.

13. Kaaks R, Lukanova A, Kurzer MS. Obesity, endogenous hormones, and endometrial cancer risk: a synthetic review. *Cancer Epidemiol Biomarkers Prev.* (2002) 11:1531–43.
14. Suba Z. Interplay between insulin resistance and estrogen deficiency as co- activators in carcinogenesis. *Pathol Oncol Res.* (2012) 18:123–33. doi: 10.1007/s12253-011-9466-8
15. Ashrafian H, Ahmed K, Rowland SP, Patel VM, Gooderham NJ, Holmes E, et al. Metabolic surgery and cancer: protective effects of bariatric procedures. *Cancer.* (2011) 117:1788–99. doi: 10.1002/cncr.25738
16. Castagneto Gissey L, Casella Mariolo J, Mingrone G. Intestinal peptide changes after bariatric and minimally invasive surgery: Relation to diabetes remission. *Peptides.* (2018) 100:114–122. doi: 10.1016/j.peptides.2017.12.010
17. Arnold M, Pandeya N, Byrnes G, Renehan PAG, Stevens GA, Ezzati PM, et al. Global burden of cancer attributable to high body-mass index in 2012: a population-based study. *Lancet Oncol.* (2015) 16:36–46. doi: 10.1016/S1470-2045(14)71123-4
18. International Agency for Research on Cancer. *World Health Organization. GLOBOCAN. Cancer Attributable to Obesity.* (2018). Available online at: https://gco.iarc.fr/causes/obesity/tools-pie.
19. Lim SS, Vos T, Flaxman AD, Danaei G, Shibuya K, Adair-Rohani H, et al. A comparative risk assessment of burden of disease and injury attributable to 67 risk factors and risk factor clusters in 21 regions, 1990-2010: a systematic analysis for the Global Burden of Disease Study (2010). *Lancet.* (2012) 380:2224–60. doi: 10.1016/S0140-6736(12)61766-8
20. Odutola MK, Olukomogbon T, Igbinoba F, Otu TI, Ezeome E, Hassan R, et al. Cancers attributable to overweight and obesity from 2012 to 2014 in Nigeria: a population-based cancer registry study. *Front Oncol.* (2019) 9:460. doi: 10.3389/fonc.2019.00460
21. Deng T, Lyon CJ, Bergin S, Caligiuri MA, Hsueh WA. Obesity, inflammation, and cancer. *Annu Rev Pathol.* (2016) 11:421–49. doi: 10.1146/annurev-pathol-012615-044359
22. Hanahan D, Coussens LM. Accessories to the crime: functions of cells recruited to the tumor microenvironment. *Cancer Cell.* (2012) 21:309–22. doi: 10.1016/j.ccr.2012.02.022
23. Martinez-Santibañez G, Cho KW, Lumeng CN. Imaging white adipose tissue with confocal microscopy. *Methods Enzymol.* (2014) 537:17–30. doi: 10.1016/B978-0-12-411619-1.00002-1
24. Kim S, Karin M. Role of TLR2-dependent inflammation in metastatic progression. *Ann N Y Acad Sci.* (2011) 1217:191–206. doi: 10.1111/j.1749-6632.2010.05882.x
25. Mathis D. Immunological goings-on in visceral adipose tissue. *Cell Metab.* (2013) 17:851–9. doi: 10.1016/j.cmet.2013.05.008
26. Horsburgh S, Robson-Ansley P, Adams R, Smith C. Exercise and inflammation-related epigenetic modifications: focus on DNA methylation. *Exerc Immunol Rev.* (2015) 21:26–41.
27. Berger NA, Scacheri PC. Targeting epigenetics to prevent obesity promoted cancers. *Cancer Prev Res.* (2018) 11:125–8. doi: 10.1158/1940-6207
28. Moore LL, Bradlee ML, Singer MR, Splansky GL, Proctor MH, Ellison RC, et al. BMI and waist circumference as predictors of lifetime colon cancer risk in Framingham Study adults. *Int J Obes Relat Metab Disord.* (2004) 28:559–67. doi: 10.1038/sj.ijo.0802606
29. Palou M, Priego T, Sánchez J, Rodríguez AM, Palou A, Picó C. Gene expression patterns in visceral and subcutaneous adipose depots in rats are linked to their morphologic features. *Cell Physiol Biochem.* (2009) 24:547–56. doi: 10.1159/000257511
30. Mingrone G, Castagneto-Gissey L. Type 2 diabetes mellitus in 2013: A central role of the gut in glucose homeostasis. *Nat Rev Endocrinol.* (2014) 10:73–4. doi: 10.1038/nrendo.2013.241
31. Pollak M. Insulin and insulin-like growth factor signalling in neoplasia. *Nat Rev Cancer.* (2008) 8:915–28. doi: 10.1038/nrc2536
32. Tsugane S, Inoue M. Insulin resistance and cancer: epidemiological evidence. *Cancer Sci.* (2010) 101:1073–9. doi: 10.1111/j.1349-7006.2010.01521.x
33. Key TJ, Appleby PN, Reeves GK, Roddam A, Dorgan JF, Longcope C, et al. Endogenous Hormones Breast Cancer Collaborative Group. Body mass index, serum sex hormones, and breast cancer risk in postmenopausal women. *J Natl Cancer Inst.* (2003) 95:1218–26. doi: 10.1093/jnci/djg022
34. Vona-Davis L, Rose DP. The obesity-inflammation-eicosanoid axis in breast cancer. *J Mammary Gland Biol Neoplasia.* (2013) 18:291–307. doi: 10.1007/s10911-013-9299-z
35. Gérard C, Brown KA. Obesity and breast cancer - role of estrogens and the molecular underpinnings of aromatase regulation in breast adipose tissue. *Mol Cell Endocrinol.* (2018) 466:15–30. doi: 10.1016/j.mce.2017.09.014
36. Genser L, Casella Mariolo JR, Castagneto-Gissey L, Panagiotopoulos S, Rubino F. Obesity, type 2 diabetes, and the metabolic syndrome: pathophysiologic relationships and guidelines for surgical intervention. *Surg Clin North Am.* (2016) 96:681–701. doi: 10.1016/j.suc.2016.03.013
37. Cani PD, Jordan BF. Gut microbiota-mediated inflammation in obesity: a link with gastrointestinal cancer. *Nat Rev Gastroenterol Hepatol.* (2018) 15:671–82. doi: 10.1038/s41575-018-0025-6
38. Huang TD, Behary J, Zekry A. Non-alcoholic fatty liver disease (NAFLD): a review of epidemiology, risk factors, diagnosis management. *Intern Med J.* (2019). doi: 10.1111/imj.14709. [Epub ahead of print].
39. Wong RJ, Cheung R, Ahmed A. Nonalcoholic steatohepatitis is the most rapidly growing indication for liver transplantation in patients with hepatocellular carcinoma in the U.S. *Hepatology.* (2014) 59:2188–95. doi: 10.1002/hep.26986
40. Lassailly G, Caiazzo R, Buob D, Pigeyre M, Verkindt H, Labreuche J, et al. Bariatric surgery reduces features of nonalcoholic steatohepatitis in morbidly obese patients. *Gastroenterology.* (2015) 149:379–88; quiz e15–6. doi: 10.1053/j.gastro.2015.04.014
41. Mathurin P, Hollebecque A, Arnalsteen L, Buob D, Leteurtre E, Caiazzo R, et al. Prospective study of the long-term effects of bariatric surgery on liver injury in patients without advanced disease. *Gastroenterology.* (2009) 137:532–40. doi: 10.1053/j.gastro.2009.04.052
42. Lee Y, Doumouras AG, Yu J, Brar K, Banfield L, Gmora S, et al. Complete resolution of nonalcoholic fatty liver disease after bariatric surgery: a systematic review and meta-analysis. *Clin Gastroenterol Hepatol.* (2019) 17:1040–60.e11. doi: 10.1016/j.cgh.2018.10.017
43. Sjöström L, Gummesson A, Sjöström CD, Narbro K, Peltonen M, Wedel H. Swedish obese subjects study. Effects of bariatric surgery on cancer incidence in obese patients in Sweden (Swedish Obese Subjects Study): a prospective, controlled intervention trial. *Lancet Oncol.* (2009) 10:653–62. doi: 10.1016/S1470-2045(09)70159-7
44. Adams TD, Stroup AM, Gress RE, Adams KF, Calle EE, Smith SC, et al. Cancer incidence and mortality after gastric bypass surgery. *Obesity.* (2009) 17:796–802. doi: 10.1038/oby.2008.610
45. Christou NV, Lieberman M, Sampalis F, Sampalis JS. Bariatric surgery reduces cancer risk in morbidly obese patients. *Surg Obes Relat Dis.* (2008) 4:691–5. doi: 10.1016/j.soard.2008.08.025
46. Hunsinger MA, Wood GC, Still C, Petrick A, Blansfield J, Shabahang M, et al. Maximizing weight loss after roux-en-Y gastric bypass may decrease risk of incident organ cancer. *Obes Surg.* (2016) 26:2856–61. doi: 10.1007/s11695-016-2206-0
47. McCawley GM, Ferriss JS, Geffel D, Northup CJ, Modesitt SC. Cancer in obese women: potential protective impact of bariatric surgery. *J Am Coll Surg.* (2009) 208:1093–8. doi: 10.1016/j.jamcollsurg.2009.01.045
48. Tee MC, Cao Y, Warnock GL, Hu FB, Chavarro JE. Effect of bariatric surgery on oncologic outcomes: a systematic review and meta-analysis. *Surg Endosc.* (2013) 27:4449–56. doi: 10.1007/s00464-013-3127-9
49. Argenta PA, Kassing M, Truskinovsky AM, Svendsen CA. Bariatric surgery and endometrial pathology in asymptomatic morbidly obese women: a prospective, pilot study. *BJOG.* (2013) 120:795–800. doi: 10.1111/1471-0528.12100
50. Ostlund MP, Lu Y, Lagergren J. Risk of obesity-related cancer after obesity surgery in a population-based cohort study. *Ann Surg.* (2010) 252:972–6. doi: 10.1097/SLA.0b013e3181e33778
51. Afshar S, Kelly SB, Seymour K, Lara J, Woodcock S, Mathers JC. The effects of bariatric surgery on colorectal cancer risk: systematic review and meta-analysis. *Obes Surg.* (2014) 24:1793–9. doi: 10.1007/s11695-014-1359-y
52. Derogar M, Hull MA, Kant P, Östlund M, Lu Y, Lagergren J. Increased risk of colorectal cancer after obesity surgery. *Ann Surg.* (2013) 258:983–8. doi: 10.1097/SLA.0b013e318288463a

53. Kant P, Hull MA. Excess body weight and obesity–the link with gastrointestinal and hepatobiliary cancer. *Nat Rev Gastroenterol Hepatol.* (2011) 8:224–38. doi: 10.1038/nrgastro.2011.23
54. Li JV, Ashrafian H, Bueter M, Kinross J, Sands C, le Roux CW, et al. Metabolic surgery profoundly influences gut microbial-host metabolic cross-talk. *Gut.* (2011) 60:1214–23. doi: 10.1136/gut.2010.234708
55. Candela M, Guidotti M, Fabbri A, Brigidi P, Franceschi C, Fiorentini C. Human intestinal microbiota: cross-talk with the host and its potential role in colorectal cancer. *Crit Rev Microbiol.* (2011) 37:1–14. doi: 10.3109/1040841X.2010.501760
56. Yang P, Zhou Y, Chen B, Wan HW, Jia GQ, Bai HL, et al. Overweight, obesity and gastric cancer risk: results from a meta-analysis of cohort studies. *Eur J Cancer.* (2009) 45:2867–73. doi: 10.1016/j.ejca.2009.04.019
57. Hampel H, Abraham NS, El-Serag HB. Meta-analysis: obesity and the risk for gastroesophageal reflux disease and its complications. *Ann Intern Med.* (2005) 143:199–211. doi: 10.7326/0003-4819-143-3-200508020-00006
58. Nilsson M, Lagergren J. The relation between body mass and gastro-oesophageal reflux. *Best Pract Res Clin Gastroenterol.* (2004) 18:1117–23. doi: 10.1016/j.bpg.2004.08.002
59. Dantas AC, Santo MA, de Cleva R, Sallum RA, Cecconello I. Influence of obesity and bariatric surgery on gastric cancer. *Cancer Biol Med.* (2016) 13:269–76. doi: 10.20892/j.issn.2095-3941.2016.0011
60. Näslund E, Stockeld D, Granström L, Backman L. Six cases of barrett's esophagus after gastric restrictive surgery for massive obesity: an extended case report. *Obes Surg.* (1996) 6:155–8. doi: 10.1381/096089296765557114
61. Scozzari G, Trapani R, Toppino M, Morino M. Esophagogastric cancer after bariatric surgery: systematic review of the literature. *Surg Obes Relat Dis.* (2013) 9:133–42. doi: 10.1016/j.soard.2012.10.002
62. Snook KL, Ritchie JD. Carcinoma of esophagus after adjustable gastric banding. *Obes Surg.* (2003) 13:800–2. doi: 10.1381/096089203322509444
63. Negri M, Bendet N, Halevy A, Halpern Z, Reif R, Bogokovsky H, et al. Gastric mucosal changes following gastroplasty: a comparative study between vertical banded gastroplasty and silastic ring vertical gastroplasty. *Obes Surg.* (1995) 5:383–6. doi: 10.1381/096089295765557458
64. Hackert T, Dietz M, Tjaden C, Sieg A, Buchler MW, Schmidt J. Band erosion with gastric cancer. *Obes Surg.* (2004) 14:559–61. doi: 10.1381/096089204323013622
65. Chiu S, Birch DW, Shi X, Sharma AM, Karmali S. Effect of sleeve gastrectomy on gastroesophageal reflux disease: a systematic review. *Surg Obes Relat Dis.* (2011) 7:510–5. doi: 10.1016/j.soard.2010.09.011
66. Genco A, Soricelli E, Casella G, Maselli R, Castagneto-Gissey L, Di Lorenzo N, et al. Gastroesophageal reflux disease and Barrett's esophagus after laparoscopic sleeve gastrectomy: a possible, underestimated long-term complication. *Surg Obes Relat Dis.* (2017) 13:568–4. doi: 10.1016/j.soard.2016.11.029
67. Castagneto Gissey L, Casella Mariolo JR, Genco A, Troisi A, Basso N, Casella G. 10-year follow-up after laparoscopic sleeve gastrectomy: Outcomes in a monocentric series. *Surg Obes Relat Dis.* (2018) 14:1480–7. doi: 10.1016/j.soard.2018.06.021
68. Soricelli E, Casella G, Baglio G, Maselli R, Ernesti I, Genco A. Lack of correlation between gastroesophageal reflux disease symptoms and esophageal lesions after sleeve gastrectomy. *Surg Obes Relat Dis.* (2018) 14:751–6. doi: 10.1016/j.soard.2018.02.008
69. Kauer WK, Peters JH, DeMeester TR, Ireland AP, Bremner CG, Hagen JA. Mixed reflux of gastric and duodenal juices is more harmful to the esophagus than gastric juice alone. The need for surgical therapy re-emphasized. *Ann Surg.* (1995) 222:525–31. doi: 10.1097/00000658-199522240-00010
70. Sebastianelli L, Benois M, Vanbiervliet G, Bailly L, Robert M, Turrin N. Systematic endoscopy 5 years after sleeve gastrectomy results in a high rate of barrett's esophagus: results of a multicenter study. *Obes Surg.* (2019) 29:1462–9. doi: 10.1007/s11695-019-03704-y
71. Sinar DR, Flickinger EG, Park HK, Sloss RR. Retrograde endoscopy of the bypassed stomach segment after gastric bypass surgery: unexpected lesions. *South Med J.* (1985) 78:255–8. doi: 10.1097/00007611-198503000-00006
72. Inoue H, Rubino F, Shimada Y, Lindner V, Inoue M, Riegel P, et al. Risk of gastric cancer after Roux-en-Y gastric bypass. *Arch Surg.* (2007) 142:947–53. doi: 10.1001/archsurg.142.10.947
73. Kuga R, Safatle-Ribeiro AV, Faintuch J, Ishida RK, Furuya CK Jr, Garrido AB Jr, et al. Endoscopic findings in the excluded stomach after Roux-en-Y gastric bypass surgery. *Arch Surg.* (2007) 142:942–6. doi: 10.1001/archsurg.142.10.942
74. Schnapka G, Hofstaedter F, Schwamberger K, Reissigl H. Gastric stump carcinoma following Billroth II resection for peptic ulcer disease. Comparison with cancer in non-operated stomach. *Endoscopy.* (1984) 16:171–4. doi: 10.1055/s-2007-1018572
75. Csendes A, Burgos AM, Smok G, Burdiles P, Braghetto I, Díaz JC. Latest results (12-21 years) of a prospective randomized study comparing Billroth II and Roux-en-Y anastomosis after a partial gastrectomy plus vagotomy in patients with duodenal ulcers. *Ann Surg.* (2009) 249:189–94. doi: 10.1097/SLA.0b013e3181921aa1
76. Guirat A, Addossari HM. One anastomosis gastric bypass and risk of cancer. *Obes Surg.* (2018) 28:1441–4. doi: 10.1007/s11695-018-3156-5
77. Musella M, Berardi G, Bocchetti A, Green R, Cantoni V, Velotti N, et al. Esophagogastric neoplasms following bariatric surgery: an updated systematic review. *Obes Surg.* (2019) 29:2660–9. doi: 10.1007/s11695-019-03951-z
78. Castagneto Gissey L, Casella Mariolo JR, Mingrone G. How to Choose the Best Metabolic Procedure? *Curr Atheroscler Rep.* (2016) 18:43. doi: 10.1007/s11883-016-0590-5
79. Ali M, El Chaar M, Ghiassi S, Rogers AM, American Society for Metabolic and Bariatric Surgery Clinical Issues Committee. American society for metabolic and bariatric surgery updated position statement on sleeve gastrectomy as a bariatric procedure. *Surg Obes Relat Dis.* (2017) 13:1652–7. doi: 10.1016/j.soard.2017.08.007

3

Metabolic Surgery to Treat Obesity in Diabetic Kidney Disease, Chronic Kidney Disease and End-Stage Kidney Disease: What Are the Unanswered Questions?

William P. Martin[1]*, *James White*[1], *Francisco J. López-Hernández*[2], *Neil G. Docherty*[1] *and Carel W. le Roux*[1,3]

[1] *Diabetes Complications Research Centre, School of Medicine, Conway Institute of Biomolecular and Biomedical Research, University College Dublin, Dublin, Ireland,* [2] *Instituto de Estudios de Ciencias de la Salud de Castilla y León-Instituto de Investigación Biomédica de Salamanca (IECSCYL-IBSAL), Hospital Virgen Vega, Salamanca, Spain,* [3] *Division of Investigative Science, Imperial College London, London, United Kingdom*

***Correspondence:**
William P. Martin
william.martin@ucd.ie

Obesity is a major factor in contemporary clinical practice in nephrology. Obesity accelerates the progression of both diabetic and non-diabetic chronic kidney disease and, in renal transplantation, both recipient and donor obesity increase the risk of allograft complications. Obesity is thus a major driver of renal disease progression and a barrier to deceased and living donor kidney transplantation. Large observational studies have highlighted that metabolic surgery reduces the incidence of albuminuria, slows chronic kidney disease progression, and reduces the incidence of end-stage kidney disease over extended follow-up in people with and without type 2 diabetes. The surgical treatment of obesity and its metabolic sequelae has therefore the potential to improve management of diabetic and non-diabetic chronic kidney disease and aid in the slowing of renal decline toward end-stage kidney disease. In the context of patients with end-stage kidney disease, although complications of metabolic surgery are higher, absolute event rates are low and it remains a safe intervention in this population. Pre-transplant metabolic surgery increases access to kidney transplantation in people with obesity and end-stage kidney disease. Metabolic surgery also improves management of metabolic complications post-kidney transplantation, including new-onset diabetes. Procedure selection may be critical to mitigate the risks of oxalate nephropathy and disruption to immunosuppressant pharmacokinetics. Metabolic surgery may also have a role in the treatment of donor obesity, which could increase the living kidney donor pool with potential downstream impact on kidney paired exchange programmes. The present paper provides a comprehensive coverage of the literature concerning renal outcomes in clinical studies of metabolic surgery and integrates findings from relevant mechanistic pre-clinical studies. In so doing the key unanswered questions for the field are brought to the fore for discussion.

Keywords: obesity, metabolic surgery, type 2 diabetes mellitus, diabetic kidney disease, chronic kidney disease, end-stage kidney disease, kidney transplantation, dialysis

OBESITY IS A DISEASE

Clinicians understand the risks of being obese and encourage patients to lose weight to prevent the complications of obesity. Thus, far, it has been very difficult to treat obesity as the aetiology has been misunderstood. Logically, if clinicians can convince themselves that obesity is a disease that requires treatment then progress can be made. Most human diseases are characterised by a set of reproducible symptoms and signs which affect a particular group of people and follow a predictable clinical trajectory (1). Our understanding of disease is enhanced when its aetiology and complications are well defined. Obesity can now be defined as a disease characterised by the pathognomonic symptoms of excess hunger and/or reduced satiation after a meal and the pathognomonic sign of increased adiposity, resulting in a state of dysregulated energy homeostasis that substantially increases mortality (2). Subcortical brain regions, especially the hypothalamus, integrate a diverse array of endocrine, neural, and neuroendocrine afferent signals from the viscera and external cues to govern human feeding behaviours (3). Evidence has been mounting that will help clinicians understand that by approaching obesity as a disease of the subcortical brain regions, more effective and compassionate treatments can be provided to our patients.

DIABETIC KIDNEY DISEASE AND OBESITY-RELATED GLOMERULOPATHY: AN OVERVIEW OF THE 2 MAJOR DRIVERS OF CHRONIC KIDNEY DISEASE IN PEOPLE WITH OBESITY

Diabetic Kidney Disease (DKD)

The obesity pandemic has contributed to an increased prevalence of type 2 diabetes and its attendant microvascular complications, including diabetic kidney disease (DKD) (4). DKD develops in ~40% of people with type 2 diabetes, with higher prevalence among non-Caucasian ethnicities (5). DKD is associated with significant increases in cardiovascular and all-cause mortality, with the majority of excess cardiovascular and all-cause mortality attributable to diabetes occurring in those with kidney disease (6). Compared with people with diabetes but no kidney disease, DKD [defined as eGFR ≤60 mL/min/BSA and/or urine albumin-to-creatinine ratio (uACR) ≥3 mg/mmol] increased the absolute risk of 10-year all-cause mortality by 19.6% in the Third National Health and Nutrition Examination Survey (6). The pathophysiology of DKD is primarily driven by metabolic dysregulation accompanying diabetes (hyperglycaemia, dyslipidaemia, and hypertension), and clinical management of DKD focuses on control of these inciting factors through blood pressure control, renin-angiotensin-aldosterone system (RAAS) blockade, and intensification of glycaemic and lipid control to minimise proteinuria and slow eGFR decline (7). Two recent additions to the DKD treatment paradigm include sodium-glucose co-transporter-2 inhibitors (SGLT2is) and GLP-1 receptor analogues (GLP1RAs), which independently of improvements in glycaemic control and blood pressure, have been demonstrated to improve renal outcomes in people with type 2 diabetes (8, 9). Obesity is now recognized as a risk factor for the onset and progression of type 2 DKD (7), yet obesity treatments are not currently offered to people with type 2 DKD in routine clinical practice.

Pathophysiological alterations which perpetuate DKD can be considered separately as haemodynamic (RAAS activation, endothelial dysfunction), metabolic (accumulation of advanced glycation end-products), pro-inflammatory (reactive oxygen species generation, tumour necrosis factor-α activation), and pro-fibrotic (stimulation of transforming growth factor-β signaling) (7), but in reality these elements interact locally and systemically to form a complex and dynamic interplay resulting in functional and structural changes to the kidney (10). Structural kidney changes are more heterogeneous in type 2 compared with type 1 DKD and include arteriolar hyalinosis, glomerular and tubular basement membrane thickening, mesangial matrix expansion, and podocyte foot process effacement (11). In later stages, extreme mesangial expansion may lead to nodular glomerulosclerosis and formation of pathognomonic Kimmelstiel-Wilson lesions (11). Tubular atrophy and interstitial fibrosis also occur late in the disease process (11).

A diagnosis of DKD is assigned in the presence of persistent albuminuria (uACR ≥3 mg/mmol) and/or sustained reduction in eGFR ≤60 mL/min/BSA in patients with suggestive clinical features, including presence of other diabetes microvascular complications (e.g., diabetic retinopathy), negative autoimmune serology, and absence of an active urinary sediment (e.g., dysmorphic red blood cells or red blood cell casts) (7). The natural history of type 2 DKD remains incompletely elucidated. Previously, most patients were considered to progress sequentially through phases including glomerular hyperfiltration, microalbuminuria, and macroalbuminuria with progressive eGFR decline (12). It is now recognized that a significant number of people with DKD experience progressive eGFR decline in the absence of albuminuria (13), highlighting the need for biomarkers which facilitate earlier diagnosis and prognostication of cardiovascular disease and end-stage kidney disease (ESKD) risk among people with DKD.

Obesity-Related Glomerulopathy (ORG)

The obesity pandemic has also fueled an increased incidence of obesity-related glomerulopathy (ORG), a distinct cause of chronic kidney disease (CKD) characterized by sub-nephrotic

---

Abbreviations: AGB, adjustable gastric banding; BMI, body-mass index; BPD/DS, biliopancreatic diversion/duodenal switch; BSA, body surface area; CI, confidence interval; CKD, chronic kidney disease; CKD-EPI, Chronic Kidney Disease-Epidemiology Collaboration; DKD, diabetic kidney disease; eGFR, estimated glomerular filtration rate; ESKD, end-stage kidney disease; FSGS, focal segmental glomerulosclerosis; GLP1RA, glucagon-like peptide-1 receptor analogue; GORD, gastro-oesophageal reflux disease; KDIGO, Kidney Disease Improving Global Outcomes; mGFR, measured glomerular filtration rate; NODAT, new-onset diabetes after transplantation; ORG, obesity-related glomerulopathy; PRFT, peri-renal fat thickness; PUFT, para-renal and peri-renal ultrasonographic fat thickness; RAAS, renin-angiotensin-aldosterone system; RCT, randomised controlled trial; RSF, renal sinus fat; RSNS, renal sympathetic nervous system; RYGB, Roux-en-Y gastric bypass; SGLT2i, sodium-glucose co-transporter-2 inhibitor; SOS, Swedish Obese Subjects; uACR, urinary albumin-to-creatinine ratio; VAT, visceral adipose tissue; VSG, vertical sleeve gastrectomy.

range proteinuria, glomerulomegaly, and progressive renal functional loss (14). Histological evidence of glomerulomegaly is the defining feature of ORG and is present in all biopsy-proven cases (14). In the absence of confirmation by kidney biopsy, and where other kidney diseases are not suspected based on features such as accelerated renal functional decline or an active urinary sediment, persistent proteinuria in obese patients without diabetes is generally considered diagnostic of ORG (14). Obesity increases afferent arteriolar ultrafiltration pressure to cause glomerular hyperfiltration (15); as a result, many patients with ORG also develop an adaptive form of focal segmental glomerulosclerosis (FSGS) (16). FSGS is defined as segmental solidification of the glomerular tuft by extracellular matrix and/or hyaline, with obliteration of capillaries in sclerosed segments (16). Six forms (primary, adaptive, APOL1-associated, high-penetrance genetic, virus-associated, medication-associated) and five histologic subtypes (perihilar, cellular, tip, collapsing, not otherwise specified) of FSGS are recognized (16). FSGS complicating ORG is considered an adaptive response to a mismatch between glomerular load and capacity, has a predilection for perihilar sclerosis, and generally affects fewer glomeruli and results in less podocyte foot process effacement than primary FSGS (14). As a result, adaptive FSGS accompanying ORG rarely causes full-blown nephrotic syndrome and runs a more indolent course than primary FSGS, although renal survival at 10 years from diagnosis is only 50% (17).

Similar to DKD, multiple pathophysiological disruptions, both systemically and locally in the kidney, provoke and perpetuate ORG. Indeed, many parallels exist between DKD and ORG pathogenesis, including glomerular hyperfiltration, RAAS overactivation, enhanced tubular sodium reabsorption, hypoadiponectinaemia, renal lipotoxicitiy, and impaired tubular fatty acid β-oxidation. The potential of metabolic surgery to reverse many of these phenomena simultaneously [discussed further below in the section Mechanisms Underpinning Renoprotection and in other recent reviews from our group (18)] supports a growing interest in the potential utility of metabolic surgery to treat both DKD and ORG. Glomerular hyperfiltration in ORG occurs via afferent arteriolar dilatation, resulting in abnormal transmission of increased arterial pressure to glomerular capillaries in individuals with systemic hypertension (15). Enhanced proximal tubular sodium reabsorption occurs in people with obesity, which in turn decreases distal tubular sodium delivery to the macula densa, diminishes tubuloglomerular feedback, and leads to compensatory afferent arteriolar vasodilatation to result in glomerular hyperfiltration (19). Adipose tissue synthesizes RAAS components, and obese individuals demonstrate RAAS overactivation (20). Increased leptin and decreased adiponectin synthesis by adipose tissue in obese individuals also activates the renal sympathetic nervous system (RSNS) (21). RAAS and RSNS overactivation, along with hyperinsulinaemia, further perpetuate tubular sodium reabsorption, glomerular hyperfiltration, and systemic hypertension in obese individuals (14). Obesity-associated hypoadiponectinaemia may worsen proteinuria through a direct action on podocytes (22). Beyond haemodynamic alterations, expansion of specific visceral adipose tissue depots including peri-renal fat and renal sinus fat may mechanically compress the kidney in obese individuals, while renal lipotoxicity arising from renal triglyceride and cholesterol accumulation may also exacerbate ORG (23).

The true prevalence of ORG is unknown, although the prevalence of significant proteinuria (≥1+ by urine dipstick or uACR ≥30 mg/mmol) is 4–10% amongst obese patients (24, 25). Importantly, over 45% of patients with histologically confirmed ORG in a single-centre study in the United States had a BMI <40 kg/m^2 (26). Therefore, ORG is not restricted to those with extreme BMIs and should be highly prevalent in those attending routine weight management services. Furthermore, in a study of 95 patients with BMI ≥40 kg/m^2 without overt kidney disease (normal serum creatinine and <0.2 grams proteinuria/day) who underwent kidney biopsy at the time of metabolic surgery, a wide range of histological glomerular abnormalities were present including glomerulomegaly, mesangial matrix expansion, podocyte hypertrophy, and glomerulosclerosis (27). Therefore, subclinical kidney disease with established glomerular structural abnormalities is likely severely under-recognised in patients attending weight management services. Non-invasive serum and urinary biomarkers which accurately identify such patients with subclinical ORG are urgently needed. RAAS blockade, which reduces efferent arteriolar resistance to lower glomerular hydrostatic pressure, is the main approach to ORG management (16). Dietary sodium restriction, thiazide diuretics, and aldosterone antagonists may be used to potentiate the anti-proteinuric effects of RAAS blockade, although such regimens require further study (16). Prospective, controlled studies of metabolic surgery in individuals with biopsy-proven ORG and proteinuric CKD are required.

THE OBESITY PANDEMIC IS CONTRIBUTING TO INCREASING CHRONIC KIDNEY DISEASE AND END-STAGE KIDNEY DISEASE PREVALENCE: EVIDENCE FROM OBSERVATIONAL STUDIES AND SYSTEMATIC REVIEWS AND META-ANALYSES

Obesity complications are well defined and their rising prevalence presents one of the foremost challenges to healthcare delivery in the 21st century. Importantly, many complications including hypertension (28), type 2 diabetes (29), obstructive sleep apnoea (30), idiopathic intracranial hypertension (31), polycystic ovarian syndrome (32), and non-alcoholic fatty liver disease (33) can be reversed with intentional weight loss. Compared with other obesity complications, comparatively little is known about kidney disease as a complication of obesity. The increasing prevalence of obesity, CKD, and ESKD are inter-related (34). Obesity increases risk of CKD onset and of progression of existing CKD to ESKD (34).

Chang et al. performed a meta-analysis of individual participant data to investigate relationships between adiposity measures (body-mass index, waist circumference, and waist-to-height ratio), glomerular filtration rate (GFR) decline, and all-cause mortality (35). Over mean 8-year follow-up in n = 39 general population cohorts (n = 5,459,014 participants), hazard ratios for BMIs 30, 35, and 40 were 1.18 (95% CI 1.09–1.27), 1.69 (95% CI 1.51–1.89), and 2.02 (95% CI 1.80–2.27), respectively, for increased risk of GFR decline compared with BMI of 25. The impact of BMI on subsequent GFR decline in people with established CKD was smaller. Across 18 CKD cohorts (n = 91,607 participants) over mean follow-up of 4 years, the hazard ratio for GFR decline for BMI 35 vs. 25 was 1.17 (95% CI 1.04–1.31). Similar to BMI, increasing waist circumference and waist-to-height ratio were strongly associated with GFR decline in general population cohorts and more weakly associated with GFR decline in CKD cohorts. Increasing BMI and waist circumference, but not waist-to-height ratio, were also associated mortality risk in people with CKD. Independent of relationships between obesity and type 2 diabetes, this data provides a rationale to pursue dedicated obesity treatments to reduce CKD prevalence and progression.

Similarly, Garofalo et al. performed a systematic review and meta-analysis to investigate relationships between BMI and both impaired eGFR (<60 mL/min/BSA) and/or albuminuria (1+ on urinary dipstick or uACR ≥3.4 mg/mmol) (36). Across 39 cohorts (n = 630,677 participants) with mean follow-up of 6.8 years, obesity but not overweight increased the relative risk of onset of low eGFR (1.28, 95% CI 1.07–1.54) and albuminuria (1.51, 95% CI 1.36–1.67). Each unit increase in BMI (kg/m^2) increased the relative risk of onset of both eGFR <60 mL/min/BSA and albuminuria by 2%.

Multiple epidemiologic studies have also demonstrated that obesity strongly and independently increases the risk of ESKD. Hsu et al. demonstrated that increasing severity of obesity incrementally increased the risk of ESKD compared with controls with normal BMI (18.5–24.9 kg/m^2) in n = 320,252 adults with and without baseline CKD (37). Adjusted relative risks for ESKD were 1.87 (95% CI 1.64–2.14), 3.57 (95% CI 3.05–4.18), 6.12 (95% CI 4.97–7.54), and 7.07 (95% CI 5.37–9.31) for individuals with overweight, class 1 obesity, class 2 obesity, and class 3 obesity, respectively. Similarly, Lu et al. demonstrated that BMI ≥35 kg/m^2 independently increased risk of adverse renal outcomes (steeper eGFR slope, doubling of serum creatinine, and incident ESKD) in n = 453,946 United States veterans with baseline CKD (eGFR < 60 mL/min/BSA), although associations weakened in those with more advanced CKD (38).

METABOLIC SURGERY REARRANGES THE GUT TO EFFECTIVELY TREAT OBESITY

Figure 1 outlines the four main metabolic surgery types discussed in the context of CKD and ESKD management in this review: vertical sleeve gastrectomy (VSG), Roux-en-Y gastric bypass (RYGB), adjustable gastric banding (AGB), and biliopancreatic diversion/duodenal switch (BPD/DS). All procedures can be performed laparoscopically (39). Description of the rearranged gastrointestinal anatomy for each of the four procedures is summarized below:

- VSG (**Figure 1A**) (39)
  - The stomach is excised (70–80%) along the greater curvature. The remnant tubular stomach contains the lesser curvature that is resistant to stretching due to the absence of the fundus, creating a high-pressure chamber that causes rapid gastric emptying and early delivery of ingested food to the small intestine.
- RYGB (**Figure 1B**) (39, 40):
  - The stomach is transected to create a small gastric pouch (15–30 mL volume) and a gastric remnant excluded from direct contact with food.
  - A jejunotomy is performed in the mid-jejunum, 50–75 cm distal to the ligament of Treitz.
  - An alimentary/Roux limb (100–150 cm length) is created by anastomosing the gastric pouch to the distal limb of the jejunotomy, allowing ingested food to bypass the duodenum and proximal jejunum and directly enter the mid-jejunum.
  - The small intestine proximal to the jejunotomy forms the biliopancreatic limb, which transports secretions from the remnant stomach, biliary tree, and pancreas.
  - The common channel is formed by side-to-side anastomosis of the biliopancreatic and alimentary limbs 100–150 cm distal to the gastrojejunostomy, and major absorption and digestion of nutrients occurs downstream of this juncture.
  - An alimentary limb of length 150 cm does not increase the risk of nutritional complications but does improve metabolic control compared with shorter limb lengths (41); alimentary limb lengths up to 150 cm are now the standard form of RYGB employed in clinical practice. Modification of the length of the alimentary limb beyond 150 cm ("long-limb RYGB") may be used to achieve even greater weight loss and metabolic control, although the risk for nutritional deficiencies, enteric hyperoxaluria, and suboptimal absorption of immunosuppressive agents also increases (42).
- AGB (**Figure 1C**) (39):
  - A silicone ring (band) is inserted around the stomach, immediately below the gastro- oesophageal junction, to create a 30 mL upper gastric pouch and a narrow passage to the remaining stomach.
  - The band is connected to a subcutaneous infusion port, wherein the volume of saline can be adjusted to control the band diameter.
- BPD/DS (**Figure 1D**) (39):
  - A VSG is combined with a proximal duodenoileostomy, causing ingested food to rapidly enter the small intestine and then bypass the duodenum and jejunum.

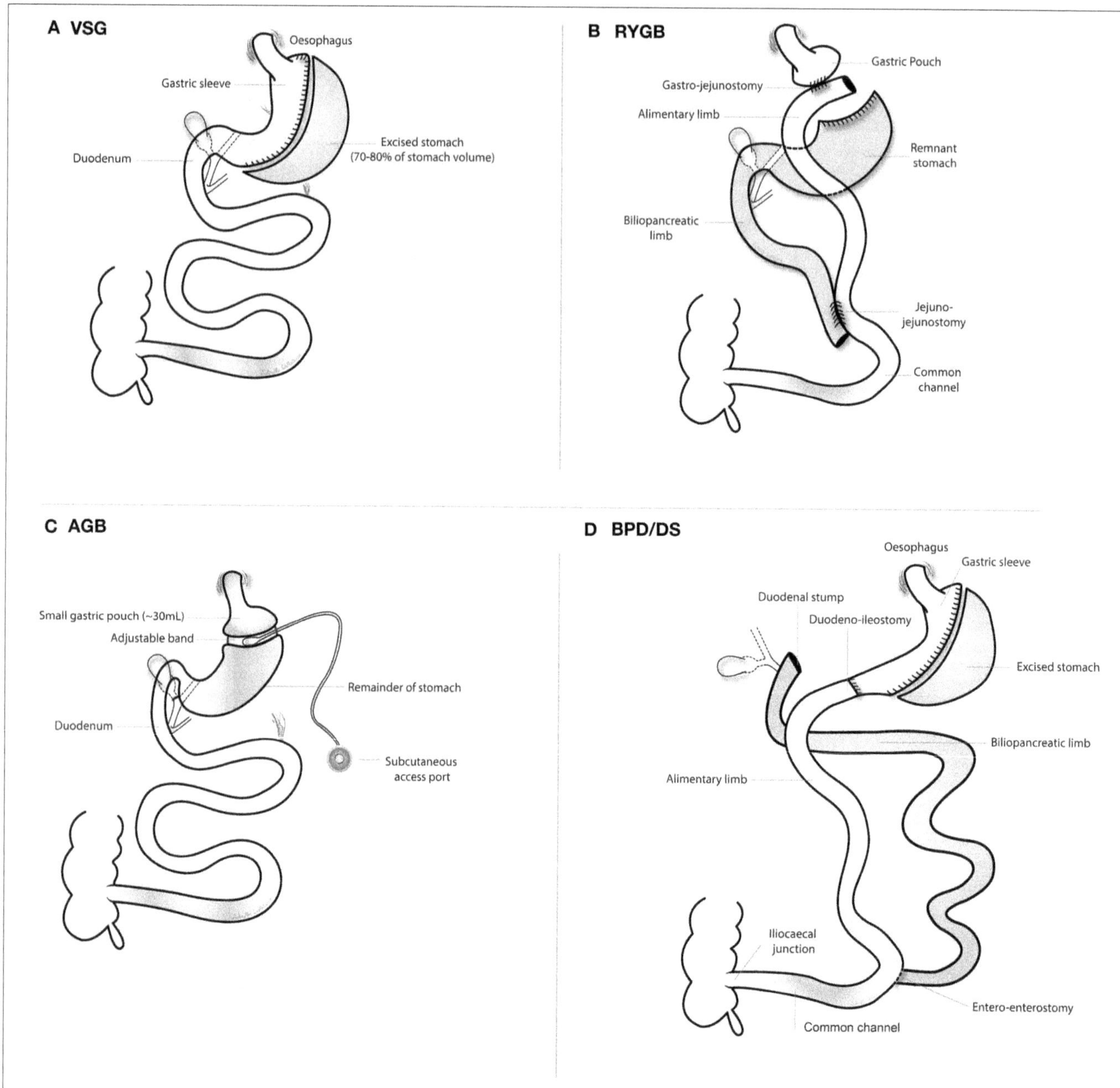

FIGURE 1 | Overview of the four principal metabolic surgery types. AGB, adjustable gastric banding; BPD/DS, biliopancreatic diversion with duodenal switch; RYGB, Roux-en-Y gastric bypass surgery; VSG, vertical sleeve gastrectomy. **(A)** vertical sleeve gastrectomy; **(B)** Roux-en-Y gastric bypass surgery; **(C)** adjustable gastric banding; **(D)** biliopancreatic diversion with duodenal switch.

AGB has declined in popularity, accounting for 5–10% of metabolic surgeries performed in the United States, due to modest efficacy and high complication rates requiring band revisions and/or removal (43). In the 2018 IFSO Global Bariatric Surgery Registry Report, which amalgamated data from 51 countries, AGB accounted for 5.0% of all metabolic surgeries performed since 2014 (44). BPD/DS is now infrequently performed due to the high burden of postoperative nutritional deficiencies resulting from the more extensive intestinal bypass (45). VSG and RYGB are the 2 most commonly performed metabolic surgeries. VSG has supplanted RYGB as the most commonly performed metabolic surgery procedure worldwide over the past decade (43, 46). Nevertheless, RYGB remains the most commonly performed metabolic surgery in South America and comprises ~40% of metabolic surgeries performed in the United States (43, 47). Compared with VSG, RYGB induces superior weight loss and metabolic control (29), and a much larger body of evidence with extended follow-up supports its efficacy in controlling diabetes complications (48). Nevertheless, VSG has dramatically increased in popularity as it is a relatively simple procedure with lower operative morbidity, and reduces the risks of internal herniation and micronutrient deficiency. At 1-year post-metabolic surgery in people with obesity and type 2 diabetes, RYGB reduced mean body weight by 4.3 kg more than VSG (49). Although further head-to-head comparisons between RYGB and VSG should be conducted in a randomised fashion, it appears that weight loss after VSG ranges between that of RYGB and AGB (50). Beyond anticipated metabolic benefits, other individual patient characteristics influence choice of metabolic surgery procedure. For example, gastro-oesophageal reflux disease (GORD) is common in obese individuals (51). *De novo* GORD and aggravation of pre-existing GORD is more common after VSG than RYGB (52), and given the relationship between obesity, GORD, and increasing incidence of oesophageal adenocarcinoma (53), RYGB may be preferable in this setting. Indeed, several large observational studies have highlighted that proton-pump inhibitors increase risk for acute interstitial nephritis and CKD onset and progression (54–56); therefore, minimising proton-pump inhibitor exposure after metabolic surgery by favouring RYGB in those at high-risk for *de novo* or aggravated GORD postoperatively may also be beneficial for kidney health.

Metabolic surgery achieves sustained weight loss and substantially lowers mortality in people with obesity (57, 58). Obesity is increasingly recognised as an important driver of CKD progression and is an important barrier to kidney transplantation, yet obesity is not specifically addressed during routine management of CKD and ESKD despite evidence of benefit (59). We herein summarise evidence supporting the potentially diverse roles of metabolic surgery in slowing DKD and CKD progression, as well as facilitating access to kidney transplantation and management of post-transplant metabolic complications. The primary purpose of the current review is to critically review clinical studies investigating the role of metabolic surgery in the management of patients with kidney disease of all stages. A limited discussion of mechanisms underpinning renoprotection conferred by metabolic surgery is provided in the section Mechanisms Underpinning Renoprotection. We refer the reader interested in mechanisms of renoprotection after metabolic surgery to a related recent review from our group (18).

WHAT IS THE ROLE OF METABOLIC SURGERY IN THE MANAGEMENT OF TYPE 2 DIABETIC KIDNEY DISEASE?

RCTs

Evidence supporting a role of metabolic surgery in the management of type 2 DKD is currently derived from RCTs of metabolic surgery for type 2 diabetes control, and observational studies investigating changes in renal parameters after metabolic surgery in people with obesity and type 2 diabetes. **Table 1** provides an overview of the major metabolic surgery RCTs which have investigated type 2 diabetes control and remission in obese individuals (29, 49, 60–67). Partial and complete diabetes remission were defined as HbA_{1c} < 6.5% and <6.0% without hypoglycaemic medication usage, respectively, although Dixon et al. defined diabetes remission as HbA_{1c} < 6.2% and fasting plasma glucose <126 mg/dL (67). All studies used intensive medical intervention as a control arm. In the largest head-to-head study (STAMPEDE RCT), RYGB achieved superior weight loss at 5 years compared with VSG (29). Additionally, complete and partial type 2 diabetes remission rates were higher in the RYGB arm compared with the VSG arm at 5 years (29). BPD/DS resulted in higher rates of partial and complete diabetes remission at 5 years than RYGB, despite similar weight loss in both groups (65).

Despite the early diabetes-remitting effects of metabolic surgery, high rates of type 2 diabetes recurrence over longer follow-up are now recognized. In the STAMPEDE RCT, of the 20 patients that achieved complete diabetes remission at 1 year post-RYGB, 10/20 (50%) experienced diabetes relapse by 5 years (29). Similarly, of the 12 patients that achieved complete diabetes remission at 1 year post-VSG, 5/12 (41.7%) experienced diabetes relapse by 5 years (29). Miras et al. randomised people with persistent or recurrent type 2 diabetes after metabolic surgery (HbA_{1c} > 6.5% at 1 year post-RYGB or VSG) to liraglutide 1.8 mg once daily or placebo, combined with a reduced-calorie diet and increased physical activity (68). Liraglutide reduced HbA_{1c} by 1.2% and body weight by 4.2 kg compared with the placebo arm at 26 weeks, with no difference in treatment response by surgery type. Thus, liraglutide may be used to optimize metabolic outcomes after metabolic surgery. Semaglutide achieved even greater reductions in body weight and glycaemia than liraglutide in the SUSTAIN clinical trial programme (69), and could also be potentially used to improve type 2 diabetes control after metabolic surgery. Liraglutide reduced DKD onset and progression in the LEADER RCT (9); thus, its use post-metabolic surgery may also confer additional renoprotective benefits. While questions remain as to the optimal type 2 diabetes medication algorithm post-metabolic surgery, it is clear that combined surgical and medical treatment approaches offer the most intensive control and should be used to optimize renal outcomes in those with type 2 DKD.

Two RCTs of metabolic surgery for type 2 diabetes reported changes in albuminuria postoperatively (29, 65) (**Table 1**). Although numbers with baseline albuminuria were small in Mingrone et al.'s RCT (n = 3 RYGB, n = 2 BPD/DS), both surgeries achieved sustained remission of albuminuria in all patients at 5 years (65). Prevalence of baseline albuminuria was higher in the STAMPEDE RCT, with RYGB reducing the proportion of patients with albuminuria from n = 17 (34%) at baseline to n = 9 (19%) at 5 years (29). Similarly, VSG reduced albuminuria prevalence from n = 12 (24%) at baseline to n = 5 (11.1%) at 5 years. Despite the low numbers of patients with albuminuria recruited to these studies, such data highlights the potent albuminuria-lowering effect of metabolic surgery. No RCTs have yet assessed the impact of metabolic surgery on primary renal outcomes in people with type 2 DKD. The Microvascular Outcomes after Metabolic Surgery (MOMS) clinical trial, which randomised people with obesity (BMI 30–34.9 kg/m^2), type 2 diabetes and moderately increased albuminuria to best medical care plus Roux-en-Y gastric bypass surgery or best medical care alone, finished recruiting in 2016; 1, 2, and 5 year outcomes are awaited (40). Individuals with

TABLE 1 | Anthropometry, type 2 diabetes control, and albuminuria in metabolic surgery RCTs in patients with obesity and type 2 diabetes.

Study	Study arms	Follow-up (months)	Body weight (kg)	BMI (kg/m^2)	T2D duration (years)	HbA$_{1c}$ (%)	HbA$_{1c}$ ≤6.5% without diabetes medications [*n* (%)]	HbA$_{1c}$ ≤6% without diabetes medications [*n* (%)]	Albuminuria[a] [*n* (%)]
Schauer et al. (STAMPEDE) (29, 49, 60)									
	RYGB + IMT	0	107 ± 15	37 ± 3	8 ± 6	9 ± 1	–	–	17 (34)
		12	77 ± 13	27 ± 3	–	6 ± 1	–	21 (42)	–
		36	81 ± 16	28	–	7 ± 1	22 (46)	17 (35)	–
		60	83 ± 15	29	–	7 ± 2	15 (31)	11 (22)	9 (19)
	VSG + IMT	0	101 ± 16	36 ± 4	9 ± 5	10 ± 2	–	–	12 (24)
		12	76 ± 13	27 ± 4	–	7 ± 1	–	13 (27)	–
		36	79 ± 15	29	–	7 ± 1	14 (29)	10 (20)	–
		60	82 ± 15	29	–	7 ± 2	11 (23)	7 (15)	5 (11)
	IMT	0	107 ± 15	37 ± 3	9 ± 6	9 ± 1	–	–	10 (20)
		12	99 ± 16	34 ± 4	–	8 ± 2	–	0 (0)	–
		36	100 ± 17	35	–	8 ± 2	0 (0)	0 (0)	–
		60	99 ± 17	34	–	9 ± 2	0 (0)	0 (0)	8 (22)
Ikramuddin et al. (DSS) (61–63)									
	RYGB + IMT	0	99 ± 14	35 (34-36)	9 ± 6	10 ± 1	–	–	–
		12	73 ± 14	26 (25-27)	–	6 ± 1	0 (0)	0 (0)	–
		24	–	27 (26-27)	–	7 ± 2	25 (42)	15 (25)	–
		60	–	27 (27-28)	–	7 (7-8)	9 (16)	4 (7)	–
	IMT	0	98 ± 17	34 (34-35)	9 ± 6	10 ± 1	–	–	–
		12	90 ± 17	32 (31-32)	–	8 ± 2	0 (0)	0 (0)	–
		24	–	32 (31-33)	–	8 ± 3	0 (0)	0 (0)	–
		60	–	31 (30-32)	–	9 (8-9)	0 (0)	0 (0)	–
Mingrone et al. (64, 65)									
	RYGB + IMT	0	130 ± 23	45 ± 5	6 ± 1	9 ± 1	–	–	3 (16)
		24	84 ± 13	29 ± 3	–	6 ± 1	15 (75)	–	–
		60	90 ± 13	31 ± 3	–	7 ± 1	8 (42)	1 (5)	0 (0)
	BPD/DS + IMT	0	138 ± 30	45 ± 8	6 ± 1	9 ± 2	–	–	2 (11)
		24	90 ± 18	29 ± 5	–	5 ± 0.5	19 (95)	–	–
		60	93 ± 14	30 ± 4	–	6 ± 0.4	13 (68)	7 (37)	0 (0)
	IMT	0	136 ± 22	46 ± 6	6 ± 1	9 ± 1	–	–	4 (27)
		24	128 ± 20	43 ± 6	–	8 ± 1	0 (0)	0 (0)	–
		60	127 ± 21	42 ± 6	–	7 ± 1	0 (0)	0 (0)	4 (27)
Cummings et al. (CROSSROADS) (66)									
	RYGB + IMT	0	109 ± 15	38 ± 4	11 ± 5	8 ± 1	–	–	–
		12	–	–	–	6 ± 2	9 (60)	9 (60)	–
	ILMI	0	113 ± 17	37 ± 4	7 ± 5	7 ± 1	–	–	–
		12	–	–	–	7 ± 1	1 (6)	1 (6)	–

(Continued)

TABLE 1 | Continued

Study	Study arms	Follow-up (months)	Body weight (kg)	BMI (kg/m^2)	T2D duration (years)	HbA_{1c} (%)	HbA_{1c} ≤6.5% without diabetes medications [n (%)]	HbA_{1c} ≤6% without diabetes medications [n (%)]	Albuminuria[a] [n (%)]
Dixon et al. (67)									
	AGB + IMT	0	106 ± 14	37 ± 3	–	8 ± 1	–	–	–
		24	85 ± 16	–	–	6 ± 1	–	22 (73)[b]	–
	IMT	0	106 ± 14	37 ± 3	–	8 ± 1	–	–	–
		24	105 ± 15	–	–	7 ± 1	0 (0)	4 (13)[b]	–

[a]Albuminuria, urine albumin/creatinine ratio ≥3 mg albumin per mmol of creatinine.
[b]Type 2 diabetes remission defined as HbA_{1c} <6.2% and fasting plasma glucose <126 mg/dL without hypoglycaemic medication usage in this study.
Mean ± SD or mean (95% CI) are presented for normally distributed continuous variables; n (%) are presented for categorical variables.
AGB, adjustable gastric banding; BMI, body-mass index; BPD/DS, biliopancreatic diversion/duodenal switch; DSS, Diabetes Surgery Study; $HbA1_c$, glycated haemoglobin; ILMI, intensive lifestyle and medical intervention; IMT, intensive medical therapy; RYGB, Roux-en-Y gastric bypass; T2D, type 2 diabetes mellitus; VSG, vertical sleeve gastrectomy.

baseline eGFR <30 mL/min/BSA were excluded from the MOMS RCT and baseline eGFR was >60 mL/min/BSA in both study arms (40). An RCT which randomizes individuals with obesity, type 2 diabetes, severely increased albuminuria, and eGFR 30–60 mL/min/BSA to metabolic surgery plus best medical care or best medical care alone and assesses mGFR in a longitudinal fashion is required to determine the impact of metabolic surgery in those with more advanced type 2 DKD.

Observational Studies

Incidence of DKD

Several large scale-observational studies have examined the impact of metabolic surgery on subsequent incidence of microvascular complications of diabetes, including type 2 DKD. O'Brien et al. performed a retrospective observational cohort study of 4,024 people with type 2 diabetes who underwent metabolic surgery between 2005 and 2011 across one of four health care systems in the United States, and 11,059 matched non-surgically treated controls (70). Metabolic surgery reduced incident nephropathy (defined as sustained CKD-EPI eGFR <60 mL/min/BSA over ≥90 days) at 7-year follow-up, with kidney disease developing in 6.4% [95% CI 5.3–7.6%] of surgically treated patients and 14% [95% CI 13–15.1%] of non-surgical controls (adjusted hazard ratio 0.45 [95% CI 0.29–0.71]).

Madsen et al. performed a matched cohort study to examine the impact of RYGB on type 2 diabetes remission and micro- and macro-vascular complications of diabetes in an obese (BMI ≥35 kg/m^2), Northern Danish population (71). RYGB-operated subjects (n = 1,111) and were compared to 1,074 matched controls. Type 2 diabetes remission occurred in 74% of RYGB-operated individuals at 1 year postoperatively; however, 27% of these relapsed at 5-year follow-up. RYGB reduced the risk of microvascular complications of type 2 diabetes over 5.3 year follow-up (HR 0.53 [95% CI 0.38–0.73]). Similarly, reduction in incident microvascular complications was greater in those that achieved type 2 diabetes remission at 1-year follow-up compared with those that did not (HR 0.43 [95% CI 0.25–0.72]). RYGB reduced the development of type 2 DKD compared with matched controls (incidence rate ratio 0.54 [95% CI 0.31–0.94]).

A subgroup analysis of people with baseline type 2 diabetes in the Swedish Obese Subjects (SOS) cohort study also identified reduced incidence of microvascular complications of diabetes after metabolic surgery (n = 343) compared with controls who received usual care (n = 260) (hazard ratio 0.44 [95% CI 0.34–0.56]) (48). Although the impact of metabolic surgery on renal endpoints is not specifically reported in this paper, a subsequent publication from the SOS study highlighted that metabolic surgery (n = 187) reduced the subsequent incidence of albuminuria in those with baseline type 2 diabetes compared with controls (n = 157) over median 10-year follow-up (hazard ratio 0.35 [95% CI 0.21–0.59]) (72). Similarly, Shulman et al. demonstrated that metabolic surgery (n = 344) in the SOS cohort reduced the incidence of a composite of CKD stage 4/ESKD in those with baseline type 2 diabetes compared with usual care controls (n = 263) over median 18-year follow-up (hazard ratio 0.35 [95% CI 0.15–0.81]) (73). Numbers needed to treat with metabolic surgery to prevent one case of albuminuria and CKD stage 4/ESKD were 4 and 46, respectively, in those with baseline type 2 diabetes (72, 73). Considering that DKD often progresses to ESKD which is costly to manage (74, 75), metabolic surgery for the prevention of ESKD is likely cost-effective although formal cost-effectiveness analysis is required.

Remission/Control of Existing DKD

Heneghan et al. investigated changes in albuminuria 5 years after metabolic surgery in 52 people with type 2 diabetes at a single centre ($n = 36$ RYGB, $n = 13$ AGB, $n = 3$ VSG) (76). Of those with baseline albuminuria (31.3 and 6.3% with moderately and severely increased albuminuria, respectively), 58.3% achieved remission of albuminuria at 5-year follow-up. Conversely, moderately increased albuminuria developed over 5 years in only 25% of those without baseline albuminuria, while no patients developed severely increased albuminuria during follow-up. The anti-albuminuric effect of metabolic surgery associated with postoperative improvement or remission of type 2 diabetes.

Canney et al. investigated the impact of RYGB in addition to optimal medical therapy in 105 individuals with type 2 diabetes (mean duration 13 ± 3 years) and moderately or severely increased albuminuria (77). At mean 13-month follow-up, mean BMI reduced from 38 to 27 kg/m^2, mean HbA$_{1c}$ decreased from 8 to 6%, and median uACR decreased by 81% from 88 to 14 mg/g. Remission of albuminuria (uACR <30 mg/g) occurred in 82 (78%) people postoperatively. Reductions in albuminuria were seen across all tertiles of baseline albuminuria indicating that RYGB is an effective anti-proteinuric strategy across the spectrum of baseline DKD severity. A parallel pre-clinical study of RYGB in the Zucker Diabetic Fatty rat model of obesity and DKD identified similar reductions in albuminuria postoperatively (mean 86% reduction in uACR) (77). Moreover, RYGB reduced glomerular volume, podocyte stress (desmin expression), and podocyte dedifferentiation (podocyte foot process effacement assessed by transmission electron microscopy) indicating that the anti-proteinuric effect of RYGB is accompanied by concordant improvements in glomerular structure and ultrastructure.

Future Directions

Thus, several RCTs indicate that metabolic surgery combined with medical therapy significantly improves type 2 diabetes control while multiple, large observational studies indicate that such metabolic benefits result in improved renal outcomes over the longer term. With recent advances in medical care of diabetes, including SGLT2is and GLP1RAs, opportunities to optimise metabolic parameters and end-organ damage in the kidney abound through combined metabolic surgery plus intensive medical care. Metabolic surgery will not serve as a sole and primary treatment modality for DKD, but rather serve as adjunct to optimal medical therapy to halt progressive DKD. Definitive RCTs investigating the impact of metabolic surgery in people with type 2 diabetes, impaired glomerular filtration, and progressive renal functional decline despite optimal medical therapy are necessary to define its role across the spectrum of CKD severity.

WHAT IS THE ROLE OF METABOLIC SURGERY FOR SLOWING THE PROGRESSION OF CHRONIC KIDNEY DISEASE?

Although metabolic surgery dramatically improves diabetes control in many patients, its renoprotective effects occur independently of improvements in glycaemia and BMI (78). Scheurlen et al. performed a systematic review and meta-analysis of changes in albuminuria after metabolic surgery in people with type 2 diabetes, and their correlation with changes in HbA$_{1c}$, BMI, and systolic blood pressure (79). The authors identified 15 suitable studies of mixed study design (five retrospective cohort studies, eight prospective cohort studies, one prospective case-control study, and one randomised controlled trial). No relationship between change in albuminuria and changes in BMI, HbA$_{1c}$, and systolic blood pressure after metabolic surgery were identified. Such observations emphasise the importance of pre-clinical studies of metabolic surgery with direct access to kidney tissue, wherein weight-independent and glycaemia-independent mediators of renoprotection can be interrogated.

An increasing body of observational evidence indicates that metabolic surgery also improves renal outcomes in people without diabetes. The major observational studies are summarized below. No RCTs have yet investigated the impact of metabolic surgery in those with non-diabetic CKD. Future prospective studies should ideally be conducted in a randomized fashion, using 24-h urinary protein excretion rates and measured glomerular filtration rate as primary outcomes, to investigate renoprotective effects of metabolic surgery in this setting.

Observational Studies

Matched Observational Cohort Studies (No Baseline CKD)

Chang et al. investigated the impact of metabolic surgery on renal outcomes in 985 people (baseline type 2 diabetes in 37.8%; RYGB 96.5%, VSG 3.5%) and an equal number of matched controls (80). The surgery and control cohorts were followed for a median of 4.4 and 3.8 years, respectively. Metabolic surgery reduced the risk of ≥30% eGFR decline by 58% (hazard ratio 0.42 [95% CI 0.32–0.55]). Similarly, metabolic surgery also lowered a composite endpoint of doubling of serum creatinine or ESKD by 57% (hazard ratio 0.43 [95% CI 0.26–0.71]).

Risk reductions in renal outcomes of similar magnitude were also reported in the SOS study, in which the baseline type 2 diabetes prevalence was significantly smaller and in which a much lower proportion of patients underwent RYGB. Carlsson et al. investigated the incidence of albuminuria over median 10-year follow-up in 1,498 surgically treated patients (baseline diabetes in 12.5%; gastric banding 18%, vertical banded gastroplasty 69%, RYGB 13%) and 1,610 matched controls (72). Metabolic surgery reduced the incidence of albuminuria by 63% (adjusted hazard ratio 0.37 [95% CI 0.30–0.47]), with the greatest reductions seen in those who received RYGB (69% reduction in albuminuria incidence). Shulman et al. highlighted that metabolic surgery reduced the incidence of ESKD after median 18-year follow-up in the SOS study by over 70% (adjusted hazard ratio 0.27 [95% CI 0.12–0.60]) (73). No matched observational cohort studies of metabolic surgery have selectively recruited people with CKD at baseline.

Observational Studies in Those With Baseline CKD

Friedman et al. investigated the impact of metabolic surgery (RYGB 71%, AGB 24%, remaining VSG, BPD/DS, and banded gastric bypass) on KDIGO CKD risk classification over up to 7 years in the Longitudinal Assessment of Bariatric Surgery (LABS)-2 cohort (81). At baseline, the majority of people were at low CKD risk (1,788, 83%), while 254 (12%), 73 (3%), and 29 (1%) were at moderate, high, and very high CKD risk, respectively, and by definition had CKD. Diabetes prevalence ranged from 28% in those with low CKD risk to 83% in those with very high CKD risk. CKD risk categories reduced for a majority of people with moderate (53% improved categories) and high (56% improved categories) CKD risk at 7 years postoperatively. Furthermore, 23% of those with very high baseline CKD risk improved their risk category by 7 years, indicating that metabolic surgery continues to have renoprotective benefits, albeit less pronounced, across the spectrum of CKD severity.

Romero-Funes et al. studied changes in CKD-EPI$_{creatinine}$ eGFR, albuminuria, and kidney failure risk before and at 12 months after metabolic surgery in $n = 69$ people (VSG 61%, RYGB 39%; 93% diabetes) at Cleveland Clinic, Florida, United States (82). In $n = 20$ (29%) people with CKD stage 3 or greater, uACR decreased from 66.5 [35.1–465.4] to 47 [25.1–66] mg/g at 12-month follow-up. Similarly, in $n = 37$ (54%) people with moderately or severely increased albuminuria, uACR decreased from 80 [47.5–389.1] to 46 [30–89.7] mg/g at 12 months. In those with CKD stage 3 or greater, these reductions in proteinuria contributed to 70 and 60% relative reductions in estimated risk of kidney failure at 2 and 5 years, respectively. However, these kidney failure risk estimates also included postoperative changes in CKD-EPI$_{creatinine}$ eGFR, which are not reliable in the setting of lean muscle loss post-metabolic surgery (83). Nevertheless, metabolic surgery in people with established CKD effectively reduces proteinuria and subsequent risk of ESKD.

Minimising the Potential for Enteric Hyperoxaluria

Enteric hyperoxaluria is common post-RYGB but not VSG. Untreated obesity itself increases the risk of kidney stones (84), but stone formation rates increase after metabolic surgery and are higher after RYGB than VSG. Lieske et al. investigated stone formation rates after metabolic surgery ($n = 762$; 78% RYGB, 14% long-limb RYGB or BPD/DS, 7% VSG or AGB) compared with non-surgical controls ($n = 759$) matched by BMI in Olmsted County, Minnesota, United States (85). Baseline CKD and nephrolithiasis prevalence were ~10 and 4% in both groups, respectively. Over mean 6-year follow-up, incident stone events were more common in metabolic surgery patients than obese controls (11 vs. 4%, $p < 0.01$) and a very high proportion of stones post-metabolic surgery were composed of calcium oxalate (94%). Stone risk was highest after long-limb RYGB or BPD/DS, intermediate after standard RYGB, and lowest after VSG or AGB. Amongst individuals who underwent metabolic surgery, those with stones preoperatively were more likely to form further stones postoperatively (42 vs. 14% at 10 years, $p < 0.001$), reflecting the known phenomenon that stone event risk increases with the number of prior events (86). Amongst people who formed stones post-metabolic surgery, urinary oxalate excretion almost doubled, urinary citrate excretion decreased by 30%, and calcium oxalate supersaturation increased by 25% beyond 8 months postoperatively.

Thus, kidney stones are common after metabolic surgery and the increased incidence is driven by hyperoxaluria, hypocitraturia, and consequently urinary calcium oxalate supersaturation (85). Usually, dietary calcium and oxalate bind in the gut lumen, precipitate as calcium oxalate, and are excreted in stool (87). Faecal fat excretion increases after RYGB (88); non-absorbed fatty acids preferentially bind calcium in the gut lumen minimising the amount of dietary calcium available to bind oxalate (87). The concentration of soluble oxalate increases in the colon, where it passively diffuses into the bloodstream. Postoperative increases in luminal fatty acids and bile acids may increase colonic permeability to oxalate (89, 90). Modifying gut microbial flora after RYGB, specifically increasing colonisation with *Oxalobacter formigenes* which protects from hyperoxaluria by degrading luminal oxalate, holds promise as a means of decreasing enteric oxalate absorption (91). Oxalate is filtered by the kidneys and excreted unchanged in the urine. The risk of urinary supersaturation with oxalate may be further increased post-RYGB by suboptimal fluid intake and hypocitraturia (85).

However, enteric hyperoxaluria is eminently controllable after standard RYGB when multi-disciplinary care is delivered with pre- and post-operative dietary education. Reduced dietary oxalate consumption and oral calcium supplementation minimise intestinal oxalate absorption (92). A low-fat diet can also minimise intestinal oxalate absorption (92), although may be nutritionally inadequate for some people postoperatively. Increased fluid intake (reduced supersaturation of stone-forming salts) and oral citrate supplementation in those with hypocitraturia (crystallisation inhibitor) also reduce stone events (93). While long-limb RYGB significantly increases stone events (85), the differential impact of shortening of the alimentary limb in a standard RYGB on metabolic control, stone event rates, and net renal outcomes remains an open question which should be addressed through a prospective, randomised study. A head-to-head comparison of the impact of RYGB with 150 vs. 75 cm alimentary limb length on weight loss, metabolic control, 24-h urinary supersaturation profiles, and mGFR in people with CKD could prove valuable in the refinement of surgical practice for RYGB in patients with extant renal disease in order to maximise benefit. In the meantime, given the high rate of new kidney stone formation post-metabolic surgery in those with baseline nephrolithiasis (85), it may be prudent to favour VSG to minimise hyperoxaluria in this group of patients for now.

Mechanisms Underpinning Renoprotection

Figure 2 summarises mechanisms underpinning weight loss, improved glycaemia, and renoprotection after metabolic surgery.

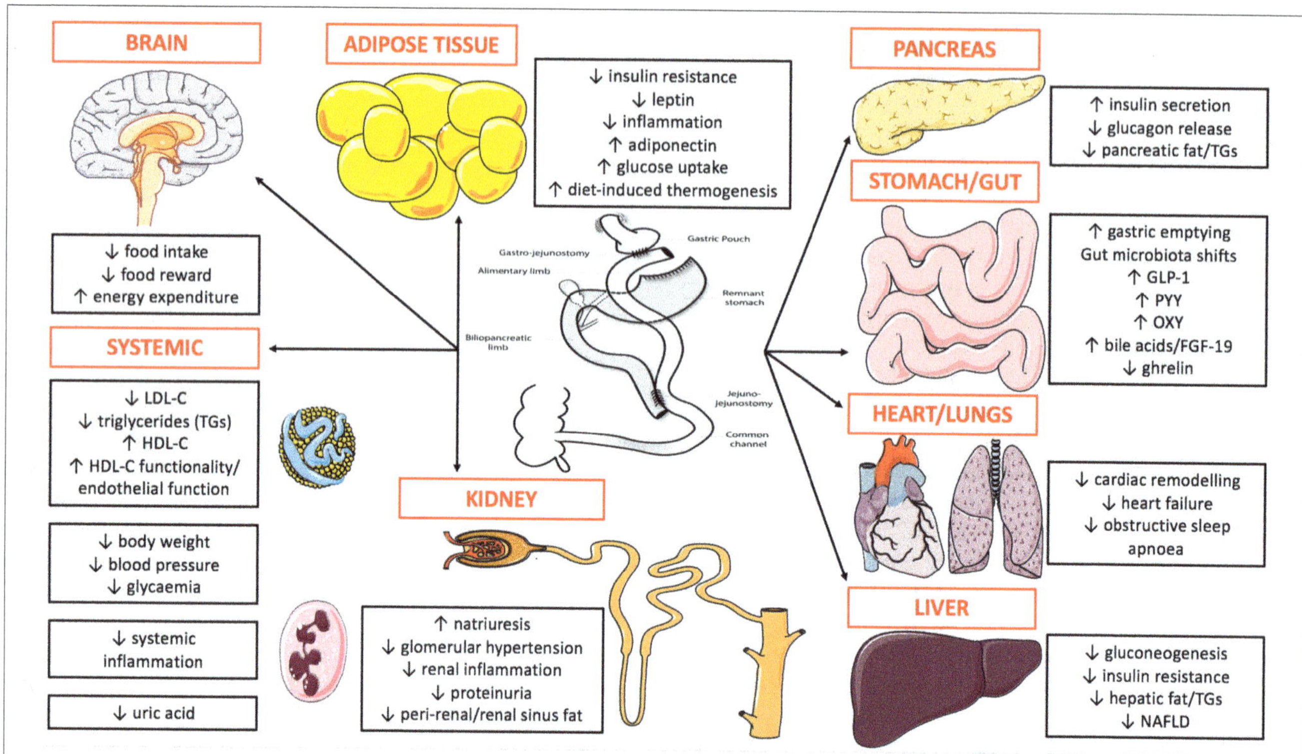

FIGURE 2 | Overview of mechanisms underpinning weight loss, improved glycaemia, and renoprotection after metabolic surgery. RYGB is depicted in the figure as more mechanistic data supports its weight loss, glycaemic, and renoprotective benefits compared with other metabolic surgery procedures. FGF-19, fibroblast growth factor-19; GLP-1, glucagon-like peptide-1; HDL-C, high-density lipoprotein-cholesterol; LDL-C, low-density lipoprotein-cholesterol; NAFLD, non-alcoholic fatty liver disease; OXY, oxyntomodulin; PYY, peptide YY; TGs, triglycerides. **Figure 2** was created by adapting images downloaded from the image bank of Servier Medical Art.

We have recently reviewed these mechanisms in detail (18, 94). More recently developed mechanistic insights include reductions in serum uric acid and increases in serum uromodulin post-metabolic surgery (95, 96). It is clear that metabolic surgery exerts diverse effects across multiple organ systems and systemically in a simultaneous fashion to exert renoprotective effects. While it is intuitive to focus on improved metabolic control as the primary driver of renoprotection post-metabolic surgery, renoprotective effects occur independently of these changes and so interrogation of weight-independent mediators is of critical importance (78). Increased glucagon-like peptide-1 post-metabolic surgery may be central to its renoprotective effects, contributing to the metabolic, antihypertensive, anti-inflammatory, and natriuretic benefits of the procedure (94, 97). We herein summarise the pathogenic role of ectopic renal fat accumulation in people with obesity, and the potential contribution of changes in these visceral fat depots after metabolic surgery to its renoprotective effects.

In obesity, ectopic fat accumulation on, around, and within abdominal viscera, may occur and contribute to pathologies (98). The left and right kidneys have a thick and multi-layered covering of adipose tissue. With reference to the kidneys, the para-renal fat lies external to the renal fascia, whilst deep to the renal fascia and external to the renal capsule lies the peri-renal fat which extends into the renal sinus at the hilum wherein it invests the renal vasculature. With increasing abdominal adiposity, increased fat deposition occurs within the renal sinus and surrounding the kidney. Obesity and visceral adiposity are established risk factors for CKD, but specific fat depots such as extra- and intra-renal fat have gained attention recently for their local and systemic contributions to disease (99–101).

With the use of magnetic resonance, computed tomography, and ultrasound imaging modalities, multiple adipose tissue compartments can be quantified (102, 103). With these tools cross-sectional population studies and longitudinal studies have investigated what contribution kidney fat expansion makes to kidney function and CKD development. Renal sinus fat (RSF) is significantly correlated with visceral adipose tissue volume (104). RSF volume is greater in males than females, and the left kidney has a significantly larger volume of RSF than the right kidney in both genders (102). In a large community population from the Framingham Heart Study, 30% of the population were described as having a high presence of RSF, termed "fatty kidney" (104). In this population, fatty kidney was associated with CKD. This association remained significant after adjustment for visceral adipose tissue (VAT) and BMI, indicating RSF may have a contribution to CKD that is independent of other fat compartments. RSF has been correlated with other markers of kidney function such as serum creatinine, serum kidney injury molecule-1 and serum fibroblast growth factor-21 (102, 105). In a cross-sectional exercise study RSF was not associated with eGFR or uACR at baseline, but had a significant association with uACR post-exercise, after adjustment for multiple variables including VAT (106). In a study of people with type 2 diabetes, RSF had an association with mGFR that remained significant after adjustment for BMI and VAT, but not after adjustment for age (107).

Similar to RSF, peri-renal fat volume is also greater in males and on the left side (108). Para-renal and peri-renal ultrasonographic fat thickness (PUFT) was associated with CKD-EPI eGFR, renal resistance index, and serum urate levels in people with type 2 diabetes (109). PUFT predicted these outcomes independently of waist circumference and BMI by multivariable regression analysis, and was a stronger predictor than waist circumference and BMI. Incidence of CKD also increased significantly across tertiles of increasing PUFT (109). In people with CKD, peri-renal fat thickness (PRFT) associates with metabolic risk factors for CKD progression such as higher fasting blood glucose, elevated blood triglycerides and hyperuricemia (110).

Several mechanisms have been suggested to explain ectopic kidney fat's association with metabolic dysfunction and CKD. One mechanism is that ectopic kidney fat exerts a physical force upon the kidney. RSF may compress the renal medulla (98). The renal vein and renal lymph vessels may be compressed by surrounding RSF, leading to decreased flow and an increase in pressure and size of the kidney. Animal studies have reported increased extracellular matrix in the medulla and increased renal interstitial hydrostatic pressure in obesity models (19, 111, 112). Hall et al. describes how this increased pressure compresses the vasa recta and loop of Henle to increase tubular reabsorption of sodium (113). This mechanism is supported by an association in humans between RSF and kidney size that persists after adjustment for age, sex, BMI and height (105).

Peri-renal fat is usually measured on images as the fat pad between the posterior surface of the kidney and the abdominal wall musculature (109, 114). Unlike the RSF, it is separated from the renal parenchyma by the fibrous renal capsule. It still may however contribute toward increasing intra-abdominal pressure and physical compression upon the kidney (115). Peri-renal fat shares the same vascularization as the renal cortex which may permit adipokines and cytokines from the fat depot to have a paracrine effect on the kidney (114). Infiltration of macrophages into peri-renal fat tissue and polarisation of macrophages toward a pro-inflammatory state has been documented in high-fat diet mice (116, 117). A paracrine effect of RSF mediated through locally secreted cytokines and vasoconstrictive factors has also been suggested as a link between RSF and renal function. One study found an association between RSF, mGFR and renal vascular resistance, a parameter implicated in the progression of CKD (107). Spit et al. hypothesize that the increased inflammation and reduced adiponectin from obese adipose tissue may mediate reduced renal vasorelaxation (107). However, when blood markers of inflammation were measured no association with RSF was found, suggesting that peri-renal fat and RSF depots are too small to have independent associations with systemic inflammation (102).

As adipose tissue expands in obesity its ability to store energy may become impaired, causing lipolysis and fatty acid release to occur (118). In their proximity to the kidney, dysfunction in the renal sinus and peri-renal fat depots may lead to lipid deposition and lipotoxicity in the kidney. Parenchymal lipid accumulation in kidney glomeruli and proximal tubules is observed in mice when fed a high-fat, but not a low-fat, diet (119). Zucker diabetic fatty rats, a model of obesity and type 2 diabetes, display intra-renal lipid accumulation (mostly in the proximal tubules) whereas lean control animals display no intra-renal lipid accumulation (120). Intra-glomerular lipid deposition and intracellular accumulation of fat are common in routine human kidney biopsies (121). Increased lipid accumulation and alterations in fatty acid beta-oxidation in proximal tubular cells promotes renal inflammation and fibrogenesis (122). Lipid accumulation in podocytes has been shown to induce insulin resistance and alterations to the actin cytoskeleton (123).

Several longitudinal studies have been performed to investigate what contribution ectopic renal fat reduction has on renal function. In a study where diet-induced weight loss occurred over 18 months, RSF correlated with eGFR and microalbuminuria at baseline (124). RSF decreased by 8.6% after 18 months and correlated with total body weight loss. Decreased RSF was associated with improvements in dyslipidaemia and glycaemic control. Improvements in uACR and uric acid associated with decreased RSF, but the association was no longer significant after adjusting for VAT. In a study of people with severe obesity, PRFT was significantly higher in hypertensive patients than those with normal blood pressure, and was significantly associated with systolic blood pressure (114). At 12 months after VSG, PRFT was significantly decreased (114). In the hypertensive group, those with higher baseline PRFT showed greater reduction in antihypertensive medications. Similarly, RSF has been found to be associated with number of prescribed antihypertensive medications and more severe hypertension (105).

The term "fatty kidney disease" has recently been coined to describe the accumulation of ectopic fat on and within the kidney. It is hoped that designating fatty kidney as a distinct clinical entity will help to focus research efforts (125). In longitudinal studies of changes in renal ectopic fat depots after metabolic surgery, it remains a challenge to separate the effect of RSF reduction from concomitantly occurring VAT and total body fat reductions (107). Despite this, future studies of metabolic surgery should include measurements of renal sinus and peri-renal fats pre- and post-intervention to further characterise the contribution of ectopic kidney fat reduction to its renoprotective effects.

Future Directions

The impact of metabolic surgery on kidney function and injury extends beyond corrections in metabolic parameters, supporting its potential utility in people with non-diabetic CKD. Obesity-related glomerulopathy is under-recognised yet increasing in prevalence (26). Even in obese people with apparently normal kidney function, distinct renal histopathological lesions including glomerulosclerosis, glomerulomegaly mesangial matrix expansion, and podocyte hypertrophy are highly prevalent, and can potentially be improved with metabolic surgery (27, 126). Furthermore, routine care of people with non-immune-mediated CKD centres on control of blood pressure and proteinuria but does not usually involve obesity treatment (127). Metabolic surgery may serve as an adjunct to intensify control of renal parameters in obese people with persistent renal functional decline and/or proteinuria despite treatment with a maximally tolerated dose of a RAAS inhibitor and/or SGLT2i (if subsequently approved for non-diabetic CKD) (128, 129). Thus, metabolic surgery may have an increasing role in outpatient nephrology care.

Reductions in proteinuria after metabolic surgery occur independently of postoperative improvements in body weight, blood pressure, and glycaemic control, suggesting that metabolic surgery has distinct renoprotective effects beyond correction of conventional risk factors for CKD progression (78). Elucidation of these mechanisms is a priority for successful translation of metabolic surgery to nephrology practice, and also to potentially non-invasively mimic and harness metabolic surgery's renoprotective benefits. The majority of evidence supporting the renoprotective effects of metabolic surgery pertains to RYGB. However, VSG is now the most commonly performed metabolic surgery procedure worldwide (43, 46) and, while adverse renal effects including enteric hyperoxaluria and kidney stones are less common after VSG, it is important to determine if VSG shares all or some of RYGB's renoprotective effects. The impact of modification of the length of the standard RYGB alimentary limb should be investigated to determine if a shorter limb length can achieve comparable metabolic control and weight-independent renoprotective benefits while minimising hyperoxaluria risk to improve net renal outcomes. Additionally, nutritional deficiencies in iron, calcium, and vitamin D after metabolic surgery may exacerbate anaemia and mineral bone disease as complications of CKD (130). Oxalosis as a consequence of enteric hyperoxaluria may also result in erythopoeitin-stimulating agent resistant anaemia (131). Thus, strategies to mitigate nutritional complications of metabolic surgery to minimise adverse impact on anaemia and bone health parameters in people with CKD should be sought.

WHAT IS THE ROLE OF METABOLIC SURGERY IN PEOPLE WITH END-STAGE KIDNEY DISEASE?

Although higher BMI is associated with lower mortality in people with ESKD on maintenance dialysis (132), the so-called obesity paradox, obesity is also a major barrier to kidney transplantation in people with ESKD as recipient obesity increases the risk of kidney allograft complications (133). Almost all kidney transplant centres avoid kidney transplantation in prospective recipients with a BMI ≥ 40 kg/m^2, while most centres consider a BMI ≥ 35 kg/m^2 a relative contraindication (134). Some centres employ a more stringent BMI cutoff of ≤ 30 kg/m^2 for transplant waitlisting (134). Survival and quality of life for people with ESKD on dialysis, particularly with diabetes, is extremely poor (135, 136). Quality of life and survival significantly improve after kidney transplantation, irrespective of BMI (137). Therefore, intentional weight loss strategies hold promise as a means of decreasing mortality rates of people with obesity, type 2 diabetes, and ESKD by increasing successful kidney transplantation listing rates.

What Evidence Supports Medical Weight Management Options in People With Obesity and End-Stage Kidney Disease?

Experience with medical treatment of obesity in people with ESKD is limited. MacLaughlin et al. investigated the impact of orlistat plus exercise and dietary advice ($n = 32$) vs. usual care ($n = 20$) over 24 months in people with advanced CKD (31.3% type 2 diabetes, 37.5% stage 3/4 CKD, and 62.5% on dialysis in orlistat group) (138). Baseline BMIs were 35.7 ± 4.5 and 34.1 ± 4.2 kg/m^2 in the orlistat and usual care groups, respectively. At 24 months, body weight significantly decreased in the orlistat group compared with the usual care group (94.6 ± 16.1 vs. 101.0 ± 26.8 kg, $p < 0.001$). Comparing the orlistat and usual care groups, more people were accepted for kidney transplant listing (35 vs. 6%) and were transplanted (3 vs. 1). Predictably, orlistat caused gastrointestinal side effects but these were not severe enough to result in participant withdrawal. No patients developed hyperoxaluria, although this remains a concern given the fat malabsorption caused by orlistat (one of the same mechanisms implicated in the enteric hyperoxaluria accompanying RYGB) (139, 140).

Idorn et al. randomised 20 people with type 2 diabetes and ESKD and 20 control subjects with type 2 diabetes but no kidney disease in a 1:1 fashion to liraglutide or placebo (141). Participants were followed for 12 weeks and liraglutide was titrated to a maximum dose of 1.8 mg once daily as tolerated. Liraglutide improved glycaemic control and reduced insulin requirements in people with and without ESKD. Liraglutide-induced weight loss was greater in people without kidney disease than in those with ESKD, with body weight decreasing by 2.4 ± 0.8 kg in those with ESKD ($p = 0.22$). Plasma trough liraglutide concentrations were increased by 49% in the ESKD group compared with the control group by 12 weeks, and gastrointestinal adverse effects were more pronounced in the ESKD group. Thus, liraglutide appears to retain glycaemic and weight management efficacy in people with ESKD, although tolerability diminishes somewhat and slower titration may be preferable. Liraglutide-induced constipation is common (~20% incidence in phase 3 RCTs of liraglutide in people without kidney disease) (142); no studies have yet investigated the tolerability of liraglutide in people on peritoneal dialysis in whom avoidance of constipation is of paramount importance (143).

Can Metabolic Surgery Facilitate Access to Kidney Transplantation for People With Dialysis-Dependent End-Stage Kidney Disease?

Compared with patients without ESKD, metabolic surgery in ESKD does not increase the relative risk of postoperative complications, but does slightly prolong length of hospital stay and increases 30-day hospital readmission rates (144). Absolute complication rates remain relatively low (2.5–6.4%) in people with ESKD, and metabolic surgery appears to be a safe and efficacious option for weight management in ESKD (144). Indeed, Sheetz et al. analysed United States Medicare claims data between 2006 and 2016 and identified a 9-fold increase in all metabolic surgeries performed in ESKD patients over this time period, largely driven by a profound increase in VSG use (144). **Figure 3** outlines the potential roles of metabolic surgery in facilitating access to kidney transplantation and improving allograft outcomes in people with obesity and ESKD.

Table 2 provides an overview of studies which have assessed the impact of metabolic surgery on transplant candidacy in people with advanced non-dialysis dependent CKD or ESKD (145–156). Most studies were small, single-centre retrospective reviews, and without control groups. Study follow-up was generally short (<5 years). VSG was the most studied metabolic surgery type, reflecting its surge in popularity over the past decade (43). BMI <35 kg/m^2, a threshold below which patients are waitlisted for kidney transplantation at many centres (134), was achieved in >50% of people in all studies in which this outcome was reported. Nevertheless, Cohen et al.'s report of 43 people is the largest observational study of pre-kidney transplant metabolic surgery to date (147). Compared with non-metabolic surgery controls with obesity, pre-transplant metabolic surgery reduced the risks of graft failure and overall mortality by almost 70% (adjusted hazard ratio 0.31 [95% CI 0.29–0.33]) and 45% (adjusted hazard ratio 0.57 [95% CI 0.53–0.61]), respectively (147). Evidence to date supports a growing role for metabolic surgery in addressing obesity as a barrier to kidney transplantation in people with ESKD, and this practice may also improve renal allograft outcomes, although larger studies with longer prospective observational follow-up are needed.

The optimal choice of pre-transplant metabolic surgery type in people with ESKD is unknown. VSG is now the most commonly performed metabolic surgery and may be preferable for people with ESKD given the complexities of immunosuppressive medication management in people post-RYGB (mycophenolate mofetil is primarily absorbed in the stomach; the duodenum is the main site of absorption and metabolism of both tacrolimus and sirolimus) (157). Indeed, Thomas et al. demonstrated that people who had RYGB performed pre-transplant required higher tacrolimus doses to achieve comparable trough levels compared with controls with obesity, and were at higher risk of biopsy-proven acute rejection

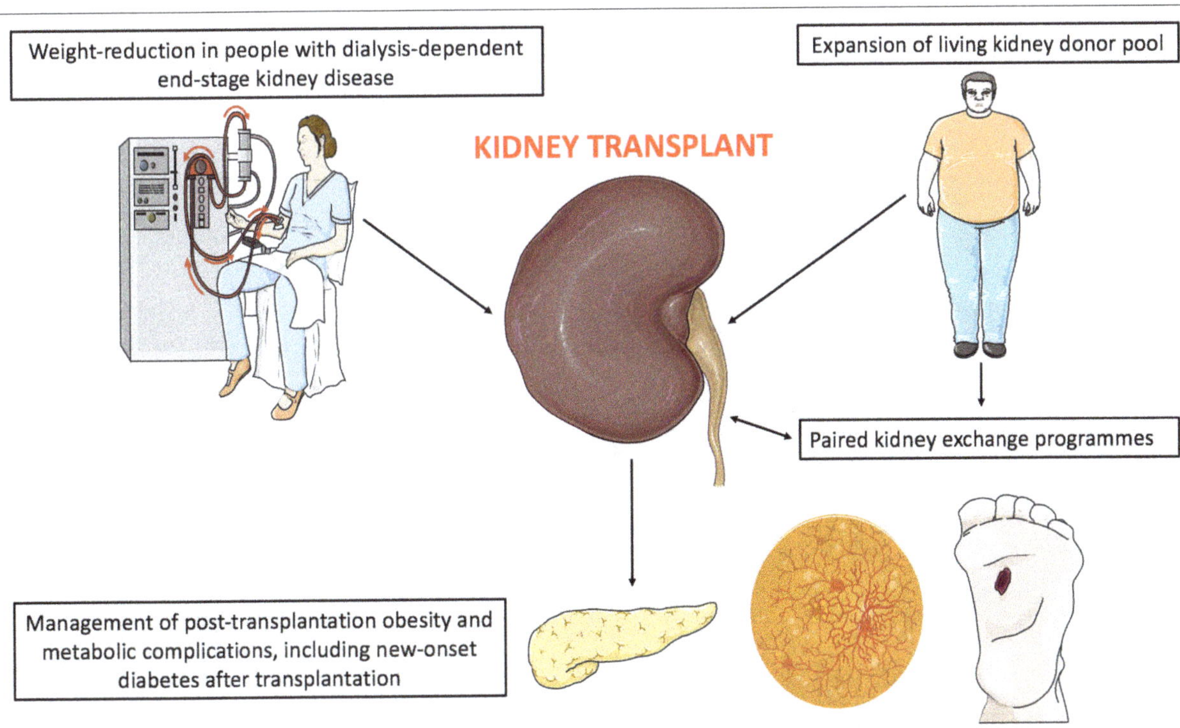

FIGURE 3 | Potential roles of metabolic surgery in facilitating access to kidney transplantation and improving allograft outcomes in people with obesity and end-stage kidney disease. Although not visually represented, pre-transplant laparoscopic metabolic surgery has been successfully performed in people on peritoneal dialysis without necessitating temporary haemodialysis. However, reports to date are limited and further study is warranted to determine surgical and dialysis complication rates in this population. **Figure 3** was created by adapting images downloaded from the image bank of Servier Medical Art.

TABLE 2 | Observational studies assessing metabolic surgery in people with advanced CKD or ESKD (prior to kidney transplantation).

Study	Year	*n*	Surgery type (*n*)	Control arm	Follow-up (years)	T2D [*n* (%)]	NDD-CKD [*n* (%)]	ESKD [*n* (%)]	Dialysis modality (*n*)		BMI (kg/m²)		BMI <35 kg/m² [*n* (%)]	KTx (*n*)	Deceased KTx (*n*)	Living KTx (*n*)	Mortality (*n*)
									HD	PD	Baseline	Last F/u					
Kim et al. (145)	2019	41	VSG	No	1.8 ± 1.35	23 (56)	2 (5)	39 (95)	–	–	41 ± 5	32 ± 5	–	41	25	16	0
Yemini et al. (146)	2019	24	VSG (17) RYGB (7)	No	3.9 ± 0.5	16 (67)	7 (29)	17 (71)	16	1	42 ± 1	29 ± 1	–	16	5	11	2
Cohen et al. (147)	2019	43	RYGB (27) VSG (9) AGB (6) Unspecified (1)	Yes	3.6 (median)	19 (44)	34 (79)	9 (21)	8	1	43 (median)	32 (median)	–	43	–	–	3
Thomas et al. (148)	2018	31	RYGB	Yes	8 (total)[a]	17 (55)	1 (3)	30 (97)	25	5	44 ± 1	28 ± 1	27 (87)	14	13	1	–
Kim et al. (149)	2017	20	VSG	Yes	3.3	12 (60)	0	20 (100)	–	–	42 ± 4	34 ± 5	–	20	14	6	0
Kienzl-Wagner et al. (150)	2017	8	VSG	No	3.2 ± 1.4	4 (50)	0 (0)	8 (100)	–	–	39 ± 4	31 ± 6	8 (100)	7	7	0	0
Carandina et al. (151)	2017	9	VSG	No	1.3	6 (67)	0 (0)	9 (100)	9	0	46	36	6 (67)	1	–	–	0
Al-Bahri et al. (152)	2017	16	RYGB (12) AGB (3) VSG (1)	No	4 ± 3	–	0 (0)	16 (100)	16	0	48 ± 8	31 ± 7	12 (75)	4	3	1	2
Freeman et al. (153)	2015	52	VSG	No	0.6 ± 0.4	28 (53)	5 (10)	47 (90)	47	0	43 ± 5	36 ± 5	29 (56)	6	3	3	3
Jamal et al. (154)	2015	21	RYGB (18) VSG (2) AGB (1)	No	2.3 ± 1.9	14 (67)	0 (0)	21 (100)	–	–	47 ± 6	35.3 ± 8	–	2	–	–	1
Lin et al. (155)	2013	6	VSG (6)	No	0.5–4[b]	–	1 (17)	5 (83)	5	0	–	–	–	2	–	–	–
Alexander et al. (156)	2007	41	RYGB (41)	No	13 (total)[a]	22 (54)	–	–	–	–	48	–	–	9	–	–	6

[a] *Total study duration reported where mean follow-up not reported.*
[b] *Range of follow-up reported where mean follow-up not reported.*
Mean ± SD are presented for normally distributed continuous variables; n (%) are presented for categorical variables.
AGB, adjustable gastric banding; BMI, body-mass index; ESKD, end-stage kidney disease; F/u, follow-up; HD, haemodialysis; KTx, kidney transplant; NDD-CKD, non-dialysis-dependent chronic kidney disease; PD, peritoneal dialysis; RYGB, Roux-en-Y gastric bypass; T2D, type 2 diabetes mellitus; VSG, vertical sleeve gastrectomy.

in the post-transplant period (148). The higher biopsy-proven acute rejection rate in RYGB-operated people associated with subtherapeutic tacrolimus trough levels (<4 ng/mL), although several RYGB-operated people were also non-compliant with immunosuppressive medications (148). Similarly, Cohen et al. demonstrated that pre-transplant metabolic surgery ($n = 38$ total, >50% RYGB) increased the risk of acute rejection within the first-year post-transplant by almost 20% compared with non-metabolic surgery controls with obesity (147). As discussed above, urinary oxalate excretion increases post-RYGB with potential for increased stone events and enteric oxalate nephropathy in the renal allograft (158), another factor which has driven the use of VSG in people with ESKD. AGB is a less studied and likely a less favourable surgical option in people with ESKD as the implanted foreign body may increase intra-abdominal infection risks post-transplantation (159). Head-to-head studies between RYGB and VSG in people with ESKD, and between surgical and medical obesity treatment options, would be ideal. Pharmacokinetic studies of immunosuppressive agents post-metabolic surgery are limited (157); larger studies are required, along with clarification of whether acute rejection rates are higher post-RYGB compared with other forms of metabolic surgery.

Does the Feasibility of Metabolic Surgery Differ With Dialysis Modality?

From **Table 2**, it is clear that very few people on peritoneal dialysis have been included in studies of pre-transplant metabolic surgery in ESKD to date. Many studies conducted to date have not outlined the dialysis modalities of included patients, although it is assumed that most included patients have been on haemodialysis where not specifically stated. Surgical interventions pose unique challenges in people on peritoneal dialysis, with potential for surgical damage of the peritoneum requiring interruption of peritoneal dialysis and temporary switching to haemodialysis (with the possibility of haemodialysis catheter complications), dialysate fluid leaks, and peritonitis (160). Conversely, peritoneal thickening and adhesions as a result of long-term dialysis may increase surgical complexity and operative morbidity (160).

The rate of peritoneal dialysis failure as a result of surgery increased as a consequence of open laparotomies (161, 162). Reports of laparoscopic surgical interventions in people on peritoneal dialysis remain limited, although laparoscopic approaches hold promise as a means of maximally preserving peritoneal structural integrity (160). Metabolic surgery procedures are now routinely performed laparoscopically in the general population (39). Valle et al. were the first to report a case series of pre-transplant laparoscopic metabolic surgery in 5 people on peritoneal dialysis in 2012 (163). Imam et al. reported a case of laparoscopic VSG in a 27-year old male on peritoneal dialysis for 3.6 years which did not require perioperative interruption of peritoneal dialysis (164). No perioperative surgical complications occurred and the patient was able to resume his pre-operative dialysis regimen after 4 weeks. Thomas et al. included five people on peritoneal dialysis in their study of pre-transplant RYGB (148), while Yemini et al. and Cohen et al. each included one person on peritoneal dialysis in their studies of pre-transplant metabolic surgery (146, 147). Nevertheless, fewer than 20 cases of pre-transplant metabolic surgery in people on peritoneal dialysis have been reported to date. Further study of the feasibility and efficacy of laparoscopic metabolic surgery is required in this population, particularly to determine if operative morbidity and dialysis complication rates are acceptable and comparable to people on haemodialysis (165).

Should Metabolic Surgery Be Used to Expand the Living Kidney Donor Pool?

Kidney allograft survival is superior for living compared with deceased donor kidneys (166). Metabolic surgery may increase the living kidney donor pool by addressing donor obesity. As a consequence of the obesity pandemic, >25% of contemporary living kidney donors are obese, compared with <8% in the 1970s (167), and living kidney donation rates have declined by 13% in the United States since 2004 (168). KDIGO recommend that approval of people with BMI $\geq$30 kg/m^2 for living kidney donation should be individualized on a case-by case basis and based on the transplant centre's acceptable risk threshold due to higher rates of *de novo* diabetes, hypertension, and ESKD post-donation compared with non-obese donors (169). Additionally, delayed graft function is more common after donation from people with obesity (170). Locke et al. investigated long-term mortality rates in nearly 120,000 living kidney donors with obesity in the United States over 10.7-year median follow-up (171). Obesity increased the relative risk of 20-year mortality by 30% compared with non-obese donors, and although absolute risk of post-donation mortality was low, these findings justify the caution exerted by transplant centres in limiting kidney donation by obese individuals.

Metabolic surgery could potentially improve both donor and recipient outcomes in prospective, obese living kidney donors. Kidney donation is an altruistic act which offers no medical benefit to the donor. However, addressing obesity identified during the donor evaluation process could add tangible medical benefit to donors and potentially reduce post-donation diabetes, hypertension, ESKD, and mortality (57, 58). Nguyen et al. recently provided proof-of-principle that pre-donation metabolic surgery is safe and feasible (172). They performed a case series of 22 people who underwent metabolic surgery prior to living kidney donation across 2 centres in the United States (8 RYGB, 7 VSG, 6 AGB, and 1 BPD/DS). Importantly, none of the metabolic surgeries were performed specifically in preparation for living kidney donation but rather purely for obesity treatment in the donors. Mean pre-operative BMI was 46 kg/m^2 and 17 donors achieved a post-operative BMI <35 kg/m^2. Prior metabolic surgery did not impact the donor nephrectomy procedure or early post-donation outcomes. Longer-term donor outcomes and recipient outcomes were not reported.

Thus, it appears that metabolic surgery could be used to expand the living kidney donor pool and potentially improve both donor and recipient outcomes after living kidney donation (**Figure 3**). Conceivably, this could have even wider downstream impact on paired kidney exchange programmes to circumvent issues of blood group and human leucocyte antigen incompatibility (173). However, many questions remain. Long-term donor and recipient outcomes after pre-donation metabolic surgery have not been characterized (50). The preferred metabolic surgery procedure in this setting is unknown and would ideally be defined through prospective, head-to head studies. Increased kidney stone and oxalate nephropathy risk after RYGB are pertinent to both the donor and recipient in this setting, although the superior metabolic outcomes with RYGB could improve net renal outcomes compared with VSG overall (29, 158).

Metabolic surgery could be performed before, concurrently with, or after kidney donation, and the optimal timing is unknown (174). It seems logical to favour pre-donation metabolic surgery so that benefits of the surgery could also extend to the recipient. Pre-donation metabolic surgery could improve recipient outcomes by reducing glomerular hyperfiltration and other adverse renal consequences of obesity in the transplanted kidney (126). It would also ensure that the prospective donor had adequately responded in terms of weight loss and/or remission of obesity complications such as hypertension prior to proceeding with donation (28). However, laparoscopic metabolic surgery performed concurrently with donor nephrectomy could minimise operative morbidity and recovery time for the donor. An acceptable level of obesity-related comorbidities will need to be defined prior to proceeding with metabolic surgery for prospective living kidney donors (174). While metabolic surgery effectively treats both hypertension and type 2 diabetes (28, 29), given the high rates of type 2 diabetes recurrence at 5 years, it would seem logical to exclude people with type 2 diabetes from studies of peri-donation metabolic surgery for now.

Can Metabolic Surgery Assist in the Management of Post-Kidney Transplantation Obesity and Metabolic Complications?

Treatment of obesity, hypertension, dyslipidaemia, and diabetes to prevent cardiovascular disease is challenging post-kidney transplantation, partly due to the metabolic side effects of commonly used immunosuppressant drugs. Both cyclosporine and tacrolimus cause hypertension, dyslipidaemia, and pancreatic β-cell toxicity; hypertension and dyslipidaemia are more common with cyclosporine while dysglycaemia and new-onset diabetes after transplantation (NODAT) are more commonly induced by tacrolimus (175). Although steroid-free regimens are sometimes used in allografts of lower immunologic risk, many patients still take a maintenance dose of low-dose glucocorticoid which exacerbates dyslipidaemia and dysglycaemia, and contributes to post-transplant weight gain (176, 177). Mammalian target of rapamycin inhibitors, everolimus and sirolimus, cause dyslipidaemia and may also be toxic to pancreatic β-cells (178). Accordingly, cardiovascular disease remains a leading cause of death post-kidney transplantation, and diabetes is the strongest modifiable risk factor in this setting (179, 180). Furthermore, diabetes is a common cause of renal functional decline in the allograft; over mean 5.4-year follow-up, diabetes accounted for 11% of recurrent and *de novo* glomerular diseases in a large Renal Allograft Disease Registry cohort (181). Death with a functioning allograft remains the leading cause of allograft loss (182). Therefore, better control of conventional cardiovascular risk factors through directed treatment of obesity post-kidney transplantation with metabolic surgery has the potential to improve graft survival and overall patient mortality.

Chen et al. reported a case in which VSG at 3 years post-kidney transplantation significantly improved body weight and glycaemic control in a patient with post-transplant weight gain and NODAT (183). Several small case series and observational studies have investigated the impact of post-transplant metabolic surgery on body weight, metabolic control, and graft outcomes (184–188). Viscido et al. demonstrated that VSG at mean 15 years after kidney transplantation reduced mean BMI from 42.2±6.8 to 29.8±7.3 kg/m^2 over 1.4±1-year follow-up in five patients (189). Concordant improvements in blood pressure and glycaemic control, lipid parameters, and proteinuria were observed in the majority of patients.

Cohen et al. reported renal allograft outcomes over extended follow-up for patients who underwent post-transplantation metabolic surgery (n = 21), and compared graft outcomes for n=18 patients to non-metabolic surgery registry controls (n = 180) (147). Metabolic surgery (48% VSG, 28% RYGB, 19% AGB, and 5% vertical banded gastroplasty) resulted in 71% excess weight loss at 2 years. Body weight loss did not differ when compared with a cohort of patients who had metabolic surgery performed prior to kidney transplantation. Over median 11.6-year follow-up, n = 7 patients experienced allograft failure (consistent with the national average over that time period). Importantly, compared with controls matched for BMI at the time of transplant, metabolic surgery reduced allograft failure by 15% (adjusted hazard ratio 0.85 [95% 0.85–0.86]) and overall mortality by 20% (adjusted hazard ratio 0.80 [0.79–0.82]).

Prospective studies examining the relative impact of metabolic surgery and medical management of obesity on metabolic parameters, allograft function, and mortality should be conducted to further define the role of intentional weight loss strategies in this setting. Caveats pertaining to RYGB highlighted above, including concerns regarding immunosuppressant medication absorption and enteric oxalate nephropathy resulting in allograft loss, may make VSG the metabolic surgery type of choice post-kidney transplant (157, 158). However, adequate control of enteric hyperoxaluria is feasible with appropriate dietary education and oral calcium and citrate supplementation, which may allow a greater number of patients to benefit from the superior body weight and metabolic control achieved with RYGB (29, 92). Additionally, RYGB with a shorter alimentary limb (~75 cm) has the potential to achieve superior metabolic control to VSG while minimising hyperoxaluria and improving immunosuppressive absorption (42), although this requires prospective study in the pre- and post-transplant setting. For people with BMIs close to the limit set by their transplant centre for waitlisting, the optimal timing of metabolic surgery, pre- or post-kidney transplantation, needs to be defined. Pre-transplant metabolic surgery may be preferable as it minimises the early adverse consequences of obesity on the allograft and reduces the incidence of NODAT and other adverse post-transplant metabolic consequences (145).

Future Directions

Small observational studies support the role of both medical and surgical obesity treatments in people with ESKD, although the longer-term impact of both strategies on kidney transplant waitlisting, kidney allograft outcomes, and overall mortality are unknown. It is unknown whether different metabolic surgery procedures result in differential success in kidney transplant waitlisting and in allograft function. Efforts to recruit more patients on peritoneal dialysis to studies of pre-transplant metabolic surgery should be made, as the majority of studies to date have focused on subjects on haemodialysis. RCTs comparing the impact of medical vs. surgical weight management strategies in people with ESKD would be ideal. Similar to native CKD, combined medical and surgical treatment approaches to obesity may also be set to become the new standard for care for people with ESKD (68). Given the unrelenting obesity pandemic which has increased ESKD prevalence, obesity will become a barrier to kidney transplantation for an increasing number of patients worldwide (35). Therefore, clear guidance on optimal weight management strategies in this setting is critical. Metabolic surgery could help to expand the living kidney donor pool and improve both donor and recipient outcomes, although the optimal timing of metabolic surgery as well as optimal procedure type need to be defined (174). Post-transplant metabolic surgery appears to improve allograft and overall survival (147), and may be increasingly performed to improve cardiovascular risk in those with suboptimal metabolic control, although studies to date have been small with limited longitudinal follow-up.

CONCLUSIONS

There are myriad potential roles for metabolic surgery as a means of improving outcomes for people with kidney disease. Metabolic surgery as an adjunct to medical therapy to slow the progression of diabetic kidney disease currently has the best evidence base and is closest to incorporation into clinical practice. The precise role of metabolic surgery in the diabetic kidney disease treatment algorithm should be defined through randomised controlled trials in people with type 2 diabetes and progressive renal functional decline despite treatment with RAAS inhibitors, SGLT2is, and/or GLP1RAs (8, 9, 190). Many of the mechanisms supporting metabolic surgery use in people with type 2 diabetes and CKD also apply to people with non-diabetic CKD (18); thus, metabolic surgery may assume a broader role in the control of hypertension and proteinuria in non-immune-mediated CKD.

Pre-transplant metabolic surgery improves access to kidney transplantation and improves renal allograft outcomes, decreasing allograft failure and overall mortality (147). Post-transplantation metabolic surgery also improves graft and overall survival (147). Concerns exist regarding the role of RYGB pre- and post-kidney transplantation, particularly with regard to oxalate nephropathy and increased rejection episodes due to unreliable immunosuppressant medication absorption as causes of allograft loss (157, 158). Nevertheless, weight loss and metabolic control are superior after RYGB compared with VSG (29), which may confer incremental renoprotection to the renal allograft. Shortening the length of the alimentary limb should be investigated as a means to optimise renal outcomes post-RYGB by minimising hyperoxaluria and acute rejection risks while preserving superior metabolic control to VSG (41). Finally, metabolic surgery may confer tangible medical benefit to kidney donors by addressing obesity before, concurrently with, or after kidney donation (172).

AUTHOR CONTRIBUTIONS

WM and JW wrote the manuscript with critical input from FL-H, ND, and CR. All authors reviewed and approved the final manuscript and as such are accountable for the content of the work.

ACKNOWLEDGMENTS

We are grateful to Ludmilla Dellatorre Pessanha (ludmilla.pessanha@ucd.ie) for preparing illustrations of the metabolic surgery types outlined in **Figure 1**. **Figures 2** and **3** were created by adapting images downloaded from the image bank of Servier Medical Art.

REFERENCES

1. Jones DS, Podolsky SH, Greene JA. The burden of disease and the changing task of medicine. *New Engl J Med.* (2012) 366:2333–8. doi: 10.1056/NEJMp1113569
2. Fontaine KR, Redden DT, Wang C, Westfall AO, Allison DB. Years of life lost due to obesity. *JAMA.* (2003) 289:187–93. doi: 10.1001/jama.289.2.187
3. Saper CB, Lowell BB. The hypothalamus. *Curr Biol.* (2014) 24:R1111–6. doi: 10.1016/j.cub.2014.10.023
4. Maric-Bilkan C. Obesity and diabetic kidney disease. *Med Clin North Am.* (2013) 97:59–74. doi: 10.1016/j.mcna.2012.10.010
5. Reutens AT. Epidemiology of diabetic kidney disease. *Med Clin North Am.* (2013) 97:1–18. doi: 10.1016/j.mcna.2012.10.001

6. Afkarian M, Sachs MC, Kestenbaum B, Hirsch IB, Tuttle KR, Himmelfarb J, et al. Kidney disease and increased mortality risk in type 2 diabetes. *J Am Soc Nephrol.* (2013) 24:302–8. doi: 10.1681/ASN.2012070718
7. Alicic RZ, Rooney MT, Tuttle KR. Diabetic kidney disease: challenges, progress, and possibilities. *Clin J Am Soc Nephrol.* (2017) 12:2032–45. doi: 10.2215/CJN.11491116
8. Perkovic V, Jardine MJ, Neal B, Bompoint S, Heerspink HJL, Charytan DM, et al. Canagliflozin and renal outcomes in type 2 diabetes and nephropathy. *New Engl J Med.* (2019) 380:2295–306. doi: 10.1056/NEJMoa1811744
9. Mann JFE, Orsted DD, Brown-Frandsen K, Marso SP, Poulter NR, Rasmussen S, et al. Liraglutide and renal outcomes in type 2 diabetes. *New Engl J Med.* (2017) 377:839–48. doi: 10.1056/NEJMoa1616011
10. Griffin TP, Martin WP, Islam N, O'Brien T, Griffin MD. The promise of mesenchymal stem cell therapy for diabetic kidney disease. *Curr Diab Rep.* (2016) 16:42. doi: 10.1007/s11892-016-0734-6
11. Fioretto P, Mauer M. Histopathology of diabetic nephropathy. *Semin Nephrol.* (2007) 27:195–207. doi: 10.1016/j.semnephrol.2007.01.012
12. Mogensen CE, Christensen CK, Vittinghus E. The stages in diabetic renal disease: with emphasis on the stage of incipient diabetic nephropathy. *Diabetes.* (1983) 32(Suppl. 2):64. doi: 10.2337/diab.32.2.S64
13. Robles NR, Villa J, Gallego RH. Non-proteinuric diabetic nephropathy. *J Clin Med.* (2015) 4:1761–73. doi: 10.3390/jcm4091761
14. D'Agati VD, Chagnac A, de Vries AP, Levi M, Porrini E, Herman-Edelstein M, et al. Obesity-related glomerulopathy: clinical and pathologic characteristics and pathogenesis. *Nat Rev Nephrol.* (2016) 12:453–71. doi: 10.1038/nrneph.2016.75
15. Chagnac A, Weinstein T, Korzets A, Ramadan E, Hirsch J, Gafter U. Glomerular hemodynamics in severe obesity. *Am J Physiol Renal Physiol.* (2000) 278:F817–22. doi: 10.1152/ajprenal.2000.278.5.F817
16. Rosenberg AZ, Kopp JB. Focal segmental glomerulosclerosis. *Clin J Am Soc Nephrol.* (2017) 12:502–17. doi: 10.2215/CJN.05960616
17. Praga M, Hernandez E, Morales E, Campos AP, Valero MA, Martinez MA, et al. Clinical features and long-term outcome of obesity-associated focal segmental glomerulosclerosis. *Nephrol Dial Transplant.* (2001) 16:1790–8. doi: 10.1093/ndt/16.9.1790
18. Martin WP, Docherty NG, Le Roux CW. Impact of bariatric surgery on cardiovascular and renal complications of diabetes: a focus on clinical outcomes and putative mechanisms. *Exp Rev Endocrinol Metab.* (2018) 13:251–62. doi: 10.1080/17446651.2018.1518130
19. Hall JE. Mechanisms of abnormal renal sodium handling in obesity hypertension. *Am J Hypertens.* (1997) 10:49s–55s. doi: 10.1016/S0895-7061(97)00075-7
20. Ehrhart-Bornstein M, Arakelyan K, Krug AW, Scherbaum WA, Bornstein SR. Fat cells may be the obesity-hypertension link: human adipogenic factors stimulate aldosterone secretion from adrenocortical cells. *Endocr Res.* (2004) 30:865–70. doi: 10.1081/ERC-200044122
21. Hall JE, da Silva AA, do Carmo JM, Dubinion J, Hamza S, Munusamy S, et al. Obesity-induced hypertension: role of sympathetic nervous system, leptin, and melanocortins. *J Biol Chem.* (2010) 285:17271–6. doi: 10.1074/jbc.R110.113175
22. Sharma K, Ramachandrarao S, Qiu G, Usui HK, Zhu Y, Dunn SR, et al. Adiponectin regulates albuminuria and podocyte function in mice. *J Clin Investig.* (2008) 118:1645–56. doi: 10.1172/JCI32691
23. Escasany E, Izquierdo-Lahuerta A, Medina-Gomez G. Underlying mechanisms of renal lipotoxicity in obesity. *Nephron.* (2019) 143:28–32. doi: 10.1159/000494694
24. Hashimoto Y, Tanaka M, Okada H, Senmaru T, Hamaguchi M, Asano M, et al. Metabolically healthy obesity and risk of incident CKD. *Clin J Am Soc Nephrol.* (2015) 10:578–83. doi: 10.2215/CJN.08980914
25. Lin WY, Pi-Sunyer FX, Liu CS, Li CI, Davidson LE, Li TC, et al. Central obesity and albuminuria: both cross-sectional and longitudinal studies in Chinese. *PLoS ONE.* (2012) 7:e47960. doi: 10.1371/journal.pone.0047960
26. Kambham N, Markowitz GS, Valeri AM, Lin J, D'Agati VD. Obesity-related glomerulopathy: an emerging epidemic. *Kidney Int.* (2001) 59:1498–509. doi: 10.1046/j.1523-1755.2001.0590041498.x
27. Serra A, Romero R, Lopez D, Navarro M, Esteve A, Perez N, et al. Renal injury in the extremely obese patients with normal renal function. *Kidney Int.* (2008) 73:947–55. doi: 10.1038/sj.ki.5002796
28. Schiavon CA, Bersch-Ferreira AC, Santucci EV, Oliveira JD, Torreglosa CR, Bueno PT, et al. Effects of bariatric surgery in obese patients with hypertension: the GATEWAY randomized trial (gastric bypass to treat obese patients with steady hypertension). *Circulation.* (2017) 137:1132–42. doi: 10.1161/CIRCULATIONAHA.117.032130
29. Schauer PR, Bhatt DL, Kirwan JP, Wolski K, Aminian A, Brethauer SA, et al. Bariatric surgery versus intensive medical therapy for diabetes — 5-year outcomes. *New Engl J Med.* (2017) 376:641–51. doi: 10.1056/NEJMoa1600869
30. Ashrafian H, Toma T, Rowland SP, Harling L, Tan A, Efthimiou E, et al. Bariatric surgery or non-surgical weight loss for obstructive sleep apnoea? A systematic review and comparison of meta-analyses. *Obes Surg.* (2015) 25:1239–50. doi: 10.1007/s11695-014-1533-2
31. Manfield JH, Yu KK, Efthimiou E, Darzi A, Athanasiou T, Ashrafian H. Bariatric surgery or non-surgical weight loss for idiopathic intracranial hypertension? A systematic review and comparison of meta-analyses. *Obes Surg.* (2017) 27:513–21. doi: 10.1007/s11695-016-2467-7
32. Nicholson F, Rolland C, Broom J, Love J. Effectiveness of long-term (twelve months) nonsurgical weight loss interventions for obese women with polycystic ovary syndrome: a systematic review. *Int J Women's Health.* (2010) 2:393–9. doi: 10.2147/IJWH.S13456
33. Bower G, Toma T, Harling L, Jiao LR, Efthimiou E, Darzi A, et al. Bariatric surgery and non-alcoholic fatty liver disease: a systematic review of liver biochemistry and histology. *Obes Surg.* (2015) 25:2280–9. doi: 10.1007/s11695-015-1691-x
34. Kovesdy CP, Furth SL, Zoccali C, World Kidney Day Steering C. Obesity and kidney disease: hidden consequences of the epidemic. *Can J Kidney Health Dis.* (2017) 4:2054358117698669. doi: 10.1177/2054358117698669
35. Chang AR, Grams ME, Ballew SH, Bilo H, Correa A, Evans M, et al. Adiposity and risk of decline in glomerular filtration rate: meta-analysis of individual participant data in a global consortium. *BMJ.* (2019) 364:k5301. doi: 10.1136/bmj.k5301
36. Garofalo C, Borrelli S, Minutolo R, Chiodini P, De Nicola L, Conte G. A systematic review and meta-analysis suggests obesity predicts onset of chronic kidney disease in the general population. *Kidney Int.* (2017) 91:1224–35. doi: 10.1016/j.kint.2016.12.013
37. Hsu CY, McCulloch CE, Iribarren C, Darbinian J, Go AS. Body mass index and risk for end-stage renal disease. *Ann Int Med.* (2006) 144:21–8. doi: 10.7326/0003-4819-144-1-200601030-00006
38. Lu JL, Kalantar-Zadeh K, Ma JZ, Quarles LD, Kovesdy CP. Association of body mass index with outcomes in patients with CKD. *J Am Soc Nephrol.* (2014) 25:2088–96. doi: 10.1681/ASN.2013070754
39. Pareek M, Schauer PR, Kaplan LM, Leiter LA, Rubino F, Bhatt DL. Metabolic surgery: weight loss, diabetes, and beyond. *J Am Coll Cardiol.* (2018) 71:670–87. doi: 10.1016/j.jacc.2017.12.014
40. Cohen RV, Pereira TV, Aboud CM, Caravatto PPdP, Petry TBZ, Correa JLL, et al. Microvascular Outcomes after Metabolic Surgery (MOMS) in patients with type 2 diabetes mellitus and class I obesity: rationale and design for a randomised controlled trial. *BMJ Open.* (2017) 7:e013574. doi: 10.1136/bmjopen-2016-013574
41. Brolin RE, Kenler HA, Gorman JH, Cody RP. Long-limb gastric bypass in the superobese. A prospective randomized study. *Ann Surg.* (1992) 215:387–95. doi: 10.1097/00000658-199204000-00014
42. Brolin RE. Long limb Roux en Y gastric bypass revisited. *Surg Clin North Am.* (2005) 85:807–17, vii. doi: 10.1016/j.suc.2005.03.003
43. Khorgami Z, Shoar S, Andalib A, Aminian A, Brethauer SA, Schauer PR. Trends in utilization of bariatric surgery, 2010-2014: sleeve gastrectomy dominates. *Surg Obes Relat Dis.* (2017) 13:774–8. doi: 10.1016/j.soard.2017.01.031
44. Welbourn R, Hollyman M, Kinsman R, Dixon J, Liem R, Ottosson J, et al. Bariatric surgery worldwide: baseline demographic description and one-year outcomes from the fourth IFSO global registry report 2018. *Obes Surg.* (2019) 29:782–95. doi: 10.1007/s11695-018-3593-1
45. Homan J, Betzel B, Aarts EO, Dogan K, van Laarhoven KJ, Janssen IM, et al. Vitamin and mineral deficiencies after biliopancreatic diversion and biliopancreatic diversion with duodenal switch–the rule rather than the exception. *Obes Surg.* (2015) 25:1626–32. doi: 10.1007/s11695-015-1570-5

46. Ozsoy Z, Demir E. Which bariatric procedure is the most popular in the world? A bibliometric comparison. *Obes Surg.* (2018) 28:2339–52. doi: 10.1007/s11695-018-3163-6
47. Angrisani L, Santonicola A, Iovino P, Vitiello A, Zundel N, Buchwald H, et al. Bariatric surgery and endoluminal procedures: IFSO Worldwide Survey 2014. *Obes Surg.* (2017) 27:2279–89. doi: 10.1007/s11695-017-2666-x
48. Sjostrom L, Peltonen M, Jacobson P, Ahlin S, Andersson-Assarsson J, Anveden A, et al. Association of bariatric surgery with long-term remission of type 2 diabetes and with microvascular and macrovascular complications. *JAMA.* (2014) 311:2297–304. doi: 10.1001/jama.2014.5988
49. Schauer PR, Kashyap SR, Wolski K, Brethauer SA, Kirwan JP, Pothier CE, et al. Bariatric surgery versus intensive medical therapy in obese patients with diabetes. *New Engl J Med.* (2012) 366:1567–76. doi: 10.1056/NEJMoa1200225
50. Hutter MM, Schirmer BD, Jones DB, Ko CY, Cohen ME, Merkow RP, et al. First report from the American College of Surgeons Bariatric Surgery Center Network: laparoscopic sleeve gastrectomy has morbidity and effectiveness positioned between the band and the bypass. *Ann Surg.* (2011) 254:410–20; discussion 20–2. doi: 10.1097/SLA.0b013e31822c9dac
51. Chang P, Friedenberg F. Obesity and GERD. *Gastroenterol Clin North Am.* (2014) 43:161–73. doi: 10.1016/j.gtc.2013.11.009
52. Stenard F, Iannelli A. Laparoscopic sleeve gastrectomy and gastroesophageal reflux. *World J Gastroenterol.* (2015) 21:10348–57. doi: 10.3748/wjg.v21.i36.10348
53. Long E, Beales ILP. The role of obesity in oesophageal cancer development. *Therap Adv Gastroenterol.* (2014) 7:247–68. doi: 10.1177/1756283X14538689
54. Blank ML, Parkin L, Paul C, Herbison P. A nationwide nested case-control study indicates an increased risk of acute interstitial nephritis with proton pump inhibitor use. *Kidney Int.* (2014) 86:837–44. doi: 10.1038/ki.2014.74
55. Lazarus B, Chen Y, Wilson FP, Sang Y, Chang AR, Coresh J, et al. Proton pump inhibitor use and the risk of chronic kidney disease. *JAMA Int Med.* (2016) 176:238–46. doi: 10.1001/jamainternmed.2015.7193
56. Xie Y, Bowe B, Li T, Xian H, Balasubramanian S, Al-Aly Z. Proton pump inhibitors and risk of incident CKD and progression to ESRD. *J Am Soc Nephrol.* (2016) 27:3153. doi: 10.1681/ASN.2015121377
57. Sjöström L, Narbro K, Sjöström CD, Karason K, Larsson B, Wedel H, et al. Effects of bariatric surgery on mortality in swedish obese subjects. *New Engl J Med.* (2007) 357:741–52. doi: 10.1056/NEJMoa066254
58. Adams TD, Gress RE, Smith SC, Halverson RC, Simper SC, Rosamond WD, et al. Long-term mortality after gastric bypass surgery. *New Engl J Med.* (2007) 357:753–61. doi: 10.1056/NEJMoa066603
59. Holland JA, Martin WP, Docherty NG, le Roux CW. Impact of intentional weight loss on diabetic kidney disease. *Diabetes Obes Metab.* (2019) 21:2338–41. doi: 10.1111/dom.13813
60. Schauer PR, Bhatt DL, Kirwan JP, Wolski K, Brethauer SA, Navaneethan SD, et al. Bariatric surgery versus intensive medical therapy for diabetes — 3-year outcomes. *New Engl J Med.* (2014) 370:2002–13. doi: 10.1056/NEJMoa1401329
61. Ikramuddin S, Billington CJ, Lee WJ, Bantle JP, Thomas AJ, Connett JE, et al. Roux-en-Y gastric bypass for diabetes (the Diabetes Surgery Study): 2-year outcomes of a 5-year, randomised, controlled trial. *Lancet Diabetes Endocrinol.* (2015) 3:413–22. doi: 10.1016/S2213-8587(15)00089-3
62. Ikramuddin S, Korner J, Lee WJ, Connett JE, Inabnet WB, Billington CJ, et al. Roux-en-Y gastric bypass vs intensive medical management for the control of type 2 diabetes, hypertension, and hyperlipidemia: the Diabetes Surgery Study randomized clinical trial. *JAMA.* (2013) 309:2240–9. doi: 10.1001/jama.2013.5835
63. Ikramuddin S, Korner J, Lee WJ, Thomas AJ, Connett JE, Bantle JP, et al. Lifestyle intervention and medical management with vs without roux-en-y gastric bypass and control of hemoglobin A1c, LDL cholesterol, and systolic blood pressure at 5 years in the diabetes surgery study. *JAMA.* (2018) 319:266–78. doi: 10.1001/jama.2017.20813
64. Mingrone G, Panunzi S, De Gaetano A, Guidone C, Iaconelli A, Leccesi L, et al. Bariatric surgery versus conventional medical therapy for type 2 diabetes. *New Engl J Med.* (2012) 366:1577–85. doi: 10.1056/NEJMoa1200111
65. Mingrone G, Panunzi S, De Gaetano A, Guidone C, Iaconelli A, Nanni G, et al. Bariatric-metabolic surgery versus conventional medical treatment in obese patients with type 2 diabetes: 5 year follow-up of an open-label, single-centre, randomised controlled trial. *Lancet.* (2015) 386:964–73. doi: 10.1016/S0140-6736(15)00075-6
66. Cummings DE, Arterburn DE, Westbrook EO, Kuzma JN, Stewart SD, Chan CP, et al. Gastric bypass surgery vs intensive lifestyle and medical intervention for type 2 diabetes: the CROSSROADS randomised controlled trial. *Diabetologia.* (2016) 59:945–53. doi: 10.1007/s00125-016-3903-x
67. Dixon JB, O'Brien PE, Playfair J, Chapman L, Schachter LM, Skinner S, et al. Adjustable gastric banding and conventional therapy for type 2 diabetes: a randomized controlled trial. *JAMA.* (2008) 299:316–23. doi: 10.1001/jama.299.3.316
68. Miras AD, Perez-Pevida B, Aldhwayan M, Kamocka A, McGlone ER, Al-Najim W, et al. Adjunctive liraglutide treatment in patients with persistent or recurrent type 2 diabetes after metabolic surgery (GRAVITAS): a randomised, double-blind, placebo-controlled trial. *Lancet Diabetes Endocrinol.* (2019) 7:549–59. doi: 10.1016/S2213-8587(19)30157-3
69. Capehorn MS, Catarig AM, Furberg JK, Janez A, Price HC, Tadayon S, et al. Efficacy and safety of once-weekly semaglutide 1.0mg vs once-daily liraglutide 1.2mg as add-on to 1-3 oral antidiabetic drugs in subjects with type 2 diabetes (SUSTAIN 10). *Diabetes Metab.* (2019) 46:100–109. doi: 10.1016/j.diabet.2019.101117
70. O'Brien R, Johnson E, Haneuse S, Coleman KJ, O'Connor PJ, Fisher DP, et al. Microvascular outcomes in patients with diabetes after bariatric surgery versus usual care: a matched cohort study. *Ann Int Med.* (2018) 169:300–10. doi: 10.7326/M17-2383
71. Madsen LR, Baggesen LM, Richelsen B, Thomsen RW. Effect of Roux-en-Y gastric bypass surgery on diabetes remission and complications in individuals with type 2 diabetes: a Danish population-based matched cohort study. *Diabetologia.* (2019) 62:611–20. doi: 10.1007/s00125-019-4816-2
72. Carlsson LM, Romeo S, Jacobson P, Burza MA, Maglio C, Sjoholm K, et al. The incidence of albuminuria after bariatric surgery and usual care in Swedish Obese Subjects (SOS): a prospective controlled intervention trial. *Int J Obes.* (2015) 39:169–75. doi: 10.1038/ijo.2014.72
73. Shulman A, Peltonen M, Sjostrom CD, Andersson-Assarsson JC, Taube M, Sjoholm K, et al. Incidence of end-stage renal disease following bariatric surgery in the Swedish Obese Subjects Study. *Int J Obes.* (2018) 42:964–73. doi: 10.1038/s41366-018-0045-x
74. Vanholder R, Annemans L, Brown E, Gansevoort R, Gout-Zwart JJ, Lameire N, et al. Reducing the costs of chronic kidney disease while delivering quality health care: a call to action. *Nat Rev Nephrol.* (2017) 13:393–409. doi: 10.1038/nrneph.2017.63
75. Martin WP, Griffin TP, Lappin DW, Griffin DG, Ferguson JP, O'Brien T, et al. Influence of referral to a combined diabetology and nephrology clinic on renal functional trends and metabolic parameters in adults with diabetic kidney disease. *Mayo Clin Proc Innovations Qual Outcomes.* (2017) 1:150–60. doi: 10.1016/j.mayocpiqo.2017.07.003
76. Heneghan HM, Cetin D, Navaneethan SD, Orzech N, Brethauer SA, Schauer PR. Effects of bariatric surgery on diabetic nephropathy after 5 years of follow-up. *Surg Obes Relat Dis.* (2013) 9:7–14. doi: 10.1016/j.soard.2012.08.016
77. Canney AL, Cohen RV, Elliott JA, C MA, Martin WP, Docherty NG, et al. Improvements in diabetic albuminuria and podocyte differentiation following Roux-en-Y gastric bypass surgery. *Diabetes Vasc Dis Res.* (2019) 17:1479164119879039. doi: 10.1177/1479164119879039
78. Martin WP, le Roux CW. Comment on: metabolic surgery improves renal injury independent of weight loss: a meta-analysis. *Surg Obes Relat Dis.* (2019) 15:1020–3. doi: 10.1016/j.soard.2019.04.001
79. Scheurlen KM, Probst P, Kopf S, Nawroth PP, Billeter AT, Muller-Stich BP. Metabolic surgery improves renal injury independent of weight loss: a meta-analysis. *Surg Obes Relat Dis.* (2019) 15:1006–20. doi: 10.1016/j.soard.2019.03.013
80. Chang AR, Chen Y, Still C, Wood GC, Kirchner HL, Lewis M, et al. Bariatric surgery is associated with improvement in kidney outcomes. *Kidney Int.* (2016) 90:164–71. doi: 10.1016/j.kint.2016.02.039
81. Friedman AN, Wahed AS, Wang J, Courcoulas AP, Dakin G, Hinojosa MW, et al. Effect of bariatric surgery on CKD risk. *J Am Soc Nephrol.* (2018) 29:1289–300. doi: 10.1681/ASN.2017060707

82. Funes DR, Blanco DG, Gomez CO, Frieder JS, Menzo EL, Szomstein S, et al. Metabolic surgery reduces the risk of progression from chronic kidney disease to kidney failure. *Ann Surg.* (2019) 270:511–8. doi: 10.1097/SLA.0000000000003456
83. Alba DL, Wu L, Cawthon PM, Mulligan K, Lang T, Patel S, et al. Changes in lean mass, absolute and relative muscle strength, and physical performance after gastric bypass surgery. *J Clin Endocrinol Metab.* (2019) 104:711–20. doi: 10.1210/jc.2018-00952
84. Taylor EN, Stampfer MJ, Curhan GC. Obesity, weight gain, and the risk of kidney stones. *JAMA.* (2005) 293:455–62. doi: 10.1001/jama.293.4.455
85. Lieske JC, Mehta RA, Milliner DS, Rule AD, Bergstralh EJ, Sarr MG. Kidney stones are common after bariatric surgery. *Kidney Int.* (2015) 87:839–45. doi: 10.1038/ki.2014.352
86. Rule AD, Lieske JC, Li X, Melton LJ III, Krambeck AE, Bergstralh EJ. The ROKS nomogram for predicting a second symptomatic stone episode. *J Am Soc Nephrol.* (2014) 25:2878–86. doi: 10.1681/ASN.2013091011
87. Bhatti UH, Duffy AJ, Roberts KE, Shariff AH. Nephrolithiasis after bariatric surgery: a review of pathophysiologic mechanisms and procedural risk. *Int J Surg.* (2016) 36(Pt D):618–23. doi: 10.1016/j.ijsu.2016.11.025
88. Canales BK, Ellen J, Khan SR, Hatch M. Steatorrhea and hyperoxaluria occur after gastric bypass surgery in obese rats regardless of dietary fat or oxalate. *J Urol.* (2013) 190:1102–9. doi: 10.1016/j.juro.2013.02.3229
89. Dobbins JW, Binder HJ. Effect of bile salts and fatty acids on the colonic absorption of oxalate. *Gastroenterology.* (1976) 70:1096–100. doi: 10.1016/S0016-5085(76)80318-6
90. Kumar R, Lieske JC, Collazo-Clavell ML, Sarr MG, Olson ER, Vrtiska TJ, et al. Fat malabsorption and increased intestinal oxalate absorption are common after Roux-en-Y gastric bypass surgery. *Surgery.* (2011) 149:654–61. doi: 10.1016/j.surg.2010.11.015
91. Canales BK, Hatch M. Oxalobacter formigenes colonization normalizes oxalate excretion in a gastric bypass model of hyperoxaluria. *Surg Obes Relat Dis.* (2017) 13:1152–7. doi: 10.1016/j.soard.2017.03.014
92. Asplin JR. The management of patients with enteric hyperoxaluria. *Urolithiasis.* (2016) 44:33–43. doi: 10.1007/s00240-015-0846-5
93. Zisman AL. Effectiveness of treatment modalities on kidney stone recurrence. *Clin J Am Soc Nephrol.* (2017) 12:1699–708. doi: 10.2215/CJN.11201016
94. Miras AD, le Roux CW. Mechanisms underlying weight loss after bariatric surgery. *Nat Rev Gastroenterol Hepatol.* (2013) 10:575–84. doi: 10.1038/nrgastro.2013.119
95. Martin WP, le Roux CW. Comment on: impact of serum uric acid on renal function after bariatric surgery: a retrospective study. *Surg Obes Relat Dis.* (2019) 16:295–8. doi: 10.1016/j.soard.2019.11.002
96. Scheurlen KM, Billeter AT, Kopf S, Herbst V, Block M, Nawroth PP, et al. Serum uromodulin and Roux-en-Y gastric bypass: improvement of a marker reflecting nephron mass. *Surg Obes Relat Dis.* (2019) 15:1319–25. doi: 10.1016/j.soard.2019.05.002
97. Docherty NG, Fandriks L, le Roux CW, Hallersund P, Werling M. Urinary sodium excretion after gastric bypass surgery. *Surg Obes Relat Dis.* (2017) 13:1506–14. doi: 10.1016/j.soard.2017.04.002
98. Montani JP, Carroll JF, Dwyer TM, Antic V, Yang Z, Dulloo AG. Ectopic fat storage in heart, blood vessels and kidneys in the pathogenesis of cardiovascular diseases. *Int J Obes Relat Metab Disord.* (2004) 28 (Suppl. 4):S58–65. doi: 10.1038/sj.ijo.0802858
99. Wang Y, Chen X, Song Y, Caballero B, Cheskin LJ. Association between obesity and kidney disease: a systematic review and meta-analysis. *Kidney Int.* (2008) 73:19–33. doi: 10.1038/sj.ki.5002586
100. Kang SH, Cho KH, Park JW, Yoon KW, Do JY. Association of visceral fat area with chronic kidney disease and metabolic syndrome risk in the general population: analysis using multi-frequency bioimpedance. *Kidney blood Press Res.* (2015) 40:223–30. doi: 10.1159/000368498
101. Chen YC, Lai SH, Tsai YW, Chang SS. Visceral adiposity index as a predictor of chronic kidney disease in a relatively healthy population in Taiwan. *J Renal Nutr.* (2018) 28:91–100. doi: 10.1053/j.jrn.2017.07.006
102. Krievina G, Tretjakovs P, Skuja I, Silina V, Keisa L, Krievina D, et al. Ectopic adipose tissue storage in the left and the right renal sinus is asymmetric and associated with serum kidney injury molecule-1 and fibroblast growth factor-21 levels increase. *EBioMedicine.* (2016) 13:274–83. doi: 10.1016/j.ebiom.2016.10.020
103. Caglar V, Songur A, Acar M, Uygur R, Alkoc OA, Acar T. Volumetric evaluation of fat in the renal sinus in normal subjects using stereological method on computed tomography images and its relationship with body composition. *Folia Morphol.* (2014) 73:302–8. doi: 10.5603/FM.2014.0016
104. Foster MC, Hwang SJ, Porter SA, Massaro JM, Hoffmann U, Fox CS. Fatty kidney, hypertension, and chronic kidney disease: the Framingham Heart Study. *Hypertension.* (2011) 58:784–90. doi: 10.1161/HYPERTENSIONAHA.111.175315
105. Chughtai HL, Morgan TM, Rocco M, Stacey B, Brinkley TE, Ding J, et al. Renal sinus fat and poor blood pressure control in middle-aged and elderly individuals at risk for cardiovascular events. *Hypertension.* (2010) 56:901–6. doi: 10.1161/HYPERTENSIONAHA.110.157370
106. Wagner R, Machann J, Lehmann R, Rittig K, Schick F, Lenhart J, et al. Exercise-induced albuminuria is associated with perivascular renal sinus fat in individuals at increased risk of type 2 diabetes. *Diabetologia.* (2012) 55:2054–8. doi: 10.1007/s00125-012-2551-z
107. Spit KA, Muskiet MHA, Tonneijck L, Smits MM, Kramer MHH, Joles JA, et al. Renal sinus fat and renal hemodynamics: a cross-sectional analysis. *Magma.* (2019) 33:73–80. doi: 10.1007/s10334-019-00773-z
108. Favre G, Grangeon-Chapon C, Raffaelli C, Francois-Chalmin F, Iannelli A, Esnault V. Perirenal fat thickness measured with computed tomography is a reliable estimate of perirenal fat mass. *PLoS ONE.* (2017) 12:e0175561. doi: 10.1371/journal.pone.0175561
109. Lamacchia O, Nicastro V, Camarchio D, Valente U, Grisorio R, Gesualdo L, et al. Para- and perirenal fat thickness is an independent predictor of chronic kidney disease, increased renal resistance index and hyperuricaemia in type-2 diabetic patients. *Nephrol Dialysis, Transplant.* (2011) 26:892–8. doi: 10.1093/ndt/gfq522
110. D'Marco L, Salazar J, Cortez M, Salazar M, Wettel M, Lima-Martinez M, et al. Perirenal fat thickness is associated with metabolic risk factors in patients with chronic kidney disease. *Kidney Res Clin Pract.* (2019) 38:365–72. doi: 10.23876/j.krcp.18.0155
111. Alonso-Galicia M, Dwyer TM, Herrera GA, Hall JE. Increased hyaluronic acid in the inner renal medulla of obese dogs. *Hypertension.* (1995) 25:888–92. doi: 10.1161/01.HYP.25.4.888
112. Dwyer TM, Banks SA, Alonso-Galicia M, Cockrell K, Carroll JF, Bigler SA, et al. Distribution of renal medullary hyaluronan in lean and obese rabbits. *Kidney Int.* (2000) 58:721–9. doi: 10.1046/j.1523-1755.2000.00218.x
113. Hall JE. The kidney, hypertension, and obesity. *Hypertension.* (2003) 41:625–33. doi: 10.1161/01.HYP.0000052314.95497.78
114. Ricci MA, Scavizzi M, Ministrini S, De Vuono S, Pucci G, Lupattelli G. Morbid obesity and hypertension: The role of perirenal fat. *J Clin Hypertens.* (2018) 20:1430–7. doi: 10.1111/jch.13370
115. Fujioka S, Matsuzawa Y, Tokunaga K, Tarui S. Contribution of intra-abdominal fat accumulation to the impairment of glucose and lipid metabolism in human obesity. *Metab Clin Exp.* (1987) 36:54–9. doi: 10.1016/0026-0495(87)90063-1
116. Weinberg JM. Lipotoxicity. *Kidney Int.* (2006) 70:1560–6. doi: 10.1038/sj.ki.5001834
117. Liu Y, Wang L, Luo M, Chen N, Deng X, He J, et al. Inhibition of PAI-1 attenuates perirenal fat inflammation and the associated nephropathy in high-fat diet-induced obese mice. *Am J Physiol Endocrinol Metab.* (2019) 316:E260–7. doi: 10.1152/ajpendo.00387.2018
118. Longo M, Zatterale F, Naderi J, Parrillo L, Formisano P, Raciti GA, et al. Adipose tissue dysfunction as determinant of obesity-associated metabolic complications. *Int J Mol Sci.* (2019) 20:2358. doi: 10.3390/ijm20092358
119. Deji N, Kume S, Araki S, Soumura M, Sugimoto T, Isshiki K, et al. Structural and functional changes in the kidneys of high-fat diet-induced obese mice. *Am J Physiol Renal Physiol.* (2009) 296:F118–26. doi: 10.1152/ajprenal.00110.2008
120. Bobulescu IA, Dubree M, Zhang J, McLeroy P, Moe OW. Effect of renal lipid accumulation on proximal tubule Na+/H+ exchange and ammonium secretion. *Am J Physiol Renal Physiol.* (2008) 294:F1315–22. doi: 10.1152/ajprenal.00550.2007
121. Lee HS, Lee JS, Koh HI, Ko KW. Intraglomerular lipid deposition in routine biopsies. *Clinical nephrology.* (1991) 36:67–75.

122. Simon N, Hertig A. Alteration of fatty acid oxidation in tubular epithelial cells: from acute kidney injury to renal fibrogenesis. *Front Med.* (2015) 2:52. doi: 10.3389/fmed.2015.00052
123. Martinez-Garcia C, Izquierdo-Lahuerta A, Vivas Y, Velasco I, Yeo TK, Chen S, et al. Renal lipotoxicity-associated inflammation and insulin resistance affects actin cytoskeleton organization in podocytes. *PLoS ONE.* (2015) 10:e0142291. doi: 10.1371/journal.pone.0142291
124. Zelicha H, Schwarzfuchs D, Shelef I, Gepner Y, Tsaban G, Tene L, et al. Changes of renal sinus fat and renal parenchymal fat during an 18-month randomized weight loss trial. *Clin Nutr.* (2018) 37:1145–53. doi: 10.1016/j.clnu.2017.04.007
125. Mende CW, Einhorn D. Fatty kidney disease: a new renal and endocrine clinical entity? Describing the role of the kidney in obesity, metabolic syndrome, and type 2 diabetes. *Endocr Pract.* (2019) 25:854–8. doi: 10.4158/EP-2018-0568
126. Navarro-Diaz M, Serra A, Romero R, Bonet J, Bayes B, Homs M, et al. Effect of drastic weight loss after bariatric surgery on renal parameters in extremely obese patients: long-term follow-up. *J Am Soc Nephrol.* (2006) 17(12 Suppl. 3):S213–7. doi: 10.1681/ASN.2006080917
127. Ruggenenti P, Perticucci E, Cravedi P, Gambara V, Costantini M, Sharma SK, et al. Role of remission clinics in the longitudinal treatment of CKD. *J Am Soc Nephrol.* (2008) 19:1213–24. doi: 10.1681/ASN.2007090970
128. McMurray JJV, Solomon SD, Inzucchi SE, Køber L, Kosiborod MN, Martinez FA, et al. Dapagliflozin in patients with heart failure and reduced ejection fraction. *New Engl J Med.* (2019) 381:1995–2008. doi: 10.1056/NEJMoa1911303
129. Vergara A, Jacobs-Cacha C, Soler MJ. Sodium-glucose cotransporter inhibitors: beyond glycaemic control. *Clin Kidney J.* (2019) 12:322–5. doi: 10.1093/ckj/sfz019
130. Mangan A, Le Roux CW, Miller NG, Docherty NG. Iron and vitamin D/calcium deficiency after gastric bypass: mechanisms involved and strategies to improve oral supplement disposition. *Curr Drug Metab.* (2019) 20:244–52. doi: 10.2174/1389200219666181026160242
131. Bakshi NA, Al-Zahrani H. Bone marrow oxalosis. *Blood.* (2012) 120:8. doi: 10.1182/blood-2011-12-400192
132. Kalantar-Zadeh K, Kopple JD. Obesity paradox in patients on maintenance dialysis. *Contrib Nephrol.* (2006) 151:57–69. doi: 10.1159/000095319
133. Lafranca JA, IJermans JNM, Betjes MG, Dor FJ. Body mass index and outcome in renal transplant recipients: a systematic review and meta-analysis. *BMC Med.* (2015) 13:111. doi: 10.1186/s12916-015-0340-5
134. Potluri K, Hou S. Obesity in kidney transplant recipients and candidates. *Am J Kidney Dis.* (2010) 56:143–56. doi: 10.1053/j.ajkd.2010.01.017
135. Soleymanian T, Kokabeh Z, Ramaghi R, Mahjoub A, Argani H. Clinical outcomes and quality of life in hemodialysis diabetic patients versus non-diabetics. *J Nephropathol.* (2017) 6:81–9. doi: 10.15171/jnp.2017.14
136. Villar E, Remontet L, Labeeuw M, Ecochard R. Effect of age, gender, and diabetes on excess death in end-stage renal failure. *J Am Soc Nephrol.* (2007) 18:2125–34. doi: 10.1681/ASN.2006091048
137. Krishnan N, Higgins R, Short A, Zehnder D, Pitcher D, Hudson A, et al. Kidney transplantation significantly improves patient and graft survival irrespective of BMI: a cohort study. *Am J Transplant.* (2015) 15:2378–86. doi: 10.1111/ajt.13363
138. MacLaughlin HL, Cook SA, Kariyawasam D, Roseke M, van Niekerk M, Macdougall IC. Nonrandomized trial of weight loss with orlistat, nutrition education, diet, and exercise in obese patients with CKD: 2-year follow-up. *Am J Kidney Dis.* (2010) 55:69–76. doi: 10.1053/j.ajkd.2009.09.011
139. Beyea MM, Garg AX, Weir MA. Does orlistat cause acute kidney injury? *Ther Adv Drug Saf.* (2012) 3:53–7. doi: 10.1177/2042098611429985
140. Solomon LR, Nixon AC, Ogden L, Nair B. Orlistat-induced oxalate nephropathy: an under-recognised cause of chronic kidney disease. *BMJ Case Rep.* (2017) 2017:bcr2016218623. doi: 10.1136/bcr-2016-218623
141. Idorn T, Knop FK, Jorgensen MB, Jensen T, Resuli M, Hansen PM, et al. Safety and efficacy of liraglutide in patients with type 2 diabetes and end-stage renal disease: an investigator-initiated, placebo-controlled, double-blind, parallel-group, randomized trial. *Diabetes Care.* (2016) 39:206–13. doi: 10.2337/dc15-1025
142. Mehta A, Marso SP, Neeland IJ. Liraglutide for weight management: a critical review of the evidence. *Obes Sci Pract.* (2017) 3:3–14. doi: 10.1002/osp4.84
143. McCormick BB, Bargman JM. Noninfectious complications of peritoneal dialysis: implications for patient and technique survival. *J Am Soc Nephrol.* (2007) 18:3023–5. doi: 10.1681/ASN.2007070796
144. Sheetz KH, Woodside KJ, Shahinian VB, Dimick JB, Montgomery JR, Waits SA. Trends in bariatric surgery procedures among patients with ESKD in the United States. *Clin J Am Soc Nephrol.* (2019) 14:1193–9. doi: 10.2215/CJN.01480219
145. Kim Y, Bailey AJ, Morris MC, Kassam AF, Shah SA, Diwan TS. Kidney transplantation after sleeve gastrectomy in the morbidly obese candidate: results of a 2-year experience. *Surg Obes Relat Dis.* (2019) 16:10–4. doi: 10.1016/j.soard.2019.09.069
146. Yemini R, Nesher E, Carmeli I, Winkler J, Rahamimov R, Mor E, et al. Bariatric surgery is efficacious and improves access to transplantation for morbidly obese renal transplant candidates. *Obes Surg.* (2019) 29:2373–80. doi: 10.1007/s11695-019-03925-1
147. Cohen JB, Lim MA, Tewksbury CM, Torres-Landa S, Trofe-Clark J, Abt PL, et al. Bariatric surgery before and after kidney transplantation: long-term weight loss and allograft outcomes. *Surg Obes Relat Dis.* (2019) 15:935–41. doi: 10.1016/j.soard.2019.04.002
148. Thomas IA, Gaynor JJ, Joseph T, De La Cruz-Munoz N, Sageshima J, Kupin W, et al. Roux-en-Y gastric bypass is an effective bridge to kidney transplantation: Results from a single center. *Clin Transplant.* (2018) 32:e13232. doi: 10.1111/ctr.13232
149. Kim Y, Jung AD, Dhar VK, Tadros JS, Schauer DP, Smith EP, et al. Laparoscopic sleeve gastrectomy improves renal transplant candidacy and posttransplant outcomes in morbidly obese patients. *Am J Transplant.* (2018) 18:410–6. doi: 10.1111/ajt.14463
150. Kienzl-Wagner K, Weissenbacher A, Gehwolf P, Wykypiel H, Ofner D, Schneeberger S. Laparoscopic sleeve gastrectomy: gateway to kidney transplantation. *Surg Obes Relat Dis.* (2017) 13:909–15. doi: 10.1016/j.soard.2017.01.005
151. Carandina S, Genser L, Bossi M, Montana L, Cortes A, Seman M, et al. Laparoscopic sleeve gastrectomy in kidney transplant candidates: a case series. *Obes Surg.* (2017) 27:2613–8. doi: 10.1007/s11695-017-2679-5
152. Al-Bahri S, Fakhry TK, Gonzalvo JP, Murr MM. Bariatric surgery as a bridge to renal transplantation in patients with end-stage renal disease. *Obes Surg.* (2017) 27:2951–5. doi: 10.1007/s11695-017-2722-6
153. Freeman CM, Woodle ES, Shi J, Alexander JW, Leggett PL, Shah SA, et al. Addressing morbid obesity as a barrier to renal transplantation with laparoscopic sleeve gastrectomy. *Am J Transplant.* (2015) 15:1360–8. doi: 10.1111/ajt.13116
154. Jamal MH, Corcelles R, Daigle CR, Rogula T, Kroh M, Schauer PR, et al. Safety and effectiveness of bariatric surgery in dialysis patients and kidney transplantation candidates. *Surg Obes Relat Dis.* (2015) 11:419–23. doi: 10.1016/j.soard.2014.09.022
155. Lin MY, Tavakol MM, Sarin A, Amirkiai SM, Rogers SJ, Carter JT, et al. Laparoscopic sleeve gastrectomy is safe and efficacious for pretransplant candidates. *Surg Obes Relat Dis.* (2013) 9:653–8. doi: 10.1016/j.soard.2013.02.013
156. Alexander JW, Goodman H. Gastric bypass in chronic renal failure and renal transplant. *Nutr Clin Pract.* (2007) 22:16–21. doi: 10.1177/011542650702200116
157. Rogers CC, Alloway RR, Alexander JW, Cardi M, Trofe J, Vinks AA. Pharmacokinetics of mycophenolic acid, tacrolimus and sirolimus after gastric bypass surgery in end-stage renal disease and transplant patients: a pilot study. *Clin Transplant.* (2008) 22:281–91. doi: 10.1111/j.1399-0012.2007.00783.x
158. Troxell ML, Houghton DC, Hawkey M, Batiuk TD, Bennett WM. Enteric oxalate nephropathy in the renal allograft: an underrecognized complication of bariatric surgery. *Am J Transplant.* (2013) 13:501–9. doi: 10.1111/ajt.12029
159. Eid I, Birch DW, Sharma AM, Sherman V, Karmali S. Complications associated with adjustable gastric banding for morbid obesity: a surgeon's guides. *Can J Surg.* (2011) 54:61–6. doi: 10.1503/cjs.015709
160. Mari G, Scanziani R, Auricchio S, Crippa J, Maggioni D. Laparoscopic surgery in patients on peritoneal dialysis: a review of the literature. *Surg Innovat.* (2017) 24:397–401. doi: 10.1177/1553350617708723

161. Del Peso G, Bajo MA, Costero O, Hevia C, Gil F, Diaz C, et al. Risk factors for abdominal wall complications in peritoneal dialysis patients. *Perit Dial Int.* (2003) 23:249–54. doi: 10.1177/089686080302300306
162. Keshvari A, Fazeli MS, Meysamie A, Seifi S, Taromloo MK. The effects of previous abdominal operations and intraperitoneal adhesions on the outcome of peritoneal dialysis catheters. *Perit Dial Int.* (2010) 30:41–5. doi: 10.3747/pdi.2008.00121
163. Valle GA, Kissane BE, de la Cruz-Munoz N. Successful laparoscopic bariatric surgery in peritoneal dialysis patients without interruption of their CKD6 treatment modality. *Adv Perit Dial Conf Perit Dial.* (2012) 28:134–9.
164. Imam TH, Wang J, Khayat FS. Bariatric surgery in a patient on peritoneal dialysis. *Perit Dial Int.* (2013) 33:710–1. doi: 10.3747/pdi.2012.00272
165. Andalib A, Aminian A, Khorgami Z, Navaneethan SD, Schauer PR, Brethauer SA. Safety analysis of primary bariatric surgery in patients on chronic dialysis. *Surg Endosc.* (2016) 30:2583–91. doi: 10.1007/s00464-015-4530-1
166. Nemati E, Einollahi B, Lesan Pezeshki M, Porfarziani V, Fattahi MR. Does kidney transplantation with deceased or living donor affect graft survival? *Nephrourol Mon.* (2014) 6:e12182. doi: 10.5812/numonthly.12182
167. Taler SJ, Messersmith EE, Leichtman AB, Gillespie BW, Kew CE, Stegall MD, et al. Demographic, metabolic, and blood pressure characteristics of living kidney donors spanning five decades. *Am J Transplant.* (2013) 13:390–8. doi: 10.1111/j.1600-6143.2012.04321.x
168. Rodrigue JR, Schold JD, Mandelbrot DA. The decline in living kidney donation in the United States: random variation or cause for concern? *Transplantation.* (2013) 96:767–73. doi: 10.1097/TP.0b013e318298fa61
169. Lentine KL, Kasiske BL, Levey AS, Adams PL, Alberu J, Bakr MA, et al. KDIGO clinical practice guideline on the evaluation and care of living kidney donors. *Transplantation.* (2017) 101(8S Suppl. 1):S1–109. doi: 10.1097/TP.0000000000001769
170. Reese PP, Feldman HI, Asch DA, Thomasson A, Shults J, Bloom RD. Short-term outcomes for obese live kidney donors and their recipients. *Transplantation.* (2009) 88:662–71. doi: 10.1097/TP.0b013e3181b27a17
171. Locke JE, Reed RD, Massie AB, MacLennan PA, Sawinski D, Kumar V, et al. Obesity and long-term mortality risk among living kidney donors. *Surgery.* (2019) 166:205–8. doi: 10.1016/j.surg.2019.03.016
172. Nguyen MJP, Carpenter D, Tadros J, Mathur A, Sandoval PR, Woodle ES, et al. Bariatric surgery prior to living donor nephrectomy: a solution to expand the living donor kidney pool - a retrospective study. *Transplant Int.* (2019) 32:702–9. doi: 10.1111/tri.13408
173. Cowan N, Gritsch HA, Nassiri N, Sinacore J, Veale J. Broken chains and reneging: a review of 1748 kidney paired donation transplants. *Am J Transplant.* (2017) 17:2451–7. doi: 10.1111/ajt.14343
174. Montgomery JR, Telem DA, Waits SA. Bariatric surgery for prospective living kidney donors with obesity? *Am J Transplant.* (2019) 19:2415–20. doi: 10.1111/ajt.15260
175. Marchetti P, Navalesi R. The metabolic effects of cyclosporin and tacrolimus. *J Endocrinol Investig.* (2000) 23:482–90. doi: 10.1007/BF03343761
176. Steiner RW. Steroid-free chronic immunosuppression in renal transplantation. *Curr Opin Nephrol Hypertens.* (2012) 21:567–73. doi: 10.1097/MNH.0b013e328359226c
177. Rizzari MD, Suszynski TM, Gillingham KJ, Dunn TB, Ibrahim HN, Payne WD, et al. Ten-year outcome after rapid discontinuation of prednisone in adult primary kidney transplantation. *Clin J Am Soc Nephrol.* (2012) 7:494–503. doi: 10.2215/CJN.08630811
178. Pallet N, Legendre C. Adverse events associated with mTOR inhibitors. *Exp Opin Drug Safety.* (2013) 12:177–86. doi: 10.1517/14740338.2013.752814
179. Methven S, Steenkamp R, Fraser S. UK Renal Registry 19th Annual Report: chapter 5 survival and causes of death in UK adult patients on renal replacement therapy in 2015: National and Centre-specific Analyses. *Nephron.* (2017) 137 (Suppl. 1):117–50. doi: 10.1159/000481367
180. Saran R, Robinson B, Abbott KC, Agodoa LYC, Bragg-Gresham J, Balkrishnan R, et al. US Renal Data System 2018 Annual Data Report: epidemiology of kidney disease in the United States. *Am J Kidney Dis.* (2019) 73(3S1):A7–A8. doi: 10.1053/j.ajkd.2019.01.001
181. Hariharan S, Adams MB, Brennan DC, Davis CL, First MR, Johnson CP, et al. Recurrent and de novo glomerular disease after renal transplantation: a report from Renal Allograft Disease Registry (RADR). *Transplantation.* (1999) 68:635–41. doi: 10.1097/00007890-199909150-00007
182. Burton H, Iyamu Perisanidou L, Steenkamp R, Evans R, Mumford L, Evans KM, et al. Causes of renal allograft failure in the UK: trends in UK Renal Registry and National Health Service Blood and Transplant data from 2000 to 2013. *Nephrol Dial Transplant.* (2019) 34:355–64. doi: 10.1093/ndt/gfy168
183. Chen JH, Lee CH, Chang CM, Yin WY. Successful management of new-onset diabetes mellitus and obesity with the use of laparoscopic sleeve gastrectomy after kidney transplantation-a case report. *Transplant Proc.* (2016) 48:938–9. doi: 10.1016/j.transproceed.2015.12.074
184. Gheith O, Al-Otaibi T, Halim MA, Mahmoud T, Mosaad A, Yagan J, et al. Bariatric surgery in renal transplant patients. *Exp Clin Transplant.* (2017) 15 (Suppl. 1):164–9. doi: 10.6002/ect.mesot2016.P35
185. Elli EF, Gonzalez-Heredia R, Sanchez-Johnsen L, Patel N, Garcia-Roca R, Oberholzer J. Sleeve gastrectomy surgery in obese patients post-organ transplantation. *Surg Obes Relat Dis.* (2016) 12:528–34. doi: 10.1016/j.soard.2015.11.030
186. Khoraki J, Katz MG, Funk LM, Greenberg JA, Fernandez LA, Campos GM. Feasibility and outcomes of laparoscopic sleeve gastrectomy after solid organ transplantation. *Surg Obes Relat Dis.* (2016) 12:75–83. doi: 10.1016/j.soard.2015.04.002
187. Szomstein S, Rojas R, Rosenthal RJ. Outcomes of laparoscopic bariatric surgery after renal transplant. *Obes Surg.* (2010) 20:383–5. doi: 10.1007/s11695-009-9969-5
188. Gazzetta PG, Bissolati M, Saibene A, Ghidini CGA, Guarneri G, Giannone F, et al. Bariatric surgery to target obesity in the renal transplant population: preliminary experience in a single center. *Transplant Proc.* (2017) 49:646–9. doi: 10.1016/j.transproceed.2017.02.032
189. Viscido G, Gorodner V, Signorini FJ, Campazzo M, Navarro L, Obeide LR, et al. Sleeve gastrectomy after renal transplantation. *Obes Surg.* (2018) 28:1587–94. doi: 10.1007/s11695-017-3056-0
190. Brenner BM, Cooper ME, de Zeeuw D, Keane WF, Mitch WE, Parving H-H, et al. Effects of losartan on renal and cardiovascular outcomes in patients with type 2 diabetes and nephropathy. *New Engl J Med.* (2001) 345:861–9. doi: 10.1056/NEJMoa011161

4

Glucocorticoid Metabolism in Obesity and Following Weight Loss

Elina Akalestou[1], *Laurent Genser*[1,2] *and Guy A. Rutter*[1*]

[1] *Section of Cell Biology and Functional Genomics, Division of Diabetes, Endocrinology and Metabolism, Department of Metabolism, Digestion and Reproduction, Imperial Centre for Translational and Experimental Medicine, Imperial College London, London, United Kingdom,* [2] *Department of Digestive and Hepato-Pancreato-Biliary Surgery, Liver Transplantation, Assistance Publique-Hôpitaux de Paris, Pitié-Salpêtrière University Hospital, Institut Hospitalo-Universitaire ICAN, Sorbonne Université, Paris, France*

Correspondence:
Guy A. Rutter
g.rutter@imperial.ac.uk

Glucocorticoids are steroid hormones produced by the adrenal cortex and are essential for the maintenance of various metabolic and homeostatic functions. Their function is regulated at the tissue level by 11β-hydroxysteroid dehydrogenases and they signal through the glucocorticoid receptor, a ligand-dependent transcription factor. Clinical observations have linked excess glucocorticoid levels with profound metabolic disturbances of intermediate metabolism resulting in abdominal obesity, insulin resistance and dyslipidaemia. In this review, we discuss the physiological mechanisms of glucocorticoid secretion, regulation and function, and survey the metabolic consequences of excess glucocorticoid action resulting from elevated release and activation or up-regulated signaling. Finally, we summarize the reported impact of weight loss by diet, exercise, or bariatric surgery on circulating and tissue-specific glucocorticoid levels and examine the therapeutic possibility of reversing glucocorticoid-associated metabolic disorders.

Keywords: glucocorticoids, obesity, weight loss, bariatric surgery, 11β-HSD1

GLUCOCORTICOID SECRETION

Glucocorticoid hormones are a class of corticosteroids, produced by the adrenal cortex primarily under the control of the hypothalamic-pituitary-adrenal (HPA) axis (1). Briefly, corticotropin-releasing hormone (CRH) and vasopressin are released from the hypothalamus and synergistically stimulate the secretion of stored adrenocorticotropic hormone (ACTH) from corticotrope cells in the anterior pituitary gland. Following this, ACTH is transported by the blood to the adrenal cortex, where it rapidly stimulates biosynthesis of corticosteroids such as cortisol from cholesterol (2). However, it recently became apparent (3) that the fine-tuning and regulation of the adrenal system is also controlled by ACTH-independent mechanisms. These include a temporal lag between stimulus-induced changes in circulating ACTH and in corticosteroid levels (4), adrenal corticosteroid metabolism and kinetics, and plasma protein binding (5–7). Moreover, dysregulation is observed in glucocorticoid secretion under pathological conditions (8, 9). An example of this is in obesity, where several studies in humans report (8, 10–12) an increase of cortisol secretion directly from the adrenal gland, yet the circulating plasma levels are normal, potentially due to higher metabolic clearance rate.

A variety of growth factors, neuropeptides, cytokines and adipokines have been demonstrated to affect adrenal secretions. Correspondingly, adrenocortical cells express receptors for each of these factors (13, 14). *In vitro* studies found that vital glucose regulating-peptides also have the capacity to regulate ACTH-stimulated glucocorticoid secretion. More specifically, insulin inhibits cortisol secretion from bovine adrenocortical cells (15), while glucagon inhibits cortisol secretion from human adrenocortical cells (16, 17). The satiety factor leptin was found to directly regulate adrenal secretions via its receptors on adrenocortical cells (18, 19). Likewise, the gut-derived incretin hormone glucagon-like peptide 1 (GLP-1) was also shown to inhibit glucocorticoid release from rat adrenal cortex in response to ACTH, by decreasing the activation of adenylate cyclase and by impairing the late steps of glucocorticoid synthesis (17). Nonetheless, intracerebroventricular, intravenous, and intraperitoneal administration of GLP-1 increased circulating levels of cortisol in rats, a change preceded by an increase in ACTH levels (20, 21). The mechanisms through which circulating GLP-1 activate the HPA axis remain to be elucidated, and may provide further evidence for the beneficial effect of GLP-1 receptor agonists in obesity and type 2 diabetes (T2DM) treatment.

11β-Hydroxysteroid Dehydrogenases

Although the regulation of glucocorticoid secretion is an important means of their action, the effects of glucocorticoids on target tissues such as liver and adipose tissue are dependent on metabolism by 11β-hydroxysteroid dehydrogenases (11β-HSDs), with the notable exception of pancreatic β-cells (22). 11β-HSD1 is present in most cells and tissues and acts predominantly as an NADPH-dependent reductase to regenerate the active glucocorticoid receptor (GR) ligand cortisol (or corticosterone, in rodents) from inactive cortisone (**Figure 1**) (23). Conversely, 11β-HSD2 inactivates cortisol by converting it into cortisone, thereby protecting the mineralocorticoid receptor from cortisol ligands. 11β-HSD2 is largely expressed in the kidney, placenta, and colon whereas the principle sites of 11β-HSD1 expression are liver, adipose tissue and muscle (24). The A-ring reductases, 5-reductase types 1 and 2 (5R1 and 5R2) convert cortisol and cortisone to their dihydrometabolites, and these are next converted to tetrahydrometabolites through the action of 3-hydroxysteroid dehydrogenase (25, 26). Total glucocorticoid production can be estimated by analyzing the sum of glucocorticoid metabolites in a 24 h urinary sample. The relative excretion of cortisol to cortisonemetabolites [(5a-THF + THF + a-cortol)/(THE + a-cortolone)] reflects the global activity of 11β-HSD 1 (27).

Glucocorticoid metabolism at the tissue level is dysregulated in human obesity, with increased 5-reductase activity and decreased cortisol levels in the liver (28–30). Contrariwise, 11β-HSD1 activity is increased in adipose tissue, which increases tissue glucocorticoid levels. Mice overexpressing 11β-HSD1 in adipose tissue develop visceral obesity, insulin resistance, dyslipidaemia, and hypertension (31), while liver-specific 11β-HSD1 overexpression results in insulin resistance and hypertension, but not obesity (32). Interestingly, 11β-HSD1 appears to be absent from pancreatic α and β- cells though present in other cell types in the mouse and human islet (22, 33). Selective 11β-HSD1 inhibitors have been shown to lower glucose intolerance and reduce food intake and weight gain in hyperglycaemic mouse models (34–36). 11β-HSD1 knockout mice are resistant to hyperglycaemia when fed a high-fat diet and show reduced expression of mRNA encoding the key hepatic gluconeogenic enzyme phosphoenolpyruvate carboxykinase (PCK1) (37). Overall, these studies place 11β-HSD1 in a central position of cortisol metabolism and suggest that its inhibition may be a key target for diabetes and obesity treatments, especially as a mediator of insulin sensitivity. Nonetheless, the differential regulation of11β-HSD1 between organs implies a more complex pathway that may require equal attention to be paid to 11β-HSD2.

Glucocorticoid Receptors (GR)

The function of glucocorticoids, both at a physiological and pharmacological level, is mediated by the GR. The GR is a member of the nuclear receptor superfamily of ligand-dependent transcription factors and its gene is regulated by both developmental and tissue-specific factors (38). Activated GR controls the expression of thousands of genes, either by inducing or inhibiting their transcription through DNA binding (39–41). The GR is composed of three main domains; the N-terminal transactivation, the central DNA-binding and the C-terminal ligand binding domains, with the central domain containing two zinc fingers. In the absence of glucocorticoids, GR is located primarily in the cytoplasm inside a large multi-protein complex. Once glucocorticoids are bound, GR dissociates from the complex and exposes two nuclear localization signals. GR then rapidly translocates into the nucleus through nuclear pores and, once inside, binds directly to glucocorticoid-responsive elements (GRE) and regulates the expression of target genes (**Figure 1**) (42). Our understanding of the role of the GR protein has changed dramatically within the last decade, as it is now accepted that the GR gene can be spliced into a large group of receptor isoforms, each with a different expression and function that widens the glucocorticoid diversity of GR action (43). Moreover, although this review focuses on the genomic mechanism of glucocorticoid function, several studies have demonstrated a rapid, non-genomic action mechanism that does not involve gene expression alteration and may involve an, as yet uncharacterised, receptor located at the plasma membrane (44–46).

Glucocorticoids acting through the GR regulate glucose metabolism in the liver, skeletal muscle, adipose tissue, and the pancreas, by controlling the expression of key enzymes. However, in obesity, cortisol levels remain at near normal concentrations, pointing to intracellular control of GR action in these circumstances. This suggests that GR polymorphisms might be responsible for the pathophysiology and evolution of obesity and diabetes (47, 48). The GR levels and activity have also been linked to diabetes pathogenesis, as increased hepatic GR mRNA induces activation of phosphoenolpyruvate carboxykinase (PEPCK), which results in hyperglycaemia and insulin resistance in diabetic obese mice and obese Zucker rats (49, 50). This observation was also made in human skeletal muscle, as increased GR was linked to the metabolic syndrome (51). Furthermore, general and hepatic inactivation of GR, achieved through the use of antagonists, was shown to improve glucose tolerance and insulin resistance in diabetic animals (52–54). The mass emerging observations on GR

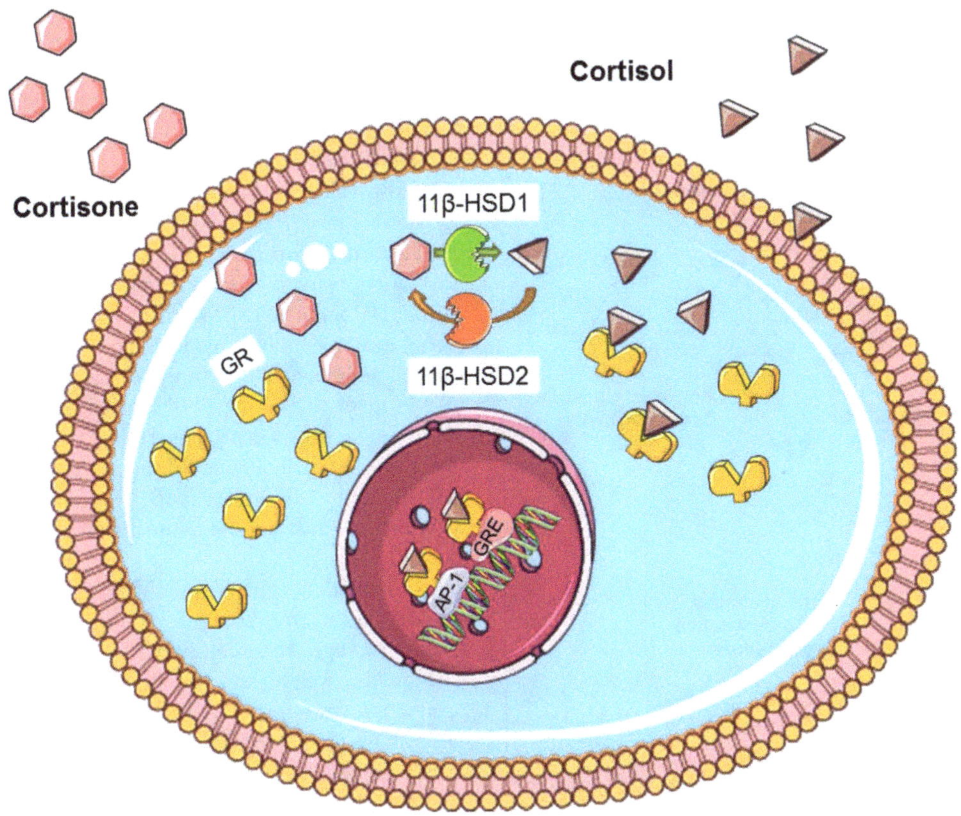

FIGURE 1 | Glucocorticoid metabolism. Cortisone is activated to cortisol by the enzyme 11β-HSD1. Conversely, 11β-HSD2 inactivates cortisol by converting it into cortisone. GR is found in the cytosol. Cortisol binds on the GR and the ligand-receptor complex translocates to the nucleus where in can bind on GRE or to different transcription factors such as AP-1. Figure was created using Servier Medical Art.

polymorphism could further indicate which receptor subtype can be a disease risk indicator, as well as improve specificity for GR antagonism treatment.

METABOLIC FUNCTION OF GLUCOCORTICOIDS

Glucocorticoids are involved in metabolic, inflammatory, cardiovascular, and behavioral processes. Thus, as mentioned above, they modulate the transcription of a variety of genes, including cytokines and chemokines, receptors, enzymes, adhesion molecules, and inhibitory proteins. Clinical observations linking high glucocorticoid levels to the metabolic syndrome provided evidence for their role on diabetes and obesity (55). The metabolic effects of glucocorticoids are linked to physiological mechanisms that are associated with hepatic and peripheral insulin resistance, hyperglycaemia, and dyslipidaemia. In the liver, glucocorticoids stimulate gluconeogenesis by activating PEPCK and glucose-6-phosphatase (G6Pase) (56). Moreover, in the fasting condition, glucocorticoids stimulate lipolysis in adipocytes, resulting in generation of glycerol to be utilized in gluconeogenesis and free fatty acids to be oxidized and get used as energy (57, 58). Although glucocorticoids are important for the maintenance of lipid homeostasis, excess glucocorticoids can result in an increase the circulating free fatty acids and induce lipid accumulation in skeletal muscle and liver, both of which are associated with insulin resistance (59–61). In rat skeletal muscle, glucocorticoid excess can also inhibit the translocation of GLUT4 glucose transporters to the plasma membrane in response to insulin, resulting in insulin resistance (**Figure 2**) (62). In human adipose tissue, glucocorticoids induce adipocyte differentiation leading to increased adiposity and insulin resistance (63–65).

The link between glucocorticoids and T2DM is strong, yet the effect of glucocorticoids on the endocrine pancreas remains controversial. The study of transgenic mice overexpressing the GR selectively in the β-cell indicated that glucocorticoids may directly inhibit insulin release *in vivo* (66). Correspondingly, several *in vitro* studies have demonstrated an inhibitory effect of glucocorticoids on mouse islets (67, 68). The function of 11β-HSD1 in mouse and human islets has been examined *in vitro*, and data suggest direct control over α-cell glucagon release and a paracrine effect on insulin secretion (69). In islets obtained from diabetic obese mice, glucocorticoid administration

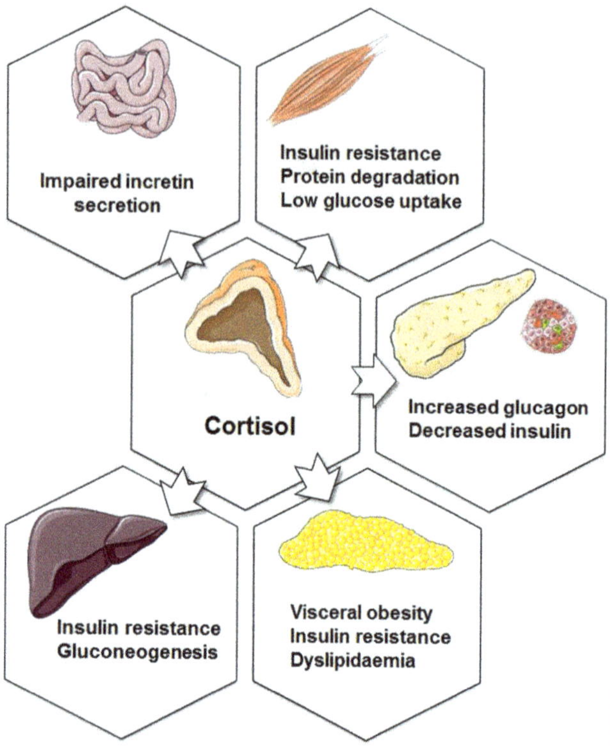

FIGURE 2 | Metabolic functions of glucocorticoids. The effects of increased cortisol secretion on the endocrine pancreas, adipose tissue, liver, muscle, and gastrointestinal system. Figure was created using Servier Medical Art.

up regulated 11β-HSD1 causing impaired insulin secretion. This effect was abolished by GR antagonist or an 11β-HSD1 inhibitor (70).

Glucocorticoids have also been associated with pancreatic development. Treatment of fetal rats with dexamethasone reduced β-cell insulin content and examination of embryonic pancreata from glucocorticoid-treated animals revealed a decrease of insulin-producing cells and an increase in exocrine cells, possibly the result of down-regulation of pancreas maturation transcription factors such as Pdx1, Pax6, and Nkx6.1 (71, 72). However, islets from Wistar rats treated with dexamethasone for 5 days showed an enhanced insulin release in response to glucose, with an increased number of insulin granules docked at the plasma membrane observed in β-cells (73). Transgenic mice overexpressing 11β-HSD1 selectively to the β-cell displayed a reversal of high fat-induced β-cell failure. This was due to the expansion of β-cell population and the function of small islets, the latter being linked to protein kinase A and p21 signaling pathways (74). Finally, corticosterone, cortisol, and cortisone suppressed voltage-dependent Ca^{2+} channel activity in human and rodent β-cells, while in parallel amplifying cAMP signals and increasing the number of membrane-docked insulin secretory granules. Interestingly, no changes were observed in glucose-stimulated insulin secretion nor in the maximal ATP/ADP responses to glucose (75).

GLUCOCORTICOIDS AND WEIGHT LOSS

Diet and Exercise

Although a link between glucocorticoids and obesity has been reported in many studies, it is still unclear what changes following weight loss. Tomlinson et al. (76) reported the effects of weight loss on glucocorticoids in patients with obesity on very low calorie diet. Even though circulating cortisol and cortisone concentrations did not change with weight loss, the 0900h cortisol/cortisone ratio increased, indicating a shift in set-point toward cortisol generation consistent with increased 11β-HSD1 activity. Expression of 11β-HSD1 in whole adipose tissue did not change with weight loss but did increase in isolated adipocytes. No other corticosteroid was affected. A follow-up of this study (77) showed that total glucocorticoid secretion in this scenario decreased post-diet-induced weight loss. However, urinary steroid metabolite ratios that reflect 11β-HSD1 activity did not change. Moreover, increased cortisol availability within adipose tissue interstitial fluid was shown after weight loss.

In men with weight loss following 6 months of dieting, cortisol production rate, free cortisol levels and metabolic clearance rate did not change when compared to baseline (78). Nonetheless, with greater weight loss and decreased body fat, both cortisol production and free cortisol levels increased, whilst adipose 11β-HSD-1 decreased, compared to baseline (78). One week of caloric restriction in men also failed to reveal any change in cortisol levels (79). These results were further investigated in overweight/obese post-menopausal women following diet-induced weight loss with contradictory results. In one study (80), 11β-HSD1 expression in adipose tissue was decreased post-weight loss and this reduction was correlated with a reduction in BMI between baseline and 6 months post-diet initiation. In contrast, a previous study showed that weight reduction did not impact gene expression levels of 11β-HSD1 in adipose tissue (81).

Glucocorticoids respond acutely to changes in nutritional status, with cortisol levels increasing within minutes following a meal (82, 83). Given the discrepancies between studies, as well as differences in human and rodent data, it became clear that the type of meal in each diet had to be specified and specific dietary macronutrients were investigated with regards to their effect on metabolism (84). A high fat-low carbohydrate diet increased whole body 11β-HSD1 activity and decreased 5a- and 5b-reductase activities in men, compared with a moderate fat-moderate carbohydrate diet, with no effect on subcutaneous adipose tissue 11β-HSD1 (84). In rodents, although there was no difference between low carbohydrate and moderate carbohydrate diets, hepatic 11β-HSD1 mRNA was reduced in both diets when compared with a high fat Western diet (85).

Apart from diet, exercise is a common treatment for weight loss. However, exercise is also a form of metabolic stress which can stimulate the HPA axis and lead to increased levels of circulating glucocorticoids (86, 87). The importance of this has been investigated by separating acute intense and chronic voluntary exercises in rats on treadmill running, where intense exercise studies have shown higher corticosterone levels in urine, enlargement of the adrenal glands and reduced adrenal sensitivity to ACTH, as indicated by low ACTH-to-glucocorticoid ratio (88, 89), whether regular and voluntary exercise increased adrenal sensitivity, demonstrating that long-term training balances glucocorticoid fluctuations (86, 90).

Although increased glucocorticoid concentration can indeed have a negative impact in pancreatic β-cells alone (91), regular exercise can improve insulin sensitivity and glucose tolerance and this could be attributed to tissular, rather than systemic, glucocorticoid metabolism. It has previously been shown that exercise can lead to reduced expression of the glucocorticoid receptor and 11β-HSD1 in muscle and liver, yet unchanged circulating cortisol, in hamsters (87). Importantly, previous studies in humans and rodents have demonstrated that various types of exercise are able to improve insulin sensitivity, by recovering the function of specific insulin signaling proteins such as Akt and IRS-1 and also augment GLUT-4 expression (92–97). Insulin-stimulated glucose uptake in muscle, impaired by exposure to glucocorticoids, can also be enhanced by exercise. The effects of exercise appear to involve increased activation of insulin signal via Akt and IRS1 in rodents, as well as slow the glucocorticoid-induced muscle atrophy. This appears to improve through a combination of increases in mTOR and its downstream target p70S6K protein, and a small increase in MuRF-1 protein level, the latter a regulator of proteasome-dependent degradation of muscle proteins (94–96). To date, studies have been able to demonstrate that exercise is able to attenuate exogenous glucocorticoid-induced hyperglycaemia, while less is known about its effect on endogenous glucocorticoids.

Overall, reporting on the relationship between cortisol levels, obesity and weight loss has been challenging, especially if cortisol was measured in the serum, urine or saliva which would provide a snapshot in time rather than continuous reporting. This is most likely due to the fact that cortisol is secreted in a pulsatile manner, affected by the circadian rhythm, environmental circumstances and stress (98), which could even be diet-induced. In addition, gender and adiposity location also appear to have an effect on results. It is therefore important to remember that not all patients with obesity will demonstrate similar cortisol secretion and metabolism, especially at baseline level. Chronic cortisol measurement may provide a more appropriate and ubiquitous way to report changes in glucocorticoid metabolism, potentially by using hair cortisol measurements (99–102), which has been shown to be a novel and accurate way to measure average systemic cortisol levels.

Bariatric Surgery

Bariatric surgery, and particularly Roux-en-Y gastric bypass (RYGB), causes sustained weight loss in individuals with morbid obesity, as well as dramatic and rapid improvement of T2DM, dyslipidaemia, hypertension and a significant reduction of cardiovascular disease and death (103). Although the effects of RYGB on diabetes were initially attributed to the substantial weight loss subsequent to post-operative restriction of nutrient intake and/or absorption, the same effect was demonstrated in rodents that did not experience weight loss, suggesting a mechanism of action that is weight independent. Moreover, the improvements are observed within hours and days, long before substantial weight loss occurred.

In an effort to understand the underlying mechanisms of diabetes remission, this observation has since led to numerous investigations on the glucoregulatory role of the gastrointestinal tract, including the role of an increase in observed post-operative GLP-1 concentration. This includes the "hindgut hypothesis" which holds that euglycaemic effects are derived from the expedited delivery of nutrients to the distal intestine, where GLP-1 is primarily secreted, and therefore enhances the insulin signal that improves glucose metabolism (104). Few data are available regarding the specific modifications in glucocorticoid metabolism after bariatric surgery in human obesity. Given the numerous endocrine changes following surgery, one might expect to have a conclusive picture of glucocorticoid metabolism post-operatively. The fact that this is the case due to different surgical procedures, as well as alterations of the same procedures, which can cause perioperative stress and different levels of caloric restriction and weight loss.

Several observations have linked bariatric surgery to glucocorticoid metabolism, notably in the context of post-operative adipose tissue reduction. Woods et al. investigated the activity and expression of 11β-HSD1 in hepatic and adipose tissue before and ~14 months after RYGB, revealing a post-operative increase in hepatic 11β-HSD1 activity, as inferred from a by raised serum cortisol/costisone ratio (F/E) (105). However, subcutaneous adipose tissue 11β-HSD1 activity was decreased, as showed by the tissue's F/E. Moreover, total urinary cortisol metabolites were reduced, suggesting a reduction in HPA axis activity (105). The decrease of subcutaneous adipose tissue 11β-HSD1 activity at 1 and 2 years after gastric bypass surgery in humans has also been reported through both mRNA expression and urine and adipose tissue F/E, along with positive changes in insulin sensitivity, circulating leptin, and adiponectin, and peripheral glucocorticoid metabolism (106–108). Additionally, intra-adipose levels of cortisone, rather than cortisol, demonstrated the most obvious changes, suggesting that the altered glucocorticoid metabolism after weight loss may be an adaptive response to insufficient levels of adipose cortisol. Of note, supplementary data in Methlie et al. (108), show that obese patients at 1 year post-RYGB demonstrated a significant reduction of adipose tissue F/E, when compared to non-obese controls. This observation points to an effect potentially caused by more than surgery-induced weight loss and may include the gastrointestinal tract manipulation itself. One potential mechanism could be the effect of post-operatively increased GLP-1 on glucocorticoid regulation, as discussed before. Taken together, the reduction in glucocorticoid exposure in subjects with obesity may represent an additional possible contribution to the health benefits of bariatric surgery.

DISCUSSION

Glucocorticoids are steroid hormones that are crucial for the preservation of homeostasis. Their physiological and therapeutic effects have made them key targets for drug development, primarily as anti-inflammatory agents. Nonetheless, their side effects can be severe, especially in terms of metabolism. In this review, we provide an overview of the physiology glucocorticoid regulation, metabolism, and signaling pathways, as well as their effects on obesity and diabetes. We also discussed the ability of weight loss to reverse some of these effects.

Overall, high glucocorticoid levels are associated with hyperglycaemia and insulin resistance and affect key metabolic organs such as the pancreas, liver, muscle and adipose tissue (28, 30, 107, 109). Of note, the exact mechanism of glucocorticoid action remains controversial in pancreatic islets, especially in insulin secretion during glucocorticoid treatment (66–68). Glucocorticoid metabolism is largely controlled by 11β-HSD1 and GR and has been shown to be strongly linked to Body Mass Index, as intra-adipose cortisol levels are increased relative to inactive cortisone in the obese state, even if circulating cortisol levels remain stable. Weight loss through diet, exercise, and bariatric surgery is linked to reduced glucocorticoid secretion and function, possibly through the recovery of insulin sensitivity and function of insulin sensitivity proteins. In all three weight loss interventions, the expression levels of 11β-HSD1 in adipose tissue and liver remains a matter of debate, as studies report both increasing and decreasing levels (78–80, 107, 108). Moreover, acute cortisol measurements are presented, through serum and plasma samples. It is therefore vital to measure chronic cortisol levels to get a longer-term picture of cortisol alterations, and investigate the role of 11β-HSD1 and GR following rapid weight loss in patients, especially following bariatric surgery which is currently the least published field. This will help us determine if the positive observations on glucocorticoid metabolism are due to weight loss or if direct or indirect gastrointestinal manipulation can also have an effect.

AUTHOR CONTRIBUTIONS

EA prepared the first draft and revised the manuscript. LG and GR revised the manuscript.

FUNDING

EA was supported by a grant from the Rosetrees Trust (M825) and from the British Society for Neuroendocrinology. GR was supported by a Wellcome Trust Investigator (212625/Z/18/Z) Award, MRC Programme grants (MR/R022259/1, MR/J0003042/1, MR/L020149/1), and Experimental Challenge Grant (DIVA, MR/L02036X/1), MRC (MR/N00275X/1), and Diabetes UK (BDA/11/0004210, BDA/15/0005275, BDA 16/0005485) grants. This project has received funding from the European Union's Horizon 2020 research and innovation programme via the Innovative Medicines Initiative 2 Joint Undertaking under grant agreement No. 115881 (RHAPSODY) to GR. LG was supported by the Institute of Cardiometabolism and Nutrition, Société Française de Chirurgie Digestive, Fondation Obélisque, APPERT Institute, and Société Française et Francophone de l'obésité et des maladies métaboliques.

REFERENCES

1. Smith SM, Vale WW. The role of the hypothalamic-pituitary-adrenal axis in neuroendocrine responses to stress. *Dialogues Clin Neurosci.* (2006) 8:383–95.
2. Adriana Del Rey GC, Besedovsky H. *The Hypothalamus-Pituitary-Adrenal Axis. The Hypothalamus-Pituitary-Adrenal Axis.* 7.1 Edn. Amsterdam: Elsevier Science (2008).
3. Bornstein SR, Engeland WC, Ehrhart-Bornstein M, Herman JP. Dissociation of ACTH and glucocorticoids. *Trends Endocrinol Metab.* (2008) 19:175–80. doi: 10.1016/j.tem.2008.01.009
4. Engeland WC, Shinsako J, Winget CM, Vernikos-Danellis J, Dallman MF. Circadian patterns of stress-induced ACTH secretion are modified by corticosterone responses. *Endocrinology.* (1977) 100:138–47. doi: 10.1210/endo-100-1-138
5. Vazquez DM, Morano MI, Taylor L, Akil H. Kinetics of radiolabeled adrenocorticotropin hormone in infant and weanling rats. *J Neuroendocrinol.* (1997) 9:529–36. doi: 10.1046/j.1365-2826.1997.00608.x
6. Dhillo WS, Kong WM, Le Roux CW, Alaghband-Zadeh J, Jones J, Carter G, et al. Cortisol-binding globulin is important in the interpretation of dynamic tests of the hypothalamic–pituitary–adrenal axis. *Eur J Endocrinol.* (2002) 146:231–5. doi: 10.1530/eje.0.1460231
7. Gardner DS, Fletcher AJ, Fowden AL, Giussani DA. Plasma adrenocorticotropin and cortisol concentrations during acute hypoxemia after a reversible period of adverse intrauterine conditions in the ovine fetus during late gestation. *Endocrinology.* (2001) 142:589–98. doi: 10.1210/endo.142.2.7980
8. Vierhapper H, Nowotny P, Waldhausl W. Production rates of cortisol in obesity. *Obes Res.* (2004) 12:1421–5. doi: 10.1038/oby.2004.178
9. Stewart PM, Boulton A, Kumar S, Clark PM, Shackleton CH. Cortisol metabolism in human obesity: impaired cortisone–>cortisol conversion in subjects with central adiposity. *J Clin Endocrinol Metab.* (1999) 84:1022–7. doi: 10.1210/jc.84.3.1022
10. Andrew R, Phillips DI, Walker BR. Obesity and gender influence cortisol secretion and metabolism in man. *J Clin Endocrinol Metab.* (1998) 83:1806–9. doi: 10.1210/jcem.83.5.4951
11. Phillips DIW, Barker DJP, Fall CHD, Seckl JR, Whorwood CB, Wood PJ, et al. Elevated plasma cortisol concentrations: a link between low birth weight and the insulin resistance syndrome? *J Clin Endocr Metab.* (1998) 83:757–60. doi: 10.1210/jcem.83.3.4634
12. Strain GW, Zumoff B, Kream J, Strain JJ, Levin J, Fukushima D. Sex Difference in the influence of obesity on the 24-hr mean plasma-concentration of cortisol. *Metabolism.* (1982) 31:209–12. doi: 10.1016/0026-0495(82)90054-3
13. Bornstein SR, Chrousos GP. Clinical review 104: Adrenocorticotropin (ACTH)- and non-ACTH-mediated regulation of the adrenal cortex: neural and immune inputs. *J Clin Endocrinol Metab.* (1999) 84:1729–36. doi: 10.1210/jcem.84.5.5631
14. Lamounier-Zepter V, Ehrhart-Bornstein M, Bornstein SR. Metabolic syndrome and the endocrine stress system. *Horm Metab Res.* (2006) 38:437–41. doi: 10.1055/s-2006-947837
15. Klein NA, Andersen RN, Casson PR, Buster JE, Kramer RE. Mechanisms of insulin-inhibition of acth-stimulated steroid-secretion by cultured bovine adrenocortical-cells. *J Steroid Biochem.* (1992) 41:11–20. doi: 10.1016/0960-0760(92)90219-9
16. Andreis PG, Malendowicz LK, Neri G, Tortorella C, Nussdorfer GG. Effects of glucagon and glucagon-like peptide-1 on glucocorticoid secretion of dispersed rat adrenocortical cells. *Life Sci.* (1999) 64:2187–97. doi: 10.1016/S0024-3205(99)00170-8
17. Mazzocchi G, Gottardo L, Aragona F, Albertin G, Nussdorfer GG. Glucagon inhibits ACTH-stimulated cortisol secretion from dispersed human adrenocortical cells by activating unidentified receptors negatively

coupled with the adenylate cyclase cascade. *Horm Metab Res.* (2000) 32:265–8. doi: 10.1055/s-2007-978633

18. Bornstein SR, Uhlmann K, Haidan A, EhrhartBornstein M, Scherbaum WA. Evidence for a novel peripheral action of leptin as a metabolic signal to the adrenal gland - Leptin inhibits cortisol release directly. *Diabetes.* (1997) 46:1235–8. doi: 10.2337/diab.46.7.1235
19. Glasow A, Bornstein SR. Leptin and the adrenal gland. *Eur J Clin Invest.* (2000) 30:39–45. doi: 10.1046/j.1365-2362.2000.0300s3039.x
20. Kinzig KP, D'Alessio DA, Herman JP, Sakai RR, Vahl TP, Figueredo HF, et al. CNS glucagon-like peptide-1 receptors mediate endocrine and anxiety responses to interoceptive and psychogenic stressors. *J Neurosci.* (2003) 23:6163–70. doi: 10.1523/JNEUROSCI.23-15-06163.2003
21. Gil-Lozano M, Perez-Tilve D, Alvarez-Crespo M, Martis A, Fernandez AM, Catalina PAF, et al. GLP-1(7-36)-amide and exendin-4 stimulate the HPA axis in rodents and humans. *Endocrinology.* (2010) 151:2629–40. doi: 10.1210/en.2009-0915
22. Pullen TJ, Huising MO, Rutter GA. Analysis of purified pancreatic islet beta and alpha cell transcriptomes reveals 11beta-hydroxysteroid dehydrogenase (Hsd11b1) as a novel disallowed gene. *Front Genet.* (2017) 8:41. doi: 10.3389/fgene.2017.00041
23. Rebuffescrive M, Bronnegard M, Nilsson A, Eldh J, Gustafsson JA, Bjorntorp P. Steroid-hormone receptors in human adipose tissues. *J Clin Endocr Metab.* (1990) 71:1215–9. doi: 10.1210/jcem-71-5-1215
24. Liu YJ, Nakagawa Y, Ohzeki T. Gene expression of 11 beta-hydroxysteroid dehydrogenase type 1 and type 2 in the kidneys of insulin-dependent diabetic rats. *Hypertension.* (1998) 31:885–9. doi: 10.1161/01.HYP.31.3.885
25. Palermo M, Shackleton CHL, Mantero F, Stewart PM. Urinary free cortisone and the assessment of 11 beta-hydroxysteroid dehydrogenase activity in man. *Clin Endocrinol.* (1996) 45:605–11. doi: 10.1046/j.1365-2265.1996.00853.x
26. Rogers SL, Hughes BA, Jones CA, Freedman L, Smart K, Taylor N, et al. Diminished 11 beta-hydroxysteroid dehydrogenase type 2 activity is associated with decreased weight and weight gain across the first year of life. *J Clin Endocr Metab.* (2014) 99:E821–E31. doi: 10.1210/jc.2013-3254
27. Andrew R, Smith K, Jones GC, Walker BR. Distinguishing the activities of 11 beta-hydroxysteroid dehydrogenases *in vivo* using isotopically labeled cortisol. *J Clin Endocr Metab.* (2002) 87:277–85. doi: 10.1210/jc.87.1.277
28. Livingstone DE, Jones GC, Smith K, Jamieson PM, Andrew R, Kenyon CJ, et al. Understanding the role of glucocorticoids in obesity: tissue-specific alterations of corticosterone metabolism in obese Zucker rats. *Endocrinology.* (2000) 141:560–3. doi: 10.1210/endo.141.2.7297
29. Rask E, Olsson T, Soderberg S, Andrew R, Livingstone DE, Johnson O, et al. Tissue-specific dysregulation of cortisol metabolism in human obesity. *J Clin Endocrinol Metab.* (2001) 86:1418–21. doi: 10.1210/jcem.86.3.7453
30. Stomby A, Andrew R, Walker BR, Olsson T. Tissue-specific dysregulation of cortisol regeneration by 11betaHSD1 in obesity: has it promised too much? *Diabetologia.* (2014) 57:1100–10. doi: 10.1007/s00125-014-3228-6
31. Masuzaki H, Paterson J, Shinyama H, Morton NM, Mullins JJ, Seckl JR, et al. A transgenic model of visceral obesity and the metabolic syndrome. *Science.* (2001) 294:2166–70. doi: 10.1126/science.1066285
32. Paterson JM, Morton NM, Fievet C, Kenyon CJ, Holmes MC, Staels B, et al. Metabolic syndrome without obesity: hepatic overexpression of 11 beta-hydroxysteroid dehydrogenase type 1 in transgenic mice. *Proc Natl Acad Sci USA.* (2004) 101:7088–93. doi: 10.1073/pnas.0305524101
33. Fine NHF, Doig CL, Elhassan YS, Vierra NC, Marchetti P, Bugliani M, et al. Glucocorticoids reprogram beta-cell signaling to preserve insulin secretion. *Diabetes.* (2018) 67:278–90. doi: 10.2337/db16-1356
34. Alberts P, Nilsson C, Selen G, Engblom LOM, Edling NHM, Norling S, et al. Selective inhibition of 11 beta-hydroxysteroid dehydrogenase type 1 improves hepatic insulin sensitivity in hyperglycemic mice strains. *Endocrinology.* (2003) 144:4755–62. doi: 10.1210/en.2003-0344
35. Wang SJY, Birtles S, de Schoolmeester J, Swales J, Moody G, Hislop D, et al. Inhibition of 11 beta-hydroxysteroid dehydrogenase type 1 reduces food intake and weight gain but maintains energy expenditure in diet-induced obese mice. *Diabetologia.* (2006) 49:1333–7. doi: 10.1007/s00125-006-0239-y
36. Liu YJ, Nakagawa Y, Wang Y, Liu LM, Du HW, Wang W, et al. Reduction of hepatic glucocorticoid receptor and hexose-6-phosphate dehydrogenase expression ameliorates diet-induced obesity and insulin resistance in mice. *J Mol Endocrinol.* (2008) 41:53–64. doi: 10.1677/JME-08-0004
37. Kotelevtsev Y, Holmes MC, Burchell A, Houston PM, Schmoll D, Jamieson P, et al. 11 beta-hydroxysteroid dehydrogenase type 1 knockout mice show attenuated glucocorticoid-inducible responses and resist hyperglycemia on obesity or stress. *Proc Natl Acad Sci USA.* (1997) 94:14924–9. doi: 10.1073/pnas.94.26.14924
38. Kalinyak JE, Griffin CA, Hamilton RW, Bradshaw JG, Perlman AJ, Hoffman AR. Developmental and hormonal-regulation of glucocorticoid receptor messenger-RNA in the rat. *J Clin Invest.* (1989) 84:1843–8. doi: 10.1172/JCI114370
39. Evans RM. The steroid and thyroid-hormone receptor superfamily. *Science.* (1988) 240:889–95. doi: 10.1126/science.3283939
40. Oakley RH, Cidlowski JA. The biology of the glucocorticoid receptor: new signaling mechanisms in health and disease. *J Allergy Clin Immunol.* (2013) 132:1033–44. doi: 10.1016/j.jaci.2013.09.007
41. Scheschowitsch K, Leite JA, Assreuy J. New insights in glucocorticoid receptor signaling-more than just a ligand-binding receptor. *Front Endocrinol.* (2017) 8:16. doi: 10.3389/fendo.2017.00016
42. Beato M. Gene-Regulation by Steroid-Hormones. *Cell.* (1989) 56:335–44. doi: 10.1016/0092-8674(89)90237-7
43. van Rossum EFC, Lamberts SWJ. Polymorphisms in the glucocorticoid receptor gene and their associations with metabolic parameters and body composition. *Recent Prog Horm Res.* (2004) 59:333–57. doi: 10.1210/rp.59.1.333
44. Johnstone WM 3rd, Honeycutt JL, Deck CA, Borski RJ. Nongenomic glucocorticoid effects and their mechanisms of action in vertebrates. *Int Rev Cell Mol Biol.* (2019) 346:51-96. doi: 10.1016/bs.ircmb.2019.03.004
45. Borski RJ. Nongenomic membrane actions of glucocorticoids in vertebrates. *Trends Endocrinol Metab.* (2000) 11:427–36. doi: 10.1016/S1043-2760(00)00325-8
46. Song IH, Buttgereit F. Non-genomic glucocorticoid effects to provide the basis for new drug developments. *Mol Cell Endocrinol.* (2006) 246:142–6. doi: 10.1016/j.mce.2005.11.012
47. Moraitis AG, Block T, Nguyen D, Belanoff JK. The role of glucocorticoid receptors in metabolic syndrome and psychiatric illness. *J Steroid Biochem.* (2017) 165:114–20. doi: 10.1016/j.jsbmb.2016.03.023
48. Majer-Lobodzinska A, Adamiec-Mroczek J. Glucocorticoid receptor polymorphism in obesity and glucose homeostasis. *Adv Clin Exp Med.* (2017) 26:143–8. doi: 10.17219/acem/41231
49. Liu YJ, Nakagawa Y, Wang Y, Sakurai R, Tripathi PV, Lutfy K, et al. Increased glucocorticoid receptor and 11 beta-hydroxysteroid dehydrogenase type 1 expression in hepatocytes may contribute to the phenotype of type 2 diabetes in db/db mice. *Diabetes.* (2005) 54:32–40. doi: 10.2337/diabetes.54.1.32
50. Jenson M, Kilroy G, York DA, Braymer D. Abnormal regulation of hepatic glucocorticoid receptor mRNA and receptor protein distribution in the obese Zucker rat. *Obes Res.* (1996) 4:133–43. doi: 10.1002/j.1550-8528.1996.tb00525.x
51. Whorwood CB, Donovan SJ, Flanagan D, Phillips DIW, Byrne CD. Increased glucocorticoid receptor expression in human skeletal muscle cells may contribute to the pathogenesis of the metabolic syndrome. *Diabetes.* (2002) 51:1066–75. doi: 10.2337/diabetes.51.4.1066
52. Watts LM, Manchem VP, Leedom TA, Rivard AL, McKay RA, Bao DJ, et al. Reduction of hepatic and adipose tissue glucocorticoid receptor expression with antisense oligonucleotides improves hyperglycemia and hyperlipidemia in diabetic rodents without causing systemic glucocorticoid antagonism. *Diabetes.* (2005) 54:1846–53. doi: 10.2337/diabetes.54.6.1846
53. Opherk C, Tronche F, Kellendonk C, Kohlmuller D, Schulze A, Schmid W, et al. Inactivation of the glucocorticoid receptor in hepatocytes leads to fasting hypoglycemia and ameliorates hyperglycemia in streptozotocin-induced diabetes mellitus. *Mol Endocrinol.* (2004) 18:1346–53. doi: 10.1210/me.2003-0283
54. John K, Marino JS, Sanchez ER, Hinds TD, Jr. The glucocorticoid receptor: cause of or cure for obesity? *Am J Physiol Endocrinol Metab.* (2016) 310:E249–57. doi: 10.1152/ajpendo.00478.2015
55. Andrew R, Gale CR, Walker BR, Seckl JR, Martyn CN. Glucocorticoid metabolism and the metabolic syndrome: associations in an elderly cohort. *Exp Clin Endocr Diab.* (2002) 110:284–90. doi: 10.1055/s-2002-34591
56. Argaud D, Zhang Q, Pan WS, Maitra S, Pilkis SJ, Lange AJ. Regulation of rat liver glucose-6-phosphatase gene expression in different nutritional and

hormonal states—Gene structure and 5'-flanking sequence. *Diabetes*. (1996) 45:1563–71. doi: 10.2337/diab.45.11.1563
57. Berdanier CD. Role of glucocorticoids in the regulation of lipogenesis. *FASEB J*. (1989) 3:2179–83. doi: 10.1096/fasebj.3.10.2666232
58. Xu C, He J, Jiang H, Zu L, Zhai W, Pu S, et al. Direct effect of glucocorticoids on lipolysis in adipocytes. *Mol Endocrinol*. (2009) 23:1161–70. doi: 10.1210/me.2008-0464
59. Samuel VT, Petersen KF, Shulman GI. Lipid-induced insulin resistance: unravelling the mechanism. *Lancet*. (2010) 375:2267–77. doi: 10.1016/S0140-6736(10)60408-4
60. Petersen KF, Shulman GI. Etiology of insulin resistance. *Am J Med*. (2006) 119(5 Suppl 1):S10–6. doi: 10.1016/j.amjmed.2006.01.009
61. Dourakis SP, Sevastianos VA, Kaliopi P. Acute severe steatohepatitis related to prednisolone therapy. *Am J Gastroenterol*. (2002) 97:1074–5. doi: 10.1111/j.1572-0241.2002.05644.x
62. Dimitriadis G, Leighton B, ParryBillings M, Sasson S, Young M, Krause U, et al. Effects of glucocorticoid excess on the sensitivity of glucose transport and metabolism to insulin in rat skeletal muscle. *Biochem J*. (1997) 321:707–12. doi: 10.1042/bj3210707
63. Hauner H, Entenmann G, Wabitsch M, Gaillard D, Ailhaud G, Negrel R, et al. Promoting effect of glucocorticoids on the differentiation of human adipocyte precursor cells cultured in a chemically defined medium. *J Clin Invest*. (1989) 84:1663–70. doi: 10.1172/JCI114345
64. Hauner H, Schmid P, Pfeiffer EF. Glucocorticoids and insulin promote the differentiation of human adipocyte precursor cells into fat-cells. *J Clin Endocr Metab*. (1987) 64:832–5. doi: 10.1210/jcem-64-4-832
65. Gathercole LL, Morgan SA, Bujalska IJ, Hauton D, Stewart PM, Tomlinson JW. Regulation of lipogenesis by glucocorticoids and insulin in human adipose tissue. *PLoS ONE*. (2011) 6:e26223. doi: 10.1371/journal.pone.0026223
66. Delaunay F, Khan A, Cintra A, Davani B, Ling ZC, Andersson A, et al. Pancreatic beta cells are important targets for the diabetogenic effects of glucocorticoids. *J Clin Invest*. (1997) 100:2094–8. doi: 10.1172/JCI119743
67. Gremlich S, Roduit R, Thorens B. Dexamethasone induces posttranslational degradation of GLUT2 and inhibition of insulin secretion in isolated pancreatic beta cells - Comparison with the effects of fatty acids. *J Biol Chem*. (1997) 272:3216–22. doi: 10.1074/jbc.272.6.3216
68. Lambillotte C, Gilon P, Henquin JC. Direct glucocorticoid inhibition of insulin secretion - An *in vitro* study of dexamethasone effects in mouse islets. *J Clin Invest*. (1997) 99:414–23. doi: 10.1172/JCI119175
69. Swali A, Walker EA, Lavery GG, Tomlinson JW, Stewart PM. 11 beta-hydroxysteroid dehydrogenase type 1 regulates insulin and glucagon secretion in pancreatic islets. *Diabetologia*. (2008) 51:2003–11. doi: 10.1007/s00125-008-1137-2
70. Ortsater H, Alberts P, Warpman U, Engblom LOM, Abrahmsen L, Bergsten P. Regulation of 11 beta-hydroxysteroid dehydrogenase type 1 and glucose-stimulated insulin secretion in pancreatic islets of Langerhans. *Diabetes-Metab Res*. (2005) 21:359–66. doi: 10.1002/dmrr.525
71. Gesina E, Tronche F, Herrera P, Duchene B, Tales W, Czernichow P, et al. Dissecting the role of glucocorticoids on pancreas development. *Diabetes*. (2004) 53:2322–9. doi: 10.2337/diabetes.53.9.2322
72. Shen CN, Seckl JR, Slack JMW, Tosh D. Glucocorticoids suppress beta-cell development and induce hepatic metaplasia in embryonic pancreas. *Biochem J*. (2003) 375:41–50. doi: 10.1042/bj20030140
73. Rafacho A, Marroqui L, Taboga SR, Abrantes JLF, Silveira LR, Boschero AC, et al. Glucocorticoids *in vivo* induce both insulin hypersecretion and enhanced glucose sensitivity of stimulus-secretion coupling in isolated rat islets. *Endocrinology*. (2010) 151:85–95. doi: 10.1210/en.2009-0704
74. Turban S, Liu XX, Ramage L, Webster SP, Walker BR, Dunbar DR, et al. Optimal elevation of beta-cell 11 beta-hydroxysteroid dehydrogenase type 1 is a compensatory mechanism that prevents high-fat diet induced beta-cell failure. *Diabetes*. (2012) 61:642–52. doi: 10.2337/db11-1054
75. Fine NHF, Doig CL, Elhassan Y, Marchetti P, Bugliani M, Piemonti L, et al. Glucocorticoids re-programme the beta cell signalling cassette to preserve functional identity and insulin secretion. *Diabetologia*. (2017) 60:S83.
76. Tomlinson JW, Moore JS, Clark PM, Holder G, Shakespeare L, Stewart PM. Weight loss increases 11beta-hydroxysteroid dehydrogenase type 1 expression in human adipose tissue. *J Clin Endocrinol Metab*. (2004) 89:2711–6. doi: 10.1210/jc.2003-031376
77. Tomlinson JW, Finney J, Hughes BA, Hughes SV, Stewart PM. Reduced glucocorticoid production rate, decreased 5 alpha-reductase activity, and adipose tissue insulin sensitization after weight loss. *Diabetes*. (2008) 57:1536–43. doi: 10.2337/db08-0094
78. Purnell JQ, Kahn SE, Samuels MH, Brandon D, Loriaux DL, Brunzell JD. Enhanced cortisol production rates, free cortisol, and 11beta-HSD-1 expression correlate with visceral fat and insulin resistance in men: effect of weight loss. *Am J Physiol Endocrinol Metab*. (2009) 296:E351–7. doi: 10.1152/ajpendo.90769.2008
79. Johnstone AM, Faber P, Andrew R, Gibney ER, Elia M, Lobley G, et al. Influence of short-term dietary weight loss on cortisol secretion and metabolism in obese men. *Eur J Endocrinol*. (2004) 150:185–94. doi: 10.1530/eje.0.1500185
80. Stomby A, Simonyte K, Mellberg C, Ryberg M, Stimson RH, Larsson C, et al. Diet-induced weight loss has chronic tissue-specific effects on glucocorticoid metabolism in overweight postmenopausal women. *Int J Obes*. (2015) 39:814–9. doi: 10.1038/ijo.2014.188
81. Engeli S, Bohnke J, Feldpausch M, Gorzelniak K, Heintze U, Janke J, et al. Regulation of 11beta-HSD genes in human adipose tissue: influence of central obesity and weight loss. *Obes Res*. (2004) 12:9–17. doi: 10.1038/oby.2004.3
82. Basu R, Singh R, Basu A, Johnson CM, Rizza RA. Effect of nutrient ingestion on total-body and splanchnic cortisol production in humans. *Diabetes*. (2006) 55:667–74. doi: 10.2337/diabetes.55.03.06.db05-1335
83. Wake DJ, Homer NZ, Andrew R, Walker BR. Acute *in vivo* regulation of 11beta-hydroxysteroid dehydrogenase type 1 activity by insulin and intralipid infusions in humans. *J Clin Endocrinol Metab*. (2006) 91:4682–8. doi: 10.1210/jc.2006-0819
84. Stimson RH, Johnstone AM, Homer NZ, Wake DJ, Morton NM, Andrew R, et al. Dietary macronutrient content alters cortisol metabolism independently of body weight changes in obese men. *J Clin Endocrinol Metab*. (2007) 92:4480–4. doi: 10.1210/jc.2007-0692
85. Stimson RH, Lobley GE, Maraki I, Morton NM, Andrew R, Walker BR. Effects of proportions of dietary macronutrients on glucocorticoid metabolism in diet-induced obesity in rats. *PLoS ONE*. (2010) 5:e8779. doi: 10.1371/journal.pone.0008779
86. Campbell JE, Rakhshani N, Fediuc S, Bruni S, Riddell MC. Voluntary wheel running initially increases adrenal sensitivity to adrenocorticotrophic hormone, which is attenuated with long-term training. *J Appl Physiol*. (1985). (2009) 106:66–72. doi: 10.1152/japplphysiol.91128.2008
87. Coutinho AE, Campbell JE, Fediuc S, Riddell MC. Effect of voluntary exercise on peripheral tissue glucocorticoid receptor content and the expression and activity of 11 beta-HSD1 in the Syrian hamster. *J Appl Physiol*. (2006) 100:1483–8. doi: 10.1152/japplphysiol.01236.2005
88. Chennaoui M, Gomez Merino D, Lesage J, Drogou C, Guezennec CY. Effects of moderate and intensive training on the hypothalamo-pituitary-adrenal axis in rats. *Acta Physiol Scand*. (2002) 175:113–21. doi: 10.1046/j.1365-201X.2002.00971.x
89. Moraska A, Deak T, Spencer RL, Roth D, Fleshner M. Treadmill running produces both positive and negative physiological adaptations in Sprague-Dawley rats. *Am J Physiol-Reg I*. (2000) 279:R1321–R9. doi: 10.1152/ajpregu.2000.279.4.R1321
90. Dishman RK, Bunnell BN, Youngstedt SD, Yoo HS, Mougey EH, Meyerhoff JL. Activity wheel running blunts increased plasma adrenocorticotrophin (ACTH) after footshock and cage-switch stress. *Physiol Behav*. (1998) 63:911–7. doi: 10.1016/S0031-9384(98)00017-1
91. Fichna M, Fichna P. Glucocorticoids and beta-cell function. *Endokrynol Pol*. (2017) 68:568–73. doi: 10.5603/EP.2017.0060
92. Tanner CJ, Koves TR, Cortright RL, Pories WJ, Kim YB, Kahn BB, et al. Effect of short-term exercise training on insulin-stimulated PI 3-kinase activity in middle-aged men. *Am J Physiol Endocrinol Metab*. (2002) 282:E147–53. doi: 10.1152/ajpendo.2002.282.1.E147
93. Luciano E, Carneiro EM, Carvalho CRO, Carvalheira JBC, Peres SB, Reis MAB, et al. Endurance training improves responsiveness to insulin and modulates insulin signal transduction through the

phosphatidylinositol 3-kinase/Akt-1 pathway. *Eur J Endocrinol.* (2002) 147:149–57. doi: 10.1530/eje.0.1470149

94. Krug ALO, Macedo AG, Zago AS, Rush JWE, Santos CF, Amaral SL. High-intensity resistance training attenuates dexamethasone-induced muscle atrophy. *Muscle Nerve.* (2016) 53:779–88. doi: 10.1002/mus.24906
95. Barel M, Perez OAB, Giozzet VA, Rafacho A, Bosqueiro JR, do Amaral SL. Exercise training prevents hyperinsulinemia, muscular glycogen loss and muscle atrophy induced by dexamethasone treatment. *Eur J Appl Physiol.* (2010) 108:999–1007. doi: 10.1007/s00421-009-1272-6
96. Hickson RC, Davis JR. Partial Prevention of Glucocorticoid-Induced Muscle Atrophy by Endurance Training. *Am J Physiol.* (1981) 241:E226–E32. doi: 10.1152/ajpendo.1981.241.3.E226
97. Holten MK, Zacho M, Gaster M, Juel C, Wojtaszewski JFP, Dela F. Strength training increases insulin-mediated glucose uptake, GLUT4 content, and insulin signaling in skeletal muscle in patients with type 2 diabetes. *Diabetes.* (2004) 53:294–305. doi: 10.2337/diabetes.53.2.294
98. Wester VL, Lamberts SW, van Rossum EF. Advances in the assessment of cortisol exposure and sensitivity. *Curr Opin Endocrinol Diabetes Obes.* (2014) 21:306–11. doi: 10.1097/MED.0000000000000077
99. Russell E, Kirschbaum C, Laudenslager ML, Stalder T, de Rijke Y, van Rossum EFC, et al. Toward standardization of hair cortisol measurement: results of the first international interlaboratory round robin. *Ther Drug Monit.* (2015) 37:71–5. doi: 10.1097/FTD.0000000000000148
100. Wester VL, Staufenbiel SM, Veldhorst MAB, Visser JA, Manenschijn L, Koper JW, et al. Long-term cortisol levels measured in scalp hair of obese patients. *Obesity.* (2014) 22:1956–8. doi: 10.1002/oby.20795
101. Jackson SE, Kirschbaum C, Steptoe A. Hair cortisol and adiposity in a population-based sample of 2,527 men and women aged 54 to 87 years. *Obesity.* (2017) 25:539–44. doi: 10.1002/oby.21733
102. Sauve B, Koren G, Walsh G, Tokmakejian S, Van Uum SHM. Measurement of cortisol in human hair as a biomarker of systemic exposure. *Clin Invest Med.* (2007) 30:E183–E91. doi: 10.25011/cim.v30i5.2894
103. Cummings DE. Endocrine mechanisms mediating remission of diabetes after gastric bypass surgery. *Int J Obes.* (2009) 33(Suppl 1):S33–40. doi: 10.1038/ijo.2009.15
104. Rubino F, Forgione A, Cummings DE, Vix M, Gnuli D, Mingrone G, et al. The mechanism of diabetes control after gastrointestinal bypass surgery reveals a role of the proximal small intestine in the pathophysiology of type 2 diabetes. *Ann Surg.* (2006) 244:741–9. doi: 10.1097/01.sla.0000224726.61448.1b
105. Woods CP, Corrigan M, Gathercole L, Taylor A, Hughes B, Gaoatswe G, et al. Tissue specific regulation of glucocorticoids in severe obesity and the response to significant weight loss following bariatric surgery (BARICORT). *J Clin Endocr Metab.* (2015) 100:1434–44. doi: 10.1210/jc.2014-4120
106. Simonyte K, Olsson T, Naslund I, Angelhed JE, Lonn L, Mattsson C, et al. Weight loss after gastric bypass surgery in women is followed by a metabolically favorable decrease in 11 beta-hydroxysteroid dehydrogenase 1 expression in subcutaneous adipose tissue. *J Clin Endocr Metab.* (2010) 95:3527–31. doi: 10.1210/jc.2009-2472
107. Rask E, Simonyte K, Lonn L, Axelson M. Cortisol metabolism after weight loss: associations with 11 beta-HSD type 1 and markers of obesity in women. *Clin Endocrinol.* (2013) 78:700–5. doi: 10.1111/j.1365-2265.2012.04333.x
108. Methlie P, Dankel S, Myhra T, Christensen B, Gjerde J, Fadnes D, et al. Changes in adipose glucocorticoid metabolism before and after bariatric surgery assessed by direct hormone measurements. *Obesity.* (2013) 21:2495–503. doi: 10.1002/oby.20449
109. Diamant S, Shafrir E. Modulation of activity of insulin-dependent enzymes of lipogenesis by glucocorticoids. *Eur J Biochem.* (1975) 53:541–6. doi: 10.1111/j.1432-1033.1975.tb04097.x

5

Eligibility and Awareness Regarding Metabolic Surgery in Patients with Type 2 Diabetes Mellitus in the Real-World Clinical Setting: Estimate of Possible Diabetes Remission

Chrysi Koliaki [1†], Evangelia Tzeravini [1†], Eleftheria Papachristoforou [1], Ioanna Severi [1], Elina El Deik [2], Melina Karaolia [1], Marina Noutsou [2], Anastasia Thanopoulou [2], Aikaterini Kountouri [3], Konstantinos Balampanis [3], Vaia Lambadiari [3], Nicholas Tentolouris [1] and Alexander Kokkinos [1]*

[1] First Department of Propaedeutic Internal Medicine and Diabetes Center, Medical School, National and Kapodistrian University of Athens, Laiko General Hospital, Athens, Greece, [2] Diabetes Center, Second Department of Internal Medicine, Medical School, Hippokratio General Hospital, National and Kapodistrian University of Athens, Athens, Greece, [3] Second Department of Internal Medicine and Research Institute, Medical School, National and Kapodistrian University of Athens, Attikon General Hospital, Athens, Greece

***Correspondence:**
Alexander Kokkinos
akokkinos@med.uoa.gr

[†] These authors have contributed equally to this work

Despite high-quality evidence highlighting metabolic surgery as an effective treatment option for type 2 diabetes mellitus (T2DM), the number of patients receiving bariatric surgery (BS) remains low. Since the introduction of the Diabetes Surgery Summit II (DSS-II) eligibility criteria, data on eligibility rates for BS in T2DM cohorts remain scarce. The aims of the present study were to examine in a real-world clinical setting: (i) what is the percentage of T2DM patients visiting diabetes outpatient clinics who meet the DSS-II eligibility criteria, (ii) how many of these have been informed about the option of BS, and (iii) what are the characteristics associated with eligibility and awareness of BS. Demographic, anthropometric, clinical and socioeconomic data were obtained for all patients with T2DM who were consecutively examined in the outpatient clinics of three large-volume university hospitals (n = 1167). A medical registry form was completed to screen for BS eligibility. Patients were considered eligible if the recommendation by DSS-II criteria was either to "consider" or "recommend" BS. Eligible patients were further inquired whether they had ever been informed about the option of BS by their physicians. The advanced DiaRem score (ADRS) was applied to eligible patients to assess their probability of achieving postoperative T2DM remission. A significant percentage of T2DM patients who are routinely assessed in outpatient clinics meet the DSS-II eligibility criteria (15.3%). Eligible patients are younger and more obese, have a shorter T2DM duration, worse glycaemic control and better renal function, compared to non-eligible ones. Among eligible patients, only 39.3% have been medically informed about the option of BS. Informed patients are younger and more severely obese than non-informed ones. A significant percentage of non-informed patients (35%) have an ADRS $\leq$10, indicating a considerable probability for T2DM remission after BS, and are thus deprived of this opportunity due to lack of appropriate medical counseling. Screening and awareness of BS remain an unmet need in current T2DM management. Future research should focus on intensifying screening for BS eligibility at every medical visit and promoting evidence-based clinical recommendations for patients expected to benefit the most.

Keywords: bariatric surgery, metabolic surgery, eligibility criteria, type 2 diabetes mellitus, obesity, diabetes surgery summit

INTRODUCTION

A large number of randomized clinical trials and high-quality prospective matched cohort studies over the past years have demonstrated the potential of bariatric or alternatively metabolic surgery to induce sustainable weight loss and provide substantial metabolic benefits in patients with obesity and type 2 diabetes mellitus (T2DM) (1–8). In the short and medium term, a significant amount of weight is lost, T2DM may completely regress, and cardiometabolic risk factors are dramatically improved. In the long term, bariatric surgery (BS) may achieve durable weight loss, prevent T2DM and cancer, mitigate life-threatening T2DM-related complications, improve overall glycaemic control minimizing the need for glucose-lowering medications, and reduce total and T2DM-related mortality (9, 10). Despite the wealth of evidence in the field of metabolic surgery and the magnitude of anticipated benefits, the number of patients receiving BS as T2DM treatment remains low. One possible reason for this low penetration of BS into diabetes care may be the failure of physicians to systematically screen for eligibility criteria and communicate efficiently the benefits of BS for appropriately selected patients (11).

Until recently, the most commonly applied eligibility criteria for BS were those established by the National Institutes of Health (NIH) in 1992 (12). Based on these criteria, eligible for BS are patients with morbid obesity, i.e., a body mass index (BMI) $\geq$40 kg/m^2 regardless of their health status, and patients with a BMI between 35 and 40 with at least one severe obesity-related comorbidity such as T2DM, cardiovascular risk factors or non-alcoholic fatty liver disease (NAFLD). Patients with a BMI <35 or 35–40 without clinically relevant comorbidities are considered non-eligible according to NIH criteria. More than two decades later, the International Federation for the Surgery of Obesity and Metabolic Disorders (IFSO) shifted the focus of eligibility away from BMI, and recommended that BS should be further indicated for patients with a BMI >30 and comorbidities such as recent onset T2DM (13, 14). According to the IFSO, any indication for BS should consider metabolic comorbidities (T2DM), psychiatric symptoms, quality of life and functional limitations related to obesity. The terms bariatric or metabolic surgery should be thus replaced by the term "surgery for obesity and weight-related diseases" to capture the fact that these surgeries can improve and even cure obesity and weight-related conditions (13). In the same direction, in a position statement released in 2018, the American Society for Metabolic and Bariatric Surgery (ASMBS) revised its 2012 recommendations and urged the consideration of BS for individuals with a BMI between 30 and 35 (15). In June 2016, a number of leading international diabetes organizations focused on T2DM and issued new guidelines for the treatment of patients with obesity and T2DM, integrating BS into the proposed T2DM treatment algorithm. These guidelines were developed during the second Diabetes Surgery Summit (DSS-II), an international consensus conference, and were endorsed by numerous scientific societies all around the world (16). According to these guidelines, BS should be recommended to treat T2DM in patients with a BMI $\geq$40 kg/m^2 (grade III obesity), regardless of their level of glycaemic control or complexity of glucose-lowering regimens, and also in patients with a BMI 35–39.9 kg/m^2 (grade II obesity), if hyperglycemia cannot be controlled despite optimal lifestyle and medical treatment. BS should be further considered as an option to treat T2DM in patients with a BMI 30–34.9 kg/m^2 (grade I obesity), if adequate glycaemic control cannot be achieved despite maximally intensified antidiabetic treatment, including injectable agents (16). Beyond BMI and glycaemic control criteria as determined by the DSS-II, eligibility for BS further requires the absence of serious life-threatening health conditions such as irreversible cardiopulmonary or other end-organ failure, metastatic or inoperable malignancy, active drug or alcohol abuse, and severe untreated psychiatric illness (17).

Since the introduction of the DSS-II criteria, data on eligibility rates for BS in T2DM cohorts are scarce. The aims of the present study were to examine in a real-world clinical setting: (i) what is the percentage of patients with T2DM visiting diabetes outpatient clinics of large university hospitals who meet the BS eligibility criteria proposed by DSS-II, (ii) how many of the eligible patients have been informed by their physicians about the option of BS, and (iii) what are the demographic, anthropometric and clinical characteristics associated with eligibility and awareness of BS among T2DM patients. We further assessed the possibility of T2DM remission in eligible patients using a recently proposed scoring system.

MATERIALS AND METHODS

Study Population and Design

We performed an observational cross-sectional study in a large number of patients with T2DM who were consecutively examined in the diabetes outpatient clinics of three large-volume university hospitals within the time period 03/2019-12/2019 (*n* = 1167). The academic hospitals participating in this study were Laiko, Hippokrateio and Attikon General Hospital of Athens (Department of Internal Medicine and Diabetes Center), all three representing certified centers of excellence for diabetes research and clinical practice. Detailed demographic, anthropometric, clinical and socioeconomic data were obtained for all patients. These data included age, gender, BMI calculated as body weight in kg divided by height in meters squared (kg/m^2), known duration of T2DM, current glycosylated hemoglobin (HbA1c) as a marker of glycaemic control, recent laboratory tests (within the last month) including serum creatinine to estimate glomerular filtration rate (GFR) based on the MDRD (Modification of Diet in Renal Disease) equation (18), current antidiabetic treatment with information on dose and frequency of glucose-lowering agents, T2DM-related comorbidities and complications, detailed drug history beyond antidiabetic treatment, presence of advanced heart failure defined as stages III and IV of the New York Heart Association (NYHA) staging system, presence of advanced renal disease using the GFR threshold of <30 ml/min, presence of advanced liver disease and alcohol abuse, history of malignancies and serious mental or psychiatric disorders requiring treatment.

All data were obtained by means of a structured registry form which was specifically designed to screen for BS eligibility. T2DM patients were considered eligible if the recommendation by DSS-II criteria was either to "consider" or "recommend" BS (based on BMI and glycaemic control). Optimal medical treatment for each patient was defined by experienced diabetologists in accordance with the updated evidence-based American Diabetes Association (ADA) clinical guidelines for T2DM pharmacologic treatment (19). Patients with age-related (>65 years old), health-related (advanced heart, liver, kidney disease, malignancy, uncontrolled mental/psychiatric disorder, eating disorders, alcohol abuse) or other socioeconomic reasons precluding surgery (lack of supporting environment, low level of education, severely impaired cognitive capacity) were considered to be non-eligible. The advanced Diabetes Remission score (Ad DiaRem), comprising pre-operative clinical variables such as age, HbA1c, insulin treatment, number of glucose-lowering agents and T2DM duration, was applied to all eligible patients to assess their probability of achieving T2DM remission after BS (20). For T2DM patients with an Ad DiaRem score of 0-5, 6-10, 11-15, 16-20, and >20, the probability of experiencing T2DM remission within the first 5 years after Roux-en-Y Gastric Bypass (RYGB) is estimated to be 100, 74.1, 28.6, 18.5, and 0%, respectively (21). The eligible patients were further inquired whether they had ever been informed about the option of BS as a treatment modality for their T2DM by their physicians in the diabetes outpatient clinics.

Before enrollment, all participants were thoroughly informed about the rationale and the aims of the study and gave written informed consent to the study protocol, which was approved by the Ethics Committees of all three participating hospitals, and conducted according to the World Medical Association's Declaration of Helsinki (amended in 2013). No patient refused to participate, so the drop-out rate was 0%.

Statistical Analysis

Descriptive statistics were applied to present the demographic, anthropometric, and clinical characteristics of the study population. For continuous quantitative variables, data are presented as mean ± SD. For non-continuous quantitative variables such as T2DM duration and Ad DiaRem score, data are presented as median values plus interquartile range [25th-75th percentile]. For categorical variables, data are presented as absolute (n) and relative (%) frequencies. Comparisons between groups were performed with the non-parametric Mann-Whitney-Wilcoxon test for independent samples for continuous, and the Pearson's chi-square test for categorical variables. The level of statistical significance was set at 0.05, as appropriate. Statistical analysis was performed with the SPSS software package version 20.0 (Chicago, IL, USA).

TABLE 1 | Demographic, anthropometric and clinical characteristics of the study population.

Descriptive characteristics	*N* = 1167 patients with T2DM
Age (years)	65 ± 11
Female gender, *n* (%)	476 (40.8)
BMI (kg/m^2)	31.3 ± 6.5
Obesity, *n* (%)	611 (52.4)
• Grade I, *n* (%)	345 (56.5)
• Grade II, *n* (%)	149 (24.4)
• Grade III, *n* (%)	117 (19.2)
Estimated GFR (ml/min)	79.7 ± 23.2
HbA1c (%)	7.0 ± 1.4
Known T2DM duration (years)	11 [5-18]
Antidiabetic treatment	
• Oral glucose-lowering medications, *n* (%)	671 (57.5)
• Treatment with insulin, *n* (%)	473 (40.5)
• Treatment with metformin, *n* (%)	990 (84.8)
• Treatment with sulfonylureas, *n* (%)	99 (8.5)
• Treatment with GLP-1RAs, *n* (%)	236 (20.2)
• Treatment with DPP-4 inhibitors, *n* (%)	417 (35.7)
• Treatment with SGLT2 inhibitors, *n* (%)	194 (16.6)
History of CHD, *n* (%)	265 (22.7)
Hypertension, *n* (%)	837 (71.7)
Dyslipidemia, *n* (%)	964 (82.6)
Heart failure NYHA III/IV, *n* (%)	33 (2.8)
Eligibility for BS by DSS-II, *n* (%)	**179 (15.3)**
Eligibility for BS among obese patients, *n* (%)	**179 (29.1)**

For quantitative variables, data are presented as mean ± SD. For categorical variables, data are presented as absolute (n) and relative (%) frequencies. Data for known duration of T2DM are presented as median value plus interquartile range [25th-75th percentile]. Hypertension and dyslipidemia were defined based on the need for anti-hypertensive and hypolipidemic drug treatment, respectively. BMI, Body Mass Index; BS, bariatric surgery; CHD, coronary heart disease; DPP-4, dipeptidyl-peptidase 4; DSS-II, Diabetes Surgery Summit II; GFR, glomerular filtration rate; GLP-1RAs, glucagon-like peptide 1 receptor agonists; HbA1c, glycosylated hemoglobin 1c; NYHA, New York Heart Association; SGLT2, sodium-glucose cotransporter 2; T2DM, type 2 diabetes mellitus.

RESULTS

Table 1 summarizes the major demographic, anthropometric and clinical characteristics of the study population. The mean age of the study participants was 65 ± 11 years. Nearly half of the studied patients (51.4%) had an advanced age, exceeding 65 years. Female patients represented 40.8% of the study population. More than half of T2DM patients in our cohort had obesity.

TABLE 2 | Comparison of demographic and clinical characteristics between eligible (E) and non-eligible (NE) diabetic patients for metabolic surgery according to DSS-II eligibility criteria.

Characteristics	Eligible patients (E) (n = 179)	Non-eligible patients (NE) (n = 988)	p-value (E vs. NE)
Age (years)	**54 ± 8**	**67 ± 10**	**<0.001**
Female sex (%)	47.5	39.8	0.055
BMI (kg/m²)	**39.5 ± 6.3**	**29.8 ± 5.3**	**<0.001**
Estimated GFR (ml/min)	**87 ± 24**	**78 ± 23**	**<0.001**
HbA1c (%)	**7.7 ± 1.8**	**6.9 ± 1.2**	**<0.001**
T2DM duration (years)	**8 [2-15]**	**12 [5-18]**	**<0.001**
Insulin treatment (%)	**48**	**39.3**	**0.03**
History of CHD (%)	20.6	23.1	0.5
Hypertension (%)	70.5	72.1	0.8
Dyslipidemia (%)	77.8	83.7	0.056
Advanced heart failure (%)	**0**	**3.2**	**0.016**
Advanced kidney disease (%)	**0**	**2.7**	**0.029**
Psychotic disorder under treatment (%)	**0**	**6.4**	**0.001**
Alcohol abuse (%)	1.1	1.3	0.9
For eligible patients only			
Informed about the option of BS (%)	39.3	NA	
Advanced DiaRem score	12 [9-18]	NA	
• Advanced DiaRem score 0-5 (%)	7.6	NA	
• Advanced DiaRem score 6-10 (%)	32.8	NA	
• Advanced DiaRem score >10 (%)	59.6	NA	

For continuous quantitative variables, data are presented as mean ± SD. For categorical variables, data are presented as relative frequencies (%). For non-continuous quantitative variables such as T2DM duration and advanced DiaRem score, data are presented as median values plus interquartile range [25th-75th percentile]. Comparisons between groups were performed with non-parametric Mann-Whitney test for independent samples. Statistically significant differences are denoted with bold font.
Advanced DiaRem score 0-5 indicates a probability of 100% for achieving T2DM remission within the next 5 years following RYGB.
Advanced DiaRem score 6-10 indicates a probability of 74.1% for achieving T2DM remission within the next 5 years after RYGB.
Advanced DiaRem score >10 indicates a probability of only 23% for achieving T2DM remission within the next 5 years after RYGB.
NA, not applicable; BMI, Body Mass Index; BS, bariatric surgery; CHD, coronary heart disease; Diarem score, diabetes remission score; DSS-II, Diabetes Surgery Summit II; GFR, glomerular filtration rate; HbA1c, glycosylated hemoglobin 1c; RYGB, Roux-en-Y gastric bypass; T2DM, type 2 diabetes mellitus.

Among obese patients, the majority had grade I obesity (BMI 30–34.9 kg/m^2), almost a fourth had grade II obesity (BMI 35–39.9 kg/m^2), and a fifth had morbid or grade III obesity (BMI ≥40 kg/m^2). With respect to antidiabetic treatment, 57.5% of patients received only oral glucose-lowering agents, and 40.5% were treated with insulin (prandial, basal or mixture). The median duration of T2DM in our cohort was 11 years, while the mean HbA1c of the enrolled patients was 7.0 ± 1.4%, reflecting a relatively short T2DM duration and adequate glycaemic control. Regarding T2DM-related comorbidities, a significant number of patients reported hypertension and dyslipidemia, and a considerable number of patients reported a history of coronary heart disease (CHD). The prevalence of advanced heart failure (NYHA III/IV) in our cohort was 2.8%. The eligibility rate for BS according to DSS-II criteria was 15.3% in the total study population (n = 179 eligible patients), whereas the eligibility rate within the subgroup of T2DM patients with obesity was 29.1%.

Comparison Between Eligible and Non-eligible Patients

Compared to non-eligible patients (NE), the eligible patients of our cohort (E) were more than a decade younger, significantly more obese by nearly 10 kg/m^2, displayed worse glycaemic control as reflected by a higher HbA1c, better renal function, and had a shorter self-reported T2DM duration (8 vs. 12 years, p < 0.001). There was a marginally significant trend for a predominance of the female gender in eligible patients (p = 0.055). Furthermore, eligible patients were more frequently insulin-treated, possibly due to their poorer metabolic control (p = 0.03), and had a significantly lower prevalence of advanced heart failure, end-stage renal disease and mental or psychiatric disorders compared to NE patients (p < 0.05 for all). Among the eligible patients, 7.6% had an Ad DiaRem score 0-5, indicating a probability of 100% for achieving T2DM remission within the next 5 years following RYGB, 32.8% had a score 6-10, suggesting a probability of 74.1% for achieving T2DM remission, and 59.7% had a score >10, corresponding to a probability of only 23% for achieving T2DM remission after BS. Within the group of eligible patients, 39.3% declared that they had been previously informed by their physicians about the treatment option of BS.

Table 2 presents the comparison of major demographic and clinical characteristics between E and NE diabetic patients for BS according to the DSS-II eligibility criteria.

TABLE 3 | Comparison of characteristics between informed (I) and non-informed (NI) eligible diabetic patients for metabolic surgery.

Characteristics	Informed patients (I) (n = 68)	Non-informed patients (NI) (n = 111)	p-value (I vs. NI)
Age (years)	**51 ± 10**	**56 ± 7**	**<0.001**
Female sex (%)	44.1	49.5	0.49
BMI (kg/m²)	**43.1 ± 7.3**	**37.1 ± 4.3**	**<0.001**
Estimated GFR (ml/min)	91 ± 26	85 ± 23	0.16
HbA1c (%)	7.5 ± 1.7	7.9 ± 1.9	0.17
T2DM duration (years)	**4 [1-14]**	**9 [5-16]**	**0.009**
Advanced DiaRem score	**10 [7-15]**	**14 [10-18]**	**0.016**
Advanced DiaRem score ≤10 (%)	**54.3**	**34.6**	**0.047**

For continuous quantitative variables, data are presented as mean ± SD. For categorical variables, data are presented as relative frequencies (%). For non-continuous quantitative variables such as T2DM duration and Advanced DiaRem score, data are presented as median values plus interquartile range [25th-75th percentile]. Comparisons between groups were performed with non-parametric Mann-Whitney test for independent samples. Statistically significant differences are denoted with bold font.
Advanced DiaRem score ≤10 indicates a probability of up to 74.1% for achieving T2DM remission within the next 5 years following bariatric surgery.
BMI, Body Mass Index; DiaRem score, diabetes remission score; GFR, glomerular filtration rate; HbA1c, glycosylated hemoglobin 1c; T2DM, type 2 diabetes mellitus.

Comparison Between Informed and Non-informed Patients

Eligible patients who had been informed about the option of BS (I) were significantly younger ($p < 0.001$), more obese ($p < 0.001$) and reported a shorter T2DM duration ($p = 0.009$), compared to eligible patients who had never been medically informed about BS (NI), as summarized in **Table 3**. Glycaemic control and renal function did not differ significantly between I and NI groups. Informed patients had a significantly lower Ad DiaRem score (10 vs. 14, $p = 0.016$) compared to non-informed patients, indicating a higher probability to achieve T2DM remission after BS. Accordingly, the percentage of patients having an Ad DiaRem score ≤10 and thus a probability of achieving post-operative T2DM remission of up to 74%, was significantly higher among informed vs. non-informed patients (54.3 vs. 34.6%, $p = 0.047$). Among the eligible patients with high probability of achieving T2DM remission after BS (Ad DiaRem score≤10), the percentage of informed patients was 40.4 vs. 23.2% among those unlikely to experience postoperative T2DM remission, as shown in **Figure 1**.

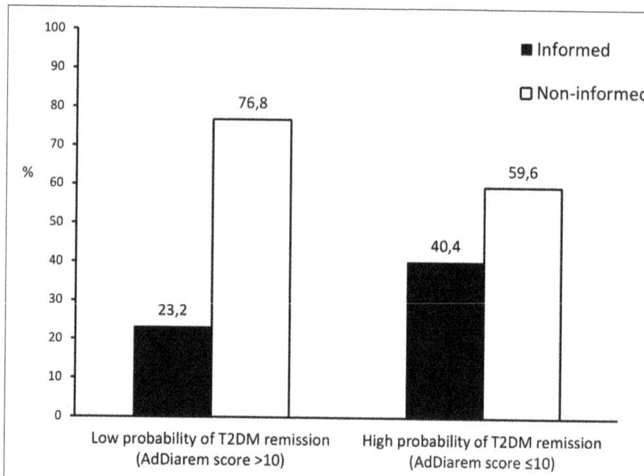

FIGURE 1 | Graphical presentation of the percentage of patients having been informed about the treatment option of metabolic surgery among those with high vs. low probability of T2DM remission within the first 5 years following bariatric surgery, stratified according to the advanced DiaRem[[Inline Image]] score. AdDiarem score, advanced diabetes remission score; T2DM, type 2 diabetes mellitus.

DISCUSSION

Summarizing the major findings of the present study, a significant number of patients with T2DM who are routinely assessed in diabetes outpatient clinics of large university hospitals meet the DSS-II eligibility criteria for BS (15.3%). Eligible patients are younger and have a higher degree of obesity, report a shorter T2DM duration and display worse glycaemic control and better renal function, compared to non-eligible patients. Among eligible patients, only around 40% have been informed by their physicians about the option of BS. Informed patients are younger and have more severe obesity than non-informed patients. A significant percentage of unaware patients (35%) have an advanced DiaRem score ≤10, indicating a considerable probability of 74% to achieve T2DM remission within the next 5 years after BS, and are thus deprived of this opportunity due to lack of appropriate medical counseling. These data highlight the fact that both screening and awareness of BS remain an unmet need in the current clinical setting of T2DM management.

We report a considerable percentage of patients with T2DM who are eligible for BS. This relates to the DSS-II eligibility criteria that we applied, which consider not only the extent of obesity but also the adequacy of glycaemic control to determine eligibility for BS in patients with T2DM. As opposed to the previously applied NIH criteria which were more BMI-centric and precluded the option of BS for patients with T2DM and mild obesity (BMI <35) (12), the DSS-II criteria expand BS eligibility to a broader spectrum of patients with obesity and T2DM who remain suboptimally controlled despite intensified medical and lifestyle treatment (16). Several studies have emphasized the need to extend BS eligibility beyond stringent BMI thresholds and instead focus on clinically relevant outcomes to maximize benefits for patients. Strict BMI cut-offs have been consistently found inappropriate for BS prioritization, considering that even non-eligible patients based on BMI may experience comparable benefits in terms of T2DM prevention, improvement of cardiovascular risk factors and mortality reduction with eligible patients (22). To date, the majority of studies addressing the epidemiology of BS eligibility have used either NIH or other evidence-based criteria sets (22, 23). Studies applying the DSS-II eligibility criteria in real-world T2DM populations are lacking, and our study aims to contribute to this literature gap.

Our study delineated the profile of eligible T2DM patients for BS by comparing demographic, anthropometric and clinical characteristics between eligible and non-eligible groups. Compared to non-eligible patients, eligible ones were found to be younger, more obese, with shorter T2DM duration, better renal function and poorer glycaemic control. The higher BMI and HbA1c found in eligible patients should be expected, considering that the degree of obesity and glycaemic control are both components of the definition of the DSS-II criteria. The younger age of eligible patients could be also expected, since advanced age (>65 years old) precludes eligibility, and a large number of T2DM patients in our cohort (nearly 50%) were considered non-eligible due to their advanced age. This also probably points to clinical inertia on the part of the medical profession, namely that doctors do not recommend BS to eligible patients for many years, until finally these patients become ineligible due to their age. The shorter reported T2DM duration in eligible patients could be partly related to their younger age. Although the duration of T2DM is not officially part of the definition of eligibility criteria for BS, it should be always considered, since patients with long-standing T2DM have a lower probability to achieve T2DM remission after BS (10). The better renal function of eligible patients could be explained by their younger age, shorter T2DM duration and fewer comorbidities.

An important finding of our study was that less than 40% of eligible T2DM patients responded positively to the question whether they had ever been informed by their physicians about the option of BS. This means that ~60% of T2DM patients who fulfill the eligibility criteria for BS and would theoretically benefit from BS in terms of T2DM treatment, overall health and quality of life improvement, are not made aware of this option due to lack of appropriate medical consultation and recommendation. Informed patients were found to be significantly younger and more obese than non-informed patients, suggesting that physicians tend to consider BS primarily for younger patients with extreme levels of adiposity. As a result of this misconception, eligible patients who are older or have less severe obesity are not promptly informed about BS, an omission which is very unfortunate for them, because as time goes by, their age will advance further, comorbidities may accumulate, T2DM duration will increase and glycaemic control may possibly deteriorate, all of which might eventually render these patients either non-eligible for BS or poor candidates for post-operative T2DM remission. An additional important observation of our study was that among eligible T2DM patients who had never been informed about the option of BS (unaware), around 35% displayed a favorable Ad DiaRem score (≤10), indicating a considerable likelihood of achieving T2DM remission within the next 5 years after BS. The significantly higher percentage of patients with a favorable prospect of T2DM regression after BS in informed vs. non-informed patients (54.3 vs. 34.6%) is definitely a positive statement, but still, a significant number of patients who are highly likely to experience T2DM remission in the next years after BS, miss this opportunity and remain diabetic and poorly controlled due to lack of awareness. Possible reasons for this huge gap in awareness are mainly related to the inadequate education of physicians about BS, ignorance of current eligibility criteria, low familiarity with BS modalities and their risks and benefits, lack of interest or confidence in BS, lack of time and reluctance to undertake the postoperative monitoring of bariatric patients (24–26), as demonstrated in a Greek study in doctors of various medical specialties, which assessed their attitudes and perceptions about BS and reported an alarmingly limited penetration of BS in the medical community (27). These data emphasize the urgent need to promote education of health care professionals in the field of obesity management and make them more knowledgeable, confident and familiar with weight management options such as BS. It would be meaningful to pursue this goal by implementing changes in the curriculum of medical schools to teach medical students how to interact with patients with obesity and optimally manage their obesity-related health conditions, as shown by innovative pilot studies in undergraduate medical students (28).

Our data reveal an unmet need in T2DM clinical management, and complement previously published data addressing several unmet needs in both obesity and T2DM management (29). Despite the indisputable weight loss efficacy of BS, only a small fraction of qualifying patients with obesity undergo BS, partly due to the associated perioperative risks, reimbursement issues, and prevalent misconceptions. Nationwide datasets suggest a huge gap between the number of patients with obesity who are eligible for BS and those who ultimately receive it, and they reveal differences in demographic parameters between eligible and operated patients, raising concerns about possible inequalities in access to BS in certain population subgroups (30). In support of these findings, an Irish study has shown that the current provision of bariatric surgical services meets much less than 0.1% of the current need based on eligibility rates in older community-dwelling adults (23). In this context, it should be emphasized that BS should be performed by experienced surgeons in specialized centers providing multidisciplinary teams and long-term follow up. Therefore, BS eligibility should be "adapted" to the capacity and availability of such units.

This study has certain limitations. Its cross-sectional design, the descriptive methodology, the subjectivity of determining individual eligibility for BS with respect to defining optimal medical treatment (based however on evidence-based clinical guidelines), and the lack of a nationally representative study sample, are the major of these. On the other hand, our study has important strengths. It adds to the limited literature applying the novel DSS-II eligibility criteria to prioritize BS in inadequately controlled diabetic patients, reflects everyday clinical practice by studying real-world patients with T2DM and varying levels of obesity assessed routinely in diabetes outpatient clinics, and conveys the simple but important message that awareness of BS remains low despite high eligibility, even among patients who are expected to benefit the most.

Taken together, the present study concludes that a significant proportion of patients with T2DM who are routinely assessed in diabetes outpatient clinics are appropriate candidates for BS, but only a minority of them have been informed by their physicians about this option. Physicians tend to recommend BS only in young patients with extreme levels of adiposity. These data highlight the fact that screening and awareness of BS in the clinical setting of T2DM management remain an unmet need possibly due to insufficient education and clinical inertia. Future research should focus on intensifying screening for BS eligibility criteria at every medical visit and promoting accurate and evidence-based clinical recommendations for patients expected to benefit the most.

AUTHOR CONTRIBUTIONS

CK analyzed data and prepared the manuscript. ET collected, tabulated and analyzed data and reviewed the manuscript. EP, IS, EE, MK, MN, AT, AKou, KB, and VL collected and tabulated data and reviewed the manuscript. NT analyzed data and reviewed the manuscript. AKok designed and coordinated the study, analyzed data and reviewed the manuscript. All authors approved the final version of the submitted manuscript.

REFERENCES

1. Mingrone G, Panunzi S, De Gaetano A, Guidone C, Iaconelli A, Leccesi L, et al. Bariatric surgery versus conventional medical therapy for type 2 diabetes. *N Engl J Med.* (2012) 366:1577–85. doi: 10.1056/NEJMoa1200111
2. Schauer PR, Kashyap SR, Wolski K, Brethauer SA, Kirwan JP, Pothier CE, et al. Bariatric surgery versus intensive medical therapy in obese patients with diabetes. *N Engl J Med.* (2012) 366:1567–76. doi: 10.1056/NEJMoa1200225
3. Mingrone G, Panunzi S, De Gaetano A, Guidone C, Iaconelli A, Nanni G, et al. Bariatric-metabolic surgery versus conventional medical treatment in obese patients with type 2 diabetes: 5 year follow-up of an open-label, single-centre, randomised controlled trial. *Lancet.* (2015) 386:964–73. doi: 10.1016/S0140-6736(15)00075-6
4. Cummings DE, Arterburn DE, Westbrook EO, Kuzma JN, Stewart SD, Chan CP, et al. Gastric bypass surgery vs intensive lifestyle and medical intervention for type 2 diabetes: the CROSSROADS randomised controlled trial. *Diabetologia.* (2016) 59:945–53. doi: 10.1007/s00125-016-3903-x
5. Halperin F, Ding SA, Simonson DC, Panosian J, Goebel-Fabbri A, Wewalka M, et al. Roux-en-Y gastric bypass surgery or lifestyle with intensive medical management in patients with type 2 diabetes: feasibility and 1-year results of a randomized clinical trial. *JAMA Surg.* (2014) 149:716–26. doi: 10.1001/jamasurg.2014.514
6. Ikramuddin S, Korner J, Lee WJ, Connett JE, Inabnet WB, Billington CJ, et al. Roux-en-Y gastric bypass vs intensive medical management for the control of type 2 diabetes, hypertension, and hyperlipidemia: the Diabetes Surgery Study randomized clinical trial. *JAMA.* (2013) 309:2240–9. doi: 10.1001/jama.2013.5835
7. Courcoulas AP, Goodpaster BH, Eagleton JK, Belle SH, Kalarchian MA, Lang W, et al. Surgical vs medical treatments for type 2 diabetes mellitus: a randomized clinical trial. *JAMA Surg.* (2014) 149:707–15. doi: 10.1001/jamasurg.2014.467
8. Courcoulas AP, Belle SH, Neiberg RH, Pierson SK, Eagleton JK, Kalarchian MA, et al. Three-Year outcomes of bariatric surgery vs lifestyle intervention for type 2 diabetes mellitus treatment: a randomized clinical trial. *JAMA Surg.* (2015) 150:931–40. doi: 10.1001/jamasurg.2015.1534
9. Koliaki C, Liatis S, le Roux CW, Kokkinos A. The role of bariatric surgery to treat diabetes: current challenges and perspectives. *BMC Endocr Disord.* (2017) 17:50. doi: 10.1186/s12902-017-0202-6
10. Tsilingiris D, Koliaki C, Kokkinos A. Remission of type 2 diabetes mellitus after bariatric surgery: fact or fiction? *Int J Environ Res Public Health.* (2019) 16:16173171. doi: 10.3390/ijerph16173171
11. Baxter J. Obesity surgery-another unmet need. *BMJ.* (2000) 321:523–4. doi: 10.1136/bmj.321.7260.523
12. NIH conference. Gastrointestinal surgery for severe obesity. Consensus Development Conference Panel. *Ann Intern Med.* (1991) 115:956–61. doi: 10.7326/0003-4819-115-12-956
13. De Luca M, Angrisani L, Himpens J, Busetto L, Scopinaro N, Weiner R, et al. Indications for surgery for obesity and weight-related diseases: position statements from the international federation for the surgery of obesity and metabolic disorders (IFSO). *Obes Surg.* (2016) 26:1659–96. doi: 10.1007/s11695-016-2271-4
14. Dixon JB, Zimmet P, Alberti KG, Rubino F, International Diabetes Federation Taskforce on Epidemiology and Prevention. Bariatric surgery: an IDF statement for obese Type 2 diabetes. *Diabet Med.* (2011) 28:628–42. doi: 10.1111/j.1464-5491.2011.03306.x
15. Aminian A, Chang J, Brethauer SA, Kim JJ, American Society for Metabolic and Bariatric Surgery Clinical Issues Committee. ASMBS updated position statement on bariatric surgery in class I obesity (BMI 30-35 kg/m2). *Surg Obes Relat Dis.* (2018) 14:1071–87. doi: 10.1016/j.soard.2018.05.025
16. Rubino F, Nathan DM, Eckel RH, Schauer PR, Alberti KG, Zimmet PZ, et al. Metabolic surgery in the treatment algorithm for type 2 diabetes: a joint statement by international diabetes organizations. *Diabetes Care.* (2016) 39:861–77. doi: 10.2337/dc16-0236
17. Provost DA. Indications and contraindications for bariatric surgery. In: *The ASMBS Textbook of Bariatric Surgery.* (2015). p. 73–6. doi: 10.1007/978-1-4939-1206-3_6
18. Levey AS, Coresh J, Greene T, Stevens LA, Zhang YL, Hendriksen S, et al. Using standardized serum creatinine values in the modification of diet in renal disease study equation for estimating glomerular filtration rate. *Ann Intern Med.* (2006) 145:247–54. doi: 10.7326/0003-4819-145-4-200608150-00004
19. American Diabetes Association. 9. Pharmacologic Approaches to Glycemic Treatment: Standards of Medical Care in Diabetes-2020. *Diabetes Care.* (2020) 43(Suppl 1):S98–S110. doi: 10.2337/dc20-S009
20. Aron-Wisnewsky J, Sokolovska N, Liu Y, Comaneshter DS, Vinker S, Pecht T, et al. The advanced-DiaRem score improves prediction of diabetes remission 1 year post-Roux-en-Y gastric bypass. *Diabetologia.* (2017) 60:1892–902. doi: 10.1007/s00125-017-4371-7
21. Dicker D, Golan R, Aron-Wisnewsky J, Zucker JD, Sokolowska N, Comaneshter DS, et al. Prediction of long-term diabetes remission after RYGB, sleeve gastrectomy, and adjustable gastric banding using diarem and advanced-diarem scores. *Obes Surg.* (2019) 29:796–804. doi: 10.1007/s11695-018-3583-3
22. Sjöholm K, Anveden A, Peltonen M, Jacobson P, Romeo S, Svensson PA, et al. Evaluation of current eligibility criteria for bariatric surgery: diabetes prevention and risk factor changes in the Swedish obese subjects (SOS) study. *Diabetes Care.* (2013) 36:1335–40. doi: 10.2337/dc12-1395
23. O'Neill KN, Finucane FM, le Roux CW, Fitzgerald AP, Kearney PM. Unmet need for bariatric surgery. *Surg Obes Relat Dis.* (2017) 13:1052–56. doi: 10.1016/j.soard.2016.12.015
24. Bleich SN, Pickett-Blakely O, Cooper LA. Physician practice patterns of obesity diagnosis and weight-related counseling. *Patient Educ Couns.* (2011) 82:123–9. doi: 10.1016/j.pec.2010.02.018
25. Salinas GD, Glauser TA, Williamson JC, Rao G, Abdolrasulnia M. Primary care physician attitudes and practice patterns in the management of obese adults: Results from a national survey. *Postgrad Med.* (2011) 123:214–19. doi: 10.3810/pgm.2011.09.2477

26. Alexander SC, Ostbye T, Pollak KI, Gradison M, Bastian LA, Brouwer RJ. Physicians' beliefs about discussing obesity: results from focus groups. *Am J Health Promot.* (2007) 21:498–500. doi: 10.4278/0890-1171-21.6.498
27. Zacharoulis D, Bakalis V, Zachari E, Sioka E, Tsimpida D, Magouliotis D, et al. Current knowledge and perception of bariatric surgery among Greek doctors living in Thessaly. *Asian J Endosc Surg.* (2018) 11:138–45. doi: 10.1111/ases.12436
28. Roberts DH, Kane EM, Jones DB, Almeida JM, Bell SK, Weinstein AR, et al. Teaching medical students about obesity: a pilot program to address an unmet need through longitudinal relationships with bariatric surgery patients. *Surg Innov.* (2011) 18:176–83. doi: 10.1177/1553350611399298
29. Nguyen N, Champion JK, Ponce J, Quebbemann B, Patterson E, Pham B, et al. A review of unmet needs in obesity management. *Obes Surg.* (2012) 22:956–66. doi: 10.1007/s11695-012-0634-z
30. Desogus D, Menon V, Singhal R, Oyebode O. An examination of who is eligible and who is receiving bariatric surgery in england: secondary analysis of the health survey for england dataset. *Obes Surg.* (2019) 29:3246–51. doi: 10.1007/s11695-019-03977-3

6

Plasma N-Acetylaspartate is Related to Age, Obesity and Glucose Metabolism: Effects of Antidiabetic Treatment and Bariatric Surgery

*Giuseppe Daniele[1], Beatrice Campi[2], Alessandro Saba[3,4], Simone Codini[1], Annamaria Ciccarone[1], Laura Giusti[1], Stefano Del Prato[1], Russel L. Esterline[5] and Ele Ferrannini[2]**

[1] Department of Clinical and Experimental Medicine, University of Pisa, Pisa, Italy, [2] C.N.R. Institute of Clinical Physiology, Pisa, Italy, [3] Department of Surgical, Medical and Molecular Pathology and Critical Care Medicine, University of Pisa, Pisa, Italy, [4] Laboratory of Clinical Pathology, St. Chiara University Hospital, Pisa, Italy, [5] AstraZeneca Pharmaceutical, Gaithersburg, MD, United States

***Correspondence:**
Ele Ferrannini
ferranni@ifc.cnr.it

Background: N-acetylaspartate (NAA) is synthesized only by neurons and is involved in neuronal metabolism and axonal myelination. NAA is the strongest signal on brain magnetic resonance spectroscopy, and its concentration have been associated with cognitive dysfunction in neurodegenerative diseases, obesity, and type 2 diabetes (T2D).

Materials and Methods: We explored the impact of obesity and T2D on circulating NAA as well as the impact of bariatric surgery and antidiabetic treatments. We developed an LC-MS method for the accurate measurements of fasting plasma NAA levels in 505 subjects (156 subjects with normal glucose tolerance, 24 subjects with impaired glucose tolerance, and 325 patients with T2D) to examine the associations of NAA with obesity and dysglycemia. To validate cross-sectional findings, plasma NAA was measured 6 months after Roux-en-Y Gastric Bypass (RYGB) in 55 morbidly obese subjects, and after 1 year of antidiabetic treatment (with dapagliflozin, exenatide, or dapagliflozin plus exenatide) in 192 T2D patients.

Results: In the whole population, NAA was associated with age ($r = 0.31$, $p < 0.0001$) and BMI ($r = -0.20$, $p < 0.0001$). Independently of age and BMI, NAA was reciprocally related to HbA1c and fasting plasma glucose (partial $r = -0.13$, both $p = 0.01$). Surgically-induced weight loss raised NAA (by 18 nmol/L on average, $p < 0.02$). Glucose lowering treatment increased NAA in proportion to the drop in HbA1c ($r = 0.31$, $p < 0.0001$) regardless of the agent used.

Conclusions: Circulating NAA concentrations are modulated by age, obesity, and glycemic control. Whether they may mark for the corresponding metabolic effects on brain function remains to be established by joint measurements of spectroscopic signal and cognitive function.

Keywords: N-acetylaspartate, neuronal function, type 2 diabetes, obesity, dapagliflozin, exenatide, bariatric surgery, glucose metabolism

INTRODUCTION

Type 2 diabetes (T2D) and obesity increase the risk of serious complications in multiple organs, including the brain (1). Obesity and T2D are associated with a higher prevalence of cognitive dysfunction, dementia, and neurodegenerative diseases, including Alzheimer and Parkinson diseases (2–5). Microvascular disease induced by hyperglycemia is responsible for disruption of the blood-brain barrier (BBB) through pericyte depletion, possibly caused by excess superoxide produced during enhanced mitochondrial respiration (6, 7). Loss of the BBB ability to protect the brain from circulating substances results in neurotoxicity and neuronal cell death (8). Neuroimaging has documented several structural and functional alterations in numerous brain regions of patients with T2D (9–11). Magnetic resonance spectroscopy (MRS) has provided details regarding metabolite changes in the brain that might be related to functional and structural alterations. Recent MRS-based analyses carried out in humans have suggested that N-acetylaspartate (NAA), the most concentrated metabolite in the brain (~10 mM) (12–14), is significantly reduced in several diseases including Alzheimer (15, 16), Huntington disease (17), bipolar disorder (18), schizophrenia (19), multiple sclerosis (20), and T2D (21–25).

NAA is reputed to be a marker of neuronal number and viability (26) but its role in brain metabolism and function in humans is far from being fully elucidated. NAA is synthesized in neuronal mitochondria and then transported by a sodium/dicarboxylate symporter (27) to aspartoacylase-containing oligodendrocytes (28) and astrocytes. NAA has two primary roles, as a facilitator of energy metabolism in neuronal mitochondria (29) and a source of acetate for fatty acid and steroid synthesis necessary for axonal myelination by oligodendrocytes (30, 31). Astrocytes, which represent the main cell type within the BBB structure, play a role in the removal of NAA from the extracellular space; a continuous NAA efflux from the brain to the circulation has been proposed (32). Therefore, plasma NAA levels might be used as a marker of central NAA alterations in neurodegenerative diseases and T2D-related brain damage. One difficulty is that the few studies measuring circulating NAA concentrations report widely different values even in healthy controls, ranging from a mean 0.11 mmol/L (33) to 0.44 μmol/L (34), very likely due to assay differences.

To the best of our knowledge, the impact of obesity and T2D on circulating NAA has not been previously explored. We therefore set forth to measure plasma NAA in non-diabetic obese and T2D subjects and the effect of treatment on plasma NAA.

Abbreviations: NAA, N-acetylaspartate; T2DM, type 2 diabetes; IGT, impaired glucose tolerance; NGT, normal glucose tolerance; RYGB, Roux-en-Y Gastric Bypass; FPG, Fasting plasma glucose; MRS, magnetic resonance spectroscopy; BBB, blood-brain barrier; GLP-1RAs, GLP-1 receptor agonists/analogs; Dapa+Plb, dapagliflozin + placebo; EQW, exenatide once weekly; EQW+Dapa, exenatide-dapagliflozin combination.

MATERIALS AND METHODS

Study Subjects

This was a data pooling project of different cohort studies. A total of 505 study subjects included patients with T2D or impaired glucose tolerance (IGT) and non-diabetic obese subjects. Two subgroups of participants were studied: (i) to assess the impact of major weight loss on circulating NAA levels, we included obese subjects undergoing Roux-en-Y Gastric Bypass (RYGB) between 2015 and 2018; (ii) to evaluate the effect of glycemic control, we included T2D patients from the DURATION-8 study (NCT02229396), which was a 52-week, multicenter, double-blind, randomized, active-controlled phase 3 trial. In DURATION-8, participants were randomly assigned to receive once-weekly exenatide (2 mg) by subcutaneous injection plus once-daily dapagliflozin (10 mg) (EQW+Dapa), exenatide with dapagliflozin-matched oral placebo (EQW), or dapagliflozin with exenatide-matched placebo injections (Dapa+Plb) (35). Lean healthy subjects with normal glucose tolerance (NGT) were included as control group. Exclusion criteria were: type 1 diabetes, psychiatric disorders, severe cognitive impairment, neurodegenerative diseases, epilepsy, depression treatment, traumatic brain injury over the preceding months, liver function enzymes higher more than two times the upper limit, heart failure (NYHA III-IV), GFR <60 ml/min/1.73 m^2, diabetes treatment other than metformin, or sulphonylureas. The ethical committee approvals refers to specific ethical approval of each study included in the pooled analysis. All procedure performed were in accordance with the Helsinki Declaration of 1975 as revised 1983.

All plasma samples were obtained in the overnight fasted [10–14 h) state, and stored at −80°C for NAA analysis. Baseline and post-treatment samples were assayed in the same run to reduce within-subject variability.

Reagents and Materials

NAA and internal standard *N*-Acetyl-L-aspartic acid-1,2,3,4-$^{13}C_4$ (IS, $^{13}C_4$-NAA) as well as acetonitrile (LC-MS grade), ultra-pure water (LC-MS grade), formic acid (MS grade), and 3N hydrochloric acid in butan-1-ol were provided by Sigma-Aldrich (Saint Louis, MO, USA).

Equipments and Analytical Method

An Agilent 1290 Infinity UHPLC system (Santa Clara, CA, USA), including binary pump, autosampler, and column oven, fitted with a Kinetex C18 (100Å, 2.6 μm, 50 × 2.10 mm ID) HPLC column (Phenomenex, Torrance, CA, USA), protected by a KrudKatcher Ultra HPLC in-line filter (0.5 μm depth × 0.004 in ID), was used for sample injection and chromatographic separation. This latter was carried out under the gradient conditions at a flow rate of 400 μL/min, by using H_2O + 0.1% formic acid (FA) as an aqueous solvent and ACN + 20% MeOH + 0.1% FA as an organic solvent. The injection volume of samples was 5 μL.

Mass spectrometry runs were carried out by an AB Sciex API 4000 triple quadrupole mass spectrometer (Concord, ON, Canada), equipped with an electrospray (ESI) Turbo-V ion source. The MS method was based on positive ion mode selected reaction monitoring (SRM) and made use of parameters optimized in order to get the best possible sensitivity and selectivity. In particular, SRM acquisitions were based on transitions 288.2 → 143.9 Da (quantifier, Q) and 288.2 → 186.1 Da (qualifier, q) for NAA and 292 → 146.9 Da (Q), 292 → 189.1 Da (q) for $^{13}C_4$-NAA.

Sample preparation was carried out as follows: plasma samples were thawed at room temperature, vortexed (15 min), and a 100 μL aliquot was added with 300 μL of acetonitrile, formic acid 1% (V%), and internal standard. The obtained suspensions were vortexed (15 min) and centrifuged (18,620 × g, 15 min). Then, 300 μL of supernatants were collected and dried under stream of N_2 at 40°C. The samples were derivatized to butyl esters (Fischer esterification reaction) by adding 100 μL 3N 1-butanol/ HCl, vortexing (15 min), heating at 60°C for 40 min. The reaction products were dried under a gentle stream of nitrogen and the dry residues were reconstituted with 100 μL ACN/H_2O (20/80; V/V), vortexed (15 min), and 5 μL of the obtained solutions were injected into the LC-MS-MS system.

The analytical method, which is not the main subject of this paper and that will be extensively described in a paper under preparation, was validated in compliance with EMA guidelines (36) for sample stability, linearity, lower limits of detection and quantitation (LLOD and LLOQ), matrix effect, recovery, selectivity, precision, and accuracy.

Statistical Analysis

Data are given as mean ± SD. Because of their skewed distribution, plasma NAA concentrations were summarized as median [interquartile range, IQR], and logarithmically transformed for use in parametric statistical tests. Group values were compared by the Mann-Whitney *U*-test, paired values by the Wilkinson signed-rank test. Change by treatment were analyzed by MANOVA for repeated measures. Univariate and multivariate linear regressions were carried out by standard methods. Data analyses were performed using JMP® 7.0 (SAS Institute Inc., 2007); $p \leq 0.05$ was considered statistically significant.

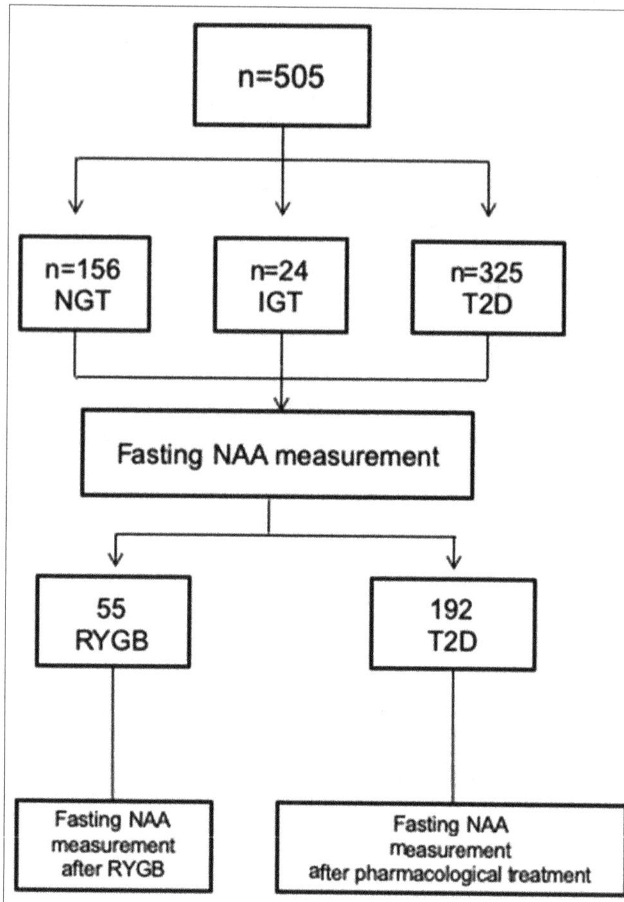

FIGURE 1 | Participants flow chart. NGT, normal glucose tolerance; IGT, Impaired glucose regulation; T2D; type 2 diabetes.

RESULTS

In the study population (259 women, 246 men), 156 subjects had normal glucose tolerance (NGT), 325 had T2D, and 24 had IGT; age ranged from 23 to 78 years, and BMI ranged from 20.1 to 57.9 kg/m^2 (**Figure 1**). In the whole data set, fasting plasma NAA concentrations ranged from 94 to 567 nmol/L, with a significantly ($p < 0.0001$) skewed distribution. Compared to NGT, T2D/IGT subjects were older ($p < 0.0001$) and more often men ($p = 0.002$) (**Table 1**). Plasma NAA concentrations were higher in men than women ($p < 0.02$), were positively associated with age, and negatively related to BMI (**Figure 2**). In the 63 NGT, normal-weight (i.e., BMI≤25 kg/m^2) subjects aged <65 years (42 women, 21 men), plasma NAA ranged 143–407 nmol/L (median 204, IQR 110 nmol/L) in men and 101–378 nmol/L (median 239, IQR 95) in women. By adjusting the entire data set for gender, age, and BMI, plasma NAA levels were inversely related to both FPG and HbA$_{1c}$ (**Figure 3**); in this model, age was still a positive ($p < 0.0001$), and BMI a negative ($p = 0.044$), covariate. To characterize the clinical phenotype of subjects with low plasma NAA levels, we split the NAA distribution into quartiles. In the lower quartile of plasma NAA levels there were more women, a younger age and higher BMI, and a worse glycemic control (**Table 2**).

In the 55 subjects (45 NGT and 10 T2D) who underwent bariatric surgery, the change in BMI at 6 months post-surgery averaged −11.5 ± 3.6 kg/m^2 ($p < 0.0001$), and was similar in NGT and T2D. Fasting plasma glucose dropped by 10 ± 16 mg/dL in NGT and by 95 ± 77 mg/dL in T2D ($p < 0.0001$ for both), and plasma NAA increased by 18 (37) μmol/L ($p < 0.02$).

Out of the 265 T2D patients, 192 individuals were randomized to receive dapagliflozin + placebo (Dapa+Plb), exenatide once weekly (EQW), or the combination (EQW+Dapa) in a 1:1:1 ratio for 1 year. At 52 weeks, NAA values were higher than at baseline [248 [94] vs. 239 [83] nmol/L, delta = 13 (38), $p = 0.0013$] across treatment. Each treatment resulted in significant reductions in BMI, fasting glucose, and HbA$_{1c}$, and an increase in plasma NAA; the changes were (for BMI, FPG, and NAA) or tended to be (for HbA$_{1c}$) accentuated with the combination as compared to

TABLE 1 | Characteristics of the study subjects*.

	NGT		T2D/IGT	
	Men	Women	Men	Women
N	60	96	186	163
Age (years)	50 ± 12	45 ± 12	58 ± 9	55 ± 10
BMI (kg/m²)	29.5 ± 8.8	37 ± 11.1	32.0 ± 5.3	33.5 ± 6.0
HbA_{1c} (%)	5.9 ± 1.7	5.7 ± 0.6	8.2 ± 1.4	8.6 ± 1.5
FPG (mg/dL)	93 ± 19	92 ± 17	158 ± 49	171 ± 61
NAA (nmol/L)	249 [113]	227 [88]	249 [67]	239 [75]

**entries are mean ± SD or median [interquartile range]; BMI, body mass index; FPG, fasting plasma glucose; NAA, N-acetylaspartate.*

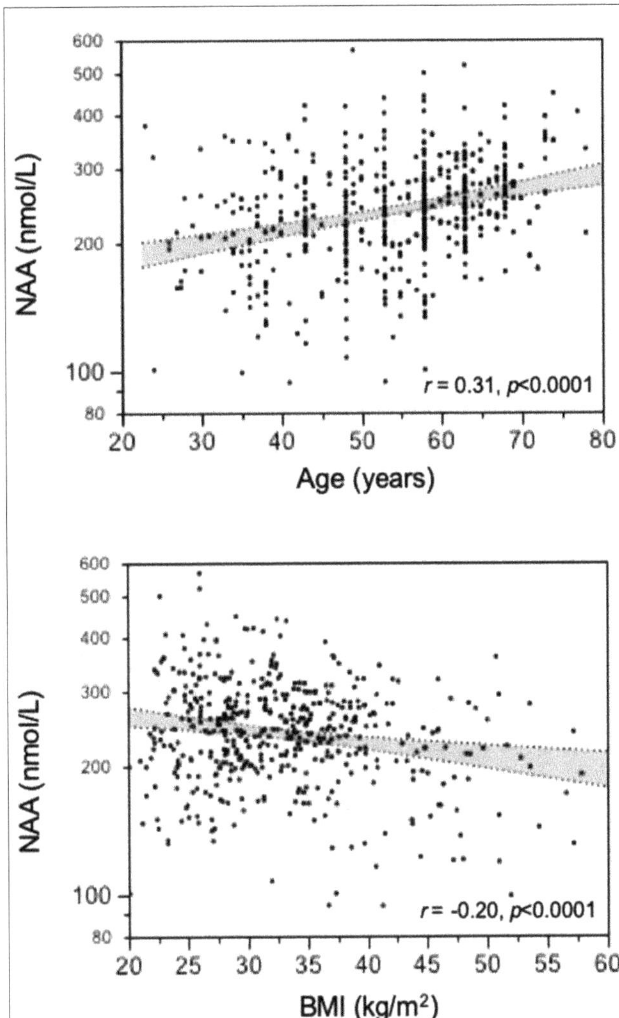

FIGURE 2 | Association of plasma N-acetylaspartate (NAA) concentrations with age and BMI.

either agent alone (**Table 3**). In the pooled data from all treatment arms, the changes in plasma NAA were inversely related to the concomitant changes in both HbA_{1c} (**Figure 4**). The regression predicts a mean NAA increase of 16 nmol/L for a 2% decrement in HbA_{1c}.

DISCUSSION

The data of this study allowed us to establish normative circulating NAA metrics, namely, median fasting concentrations of 230 nmol/L in non-obese, non-diabetic subjects below 65 years of age, and consistent, if not large, deviations with age and obesity (in opposite direction). Additionally, we report for the first time an inverse relation of plasma NAA to glycemic indices—HbA_{1c} and fasting glucose—even after controlling for sex, age, and BMI. The intervention protocols provided a prospective confirmation of this relationship by showing a consistent increase in plasma NAA concentrations following antidiabetic treatment (**Figure 3**).

It should be emphasized that no information is available on the acute changes in circulating NAA following physiological stimuli, e.g., a meal or a bout of physical exercise. More importantly, changes in plasma levels could reflect changes in NAA production/spillover from the brain into the bloodstream or changes in NAA removal from the plasma (or a combination thereof) (26). Thus, dysfunctional neurons might synthetize less NAA and/or the activity of the NAA-cleaving enzyme in glial cells [but also in brown adipocytes (39) and enterocytes (40)] might be increased: either process would reduce circulating NAA concentrations. The resulting clinical phenotype would resemble that profiled in subjects with lower NAA concentration (**Table 3**).

With regard to the effect of age, our finding of an independent, direct relationship between plasma NAA and age conflicts with two studies from the same group showing an age-related decline in serum NAA levels (41, 42). In the latter studies, however, the measured NAA concentrations were in the millimolar range, whereas reported values—including ours—are in the nanomolar range (34). Therefore, rather than a reflection of increased neuronal mass/function [i.e., an implausible correlate of aging (43)], our finding may suggest an age-related decrease in aspartoacylase, resulting in higher NAA levels. The extreme of this phenomenon would be Canavan disease, an autosomal-recessive mutation of the aspartoacylase gene associated with severe neurodegeneration (44).

The current finding of decreasing plasma NAA levels with increasing BMI is in line with the suggested role of obesity in NAA metabolism. By magnetic resonance spectroscopy (MRS), a higher BMI is associated with lower concentrations of NAA in brain frontal, parietal, and temporal white matter as well as in frontal gray matter and hippocampus (45, 46), and with progressive neuronal impairment and loss. Obesity can lead to astrogliosis, which is characterized by an increase in the number of primary astrocytic processes as well as in the length of these processes, leading to a more extensive contact between these cells and the local vasculature (47, 48). Astrocytes can be activated early after high-fat intake (49, 50) as a neuroprotective response to the rise in the concentration of fatty acids reaching the brain via the BBB (51–53). These structural changes could modify the ability of astrocytes to transport substances from the brain to the circulation, including a reduced release of

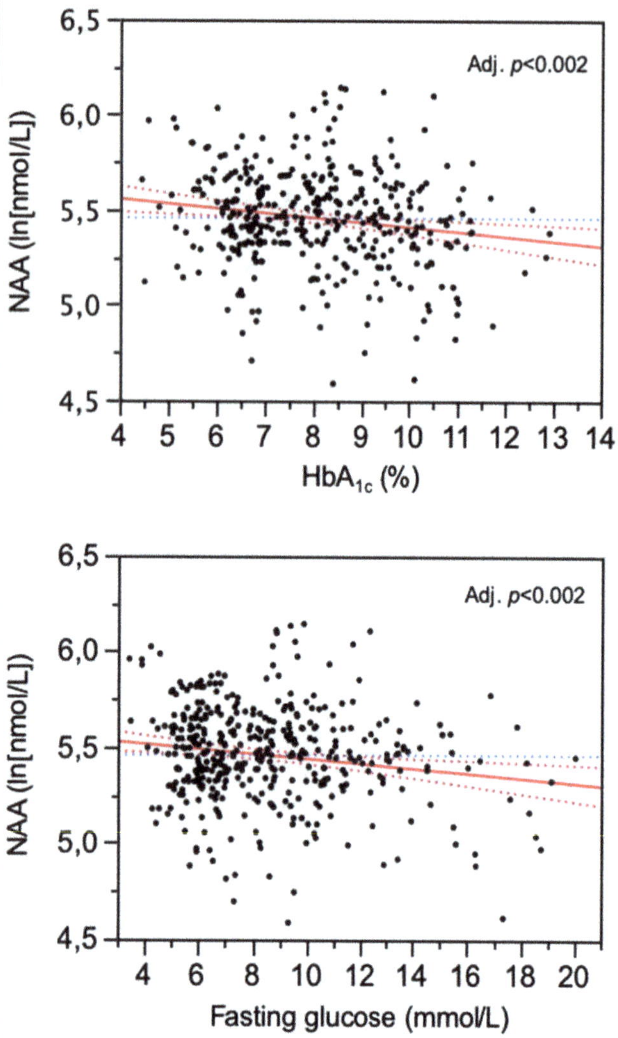

FIGURE 3 | Association of plasma N-acetylaspartate (NAA) concentrations with HbA_{1c} and fasting glucose levels. The plots are for logNAA residuals after controlling for gender, age, and BMI.

TABLE 2 | Clinical phenotype of subjects by quartile of NAA distribution*.

	Plasma NAA distribution		
	Bottom 25%	**Upper 75%**	***p***
NAA (nmol/L)	129 [41]	260 [66]	<0.0001
Women (%)	61	48	0.0138
Age (years)	48 ± 11	56 ± 11	<0.0001
BMI (kg/m^2)	34.2 ± 9.3	32.5 ± 6.6	0.07
HbA_{1c} (%)	8.2 ± 2.1	7.7 ± 1.6	0.0366
FPG (mg/dL)	158 ± 69	146 ± 53	0.09

**entries are mean ± SD or median [interquartile range]; BMI, body mass index; FPG, fasting plasma glucose; NAA, N-acetylaspartate.*

TABLE 3 | Variables by time and treatment#.

	Baseline	**1 year**	***p1***	***p2***	***p3***
Fasting glucose (mg/dL)			<0.0001	0.374	0.0214
Dapa + Plb (*n* = 70)	190 ± 42	145 ± 44			
EQW + Plb (*n* = 62)	190 ± 53	138 ± 37			
EQW + Dapa (*n* = 60)	194 ± 60	123 ± 32			
BMI (kg/m^2)			*<0.0001*	0.412	0.0004
Dapa + Plb	33.1 ± 6.1	32.3 ± 5.9			
EQW + Plb	31.6 ± 5.4	31.5 ± 5.5			
EQW + Dapa	33.6 ± 6.4	32.1 ± 6.0			
HbA1c (%)			*<0.0001*	0.249	0.084
Dapa + Plb	9.3 ± 1.0	7.7 ± 1.1			
EQW + Plb	9.3 ± 1.0	7.6 ± 1.3			
EQW + Dapa	9.3 ± 1.1	7.2 ± 1.3			
NAA (nmol/L)			*0.0005*	0.539	0.035
Dapa + Plb	242 [97]	245 [100]			
EQW + Plb	236 [82]	248 [73]			
EQW + Dapa	238 [88]	248 [110]			

#values are mean ± SD or median [IQR]; p^1 = time, p^2 = treatment, p^3 = time x treatment by MANOVA for repeated measures.

NAA (54). Several studies have documented changes in urinary NAA excretion or expression of NAA producing enzymes in association with obesity and/or diabetes (39, 40, 55–57). In the present study, the body weight reduction induced by bariatric surgery was associated to a significant increase in circulating NAA. One can therefore speculate that weight loss might have had multiple favorable consequences on central and peripheral NAA metabolism, including the reduction of brain astrogliosis.

Hyperglycemia dramatically increases neuronal glucose levels, which leads to neuronal damage, a phenomenon known as glucose neurotoxicity (58). Several mechanisms have been proposed for glucose neurotoxicity, including glucose-driven oxidative stress, and protein glycation. In line with this *in vitro* evidence, it has been shown that NAA/creatine ratio is decreased in the frontal brain cortex in diabetic patients with poor glycemic control (25). High glucose has a dramatic impact on astrocyte phenotype by inhibiting its proliferation and disrupting its energy flow (59, 60). Moreover, high glucose is associated with an increased expression and secretion of inflammatory cytokines (interleukin-6 and interleukin-8) by astrocytes (61). These hyperglycemia-induced abnormalities of astrocyte-neuron coupling may underlie the reduced central NAA concentrations and NAA spill-over into the peripheral circulation.

Although peripheral NAA levels alone cannot be taken to reflect spill-over or astrocyte-neuron coupling, our finding of consensual changes in glycemic indices and plasma NAA (**Figure 3**) does lend support to the possibility that long-term changes in circulating NAA may be markers for brain dysfunction. Clearly, simultaneous measurements of plasma NAA, brain NAA signal in relevant areas, and cognitive function before and after antihyperglycemic treatment would conclusively establish origin and value of peripheral NAA assessment.

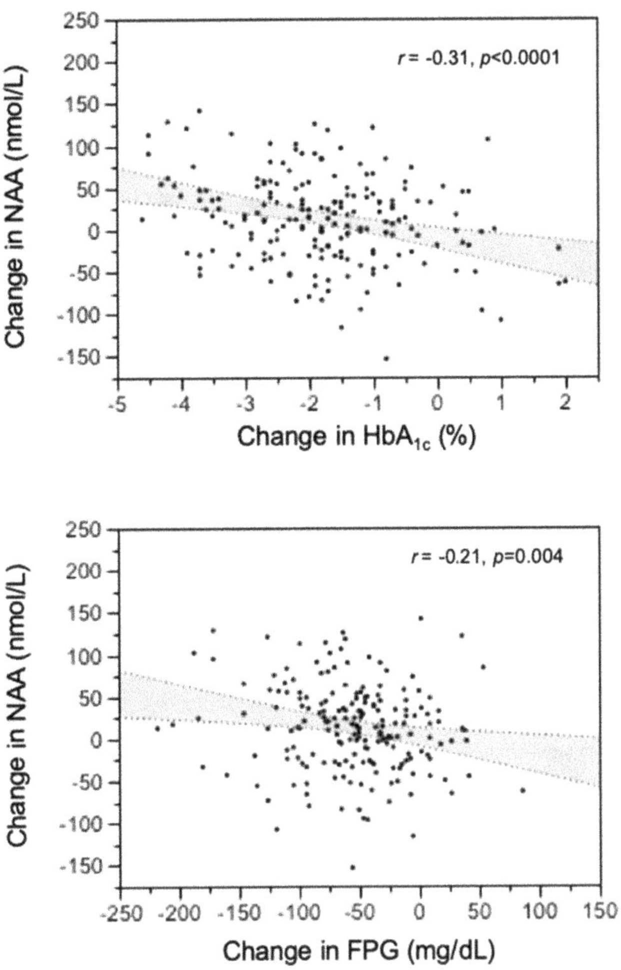

FIGURE 4 | Relation of treatment-induced changes in plasma N-acetylaspartate (NAA) concentrations to the corresponding changes in HbA_{1c} and fasting glucose levels at 1-year post-treatment.

Of note is that glucagon-like peptide 1 (GLP-1) receptors are expressed in neurons, in particular pyramidal neurons in the hippocampus and neocortex, which suggests that they may play a role in neuronal activity and synaptic transmission (62–64). Glia cells also express the receptor (65). GLP-1 analogs have demonstrated an impressive range of protective effects on neurogenesis, synaptogenesis, cell repair, and reduced inflammation, which is consistent with the profile of growth factor activity (37, 66–70). In this context, it is intriguing that patients in either EQW treatment arm showed a significantly greater change in plasma NAA than patients in the Dapa+placebo arm (**Table 2**), suggesting a potential effect of GLP-1 receptor agonists/analogs independently of the glucose lowering effect (38, 71).

The strength of the study is based on a large population including subjects with a wide range of age and body weight, and well-characterized in terms of glucose metabolism and comorbidity. In both T2D and morbidly obese groups, psychiatric disorders, intellectual disability, severe cognitive impairment, neurodegenerative diseases, epilepsy, depression treatment, and traumatic brain injury over the preceding months were exclusion criteria, which reduced the chances of NAA alterations being due to specific brain abnormalities.

The main limitation of the present study is its retrospective nature. Consequently, the NAA associations we describe, whether cross-sectional or longitudinal, do not necessarily intimate a causative role of glucose metabolism for plasma NAA or a direct relation of plasma NAA to brain NAA metabolism. The results of the study provide preliminary, inferential evidence, which remains to be confirmed by multilevel prospective studies.

AUTHOR CONTRIBUTIONS

EF and GD conceived the experimental design, analyzed the data, wrote and edited the manuscript. AS developed the tandem mass spectrometry-based assay and directed its validation. BC and SC performed LC-MS. AC and LG provided clinical samples. SD and RE provided feedback and contributed to the write-up and review of the manuscript. EF directed the study and is the guarantor of this work and, as such, had full access to all the data in the study and takes responsibility for the integrity of the data and accuracy of the data analysis. All authors read and approved the final manuscript.

ACKNOWLEDGMENTS

We thank Simona Baldi for assisting in the lab work.

REFERENCES

1. Klein JP, Waxman SG. The brain in diabetes: molecular changes in neurons and their implications for end-organ damage. *Lancet Neurol.* (2003) 2:548–54. doi: 10.1016/S1474-4422(03) 00503-9
2. Biessels GJ, Staekenborg S, Brunner E, Brayne C, Scheltens P. Risk of dementia in diabetes mellitus: a systematic review. *Lancet Neurol.* (2006) 5:64–74. doi: 10.1016/S1474-4422(05)7 0284-2
3. Gustafson D, Rothenberg E, Blennow K, Steen B, Skoog I. An 18-year follow-up of overweight and risk of Alzheimer disease. *Arch Intern Med.* (2003) 163:1524–8. doi: 10.1001/archinte.163. 13.1524
4. Whitmer RA, Gunderson EP, Barrett-Connor E, Quesenberry CP Jr, Yaffe K. Obesity in middle age and future risk of dementia: a 27-year longitudinal population based study. *BMJ.* (2005) 330:1360. doi: 10.1136/bmj.38446.466238.E0

5. Xu WL, Atti AR, Gatz M, Pedersen NL, Johansson B, Fratiglioni L. Midlife overweight and obesity increase late-life dementia risk: a population-based twin study. *Neurology.* (2011) 76:1568–74. doi: 10.1212/WNL.0b013e3182190d09
6. Shah GN, Morofuji Y, Banks WA, Price TO. High glucose-induced mitochondrial respiration and reactive oxygen species in mouse cerebral pericytes is reversed by pharmacological inhibition of mitochondrial carbonic anhydrases: implications for cerebral microvascular disease in diabetes. *Biochem Biophys Res Commun.* (2013) 440:354–8. doi: 10.1016/j.bbrc.2013.09.086
7. Liu Y, Fiskum G, Schubert D. Generation of reactive oxygen species by the mitochondrial electron transport chain. *J Neurochem.* (2002) 80:780–7. doi: 10.1046/j.0022-3042.2002.00744.x
8. Huber JD, VanGilder RL, Houser KA. Streptozotocin-induced diabetes progressively increases blood-brain barrier permeability in specific brain regions in rats. *Am J Physiol Heart Circ Physiol.* (2006) 291:H2660–8. doi: 10.1152/ajpheart.00489.2006
9. Musen G, Jacobson AM, Bolo NR, Simonson DC, Shenton ME, McCartney RL, et al. Resting-state brain functional connectivity is altered in type 2 diabetes. *Diabetes.* (2012) 61:2375–9. doi: 10.2337/db11-1669
10. Climie RE, Moran C, Callisaya M, Blizzard L, Sharman JE, Venn A, et al. Abdominal obesity and brain atrophy in type 2 diabetes mellitus. *PLoS ONE.* (2015) 10:e0142589. doi: 10.1371/journal.pone.0142589
11. Zhang Y, Lu S, Liu C, Zhang H, Zhou X, Ni C, et al. Altered brain activation and functional connectivity in working memory related networks in patients with type 2 diabetes: an ICA- based analysis. *Sci Rep.* (2016) 6:23767. doi: 10.1038/srep23767
12. Tallan HH. Studies on the distribution of N-acetyl-L-aspartic acid in brain. *J Biol Chem.* (1957) 224:41–5.
13. Tallan HH, Moore S, Stein WH. N-Acetyl-L-aspartic acid in brain. *J Biol Chem.* (1956) 219:257–64.
14. Miyake M, Kakimoto Y, Sorimachi M. A gas chromatographic method for the determination of N-acetyl-L-aspartic acid, N-acetyl-aspartylglutamic acid and beta-citryl-L-glutamic acid and their distributions in the brain and other organs of various species of animals. *J Neurochem.* (1981) 36:804–10. doi: 10.1111/j.1471-4159.1981.tb01665.x
15. Kwo-On-Yuen PF, Newmark RD, Budinger TF, Kaye JA, Ball MJ, Jagust WJ. BrainN-acetyl-L-aspartic acid in Alzheimer's disease: a proton magnetic resonance spectroscopy study. *Brain Res.* (1994) 667: 167–74. doi: 10.1016/0006-8993(94)91494-X
16. Zhu X, Schuff N, Kornak J, Soher B, Yaffe K, Kramer JH, et al. Previous magnetic resonance (MR) spectroscopy studies of Alzheimer disease (AD) reporting reduced N-acetyl aspartate (NAA), Alzheimer disease. *Assoc Disord.* (2006) 20:77–85. doi: 10.1097/01.wad.0000213809.12553.fc
17. Tsai G, Coyle JT. N-acetylaspartate in neuropsychiatric disorders, *Prog Neurobiol.* (1995) 46:531–40 doi: 10.1016/0301-0082(95)00014-M
18. Winsberg ME, Sachs N, Tate DL, Adalsteinsson E, Spielman D, Ketter TA. Decreased dorsolateral prefrontal N-acetyl aspartate in bipolar disorder. *Biol Psychiatry.* (2000) 47:475–81. doi: 10.1016/S0006-3223(99)00183-3
19. Molina V, Sánchez J, Reig S, Sanz J, Benito C, Santamarta C, et al. N-acetyl-aspartate levels in the dorsolateral prefrontal cortex in the early years of schizophrenia are inversely related to disease duration. *Schizophr Res.* (2005) 73:209–19. doi: 10.1016/j.schres.2004.02.001
20. Teunissen CE, Iacobaeus E, Khademi M, Brundin L, Norgren N, Koel-Simmelink MJA, et al. Combination of CSF N-acetylaspartate and neurofilaments in multiple sclerosis. *Neurology.* (2009) 72: 1322–9. doi: 10.1212/WNL.0b013e3181a0fe3f
21. Sinha S, Ekka M, Sharma U, Raghunandan P, Pandey RM, Jagannathan NR. Assessment of 17 changes in brain metabolites in Indian patients with type-2 diabetes mellitus 18 using proton magnetic resonance spectroscopy. *BMC Res Notes.* (2014) 7:41. doi: 10.1186/1756-0500-7-41
22. Lin Y, Zhou J, Sha L, Li Y, Qu X, Liu L, et al. Metabolite differences in the lenticular nucleus in type 2 diabetes mellitus 22 shown by proton MR spectroscopy. *AJNR Am J Neuroradiol.* (2013) 34:1692–6. doi: 10.3174/ajnr.A3492
23. Duarte JM. Metabolic alterations associated to brain dysfunction in diabetes. *Aging Dis.* (2015) 6:304–21. doi: 10.14336/AD.2014.1104
24. Duarte JM. Metabolism in the diabetic brain neurochemical profiling by 1H magnetic resonance spectroscopy. *J Diabetes Metab Disord.* (2016) 3:011. doi: 10.24966/DMD-201X/100011
25. Sahin I, Alkan A, Keskin L, Cikim A, Karakas HM, Firat AK, et al. Evaluation of in vivo cerebral metabolism on proton magnetic resonance spectroscopy in patients with impaired glucose tolerance and type 2 diabetes mellitus. *J Diabetes Complicat.* (2008) 22:254–60. doi: 10.1016/j.jdiacomp.2007.03.007
26. John R, Moffett JR, Brian Ross B, Peethambaran Arun P, Chikkathur N, Madhavarao CN, et al. N-Acetylaspartate in the CNS: from neurodiagnostics to neurobiology. *Progr Neurobiol.* (2007) 81:89–131. doi: 10.1016/j.pneurobio.2006.12.003
27. Fujita T, Katsukawa H, Yodoya E, Wada M, Shimada A, Okada N, et al. Transport characteristics of N-acetyl-L-aspartate in rat astrocytes: involvement of sodium-coupled high-affinity carboxylate transporter NaC3/ NaDC3-mediated transport system. *J Neurochem.* (2005) 93:706–14. doi: 10.1111/j.1471-4159.2005.03067.x
28. Madhavarao CN, Moffett JR, Moore RA, Viola RE, Namboodiri MA, Jacobowitz DM. Immunohistochemical localization of aspartoacylase in the rat central nervous system. *J Comp Neurol.* (2004) 472:318–29. doi: 10.1002/cne.20080
29. Clark, JB. N-acetyl aspartate: a marker for neuronal loss or mitochondrial dysfunction. *Dev Neurosci.* (1998) 20:271–6. doi: 10.1159/000017321
30. Chakraborty G, Mekala P, Yahya D, Wu G, Ledeen RW. Intraneuronal N-acetylaspartate supplies acetyl groups for myelin lipid synthesis: evidence for myelin-associated aspartoacylase. *J. Neurochem.* (2001) 78:736–45. doi: 10.1046/j.1471-4159.2001.00456.x
31. D'Adamo AF Jr, Yatsu, FM. Acetate metabolism in the nervous system. N-acetyl-L-aspartic acid and the biosynthesis of brain lipids. *J Neurochem.* (1966) 13:961–5. doi: 10.1111/j.1471-4159.1966.tb10292.x
32. Kelley RI, Stamas JN. Quantification of N-acetyl-L-aspartic acid in urine by isotope dilution gas chromatography-mass spectrometry. *J Inherit Metab Dis.* (1992) 15:97–104. doi: 10.1007/BF01800351
33. Tortorella C, Ruggieri M, Di Monte E, Ceci E, Iaffaldano P, Direnzo V, et al. Serum and CSF N-acetyl aspartate levels differ in multiple sclerosis and neuromyelitis optica. *J Neurol Neurosurg Psychiatry.* (2011) 82:1355–9. doi: 10.1136/jnnp.2011.241836
34. Jakobs C, Brink HJ, Langelaar SA, Zee T, Stellaard F, Macek M, et al. Stable isotope dilution analysis of N-acetylaspartic acid in CSF, blood, urine and amniotic fluid: accurate postnatal diagnosis and the potential for prenatal diagnosis of canavan disease. *J Inherit Metab Dis.* (1991) 14:653–60. doi: 10.1007/BF01799929
35. Frías JP, Guja C, Hardy E, Ahmed A, Dong F, Öhman P, et al. Exenatide once weekly plus dapagliflozin once daily versus exenatide or dapagliflozin alone in patients with type 2 diabetes inadequately controlled with metformin monotherapy (DURATION-8): a 28 week, multicentre, double-blind, phase 3, randomised controlled trial. *Lancet Diabetes Endocrinol.* (2016) 4:1004–16. doi: 10.1016/S2213-8587(16)30267-4
36. European Medicines Agency. *Guidelines on Bioanalytical Method Validation.* Available online at: http://www.ema.europa.eu/docs/en_GB/document_library/Scientific_guideline/2011/08/WC500109686.pdf (accessed 1 October, 2011).
37. McClean PL, Gault VA, Harriott P, Hölscher C. Glucagon-like peptide-1 analogues enhance synaptic plasticity in the brain: a link between

diabetes and Alzheimer's disease. *Eur J Pharmacol.* (2010) 630:158–62. doi: 10.1016/j.ejphar.2009.12.023

38. Gejl M, Gjedde A, Egefjord L, Moller A, Hansen SB, Vang K, et al. In Alzheimer's disease, 6-month treatment with GLP-1 analog prevents decline of brain glucose metabolism: randomized, placebo-controlled, double-blind clinical trial. *Front Aging Neurosci.* (2016) 8:108. doi: 10.3389/fnagi.2016.00108
39. Pessentheiner AR, Pelzmann HJ, Walenta E, Schweiger M, Groschner LN, Graier WF, et al. NAT8L (N-acetyltransferase 8-like) accelerates lipid turnover and increases energy expenditure in brown adipocytes. *J Biol Chem.* (2013) 288:36040–51. doi: 10.1074/jbc.M113.491324
40. Surendran S, Matalon R, Tyring SK. Upregulation of aspartoacylase activity in the duodenum of obesity induced diabetes mouse: implications on diabetic neuropathy. *Biochem Biophys Res Commun.* (2006) 345:973–5. doi: 10.1016/j.bbrc.2006.04.179
41. Ruggieri M, Tortorella C, Ceci E, Paolicelli D, Solfrizzi V, Di Bitonto G, et al. Age-related changes of serum N-acetyl-aspartate in healthy controls. *Age Ageing.* (2011) 40:391–5. doi: 10.1093/ageing/afr021
42. Simone IL, Ruggieri M, Tortelli R, Ceci E, D'Errico E, Leo A, et al. Serum N-acetylaspartate level in amyotrophic lateral sclerosis. *Arch Neurol.* (2011) 68:1308–12. doi: 10.1001/archneurol.2011.217
43. Arai H, Satake S, Kozaki K. Cognitive frailty in geriatrics. *Clin Geriatr Med.* (2018) 34:667–75. doi: 10.1016/j.cger.2018.06.011
44. Namboodiri AM, Peethambaran A, Mathew R, Sambhu PA, Hershfield J, Moffett JR, et al. Canavan disease and the role of N-acetylaspartate in myelin synthesis. *Mol Cell Endocrinol.* (2006) 252:216–23. doi: 10.1016/j.mce.2006.03.016
45. Gazdzinski S Kornak J, Weiner MW, Meyerhoff DJ. Body mass index and magnetic resonance markers of brain integrity in adults. *Ann Neurol.* (2008) 63:652–7. doi: 10.1002/ana.21377
46. Coplan JD, Fathy HM, Abdallah CG, Ragab SA, Kral JG, Mao X, et al. Reduced hippocampal N-acetyl-aspartate (NAA) as a biomarker for overweight. *Neuroimage Clin.* (2014) 4:326–35. doi: 10.1016/j.nicl.2013.12.014
47. Thaler JP, Yi CX, Schur EA, Guyenet SJ, Hwang BH, Dietrich MO, et al. Obesity is associated with hypothalamic injury in rodents and humans. *J Clin Invest.* (2012) 122:153–62. doi: 10.1172/JCI59660
48. Buckman LB, Thompson MM, Lippert RN, Blackwell TS, Yull FE, Ellacott KLJ. Evidence for a novel funcional role of astrocytes in the acute homeostatic response to HFD. *Mol Metab.* (2014) 4:58–63. doi: 10.1016/j.molmet.2014.10.001
49. Garcia-Caceres C, Fuente-Martin E, Burgos-Ramos E, Granado M, Frago LM, Barrios V, et al. Differential acute and chronic effects of leptin on hypothalamic astrocyte morphology and synaptic protein levels. *Endocrinology.* (2011) 152:1809–18. doi: 10.1210/en.2010-1252
50. Fuente-Martin E, Garcia-Caceres C, Granado M, De Ceballos ML, Sanchez-Garrido MA, Sarman B, et al. Leptin regulates glutamate and glucose transporters in hypothalamic astrocytes. *J Clin Invest.* (2012) 122:3900–13. doi: 10.1172/JCI64102
51. Dhopeshwarkar GA, Mead JF. Uptake and transport of fatty acids into the brain and the role of the blood-brain barrier system. *Adv Lipid Res.* (1973) 11:109–42. doi: 10.1016/B978-0-12-024911-4.50010-6
52. Miller JC, Gnaedinger JM, Rapoport SI. Utilization of plasma fatty acid in rat brain: distribution of [14C] palmitate between oxidative and synthetic pathways. *J Neurochem.* (1987) 49:1507–14. doi: 10.1111/j.1471-4159.1987.tb01021.x
53. Smith QR, Nagura H. Fatty acid uptake and incorporation in brain: studies with the perfusion model. *J Mol Neurosci.* (2001) 16:167–72. doi: 10.1385/JMN:16:2-3:167
54. Horvath TL, Sarman B, Garcia-Caceres C, Enriori PJ, Sotonyi P, Shanabrough M, et al. Synaptic input organization of the melanocortin system predicts diet- induced hypothalamic reactive gliosis and obesity. *Proc Natl Acad Sci USA.* (2010) 107:14875–80. doi: 10.1073/pnas.1004282107
55. Won EY, Yoon MK, Kim SW, Jung Y, Bae HW, Lee D, et al. Gender-specific metabolomic profiling of obesity in leptin-deficient ob/ob mice by 1H NMR spectroscopy. *PLoS ONE.* (2013) 8:e75998. doi: 10.1371/journal.pone.0075998
56. Hardy OT, Perugini RA, Nicoloro SM, Gallagher-Dorval K, Puri V, Straubhaar J, et al. Body mass index-independent inflammation in omental adipose tissue associated with insulin resistance in morbid obesity. *Surg Obes Relat Dis.* (2011) 7:60–7. doi: 10.1016/j.soard.2010.05.013
57. Salek RM, Maguire ML, Bentley E, Rubtsov DV, Hough T, Cheeseman M, et al. A metabolomic comparison of urinary changes in type 2 diabetes in mouse, rat, and human. *Physiol Genomics.* (2007) 29:99–108. doi: 10.1152/physiolgenomics.00194.2006
58. Tomlinson DR, Gardiner NJ. Glucose neurotoxicity. *Nat Rev Neurosci.* (2008) 9:36–45. doi: 10.1038/nrn2294
59. Jacob RJ, Fan X, Evans ML, Dziura J, Sherwin RS. Brain glucose levels are elevated in chronically hyperglycemic diabetic rats: no evidence for protective adaptation by the blood brain barrier. *Metabolism.* (2002) 51:1522–4. doi: 10.1053/meta.2002.36347
60. Salceda R, Vilchis C, Coffe V, Hernandez-Munoz R. Changes in the redox state in the retina and brain during the onset of diabetes in rats. *Neurochem Res.* (1998) 23:893–7. doi: 10.1023/A:1022467230259
61. Bahniwal M, Little JP, Klegeris A. High glucose enhances neurotoxicity and inflammatory cytokine secretion by stimulated human astrocytes. *Curr Alzheimer Res.* (2017) 14:731–41. doi: 10.2174/1567205014666170117104053
62. During MJ, Cao L, Zuzga DS, Francis JS, Fitzsimons HL, Jiao X, et al. Glucagon-likepeptide-1 receptor is involved in learning and neuroprotection. *Nat Med.* (2003) 9:1173–9. doi: 10.1038/nm919
63. Perry T, Holloway HW, Weerasuriya A, Mouton PR, Duffy K, Mattison JA, et al. Evidence of GLP-1-mediated neuroprotection in an animal model of pyridoxine-induced peripheral sensory neuropathy. *Exp Neurol.* (2007) 203:293–301. doi: 10.1016/j.expneurol.2006.09.028
64. Hamilton A, Holscher C. Receptors for the insulin-like peptide GLP-1 are expressed on neurons in the CNS. *Neuroreport.* (2009) 20:1161–6. doi: 10.1097/WNR.0b013e32832fbf14
65. Iwai T, Ito S, Tanimitsu K, Udagawa S, Oka J. Glucagon-like peptide-1 inhibits LPS-induced IL-1beta production in cultured rat astrocytes. *Neurosci Res.* (2006) 55:352–60. doi: 10.1016/j.neures.2006.04.008
66. Gengler S, McClean P, McCurtin R, Gault VA, Hölscher C. Val(8)GLP-1 rescues synaptic plasticity and reduces dense core plaques in APP/PS1 mice. *Neurobiol Aging.* (2012) 33:265–76. doi: 10.1016/j.neurobiolaging.2010.02.014
67. Wang XH, Li L, Holscher C, Pan YF, Chen XR, QI JS. Val8-glucagon-like pep- tide-1 protects against Aβ 1-40-induced impairment of hippocampal late-phase long-term potentiation and spatial learning in rats. *Neuroscience.* (2010) 170:1239–48. doi: 10.1016/j.neuroscience.2010.08.028
68. Han W-N, Holscher C, Yuan L, Yang W, Wang XH, Wu MN, et al. Liraglutide protects against amyloid-β protein-induced impairment of spatial learning and memory in rats. *Neurobiol Aging.* (2012) 34:576-88. doi: 10.1016/j.neurobiolaging.2012.04.009
69. Perry T, Haughey NJ, Mattson MP, Egan JM, Greig NH. Protection and reversal of excitotoxic neuronal damage by glucagon-like peptide-1 and exendin-4. *J Pharmacol Exp Ther.* (2002) 302:881–8. doi: 10.1124/jpet.102.037481
70. Perry T, Lahiri DK, Sambamurti K, Chen D, Mattson MP, Egan JM, et al. Glucagon-like peptide-1 decreases endogenous amyloid-beta peptide (Abeta) levels and protects hippocampal neurons from death induced by Abeta and iron. *J Neurosci Res.* (2003) 72:603–12. doi: 10.1002/jnr.10611

7

The Clinical Obesity Maintenance Model: A Theoretical Framework for Bariatric Psychology

Jayanthi Raman[1], *Dean Spirou*[1], *Lisbeth Jahren*[2] *and Trine Tetlie Eik-Nes*[3*]

[1] *Discipline of Clinical Psychology, Graduate School of Health, University of Technology Sydney, Sydney, NSW, Australia,* [2] *Library Section for Medicine and Health Sciences, NTNU University Library, NTNU–Norwegian University of Science and Technology, Trondheim, Norway,* [3] *Department of Neuromedicine and Movement Science, Faculty of Medicine and Health Sciences, NTNU–Norwegian University of Science and Technology, Trondheim, Norway*

Correspondence:
Trine Tetlie Eik-Nes
trine.t.eik-nes@ntnu.no

Ranked highly in its association with serious medical comorbidities, obesity, a rapidly growing epidemic worldwide, poses a significant socio-economic burden. While bariatric procedures offer the most efficacious treatment for weight loss, a subset of patients risk weight recidivism. Due to the heterogeneity of obesity, it is likely that there are phenotypes or sub-groups of patients that require evidence-based psychological support to produce more sustainable outcomes. So far, however, characteristics of patients have not led to a personalized treatment algorithm for bariatric surgery. Maintenance of weight loss following bariatric surgery requires long-term modification of eating behaviors and physical activity. A recent Clinical Obesity Maintenance Model (COMM) proposed a conceptual framework of salient constructs, including the role of habit, behavioral clusters, emotion dysregulation, mood, health literacy, and executive function as interconnected drivers of obesity maintaining behaviors relevant to the field of bariatric psychology. The primary aim of this concise review is to bring together emerging findings from experimental and epidemiological studies relating to the COMM constructs that may inform the assessment and follow up of bariatric surgery. We also aim to explain the phenotypes that need to be understood and screened prior to bariatric surgery to enable better pre-surgery intervention and optimum post-surgery response.

Keywords: obesity, bariatric surgery, disordered eating, executive function, depression, health literacy, emotion dysregulation, habitual cluster behaviors

INTRODUCTION

Associated with serious medical comorbidities, obesity is a major risk factor for preventable mortality and morbidity worldwide (1). Bariatric surgery has been shown to be an effective treatment for obesity resulting in greater weight loss than non-surgical treatments (2–4). Although there is a lack of consensus about what constitutes significant weight regain in bariatric surgery studies (5), there is consensus that a subset of patients risk weight recidivism (6–8), and up to 50% of patients experience weight regain within 2 years after surgery (5).

Researchers have suggested that the mechanisms that aid initial weight loss are theoretically distinct from those associated with weight loss maintenance [e.g., (9)]. A growing number of recent studies have indicated that in addition to metabolic and surgical explanations, post-surgical weight regain may be influenced by maladaptive eating, lifestyle behaviors, and psychological co-morbidities (10). Thus, the development of a sound theoretical framework will influence the design of future studies and contribute to greater pre-surgical readiness and improved treatment of post-surgical challenges that impact weight recidivism (11).

Incorporating evidence from the fields of eating disorders (ED), neuropsychology, and obesity, the Clinical Obesity Maintenance Model (COMM; 12) has highlighted the need to examine the behavioral and psychological mechanisms that underpin longer-term weight loss maintenance. The specific executive function (EF) deficits at the center of this model [**Figure 1**; (12)], can be considered to address readiness for bariatric surgery or weight recidivism following surgery. In addition, the COMM suggests that emotion dysregulation, maladaptive habits, behavioral clusters, health literacy (HL), and mood interact with executive functioning and impact eating and physical inactivity leading to maintain obesity (12). In this mini review, we aim to summarize research on the COMM constructs from the past 7 years and provide a theoretical framework of the mechanisms that may be implicated in unsuccessful outcomes following bariatric surgery. Psychological underpinnings associated with post-surgery weight regain will be elucidated and research gaps identified.

EXECUTIVE FUNCTION

The challenge of weight recidivism has prompted researchers to explore beyond the physiological and psychological aspects of obesity (9, 13). As outlined in the COMM, emerging evidence has suggested that obesity-related disordered eating behaviors (DEB) are linked to deficits in executive functioning (EF)

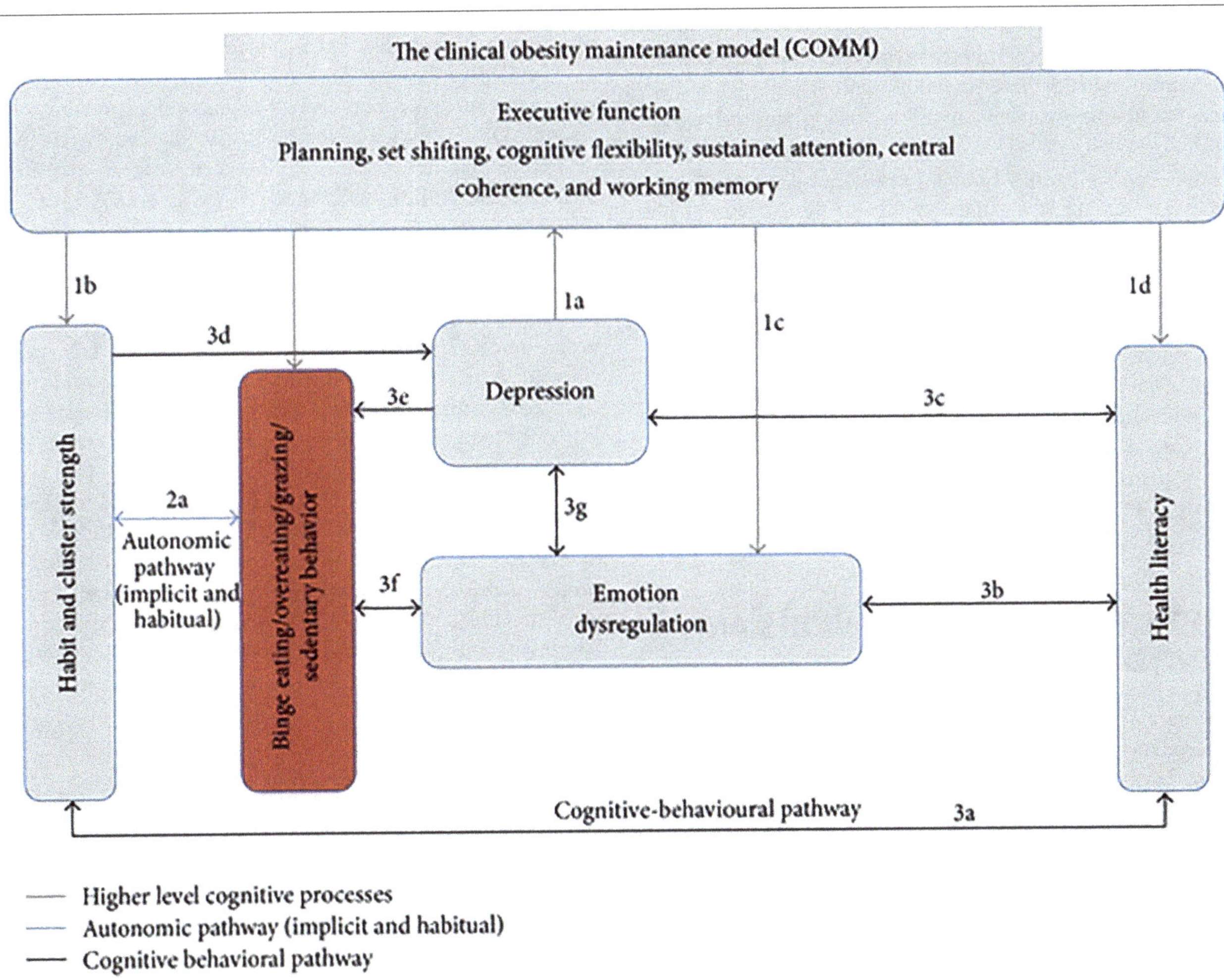

FIGURE 1 | Hypothesized model of the Clinical Obesity Maintenance Model (COMM). The letters indicate direct pathways between variables. From Raman et al. (12).

independent of differences in intelligence, level of education, and after controlling for gender, obesity severity, and age (14–18). Although not a unitary construct, EF refers to a set of cognitive processes and behavioral competencies that are involved in initiating and executing strategies, sustaining or flexibly redirecting attention, inhibiting inappropriate behavioral responses, planning, sequencing, and achievement of complex goal-oriented behavior, and cognitive flexibility (19).

A recent meta-analysis found a significant inverse relationship between obesity and EF, including cognitive flexibility, inhibition, decision-making, and planning (17). Nevertheless, the nature by which executive deficits are associated with obesity is unclear. Several plausible explanations have been proposed, including inflammation driven factors, changes in brain-derived neurotrophic factor, dopamine dysregulation implicated in hyperphagia, vascular diseases, neuroendocrine changes, and leptin [e.g., (20–22)]. Each of these factors may independently or collectively contribute to executive deficits in obesity and may influence bariatric surgery outcomes. Furthermore, the direction of this relationship remains unclear. Most studies contend that causality may occur in either direction, with impaired EF increasing the risk of obesity or obesity impacting on EF. For example, a recent systematic review found evidence of a reciprocal influence between obesity and EF (23). Supporting this interpretation, bariatric patients have demonstrated improvements in EF following surgical weight loss (24).

Executive deficits manifested through challenges in self-regulation of eating behaviors may lead to poorer weight loss maintenance after bariatric surgery (25). For example, a study of 37 bariatric surgery patients found that EF was strongly associated with adherence to post-surgical guidelines shortly after surgery (25). Supporting this notion, a recent study has shown that EF predicts a higher body mass index (BMI) 12 months after bariatric surgery (26). Similarly, poorer executive performance 12 weeks post-surgery has been found to be indicative of reduced weight loss at the 3 years follow up (27). Given this body of recent evidence, future research should further explore how best to consider executive deficits in the pre-surgery screening and follow-up of bariatric candidates.

DISORDERED EATING BEHAVIORS AND EATING DISORDERS

A substantial evidence-base supports the prevalence of disordered eating behaviors (DEB) and eating disorders (ED) in bariatric surgery outcomes [e.g., (28–31)] with two recent studies finding a higher prevalence of ED in post-surgical bariatric patients with weight regain (32, 33). In addition, Binge Eating Disorder (BED) is highly prevalent among bariatric patients (34). BED refers to eating an excessive amount of food in a discrete period of time, accompanied by a sense of LOC over eating (35). Although gastrointestinal modifications may help to restrict portion sizes post-surgery, new DEB may develop as a compensatory mechanism, with a higher frequency of energy intake (36). In support of this view, recent cross-sectional and longitudinal studies have found evidence on the association between grazing (i.e., intake of smaller portions of food over extended periods) and post-surgical weight regain [e.g., (37)]. Furthermore, researchers have emphasized the role of other DEB, such as emotional eating, night eating syndrome, and picking and nibling in bariatric surgery outcomes (37–39). One longitudinal study found that about 65% of patients with weight regain reported pre-surgery DEB (32). Thus, comprehensive pre and post-surgery assessments and intervention for ED and DEB may hold promise for optimizing bariatric outcomes.

DEPRESSION

An association between depression and obesity has been long supported by clinical and epidemiological studies (40, 41) with a recent meta-analyses providing further evidence of this relationship in bariatric surgery patients (42). A review on the psychological outcomes after bariatric surgery found that pre-surgery depression symptoms reduced at 6, 12, and 24 months after bariatric surgery; however, from 36 months onwards, depression symptoms increased and returned to pre-surgery levels (43). Similarly, a population-based study of 4,793 participants found that bariatric surgery patients had higher levels of depression than others with similar BMI and that initial reductions in depression were not maintained at the follow-up (44). Other studies have also shown that improvements in depressive symptoms following bariatric surgery may not be maintained after the initial post-surgery years (i.e., 1–3 years) and that depressive symptoms may return to baseline or worsen in some patients (45–47).

Post-surgery weight regain and depression may act as a risk factor for one another. Weight regain after surgery has been indicated as a significant risk factor for recurring or elevated depression post-surgery (48, 49). These findings are consistent with the notion that rapid post-surgery weight loss only temporarily aids the remission of depression, which later re-occurs once the surgical benefits decline (43, 50, 51). Similarly, studies have shown that depressed mood is associated with unhealthy lifestyle habits (52), emotional eating, and loss of control (LOC) eating [e.g., (53, 54)]. In particular, post-surgery depressive symptoms have been associated with ED and weight recidivism (42, 55–57). Therefore, the role of depression has important implications for post-surgery functioning and should be monitored and addressed through focused evidence-based interventions.

EMOTION DYSREGULATION

Individuals with obesity often demonstrate a dysregulated physiological response to intense emotion, known as emotional eating. Specific aspects of emotion dysregulation, such as a lowered tendency to act with emotional awareness (58), difficulty identifying emotions (59), and limited access to emotion regulation strategies (60) have been implicated. A high prevalence of emotion dysregulation in pre-surgery bariatric patients has been shown (61), and pre-surgery maladaptive eating was in one study initiated by both avoidance (of negative affect) and approach (reward sensitivity) behaviors (62). More, emotion dysregulation fully mediated the associations between emotional eating as well as eating in the absence of hunger in another study of bariatric surgery candidates (63). Distress tolerance, an aspect of emotion regulation, has been found in one study to be unrelated to 2-years post-surgical weight loss outcomes but delineated individuals opting for bariatric surgery (64). In contrast, bariatric surgery patients with greater weight loss more frequently applied emotion regulation strategies post-surgery than pre-surgery, compared to patients with lower weight loss (65). Furthermore, there is ample empirical support for a direct link between emotion dysregulation and BED (63, 65, 66), highly prevalent in bariatric patients (30, 34, 43). Accumulating evidence thus indicates that emotional regulatory factors may act as drivers to initiate and/or maintain DEB and ED in bariatric surgery patients. Consequently, future research should further explore the emotional determinants of longer-term weight loss maintenance following bariatric surgery.

HABIT

Habit has been defined as "a process by which a stimulus generates an impulse to act as a result of a learned stimulus-response association" (67). Behaviors driven by habitual automaticity require powerful intentions to override, and developing new habits involves a gradual transfer in cognitive control from purposeful actions to automatic processes (68). Poor dietary choices are likely to be perpetuated by habit (12). For example, habit strength and energy intake were significantly associated in a recent ecological momentary assessment study (69). Furthermore, researchers have asserted that grazing, a DEB described as "mindless," "distracted," and "non-anticipated," should be studied as a habitual and automatic behavior (70). This was supported in a review where a link between grazing and weight recidivism post-bariatric surgery, independent of surgery type and contextual concept of grazing was found (37). In addition, habit has been shown to partially regulate physical activity (71). More, irrespective of the amount of weight loss 6 and 12 months following bariatric surgery, patients may persist with lifestyle habits, such as physical inactivity, lower consumption of protein, fruit, and vegetables, and higher consumption of carbohydrates, sugars, and fats that place them at a high risk for weight regain (72, 73). Maladaptive pre-surgery habits and DEB may thus pose significant challenges to optimal longer-term surgical outcomes (74). Future assessments of bariatric surgery candidates should consider pre-surgery habits as a major driver of weight loss practices (75, 76).

HEALTH LITERACY

Health Literacy (HL) is another construct in the COMM that has been included as a modifiable determinant of obesity maintaining behaviors. HL has been defined as the "cognitive and social skills that determine the motivation and ability of individuals to gain access to, understand, and use information in ways which promote and maintain good health" (77). The COMM considers HL a logical prerequisite to healthy eating behaviors and an active lifestyle. Lower levels of HL are associated with excessive body weight and difficulties overcoming obesity (78) as well as increased use of unhealthy weight loss methods (79), poorer weight loss following bariatric surgery (80), and lower levels of physical activity (81). A patient's HL also contributes to decision-making regarding bariatric surgery. For example, research has found that patients with higher HL and education are more likely to elect bariatric surgery, whereas patients with lower HL and less education are less likely to opt for bariatric surgery (82). Similarly, higher pre-surgical HL is associated with successful weight loss outcomes 12 months after bariatric surgery (83). Evidence also suggests that targeting HL through primary health care interventions results in a significant reduction in weight (84). Therefore, improving one's HL may guide patients to make informed decisions about their treatment and better understand the potential implications of surgery and the barriers to longer-term weight management.

BEHAVIORAL CLUSTERS

Clustering is the co-occurrence of several risk behaviors all of which share an underlying association (85). In obesity, behavioral clusters may interact in multiple ways to maintain the condition, with potentially synergistic effects (86). In support of this view, a study found that bariatric candidates who reported pre-surgical grazing behaviors also reported more alcohol use, less physical activity, and more difficulties in post-surgery lifestyle modification (36). Similarly, longitudinal studies have indicated that pre-surgery problematic alcohol, substance, and tobacco use to be reliable correlates of post-surgery problematic alcohol and substance use in bariatric patients (87–89). Whether these maladaptive clusters are activated as coping and/or compensatory reward mechanisms in a caloric-restricted new lifestyle following bariatric surgery is yet to be explored (90). Similar to previous research that showed smoking, excessive alcohol use, unhealthy eating, and sedentary lifestyle as the salient "big four" modifiable causes of obesity (91), the above findings highlight how pattern recognition of behavioral clusters can inform future research and development of targeted interventions for bariatric surgery candidates. In addition, there is a need for bariatric research to delineate alcohol use disorder from other drug use to help identify behavioral clusters that may further inform post-surgery complications (87).

CONCLUSIONS, LIMITATIONS, AND FUTURE RESEARCH

This mini review aimed to provide a theoretical framework for bariatric psychology by summarizing emerging evidence on the psychological and behavioral constructs incorporated in the COMM. The findings of this review should be considered in light of several limitations. Firstly, a comprehensive delineation on outcome research findings from extant bariatric literature was beyond the scope of this review. For example, the magnitude and rate of weight loss outcomes and other psychological co-morbidities observed post-surgically have previously been shown to differ across types of bariatric surgeries and obesity class (92, 93). Secondly, EF, a central COMM component, has been presented as an overarching construct on account of brevity. Specific aspects of EF, in particular, cognitive flexibility may have important implications for ED and DEB and researchers have called for improved methods in pre-surgery cognitive assessment to help clarify longer term post-surgery outcomes [e.g., (94)]. Similarly, the role of depression in bariatric psychology was discussed in a broader context. Lifetime prevalence rate, type, and severity of depression and associated secondary comorbidities may play an important role in longer-term post-surgery outcomes and need to be carefully assessed at pre-surgery screening (95).

This concise review has outlined key modifiable factors and their putative pathways as interactive drivers of weight recidivism after bariatric surgery. For example, given the established links between EF and DEB, extant studies have begun to incorporate EF, binge eating, and grazing behaviors as outcome measures in the fields of eating behaviors and bariatric psychology [e.g., (36, 37, 96–98)]. Similarly, in a study comparing healthy controls and bariatric surgery patients with and without depression, obesity and depression were shown to have an additive effect on executive performance (99). This highlights the importance of addressing depression and executive deficits before and after bariatric surgery to enhance longer-term surgical outcomes. In addition, the COMM's top-down approach proposes that modification of habits rely on executive processes, which contribute to difficulties in adherence to sustainable eating following bariatric surgery. While executive processes are not typically required to perform habitual behaviors, current research has shown that EF is heavily involved when individuals aim to modify and develop new habits (100).

Under-recognized psychological difficulties and under-treated mental health may negatively impact bariatric surgery outcomes (101). To this effect, weight recidivism-specific HL, specially formulated therapies targeting ED, maladaptive habits and behavioral clusters, specific emotion regulation strategies, and evidence-based psychological therapies for depression may be offered prior to and/or following bariatric surgery. Future research could further explore these associations to gain insight into the determinants of the longer-term efficacy of bariatric surgery. The theoretical framework of COMM should also be further evaluated in bariatric studies, including the use of structural equation modeling and randomized controlled trials.

To conclude, post-surgical weight recidivism is an important public and socio-economic health issue. In addition, regaining weight after bariatric surgery has a significant impact on the patient's mental health and may lead to a recurrence of serious psychological comorbidities. A comprehensive pre-surgical psychological and behavioral assessment partnered with post-surgical management is vital in this regard. As set forth in this review, the underlying mechanisms outlined in the COMM call for a more integrative, multipronged approach in bariatric surgery assessment and care.

AUTHOR CONTRIBUTIONS

TE-N and JR conceived the study and were in charge of the overall direction and planning. LJ and DS contributed to the acquisition and screening of data. JR took the lead in writing the manuscript. All authors provided critical feedback and helped shape the review, analysis, and manuscript.

REFERENCES

1. World Health Organization. *10 Facts on Obesity*. (2017). Retrieved from: https://www.who.int/features/factfiles/obesity/en (accessed August 04, 2020).
2. Colquitt JL, Pickett K, Loveman E, Frampton GK. Surgery for weight loss in adults. *Cochrane Database Syst Rev.* (2014) 2014:CD003641. doi: 10.1002/14651858.CD003641.pub4
3. Courcoulas AP, Yanovski SZ, Bonds D, Eggerman TL, Horlick M, Staten MA, et al. Long-term outcomes of bariatric surgery: a National Institutes of Health symposium. *JAMA Surg.* (2014) 149:1323–9. doi: 10.1001/jamasurg.2014.2440
4. Adams TD, Davidson LE, Litwin SE, Kim J, Kolotkin RL, Nanjee MN, et al. Weight and metabolic outcomes 12 years after gastric bypass. *N Engl J Med.* (2017) 377:1143–55. doi: 10.1056/NEJMoa1700459
5. Karmali S, Brar B, Shi X, Sharma AM, de Gara C, Birch DW. Weight recidivism post-bariatric surgery: a systematic review. *Obes Surg.* (2013) 23:1922–33. doi: 10.1007/s11695-013-1070-4
6. Courcoulas AP, Christian NJ, Belle SH, Berk PD, Flum DR, Garcia L, et al. Weight change and health outcomes at 3 years after bariatric surgery among individuals with severe obesity. *JAMA.* (2013) 310:2416–25. doi: 10.1001/jama.2013.280928
7. King WC, Hinerman AS, Belle SH, Wahed AS, Courcoulas AP. Comparison of the performance of common measures of weight regain after bariatric surgery for association with clinical outcomes. *JAMA.* (2018) 320:1560–9. doi: 10.1001/jama.2018.14433
8. Panagiotou OA, Markozannes G, Kowalski R, Gazula A, Di M, Bond DS, et al. *Short- and Long-Term Outcomes after Bariatric Surgery in the Medicare Population*. Rockville, MD: Agency for Healthcare Research and Quality (2018).
9. Gettens KM, Gorin AA. Executive function in weight loss and weight loss maintenance: a conceptual review and novel neuropsychological model of weight control. *J Behav Med.* (2017) 40:687–701. doi: 10.1007/s10865-017-9831-5
10. Kushner RF, Sorensen KW. Prevention of weight regain following bariatric surgery. *Curr Obes Rep.* (2015) 4:198–206. doi: 10.1007/s13679-015-0146-y
11. Jumbe SE. *Post-surgical cliff after weight loss surgery: accounts of patients and their health care professionals* (Doctoral dissertation). University of the West of England, Bristol, United Kingdom (2017). Retrieved from: https://uwe-repository.worktribe.com/OutputFile/884532 (accessed August 04, 2020).
12. Raman J, Smith E, Hay P. The clinical obesity maintenance model: an integration of psychological constructs including mood, emotional regulation, disordered overeating, habitual cluster behaviours, health literacy and cognitive function. *J Obes.* (2013) 2013:240128. doi: 10.1155/2013/240128
13. Gilbert M, Raman J, Sui Z. Cognitive remediation-enabled cognitive behaviour therapy for obesity: a case series. *Eat Weight Disord.* (2019). doi: 10.1007/s40519-019-00823-4. [Epub ahead of print].
14. Jansen A, Houben K, Roefs A. A cognitive profile of obesity and its translation into new interventions. *Front Psychol.* (2015) 6:1807. doi: 10.3389/fpsyg.2015.01807

15. Lavagnino L, Arnone D, Cao B, Soares JC, Selvaraj S, Lavagnino L. Inhibitory control in obesity and binge eating disorder: a systematic review and meta-analysis of neurocognitive and neuroimaging studies. *Neurosci Biobehav Rev.* (2016) 68:714–26. doi: 10.1016/j.neubiorev.2016.06.041
16. Hayes JF, Eichen DM, Barch DM, Wilfley DE. Executive function in childhood obesity: promising intervention strategies to optimize treatment outcomes. *Appetite.* (2018) 124:10–23. doi: 10.1016/j.appet.2017.05.040
17. Yang Y, Shields GS, Guo C, Liu Y. Executive function performance in obesity and overweight individuals: a meta-analysis and review. *Neurosci Biobehav Rev.* (2018) 84:225–44. doi: 10.1016/j.neubiorev.2017.11.020
18. Segura-Serralta M, Ciscar S, Blasco L, Oltra-Cucarella J, Roncero M, Espert R, et al. Contribution of executive functions to eating behaviours in obesity and eating disorders. *Behav Cogn Psychother.* (2020). doi: 10.1017/S1352465820000260. [Epub ahead of print].
19. Robbins TW. Dissociating executive functions of the prefrontal cortex. In: Roberts AC, Robbins TW, Weiskrantz L, editors. *The Prefrontal Cortex.* Oxford: Oxford University Press (1998). p. 117–30.
20. Yao L, Bhatta A, Xu Z, Lucas R, Huo Y, Bagi Z, et al. Obesity-induced inflammation of the visceral adipose tissue is mediated by upregulation of arginase 1 in vascular endothelial cells. *Circulation.* (2016) 134:A14793. doi: 10.1161/circ.134.suppl_1.14793
21. Small DM. Dopamine adaptations as a common pathway for neurocognitive impairment in diabetes and obesity: a neuropsychological perspective. *Front Neurosci.* (2017) 11:134. doi: 10.3389/fnins.2017.00134
22. Rashidian H, Rosenblat JD, McIntyre RS, Mansur RB. Leptin, obesity, and response to ketamine. *Prog Neuropsychopharmacol Biol Psychiatry.* (2020) 98:109773. doi: 10.1016/j.pnpbp.2019.109773
23. Favieri F, Forte G, Casagrande M. The executive functions in overweight and obesity: a systematic review of neuropsychological cross-sectional and longitudinal studies. *Front Psychol.* (2019) 10:2126. doi: 10.3389/fpsyg.2019.02126
24. Handley JD, Williams DM, Caplin S, Stephens JW, Barry J. Changes in cognitive function following bariatric surgery: a systematic review. *Obes Surg.* (2016) 26:2530–7. doi: 10.1007/s11695-016-2312-z
25. Galioto R, Bond D, Gunstad J, Pera V, Rathier L, Tremont G. Executive functions predict weight loss in a medically supervised weight loss programme. *Obes Sci Pract.* (2016) 2:334–40. doi: 10.1002/osp4.70
26. Spitznagel MB, Garcia S, Miller LA, Strain G, Devlin M, Wing R, et al. Cognitive function predicts weight loss after bariatric surgery. *Surg Obes Relat Dis.* (2013) 9:453–9. doi: 10.1016/j.soard.2011.10.008
27. Spitznagel MB, Alosco M, Galioto R, Strain G, Devlin M, Sysko R, et al. The role of cognitive function in postoperative weight loss outcomes: 36-month follow-up. *Obes Surg.* (2014) 24:1078–84. doi: 10.1007/s11695-014-1205-2
28. Meule A, Heckel D, Jurowich CF, Vögele C, Kübler A. Correlates of food addiction in obese individuals seeking bariatric surgery. *Clin Obes.* (2014) 4:228–36. doi: 10.1111/cob.12065
29. Conceição EM, Utzinger LM, Pisetsky EM. Eating disorders and problematic eating behaviours before and after bariatric surgery: characterization, assessment and association with treatment outcomes. *Eur Eat Disord Rev.* (2015) 23:417–25. doi: 10.1002/erv.2397
30. Mitchell JE, King WC, Courcoulas A, Dakin G, Elder K, Engel S, et al. Eating behavior and eating disorders in adults before bariatric surgery. *Int J Eat Disord.* (2015) 48:215–22. doi: 10.1002/eat.22275
31. Parker K, Brennan L. Measurement of disordered eating in bariatric surgery candidates: a systematic review of the literature. *Obes Res Clin Pract.* (2015) 9:12–25. doi: 10.1016/j.orcp.2014.01.005
32. Conceição EM, Mitchell JE, Pinto-Bastos A, Arrojado F, Brandão I, Machado PPP. Stability of problematic eating behaviors and weight loss trajectories after bariatric surgery: a longitudinal observational study. *Surg Obes Relat Dis.* (2017) 13:1063–70. doi: 10.1016/j.soard.2016.12.006
33. Mauro MFFP, Papelbaum M, Brasil MAA, Carneiro JRI, Coutinho ESF, Coutinho W, et al. Is weight regain after bariatric surgery associated with psychiatric comorbidity? A systematic review and meta-analysis. *Obes Rev.* (2019) 20:1413–25. doi: 10.1111/obr.12907
34. Smith KE, Orcutt M, Steffen KJ, Crosby RD, Cao L, Garcia L, et al. Loss of control eating and binge eating in the 7 years following bariatric surgery. *Obes Surg.* (2019) 29:1773–80. doi: 10.1007/s11695-019-03791-x
35. American Psychiatric Association. *Diagnostic and Statistical Manual of Mental Disorders: DSM-5.* 5th ed. Washington, DC: American Psychiatric Association (2013).
36. Nicolau J, Ayala L, Rivera R, Speranskaya A, Sanchís P, Julian X, et al. Postoperative grazing as a risk factor for negative outcomes after bariatric surgery. *Eat Behav.* (2015) 18:147–50. doi: 10.1016/j.eatbeh.2015.05.008
37. Pizato N, Botelho PB, Gonçalves V, Dutra ES, de Carvalho K. Effect of grazing behavior on weight regain post-bariatric surgery: a systematic review. *Nutrients.* (2017) 9:1322. doi: 10.3390/nu9121322
38. de Zwaan M, Marschollek M, Allison KC. The night eating syndrome (NES) in bariatric surgery patients. *Eur Eat Disord Rev.* (2015) 23:426–34. doi: 10.1002/erv.2405
39. Brode CS, Mitchell JE. Problematic eating behaviors and eating disorders associated with bariatric surgery. *Psychiatr Clin North Am.* (2019) 42:287–97. doi: 10.1016/j.psc.2019.01.014
40. Rivera M, Locke AE, Corre T, Czamara D, Wolf C, Ching-Lopez A, et al. Interaction between the FTO gene, body mass index and depression: meta-analysis of 13701 individuals. *Br J Psychiatry.* (2017) 211:70–6. doi: 10.1192/bjp.bp.116.183475
41. Porras-Segovia A, Rivera M, Molina E, Lopez-Chaves D, Gutierrez B, Cervilla J. Physical exercise and body mass index as correlates of major depressive disorder in community-dwelling adults: results from the PISMA-ep study. *J Affect Disord.* (2019) 251:263–9. doi: 10.1016/j.jad.2019.01.050
42. Müller A, Hase C, Pommnitz M, de Zwaan M. Depression and suicide after bariatric surgery. *Curr Psychiatry Rep.* (2019) 21:84. doi: 10.1007/s11920-019-1069-1
43. Spirou D, Raman J, Smith E. Psychological outcomes following surgical and endoscopic bariatric procedures: a systematic review. *Obes Rev.* (2020) 21:e12998. doi: 10.1111/obr.12998
44. Gulliford MC, Charlton J, Booth HP, Fildes A, Ashworth M, Rudisill C. Costs and outcomes of increasing access to bariatric surgery for obesity: cohort study and cost-effectiveness analysis using electronic health records. *Health Serv Deliv Res.* (2016) 4:65–71. doi: 10.3310/hsdr04170
45. Booth H, Khan O, Prevost AT, Reddy M, Charlton J, Gulliford M. Impact of bariatric surgery on clinical depression. Interrupted time series study with matched controls. *J Affect Disord.* (2015) 174:644–9. doi: 10.1016/j.jad.2014.12.050
46. Ivezaj V, Grilo CM. When mood worsens after gastric bypass surgery: characterization of bariatric patients with increases in depressive symptoms following surgery. *Obes Surg.* (2015) 25:423–9. doi: 10.1007/s11695-014-1402-z
47. Ribeiro G, Giapietro H, Belarmino L, Salgado-Junior W. Depression, anxiety, and binge eating before and after bariatric surgery: problems that remain. *Arq Brasil Cirurg Digest.* (2018) 31:E1356. doi: 10.1590/0102-672020180001e1356
48. Mitchell JE, King WC, Chen JY, Devlin MJ, Flum D, Garcia L, et al. Course of depressive symptoms and treatment in the longitudinal assessment of bariatric surgery (LABS-2) study. *Obesity.* (2014) 22:1799–806. doi: 10.1002/oby.20738
49. White MA, Kalarchian MA, Levine MD, Masheb RM, Marcus MD, Grilo CM. Prognostic significance of depressive symptoms on weight loss and psychosocial outcomes following gastric bypass surgery: a prospective 24-month follow-up study. *Obes Surg.* (2015) 25:1909–16. doi: 10.1007/s11695-015-1631-9
50. Andersen JR. Quality of life following laparoscopic sleeve gastrectomy. *Surg Obes Relat Dis.* (2015) 11:76–8. doi: 10.1016/j.soard.2014.06.003
51. Lynch A. "When the honeymoon is over, the real work begins:" gastric bypass patients' weight loss trajectories and dietary change experiences. *Soc Sci Med.* (2016) 151:241–9. doi: 10.1016/j.socscimed.2015.12.024
52. Romain AJ, Marleau J, Baillot A. Impact of obesity and mood disorders on physical comorbidities, psychological well-being, health behaviours and use of health services. *J Affect Disord.* (2018) 225:381–8. doi: 10.1016/j.jad.2017.08.065
53. van Strien T, Konttinen H, Homberg JR, Engels RC, Winkens LH. Emotional eating as a mediator between depression and weight gain. *Appetite.* (2016) 100:216–24. doi: 10.1016/j.appet.2016.02.034

54. Mills JG, Larkin TA, Deng C, Thomas SJ. Weight gain in major depressive disorder: linking appetite and disordered eating to leptin and ghrelin. *Psychiatry Res.* (2019) 279:244–51. doi: 10.1016/j.psychres.2019.03.017
55. Wiedemann AA, Ivezaj V, Grilo CM. An examination of emotional and loss-of-control eating after sleeve gastrectomy surgery. *Eat Behav.* (2018) 31:48–52. doi: 10.1016/j.eatbeh.2018.07.008
56. King WC, Belle SH, Hinerman AS, Mitchell JE, Steffen KJ, Courcoulas AP. Patient behaviors and characteristics related to weight regain after Roux-en-Y gastric bypass: a multicenter prospective cohort study. *Ann Surg.* (2019). doi: 10.1097/SLA.0000000000003281. [Epub ahead of print].
57. Freire CC, Zanella MT, Segal A, Arasaki CH, Matos MIR, Carneiro G. Associations between binge eating, depressive symptoms and anxiety and weight regain after Roux-en-Y gastric bypass surgery. *Eat Weight Disord.* (2020). doi: 10.1007/s40519-019-00839-w. [Epub ahead of print].
58. Höppener MM, Larsen JK, van Strien T, Ouwens MA, Winkens LHH, Eisinga R. Depressive symptoms and emotional eating: mediated by mindfulness? *Mindfulness.* (2019) 10:670–8. doi: 10.1007/s12671-018-1002-4
59. Kass AE, Wildes JE, Coccaro EF. Identification and regulation of emotions in adults of varying weight statuses. *J Health Psychol.* (2019) 24:941–52. doi: 10.1177/1359105316689604
60. Braden A, Musher-Eizenman D, Watford T, Emley E. Eating when depressed, anxious, bored, or happy: are emotional eating types associated with unique psychological and physical health correlates? *Appetite.* (2018) 125:410–7. doi: 10.1016/j.appet.2018.02.022
61. Schäfer L, Hübner C, Carus T, Herbig B, Seyfried F, Kaiser S, et al. Identifying prebariatric subtypes based on temperament traits, emotion dysregulation, and disinhibited eating: a latent profile analysis. *Int J Eat Disord.* (2017) 50:1172–82. doi: 10.1002/eat.22760
62. Ouellette AS, Rodrigue C, Lemieux S, Tchernof A, Biertho L, Bégin C. An examination of the mechanisms and personality traits underlying food addiction among individuals with severe obesity awaiting bariatric surgery. *Eat Weight Disord.* (2017) 22:633–40. doi: 10.1007/s40519-017-0440-7
63. Baldofski S, Rudolph A, Tigges W, Herbig B, Jurowich C, Kaiser S, et al. Weight bias internalization, emotion dysregulation, and non-normative eating behaviors in prebariatric patients. *Int J Eat Disord.* (2016) 49:180–5. doi: 10.1002/eat.22484
64. Koball AM, Himes SM, Sim L, Clark MM, Collazo-Clavell ML, Mundi M, et al. Distress tolerance and psychological comorbidity in patients seeking bariatric surgery. *Obes Surg.* (2016) 26:1559–64. doi: 10.1007/s11695-015-1926-x
65. Efferdinger C, König D, Klaus A, Jagsch R. Emotion regulation and mental well-being before and six months after bariatric surgery. *Eat Weight Disord.* (2017) 22:353–60. doi: 10.1007/s40519-017-0379-8
66. Leehr EJ, Krohmer K, Schag K, Dresler T, Zipfel S, Giel KE. Emotion regulation model in binge eating disorder and obesity: a systematic review. *Neurosci Biobehav Rev.* (2015) 49:125–34. doi: 10.1016/j.neubiorev.2014.12.008
67. Gardner B. A review and analysis of the use of 'habit' in understanding, predicting and influencing health-related behaviour. *Health Psychol Rev.* (2015) 9:277–95. doi: 10.1080/17437199.2013.876238
68. Orbell S, Verplanken B. The strength of habit. *Health Psychol Rev.* (2015) 9:311–7. doi: 10.1080/17437199.2014.992031
69. Wouters S, Jacobs N, Duif M, Lechner L, Thewissen V. Negative affective stress reactivity: the dampening effect of snacking. *Stress Health.* (2018) 34:286–95. doi: 10.1002/smi.2788
70. Heriseanu AI, Hay P, Corbit L, Touyz S. Grazing in adults with obesity and eating disorders: a systematic review of associated clinical features and meta-analysis of prevalence. *Clin Psychol Rev.* (2017) 58:16–32. doi: 10.1016/j.cpr.2017.09.004
71. Gardner B, Phillips LA, Judah G. Habitual instigation and habitual execution: definition, measurement, and effects on behaviour frequency. *Br J Health Psychol.* (2016) 21:613–30. doi: 10.1111/bjhp.12189
72. King WC, Bond DS. The importance of preoperative and postoperative physical activity counseling in bariatric surgery. *Exerc Sport Sci Rev.* (2013) 41:26–35. doi: 10.1097/JES.0b013e31826444e0
73. Soares FL, Bissoni de Sousa L, Corradi-Perini C, Ramos da Cruz MR, Nunes MG, Branco-Filho AJ. Food quality in the late postoperative period of bariatric surgery: an evaluation using the bariatric food pyramid. *Obes Surg.* (2014) 24:1481–6. doi: 10.1007/s11695-014-1198-x
74. Correia Horvath JD, Dias de Castro ML, Kops N, Kruger Malinoski N, Friedman R. Obesity coexists with malnutrition? Adequacy of food consumption by severely obese patients to dietary reference intake recommendations. *Nutr Hospit.* (2014) 29:292–9. doi: 10.3305/nh.2014.29.2.7053
75. Matei R, Thuné-Boyle I, Hamer M, Iliffe S, Fox KR, Jefferis BJ, et al. Acceptability of a theory-based sedentary behaviour reduction intervention for older adults ('On Your Feet to Earn Your Seat'). *BMC Public Health.* (2015) 15:606. doi: 10.1186/s12889-015-1921-0
76. Cleo G, Isenring E, Thomas R, Glasziou P. Could habits hold the key to weight loss maintenance? A narrative review. *J Hum Nutr Dietet.* (2017) 30:655–64. doi: 10.1111/jhn.12456
77. Berkman ND, Davis TC, McCormack L. Health literacy: what is it? *J Health Commun.* (2010) 15:9–19. doi: 10.1080/10810730.2010.499985
78. Michou M, Panagiotakos DB, Costarelli V. Low health literacy and excess body weight: a systematic review. *Central Eur J Public Health.* (2018) 26:234–41. doi: 10.21101/cejph.a5172
79. Raffoul A, Hammond D. Correlates of weight-loss methods among young adults in Canada. *Obesity.* (2018) 26:1357–64. doi: 10.1002/oby.22218
80. Mahoney ST, Strassle PD, Farrell TM, Duke MC. Does lower level of education and health literacy affect successful outcomes in bariatric surgery? *J Laparoendosc Adv Surg Tech A.* (2019) 29:1011–5. doi: 10.1089/lap.2018.0806
81. Laz TH, Rahman M, Pohlmeier AM, Berenson AB. Level of nutrition knowledge and its association with weight loss behaviors among low-income reproductive-age women. *J Commun Health.* (2015) 40:542–8. doi: 10.1007/s10900-014-9969-9
82. Cayci HM, Erdogdu UE, Demirci H, Ardic A, Topak NY, Taymur I. Effect of health literacy on help-seeking behavior in morbidly obese patients agreeing to bariatric surgery. *Obes Surg.* (2018) 28:791–7. doi: 10.1007/s11695-017-2882-4
83. Erdogdu UE, Cayci HM, Tardu A, Demirci H, Kisakol G, Guclu M. Health literacy and weight loss after bariatric surgery. *Obes Surg.* (2019) 29:3948–53. doi: 10.1007/s11695-019-04060-7
84. Faruqi N, Spooner C, Joshi C, Lloyd J, Dennis S, Stocks N, et al. Primary health care-level interventions targeting health literacy and their effect on weight loss: a systematic review. *BMC Obes.* (2015) 2:6. doi: 10.1186/s40608-015-0035-7
85. Teh CH, Teh MW, Lim KH, Kee CC, Sumarni MG, Heng PP, et al. Clustering of lifestyle risk behaviours and its determinants among school-going adolescents in a middle-income country: a cross-sectional study. *BMC Public Health.* (2019) 19:1177. doi: 10.1186/s12889-019-7516-4
86. Biddle SJH, Pearson N, Salmon J. Sedentary behaviors and adiposity in young people: causality and conceptual model. *Exerc Sport Sci Rev.* (2018) 46:18–25. doi: 10.1249/jes.0000000000000135
87. Spadola CE, Wagner EF, Dillon FR, Trepka MJ, De La Cruz-Munoz N, Messiah SE. Alcohol and drug use among postoperative bariatric patients: a systematic review of the emerging research and its implications. *Alcohol Clin Exp Res.* (2015) 39:1582–601. doi: 10.1111/acer.12805
88. Li L, Wu LT. Substance use after bariatric surgery: a review. *J Psychiatr Res.* (2016) 76:16–29. doi: 10.1016/j.jpsychires.2016.01.009
89. Kanji S, Wong E, Akioyamen L, Melamed O, Taylor VH. Exploring pre-surgery and post-surgery substance use disorder and alcohol use disorder in bariatric surgery: a qualitative scoping review. *Int J Obes.* (2019) 43:1659–74. doi: 10.1038/s41366-019-0397-x
90. Blackburn AN, Hajnal A, Leggio L. The gut in the brain: the effects of bariatric surgery on alcohol consumption. *Addict Biol.* (2017) 22:1540–53. doi: 10.1111/adb.12436
91. Poortinga W. The prevalence and clustering of four major lifestyle risk factors in an English adult population. *Prev Med.* (2007) 44:124–8. doi: 10.1016/j.ypmed.2006.10.006
92. De Lorenzo A, Soldati L, Sarlo F, Calvani M, Di Lorenzo N, Di Renzo L. New obesity classification criteria as a tool for bariatric surgery indication. *World J Gastroenterol.* (2016) 22:681–703. doi: 10.3748/wjg.v22.i2.681
93. Arterburn D, Wellman R, Emiliano A, Smith S, Odegaard A, Murali S, et al. Comparative effectiveness and safety of bariatric procedures for

weight loss: a PCORnet cohort study. *Ann Intern Med.* (2018) 169:741–55. doi: 10.7326/M17-2786

94. Spitznagel MB, Hawkins M, Alosco M, Galioto R, Garcia S, Miller L, et al. Neurocognitive effects of obesity and bariatric surgery. *Eur Eat Disord Rev.* (2015) 23:488–95. doi: 10.1002/erv.2393
95. Da Silva VB, Da Silva RB, Azorin JM, Belzeaux R. Mood disorders are highly prevalent but underdiagnosed among patients seeking bariatric surgery. *Obes Surg.* (2015) 25:543–4. doi: 10.1007/s11695-014-1557-7
96. Dohle S, Diel K, Hofmann W. Executive functions and the self-regulation of eating behavior: a review. *Appetite.* (2018) 124:4–9. doi: 10.1016/j.appet.2017.05.041
97. Turton R, Nazar BP, Burgess EE, Lawrence NS, Cardi V, Treasure J, et al. To go or not to go: a proof of concept study testing food-specific inhibition training for women with eating and weight disorders. *Eur Eat Disord Rev.* (2018) 26:11–21. doi: 10.1002/erv.2566
98. Preuss H, Leister L, Pinnow M, Legenbauer T. Inhibitory control pathway to disinhibited eating: a matter of perspective? *Appetite.* (2019) 141:104297. doi: 10.1016/j.appet.2019.05.028
99. Restivo MR, McKinnon MC, Frey BN, Hall GB, Syed W, Taylor VH. The impact of obesity on neuropsychological functioningin adults with and without major depressive disorder. *PLoS ONE.* (2017) 12:e0176898. doi: 10.1371/journal.pone.0176898
100. Kwasnicka D, Dombrowski SU, White M, Sniehotta F. Theoretical explanations for maintenance of behaviour change: a systematic review of behaviour theories. *Health Psychol Rev.* (2016) 10:277–96. doi: 10.1080/17437199.2016.1151372
101. Rudolph A, Hilbert A. Cognitive-behavioral therapy for postbariatric surgery patients with mental disorders: a pilot study. *Front Psychiatry.* (2020) 11:14. doi: 10.3389/fpsyt.2020.00014

8

Bariatric Surgery and Type 1 Diabetes: Unanswered Questions

*Emmanouil Korakas [1], Aikaterini Kountouri [1], Athanasios Raptis [1], Alexander Kokkinos [2] and Vaia Lambadiari [1]**

[1] Second Department of Internal Medicine, Medical School, Attikon University Hospital, National and Kapodistrian University of Athens, Athens, Greece, [2] First Department of Propaedeutic Medicine, Medical School, Laiko General Hospital, National and Kapodistrian University of Athens, Athens, Greece

***Correspondence:**
Vaia Lambadiari
vlambad@otenet.gr

In recent decades there has been an alarming increase in the prevalence of obesity in patients with type 1 diabetes leading to the development of insulin resistance and cardiometabolic complications, with mechanisms poorly clarified. While bariatric surgery has long been considered an effective treatment option for patients with type 2 diabetes, the evidence regarding its benefits on weight loss and the prevention of complications in T1DM patients is scarce, with controversial outcomes. Bariatric surgery has been associated with a significant reduction in daily insulin requirement, along with a considerable reduction in body mass index, results which were sustained in the long term. Furthermore, studies suggest that bariatric surgery in type 1 diabetes results in the improvement of comorbidities related to obesity including hypertension and dyslipidemia. However, regarding glycemic control, the reduction of mean glycosylated hemoglobin was modest or statistically insignificant in most studies. The reasons for these results are yet to be elucidated; possible explanations include preservation of beta cell mass and increased residual function post-surgery, improvement in insulin action, altered GLP-1 function, timing of surgery, and association with residual islet cell mass. A number of concerns regarding safety issues have arisen due to the reporting of peri-operative and post-operative adverse events. The most significant complications are metabolic and include diabetic ketoacidosis, severe hypoglycemia and glucose fluctuations. Further prospective clinical studies are required to provide evidence for the effect of bariatric surgery on T1DM patients. The results may offer a better knowledge for the selection of people living with diabetes who will benefit more from a metabolic surgery.

Keywords: bariatric surgery, type 1 diabetes mellitus, obesity, weight loss, glycosylated hemoglobin, GLP-1, insulin sensitivity

INTRODUCTION

In recent decades, the prevalence of obesity and metabolic syndrome among patients with type 1 diabetes mellitus (T1DM) has alarmingly increased. In a study by Liu et al., the percentage of obesity among patients with diabetes aged 3–19 years old in the U.S. was 12.6%, with another 22.1% found to be overweight (1). The prevalence of obesity was even higher in a study by Price et al. (2), reaching up to 17.2%, with 38.3% of the 501 adults studied found to be overweight. Many other studies have shown similar results regardless of the age of the patients studied (3–6); in general, ~50% of patients with T1DM are overweight or obese, with 8–40% meeting the diagnostic criteria for metabolic syndrome (7). The reasons for this kind of epidemic have not been clarified; however, it seems that intensive insulin regimens to achieve optimal glycemic targets along with the frequent use of simple sugars by the patients to overcome hypoglycemic episodes are the main factors. Obesity is a major threat for patients with T1DM as it triggers a vicious cycle where weight gain leads to insulin resistance which, in turn, leads to increased insulin requirements to achieve glycemic control, resulting in further weight gain. Furthermore, obesity accelerates the occurrence of T1DM at a younger age in patients with a genetic predisposition to the disease (8, 9), while it is related to an increased rate of micro- and macrovascular complications (2, 10).

Bariatric surgery has long been considered an effective treatment for patients with obesity and type 2 diabetes mellitus (T2DM). In 1995, Pories et al. (11) were the first to demonstrate that 82.9% of patients with T2DM and 98.7% of patients with impaired glucose tolerance (IGT) achieved euglycemia for a follow-up period of 14 years after bariatric surgery without antidiabetic medication, and similar results were shown in a study by Buchwald et al. (12), where improvement on glycemic control or total remission of diabetes was observed in 86.6% of the patients studied. As the beneficial metabolic effects on these patients were attributed mainly to weight loss and the concomitant enhancement of insulin sensitivity, the application of bariatric surgery in patients with obesity and T1DM was discouraged, since insulin deficiency rather than insulin resistance was regarded as the main pathophysiologic mechanism of the disease. Nevertheless, the fact that improvements in glycemic control in T2DM patients take place in the course of the first few days after the surgery, before substantial weight loss is achieved, implies that other, weight-loss-independent mechanisms are also responsible for the metabolic amelioration (13). Data on the effects of bariatric surgery in T1DM is scarce, based mainly on case series with relatively few patients and several case reports, and results are conflicting. In this review, our primary end points are to present the existing data about the results of bariatric surgery on T1DM patients concerning weight loss, reduction in insulin requirements, changes in glycosylated hemoglobin (HbA1c) and metabolic comorbidities, along with the main complications and risks, especially diabetic ketoacidosis (DKA) and hypoglycemia. We then discuss the physiological pathways through which bariatric surgery exerts its beneficial effects and special concerns regarding T1DM patients.

BARIATRIC SURGERY OUTCOMES IN TYPE 1 DIABETES MELLITUS

Bariatric surgery procedures used to be classified as either restrictive or malabsorptive, depending on their mechanism of action; however, this terminology has been abandoned, as it has been shown that each procedure exerts its effects through multiple mechanisms. The main procedures include (a) adjustable gastric banding (AGB) where an adjustable gastric band is placed around the upper part of the stomach to reduce the stomach size, (b) vertical sleeve gastrectomy (VSG), where a tubular stomach is created by partial gastrectomy of the greater curvature side, (c) Roux-en-Y gastric bypass (RYGB), where a small gastric pouch is created from the proximal portion of stomach and is connected to the distal end of the small intestine by gastro-jejunal anastomosis, while entero-enteral anastomosis 100–150 cm distal to the gastro-jejunostomy site restores bowel continuity between the bilio-pancreatic limb and the alimentary limb, and (d) biliopancreatic diversion (BPD) with or without duodenal switch, where gastrectomy is done to reduce the stomach capacity, the stomach is connected to the distal small intestine and the excluded bilio-pancreatic limb is connected to the alimentary limb distally. The most commonly applied procedures are RYGB and VSG (14). However, all these techniques have been mainly studied in T2DM; studies that refer to T1DM are mostly retrospective, with a limited number of patients with heterogeneous characteristics. The most beneficial results are observed in terms of weight loss and daily insulin requirements, while data about improvements in HbA1c demonstrate modest and contradictory outcomes. The main results are summarized in **Table 1**.

Outcomes in Weight Loss

Bariatric surgery offers a significant reduction in body mass index (BMI) in patients with obesity and T1DM which is sustained in long term. Czupryniak et al. (15) were the first to show a marked improvement in the mean BMI of three women with obesity who underwent RYGB from 42.2 kg/m^2 preoperatively to 33.5 kg/m^2 post-operatively in a follow-up period of ~7 years. After an ~3-years follow-up time, mean reductions in BMI were 11.1, 8.3, and 9.4 kg/m^2 in other cohorts (20–22). In a relatively large cohort of 32 subjects with obesity studied for 4.6 years, the mean percentage of total weight loss (%TWL) at 12 months after surgery was 30.4%, with a slight decrease at 5 years, reaching 28.1% (23). Cumulatively, a meta-analysis by Chow et al. (34), including 86 patients in total, showed a reduction in BMI of 13.42 kg/m^2 post-operatively. Another meta-analysis by Ashrafian et al. (35), including 142 patients in total, showed a mean BMI decrease of 11.04 kg/m^2, in a mean follow-up time of 31.8 months. In general, similar results have been demonstrated by every study on the field regardless of the type of intervention applied, the number of patients or the follow-up period (16–19, 24–32, 36).

Outcomes in Insulin Requirements

The reduction in body weight after surgery is accompanied by a reduction in total daily insulin requirements in patients with obesity and T1DM. Middelbeek et al. (29) evaluated the post-surgical outcomes in 10 women with T1DM at 1 and 5 years after RYGB. Daily insulin requirements were decreased from 53 to 23 units/day at 1 year, with a slight increase in 31.1 units/day at 5 years, presenting a strong correlation with body weight which followed a similar trend. In accordance with weight loss outcomes, insulin requirements were reduced in the reports by Brethauer et al. (20) and Lannoo et al. (21), with a mean change of 0.34 units/kg/day and 56.33 units/day, respectively. In a study by Robert et al. (25), where the procedures applied on 10 patients with T1DM were either biliopancreatic diversion (BPD) or sleeve gastrectomy (SG), the daily insulin dose was

TABLE 1 | Effects of bariatric surgery on weight loss, daily insulin requirements and glycosylated hemoglobin in patients with obesity and type 1 diabetes mellitus.

References	Patients (n)	Mean duration of T1DM (years)	Mean duration of follow-up	Procedures (*n*)	Mean BMI loss (kg/m²)	Alteration in insulin requirements IU/day (u/kg/d)	Alterations in HbA1C
Czupryniak et al. (15)	3	11.6	75.6 months	RYGB (3)	8.7	46.4	−1.13%
Mendez et al. (16)	3	25	12 months	RYGB (3)	16.5	56.33	+0.07%
Fuertes-Zamorano et al. (17)	2	29.5	54 months	BPD (2)	23	1st patient: 0.23 u/k/d 2nd patient: 0.29 u/kg/d	−1.4%
Chuang et al. (18)	2	5.5	20 months	RYGB (1) SG (1)	18.1	1st patient: −25 IU/day (+0.1 u/kg/d) 2nd patient: −40 IU/day (no difference in u/kg/d)	1st patient: +0.2% 2nd patient: +3.7%
Tang et al. (19)	6	18	16 months	AGB (3) SG (2) RYGB (1)	11.4	Reduced in all cases	+0.1%
Brethauer et al. (20)	10	22	36.8 months	RYGB (7) AGB (2) SG (1)	11.1	0.34 u/kg/d	−1.1%
Lannoo et al. (21)	22	25.3	37.8 months	RYGB (16) SG (6)	8.3	44.5	−0.2% (non-significant)
Landau et al. (22)	26	20.2	3.5 years	SG (19) RYGB (4) AGB (3)	8.4	NA	+0.1%
Vilarrasa et al. (23)	32	20	4.6 years	SG (15) RYGB (11) BPD (6)	9	50.9	−0.6% at 12 months, return to baseline at endpoint
Raab et al. (24)	6	17.16	20 months	BPD (3) RYGB (2) SG (1)	13.8	67.4	−1.23%
Robert et al. (25)	10	23.1	55.1 months	BPD (7) SG (3)	16.56	0.65 u/kg/d	−0.4% (non-significant)
Blanco et al. (26)	7	27.3	24 months	RYGB (7)	12.1	+ 0.1 u/kg/d	−0.1% (non-significant)
Reyes- Garcia et al. (27)	1	24	10 months	RYGB (1)	14.6	Reduction	1.3%
Rottenstreich et al. (28)	13	19.1	24 months	SG (10) RYGB (3)	8.8	38	−0.8% (non-significant)
Middelbeek et al. (29)	10	24.6	5 years	RYGB (10)	9.7	21.9	+1.7%
Maraka et al. (30)	7	20.6	2 years	RYGB (9) SG (1)	13.1	19.7	−0.4%
Faucher et al. (31)	13	21	12 months	SG (7) RYGB (6)	11.5	0.35 u/kg/d	−0.7%
Al Sabah et al. (32)	10	NA	4 years	SG (10)	10.5	58.4	−0.3% (non-significant)
Moreno-Fernandez et al. (33)	6	24.2	4.5 years	RYGB (3) SG (3)	14.2	16.1	−0.6% (non-significant)

RYGB, R-n-Y gastric bypass; SG, sleeve gastrectomy; BPD, biliopancreatic diversion; AGB, adjustable gastric banding; IU, international units; NA, not applicable; HbA1c, glycosylated hemoglobin A1c; T1DM, type 1 diabetes mellitus.

diminished from 1.09 to 0.44 units/kg/day during a mean follow-up of 55.1 months. The sustained reduction in insulin dose is confirmed in the meta-analyses mentioned above (34, 35) where, irrespectively of the follow-up period, the post-operative decrease in insulin requirements was 42 units/day and 0.391 units/kg/day, respectively.

Outcomes in HbA1c

In contrast to the results concerning weight loss and insulin requirements, the effects of bariatric surgery on HbA1c seem to be inconsistent among studies. Czupryniak et al. (15) and Raab et al. (24) showed a statistically significant mean decrease in HbA1c of 1.13 and 1.23% at 7 and 1 year after surgery, respectively. Similar results were shown by Brethauer et al. (20), where the mean decrease was 1.1%, and by Fuertes-Zamorano et al. (17), who showed a mean decrease of 1% in two patients who underwent BPD at 5 years post-surgery. However, these favorable outcomes come into contradiction with those in other studies. In the study by Middelbeek et al. (29), the HbA1c was unchanged at 1 year after surgery (8.1–8.3%) and, even more interestingly, it was increased at 5 years post-operatively to 9.8%. This transient, modest improvement was observed in other studies (21–23, 26, 28). Overall, as the available meta-analyses indicate, the average mean change in HbA1c ranges from 0.64 to 0.93% (34, 35); in any case, the optimal target of ≤7% is not reached, meaning that bariatric surgery seems to be barely beneficial in terms of glycemic control. The reasons for this discrepancy are yet to be explained and are discussed below.

Outcomes in Co-morbidities

The evidence about the impact of bariatric surgery on the common metabolic co-morbidities that accompany T1DM combined with excess weight (so called "double diabetes") is scarce, as many of the already limited studies on the field did not include such risk factors in their endpoints. However, some existing data is encouraging (**Table 2**). Brethauer et al. (20) showed a reduction in the levels of low-density lipoprotein (LDL) and triglycerides (TG) of 23 and 30.5 mg/dl, respectively, along with an increase in high-density lipoprotein (HDL) of 10.8 mg/dl. Hypertension resolved in 5 out of 7 hypertensive patients and albuminuria resolved in 1 out of 2 patients who presented microalbuminuria preoperatively. Chuang et al. (18) reported on two adolescents who underwent bariatric surgery. The first one achieved a significant amelioration in his lipid profile (LDL decreased from 180 mg/dl to 81 mg/dl and HDL increased from 32 to 45 mg/dl at 12 months after surgery) and quit statin agents, while he presented with a tremendous improvement in his obstructive sleep apnea. The second patient, suffering from polycystic ovarian syndrome (PCOS) as well, presented a similar improvement in lipids (LDL decreased from 109 to 73 mg/dl and HDL increased from 41 mg/dl to 59 mg/dl at 28 months after surgery) and managed to stop oral contraceptives and restore regular menses. In a long-term cohort, the number of patients with dyslipidemia, obstructive sleep apnea, hypertension and microalbuminuria was decreased by 25, 66, 42.8, and 25%, respectively (23). A considerable decrease of 26.9 mg/dl in triglycerides was observed by Fernandez (33), who studied 6 patients who underwent either RYGB or SG for a mean follow-up of 4.5 years. In the systematic review by Ashrafian (35), it was estimated that the mean decreases in systolic blood pressure (SBP) and diastolic blood pressure (DBP) were 10.1 and 6.193 mmHg, respectively. Regarding lipid profile, LDL and TGs were reduced by a 9.54 and 11.04 mg/dl, whereas HDL was increased by a mean 13.51 mg/dl. It must be noted, however, that these results were extracted from a very limited number of studies of acceptable quality.

COMPLICATIONS OF BARIATRIC SURGERY

Bariatric surgery procedures are generally considered safe. The average perioperative mortality is <0.3%, comparable to this of appendicectomy or cholecystectomy. The 1-year complication rate varies among different procedures, being 4.6, 10.8, 14.9, and 25.7% for AGB, VSG, RYGB, and BPD, respectively (37). The factors that negatively affect the incidence of adverse events after surgery include male sex, the presence of co-morbidities, high pre-operative BMI, old age, and the lack of adequate experience of the surgical team. Among patients with T1DM, no excess in mortality has been reported (38). Apart from the common complications of bariatric surgery, however, an increased prevalence of diabetic ketoacidosis (DKA) and hypoglycemia has been observed (**Table 3**).

Diabetic Ketoacidosis

Diabetic ketoacidosis is a life-threatening condition which is not uncommon in patients with T1DM after bariatric surgery. In a study by Aminian et al. (39), the incidence of DKA in the early post-operative period (0–61 days) in T1DM patients was reported to be as high as 25%. Three out of the eight T1DM patients who developed ketoacidosis had a previous episode and all of them had poor glycemic control preoperatively with a mean HbA1c of 9.3%. In another cohort, 15% of patients had an episode of DKA within 48 h after surgery due to insufficient insulin dosage post-operatively (22). Similar results were reported by Maraka et al. (30), where 20% of T1DM patients who underwent surgery had an episode of ketoacidosis contrary to no incidents in the T2DM group, while in the group of Rottenstreich et al. (28), the incidence of DKA within the first months after surgery was 21.4%. However, DKA poses as a threat even in the long term; 3 out of a total of 32 T1DM patients studied for almost 4.5 years presented with episodes of ketoacidosis within 3 years after surgery (23). Apart from the obviously high prevalence of this complication, another interesting fact is that, in the setting of the reduced carbohydrate intake that follows surgery along with the continued insulin regimen, diabetic ketoacidosis may not necessarily present with hyperglycemia, as in the recently reported case of a 43 years-old woman who developed euglycemic diabetic ketoacidosis 10 days after she underwent sleeve gastrectomy (40). Rather than altered glucose kinetics, it seems that poor peri-operative glycemic control with discontinuation or inadequate intake of insulin is the main precipitating factor that leads to DKA; others include anesthesia, surgical stress, infection, and fluid and calorie deprivation (39).

Hypoglycemia

Hypoglycemia is a relatively frequent complication in T1DM patients undergoing bariatric surgery, reaching an incidence of even 70% (30). The majority of cases pertains to the early post-operative period; in three different cohorts, the rate of hypoglycemic episodes was 18% (32), 23% (22), and 29% (28) within the first few days to months after surgery. Altered glucose kinetics, with the rapid delivery of carbohydrates to the jejunum create an imbalance between the higher and earlier glucose excursions and the action of exogenous insulin, while the improvement in insulin sensitivity that follows weight loss renders the previously needed insulin dosages to become excessive. However, no surgical procedure seems to prevent such episodes, despite the fact that sleeve gastrectomy is considered, in general, to be safer due to a more predictable pattern of carbohydrate absorption. Among 32 patients who underwent either biliopancreatic diversion, sleeve gastrectomy

TABLE 2 | Effects of bariatric surgery on metabolic comorbidities in patients with obesity and type 1 diabetes mellitus.

References	Patients (*n*)	Mean duration of follow-up	Procedures (*n*)	Effects on co-morbidities
Czupryniak et al. (15)	3	75.6 months	RYGB (3)	Improvements in blood pressure, lipid profile, microalbuminuria
Fuertes-Zamorano et al. (17)	2	54 months	BPD (2)	1st patient: resolution of dyslipidemia 2nd patient: resolution of dyslipidemia and hypertension
Chuang et al. (18)	2	20 months	RYGB (1) SG (1)	1st patient: no treatment for dyslipidemia, sleep apnea 2nd patient: restoration of regular menses, stop OCP
Brethauer et al. (20)	10	36.8 months	RYGB (7) AGB (2) SG (1)	Improvements in LDL (−23 ± 19.3 mg/dl), HDL (10.8 ± 3.4 mg/dl), TG (−30.5 ± 17.1 mg/dl). Resolution of HTN in 5/7 patients, resolution of albuminuria in 1/2 patients.
Landau et al. (22)	26	3.5 years	SG (19) RYGB (4) AGB (3)	Improvements in hypertension, HDL increase
Vilarrasa et al. (23)	32	4.6 years	SG (15) RYGB (11) BPD (6)	Remission of HTN, dyslipidemia and OSA in 42.8, 25, and 66%, respectively. Regression of microalbuminuria to normoalbuminuria in 25%.
Robert et al. (25)	10	55.1 months	BPD (7) SG (3)	Remission of hypertension in 66.7%, dyslipidemia in 88.9%
Rottenstreich et al. (28)	13	24 months	SG (10) RYGB (3)	Resolution of hypertension in 4 patients
Middelbeek et al. (29)	10	5 years	RYGB (10)	HDL increase by 22% at 5 years. Improvements in triglycerides and SBP at 1 year but not at 5 years
Maraka et al. (30)	7	2 years	RYGB (9) SG (1)	Decrease in lipid-lowering medications
Moreno-Fernandez et al. (33)	6	4.5 years	RYGB (3) SG (3)	Remission of HTN in 1/3 patients. Improvements in TG (−26.9 ± 15.1 mg/dl)

HDL, high-density lipoprotein; OCP, oral contraceptives; SBP, systolic blood pressure; OSA, obstructive sleep apnea; HTN, hypertension; LDL, low-density lipoprotein; TG, triglycerides; RYGB, R-n-Y gastric bypass; SG, sleeve gastrectomy; BPD, biliopancreatic diversion; AGB, adjustable gastric banding.

or R-n-Y gastric bypass, three patients (9.3%) developed severe hypoglycemic episodes within the first year after surgery, one after each procedure applied (23). In a study by Faucher et al. (31), a median of four minor hypoglycemic episodes per week was reported at 6 months after surgery, with more cases being associated with sleeve gastrectomy (median 6 cases) rather than R-n-Y gastric bypass (median 3.5 cases). It is therefore evident that a close monitoring of glucose levels along with careful insulin titration according to the carbohydrate load of each meal is of vital importance in the early post-operative period in order to prevent hypoglycemic episodes regardless of the surgical method used. In this respect, sensor-augmented insulin pump therapy with automated insulin suspension has been related to more stable glycemic control in some patients (16, 26), however, adequate data regarding the most efficient type of insulin after surgery is not available.

Other Complications

As mentioned above, the rate of surgical complication ranges from 4 to 25%, depending on the procedure applied. However, these rates are constantly declining thanks to the improvement in surgical techniques and the existence of more and more experienced bariatric surgery centers. Wound infection and post-operative bleeding, which can derive from the omental or mesenteric vessels or the anastomotic site, are the most common short-term complications after surgery (41). Pulmonary embolism is another common adverse event with a risk of 2% and, along with anastomotic leak, are the leading causes of death in the early post-operative period. Among the late complications, marginal ulcers, anastomotic stenosis, cholelithiasis, and hernias are the most frequent ones. Among the T1DM population, another common concern is the presence of autonomic neuropathy and gastroparesis, which can lead to complication, such as nausea, vomiting, and acute gastric remnant dilation (38, 42).

The most common and serious complications of bariatric surgery are nutritional deficiencies, which occur mainly in malabsorptive rather than in restrictive procedures (43–46). The main nutrients affected are iron, vitamin B12, folic acid, calcium, and fat-soluble vitamins (A, D, E, K). Iron deficiency, depending on the procedure, has a risk of 13–52% within the first 5 years after surgery, and is attributed to reduced gastric acid production. Vitamin B12 deficiency can occur in up to 70% of patients after RYGB and is due to the failure of separation of B12 from food and to inadequate secretion of the intrinsic factor (47, 48). Folic acid deficiency is less frequent (up to 35% in patients after RYGB) and its causes include achlorhydria, bypassing of the duodenum, reduced dietary intake and vitamin B12 deficiency (48, 49). As calcium is preferentially absorbed in the duodenum and proximal jejunum, the exclusion of these segments leads to malabsorption and hypocalcemia, whose incidence can reach up to 10% after surgery, while the rate of vitamin D deficiency is

TABLE 3 | Incidence of diabetic ketoacidosis and hypoglycemia after bariatric surgery in patients with type 1 diabetes mellitus and obesity.

References	Patients (*n*)	Mean duration of T1DM (years)	Mean duration of follow-up	Procedures (*n*)	DKA before surgery	DKA after surgery	Hypoglycemia before surgery	Hypoglycemia after surgery
Chuang et al. (18)	2	5.5	20 months	RYGB (1) SG (1)	Patient 1: 1 episode Patient 2: (–)	Patient 1: (–) Patient 2: 1 episode	(–)	Patient 1: Mild hypoglycemic episodes 2 to 5 times per week Patient 2: Mild hypoglycemic episodes 2 to 5 times per week
Aminian et al. (39)	12	NA	90 days	RYGB (6) SG (4) AGB (2)	3 patients (25%)	Severe: 3 Moderate: 3 Mild: 6	NA	NA
Maraka et al. (30)	7	20.6	2 years	RYGB (9) SG (1)	NA	2 patients	NA	7 patients
Vilarrasa et al. (23)	32	20	4.6 years	SG (15) RYGB (11) BPD (6)	(-)	2 patients (one had a recurrent episode)	(-)	3 patients (9.3%)—severe
Landau et al. (22)	26	20.2	3.5 years	SG (19) RYGB (4) AGB (3)	NA	4 patients (within 48 h after surgery)	NA	6 patients shortly after discharge–2 patients hospitalized
Faucher et al. (31)	13	21	12 months	SG (7) RYGB (6)	NA	NA	(-)	Median number of minor episodes at 6 months: RYGB: 3.5 SG: 6 2 severe episodes
Al Sabah et al. (32)	10	NA	4 years	SG (10)	NA	NA	NA	2 patients (18.2%)

DKA, diabetic ketoacidosis; NA, not applicable; RYGB, R-n-Y gastric bypass; SG, sleeve gastrectomy; BPD, biliopancreatic diversion; AGB, adjustable gastric banding.

up to 51% (50, 51). The result is the development of secondary hyperparathyroidism, which leads to increased release of calcium from bones and, eventually, loss of bone mass and osteoporosis (52–54). Regardless of the operation performed, all patients who have undergone bariatric surgery should follow a close nutritional monitoring on a regular basis, receiving appropriate supplements when necessary.

Finally, the most recent concern regarding post-surgical complications are psychosocial disorders (55). As the gastrointestinal anatomy after RYGB and SG favors the rapid absorption of alcohol, the rate of alcohol misuse events in these patients is increased and poses as a substitute to their previous food addiction (56–58). Even more alarmingly, the risk of suicide after bariatric surgery seems to rise. In the Utah Mortality Study, a significant increase in the number of suicides, poisonings and accidental deaths after RYGB was observed, and similar were the results in the second Utah Obesity Study (59, 60). In 2010, Tindle et al. (61) reported 31 suicides in a total of 16.683 bariatric surgery operations (overall rate of 6.6/10.000), with 70% of the events occurring within the first 3 years after surgery. In a review by Peterhansel et al. (62) the suicide rate after surgery was estimated to be 4.1/10.000 person-years. A similar trend was shown in 2017 by Laggeros et al. (63), where it was also indicated that episodes of self-harm and depression were more frequent after gastric bypass in patients with a pre-existing psychiatric condition. These data underline the importance of a comprehensive evaluation of the psychiatric status of patients both prior to and after surgery by a multidisciplinary team of experienced healthcare professionals, so that timely identification and management of such conditions is achieved (64).

GLUCOSE HOMEOSTASIS AFTER BARIATRIC SURGERY AND SPECIAL CONCERNS IN T1DM

As bariatric surgery has only recently been considered as a therapeutic option for T1DM, evidence concerning the possible mechanisms through which it impacts glucose metabolism has been obtained from studies on human and animal models with T2DM. Weight loss, calorie restriction and gastrointestinal hormone modulation are some of the mechanisms which have been described to play an important role in the remission of T2DM after bariatric surgery (65). The effect of these mechanisms in T1DM has not yet been elicited due to the different pathogenesis comparing to T2DM. However, the fact that bariatric surgery results in a significant reduction of insulin requirements and an, at least modest, reduction in HbA1c in T1DM patients, implies the existence of a shared background between these two types of the disease on which surgery exerts mutually beneficial effects. The discrepancies, nevertheless, in the post-operative glycemic control in T1DM are a serious concern that needs to be elucidated. To discuss these concerns, a brief presentation of the main mechanisms through which surgery acts on glucose metabolism is required.

Mechanisms of Glycemic Improvement

Beta Cell Function and Insulin Secretion

Bariatric surgery attenuates the dysfunction of beta cells by increasing beta cell sensitivity (66). As it is obvious, in the setting of T1DM, such an action is meaningful only in cases of residual beta cell function. The physiological pathways which mediate this enhancement have been poorly clarified. Caloric restriction, removal of glucose toxicity and gastrointestinal hormone modulation have been proposed; however, it seems that a main mechanism is the enhanced glucagon-like peptide-1 (GLP-1) secretion after surgery. The rapid and early delivery of nutrients to the distal small intestine potentiates the secretion of distal gut peptides, mainly glucagon-like peptide-1 (GLP-1) and peptide YY (PYY) (67). Post-prandial concentration of GLP-1 rises almost 10-fold in the first few days after RYGB, and similar increases are observed after SG and BPD, but not after AGB (68–70). The importance of exaggerated post-prandial responses of GLP-1 post-operatively has not been studied specifically in T1DM patients after metabolic surgery, however it has been confirmed in studies where the GLP-1 receptor was blocked with exendin (9–39) and blunted insulin responses were reported after meals (71, 72). In a study by Scrocchi et al. (73), a defective glucose-stimulated insulin secretion was noted in mice which were deprived of the GLP-1 receptor in β-cells (GLP-1R$^{-/-}$), while in another murine model of diabetes, the administration of GLP-1R agonist exendin-4 attenuated translational downregulation of insulin and improved beta cell survival (74). Similarly, in a tamoxifen-inducible GLP-1R knockout mouse model, augmentation of glucose-stimulated insulin secretion during an oral glucose tolerance test (OGTT) after VSG was blunted in the knockout mice compared to the control group (75); such results were reproduced in another study on humans after RYGB, where administration of exendin 9–39 decreased insulin concentrations (12.3 ± 2.2 vs. 18.1 ± 3.1 nmol/6 h) and β-cell response to glucose post-prandially compared to controls (76). In addition, some researchers have attributed post-RYGB hyperinsulinemic hypoglycemia to GLP-1-mediated expansion of β-cell mass (nesidioblastosis) (77, 78), with reversal of the symptoms after blockade of GLP-1 receptor with exendin 9–39 (79). Contrary to these results, a human study comparing RYGB patients with a group undergoing an intensive lifestyle modification therapy showed no differences in glucose tolerance deterioration after the infusion of exendin 9–39 (80). Similar results were demonstrated in animal studies, where the infusion of exendin 9–39 in GLP-1R$^{-/-}$ and wild type mice which underwent RYGB or VSG resulted in similar glucose tolerance (81, 82). Therefore, the role of enhanced GLP-1 secretion after bariatric surgery on β-cell function remains to be clarified. As for the other major incretin, glucose-dependent insulinotropic polypeptide (GIP), evidence is inconsistent, with studies showing contradictory responses after either SG or RYGB (83–85).

Hepatic and Peripheral Insulin Resistance

The improvement of insulin sensitivity in the early post-operative period is attributed to enhanced hepatic insulin sensitivity (86). This is achieved via a reduction in the liver fat content through increased lipolysis and lipid oxidation (87). It seems that caloric restriction, which occurs immediately after all types of surgical procedures, is the main factor that leads to enhanced hepatic insulin sensitivity. In a study where patients who underwent RYGB were compared with a group who consumed the same very low-calorie diet (VLCD) of 200–300 kcal/day, the improvement in HOMA insulin resistance was 25% 4 days after surgery and similar between the two groups (88). Similar were the results in two other studies, where changes in insulin sensitivity and insulin secretion were either similar or even superior in the first days after RYGB compared to VLCD (89, 90). In another study by Gastaldelli et al. (91), insulin sensitivity was estimated in a group of 20 patients using the more precise method of the hyperinsulinemic-euglycemic clamp, conducted 1 week after a very-low-calorie diet and 1 week after RYGB or LAGB. Both types of surgery led to substantial improvements in hepatic insulin sensitivity and lipolysis compared to diet alone, while RYGB also led to enhanced adipose insulin sensitivity and M/I (peripheral insulin sensitivity divided by the steady-state plasma insulin concentration). Similar results were demonstrated in another study with human subjects, where the hyperinsulinemic-euglycemic clamp 1 week after RYGB showed enhanced hepatic insulin sensitivity and increased insulin clearance (86). On the other hand, in the late post-operative period, peripheral insulin sensitivity is augmented as a result of the substantial weight loss that has been achieved at that point, and a positive correlation has been observed (68, 87). Muscelli et al. (92), using the insulin clamp technique in patients who underwent either RYGB or BPD, showed an enhancement in peripheral insulin sensitivity both in the RYGB group (23.8 ± 6.0 μmol/min/kg at 5 months and 33.7 ± 11.3 μmol/min/kg at 16 months) and in the BPD group (52.5 ± 12.4 μmol/min/kg at 6 months and 68.7 ± 9.5 μmol/min/kg at 24 months) after comparable weight loss (53 kg on average). In agreement with these findings, Campos et al. (93) compared patients who underwent RYGB to patients who remained on diet alone at 14 days and 6 months post-surgery, and showed that peripheral glucose uptake, despite being similar at 14 days, was substantially enhanced only in the RYGB group at 6 months. This enhancement is, again, multifactorial. The increase in anorexigenic hormones (GLP-1, PYY, oxyntomodulin) induces early satiety and limited calorie intake. GLP-1 affects the brain indirectly, through vagal nerve fibers in the intestine, whereby it transmits various signals to the nucleus of the solitary tract (NTS), an area in the brain which plays a crucial role in regulating feeding patterns (94). GLP-1R signaling attenuates the release of the orexigenic neuropeptides Neuropeptide Y (NPY) and agouti-related peptide (AgRP), and enhances the release of the anorexigenic neuropeptides pro-opiomelanocortin (POMC) and cocaine- and amphetamine-regulated transcript (CART) (95, 96); it increases thermogenesis in brown adipose tissue (BAT) through enhancing sympathetic nervous system activity (97); and inhibits neuronal activity in reward processing areas as functional magnetic resonance imaging (fMRI) studies in obese and T2DM patients have shown (98). PYY levels are parallel to those of GLP-1, and therefore, are also increased after gastric bypass but not after gastric banding (99, 100). In addition, as studies in both human and animal models have shown, the levels of bile acids are increased after RYGB (but not after SG or AGB), leading to increased secretion of GLP-1 through the TGR5 receptor on L-cells, while they also induce synthesis of fibroblast growth factor 19 (FGF19) on ileal enterocytes which enhances insulin sensitivity through boosting mitochondrial activity (101–104). Finally, metabolic surgery does not contribute only to the decrease of BMI in general, but actually leads to a redistribution of overall body fat mass, while the visceral and intramuscular depot are also reduced, effects which are also mediated, at least in part, by GLP-1, which can induce increased thermogenesis in BAT through various molecular pathways (65, 94, 105). The improvement in visceral fat and glucose uptake by the skeletal muscle is a result of enhanced insulin sensitivity and the increased GLP-1 levels, which promote glycogen synthesis, glycogen synthase α (GSα) activity and glucose metabolism and, on the other hand, inhibit glycogen phosphorylase α activity, as various studies in both animal and human models have demonstrated (94), while these morphological changes in adipose tissue lead to decreased levels of leptin and other pro-inflammatory cytokines and increased levels of adiponectin (106, 107). The role of gut microbiota in insulin sensitivity is still to be elucidated (101, 108).

Glucose Metabolism

Glucose absorption is diminished after RYGB and VSG. Regarding RYGB, altered bile acids kinetics lead to the absence of sodium in the alimentary limb, which is necessary for the endoluminal absorption of glucose via the apical sodium glucose cotransporter 1 (SGLT1) (109), while regarding SG, the reduction in glucose absorption is attributed to the reduced leptin- and ghrelin-expressing cells (65). Ghrelin is an orexigenic gut hormone that is produced in gastric fundus and whose post-prandial suppression is diminished in individuals with obesity. SG decreases both fasting and post-prandial levels of ghrelin, but such suppression has been shown in RYGB as well, while other studies have shown no change or even an increase (110–112). In addition, after RYGB (but not after SG), the alimentary limb presents mucosal hypertrophy and hyperplasia, which amplifies glucose utilization from the gut (113). Finally, it has been postulated that the exclusion of nutrients from the duodenum eliminates an, unknown, "factor" with anti-incretin properties which leads to hyperglycemia (101). In a study in mice, the group which underwent RYGB presented an increased activity of phosphoenolpyruvate carboxykinase (PEPCK) and glucose-6-phosphatase (Glc6Pase) enzymes in the distal jejunum and ileum, thus promoting intestinal gluconeogenesis raising glucose concentration in the portal vein, an effect which is potentiated by GLP-1 and eventually leads to suppressed hepatic glucose production and improved glucose tolerance. These effects were not observed in mice treated with gastric banding (which does not cause redirection of nutrients), as well as in mice with downregulation of the glucose transporter 2 (GLUT2), which is essential for hepato-portal sensing and is stimulated after RYGB (114, 115).

Glycemic Control in T1DM: Who Benefits?

As the above discussed mechanisms reveal, the major pathway through which bariatric surgery beneficially affects glycemic control in T1DM is the enhancement in insulin sensitivity. "Double diabetes" (DD) is the term used to describe the type of the disease which is characterized by the occurrence of factors typical of both type 1 and type 2 diabetes; insulin resistance and autoimmunity against beta cells (116). DD can occur when a patient with T2DM develops autoantibodies against beta cells or when an individual with T1DM becomes obese and consequently develops hepatic and peripheral insulin resistance. Nevertheless, glycemic control after bariatric surgery is far from optimal, and the explanation for this is probably multifactorial. Firstly, in some studies, post-operative inhibition of glucagon secretion was not detected despite the increased GLP-1 secretion. In the study by Blanco et al. (26), where seven women with T1DM were compared with seven women with T2DM for 24 months after RYGB, the similarly enlarged post-prandial GLP-1 secretion between the two groups was not accompanied by suppression but rather by an increase in glucagon secretion. Similar were the findings by Dirksen et al. (117) in a patient at 12 months after RYGB, where the 7-fold increase in GLP-1 was accompanied by an only slight decrease in post-prandial glucagon levels. In addition, the absence of residual β-cell function in the majority of T1DM patients renders any mechanism that improves insulin secretion useless. The three available studies which directly compared the effects of surgery in T1DM and T2DM patients demonstrated impressive decreases in HbA1c in patients with C-peptide positive T2DM requiring insulin therapy but not in those with C-peptide negative T1DM (25, 26, 30). However, as a number of investigators have reported the presence of residual insulin-positive beta cells in patients with T1DM (118, 119), timing of surgery becomes crucial, as GLP-1-mediated effects can help preserve beta cell mass and delay progression to total insulin deficiency if the operation is conducted early in the course of the disease.

Another cause of "remission" of diabetes and exacerbations in glycemic control after an initial improvement in HbA1c after surgery is that the type of diabetes is often misdiagnosed, with many patients actually suffering from latent autoimmune diabetes of the adult (LADA). LADA is defined as a type of T1DM which is characterized by slow development and partial autoimmune destruction of beta cell with onset between 30 and 55 years of age (120). LADA accounts for 9–25% of adults with diabetes in the general population; in a large meta-analysis on bariatric surgery outcomes on T1DM, the rate of patients with LADA was 3.3%. The diagnosis of LADA is based on low fasting and meal-stimulated C-peptide levels and on existence of antibodies against glutamic acid decarboxylase (GAD65), insulin and/or islet cells. The secretory burden on beta cells elicited by insulin resistance leads to their subsequent apoptosis if the burden is prolonged and this is why at the early stages, adequate glycemic control can be achieved with antidiabetic oral medication, whereas in the progression of the disease insulin will be eventually required (121). Robert et al. (25) have reported a case with latent autoimmune diabetes who weaned off insulin 2 years after bariatric surgery. In the literature a case has also been reported in which sleeve gastrectomy induced remission of slowly progressive type 1 diabetes in an patient with obesity (122), with the most impressive results observed in a Japanese cohort of 5 patients with a low mean titer of anti-glutamic acid decarboxylase antibody, where mean HbA1c was reduced from 8.4 to 5.7% 1 year after sleeve gastrectomy with or without duodenojejunal bypass (123). This evidence highlights the importance of meticulous screening for LADA pre-operatively, especially in patients with poorly controlled diabetes on oral antidiabetic medication or with a history of DKA or autoimmune diseases, as early surgical intervention to preserve residual beta cell mass and function is even more important in these patients, who are the best candidates for metabolic surgery among T1DM patients. The surgery of choice is still unclear, however, even in these patients; while Robert et al. (25) showed that BPD was superior to SG in terms of weight loss, insulin requirements and resolution of dyslipidemia, other studies (124) suggest that RYGB offer the best risk-to-benefit ratio.

CONCLUSION

The prevalence of obesity and metabolic syndrome in patients with T1DM has increased significantly. The term "Double Diabetes" has been introduced to describe this type of diabetes in which factors typical of both type 1 and type 2 diabetes co-exist. Bariatric surgery has been suggested as an effective treatment for these patients, although data is scarce, based on case series and retrospective studies. Bariatric surgery results in a significant reduction in body mass index, in total daily insulin requirements and in co-morbidities related to obesity. However, its effect on glycemic control in T1DM is controversial, as sustainable and meaningful reductions in HbA1c have not been invariably achieved. Apart from the common complications of BS, diabetic ketoacidosis and hypoglycemia are life threatening conditions with increased prevalence in T1DM patients, which require special concern and whose causal mechanisms are still unclear. Improvement in beta cell function, reduction of hepatic and peripheral resistance and modifications in glucose absorption are some of the mechanisms through which BS improves glycemic control in both type 1 and type 2 diabetes suggesting that the two types of diabetes have partially a common pathophysiological pathway; however, the inadequate glycemic control post-surgery has not yet been explained. In conclusion, bariatric surgery is not yet to be recommended routinely to all T1DM patients. For the time being, those patients with LADA considered the most appropriate candidates for surgery when the operation is conducted at the early stages of the disease, as the surgical intervention preserves beta cell mass and delays progression to total insulin deficiency. For all the other T1DM patients, a careful and multidisciplinary approach is necessary, where individualized and realistic goals will be set. Randomized, prospective trials are required to conclusively evaluate the effects of surgery in T1DM both in short and long term and define the most suitable candidates who will benefit the most out of it.

AUTHOR CONTRIBUTIONS

All authors listed have made a substantial, direct and intellectual contribution to the work, and approved it for publication.

REFERENCES

1. Liu LL, Lawrence JM, Davis C, Liese AD, Pettitt DJ, Pihoker C, et al. Prevalence of overweight and obesity in youth with diabetes in USA: the SEARCH for diabetes in youth study. *Pediatr Diabetes.* (2010) 11:4–11. doi: 10.1111/j.1399-5448.2009.00519.x
2. Price SA, Gorelik A, Fourlanos S, Colman PG, Wentworth JM. Obesity is associated with retinopathy and macrovascular disease in type 1 diabetes. *Obes Res Clin Pract.* (2014) 8:178–82. doi: 10.1016/j.orcp.2013.03.007
3. Vestberg D, Rosengren A, Olsson M, Gudbjörnsdottir S, Svensson AM, Lind M. Relationship between overweight and obesity with hospitalization for heart failure in 20,985 patients with type 1 diabetes: a population-based study from the Swedish National diabetes registry. *Diabetes Care.* (2013) 36:2857–61. doi: 10.2337/dc12-2007
4. Islam ST, Abraham A, Donaghue KC, Chan AK, Lloyd M, Srinivasan S, et al. Plateau of adiposity in Australian children diagnosed with Type 1 diabetes: a 20-year study. *Diabet Med.* (2014) 31:686–90. doi: 10.1111/dme.12402
5. Baskaran C, Volkening LK, Diaz M, Laffel LM. A decade of temporal trends in overweight/obesity in youth with type 1 diabetes after the diabetes control and complications trial. *Pediatr Diabetes.* (2014) 16:263–70. doi: 10.1111/pedi.12166
6. Holt SK, Lopushnyan N, Hotaling J, Sarma AV, Dunn RL, Cleary PA, et al. Prevalence of low testosterone and predisposing risk factors in men with type 1 diabetes mellitus: findings from the DCCT/EDIC. *J Clin Endocrinol Metab.* (2014) 99:E1655–60. doi: 10.1210/jc.2014-1317
7. Chillarón JJ, Goday A, Flores-Le-Roux JA, Benaiges D, Carrera MJ, Puig J, et al. Estimated glucose disposal rate in assessment of the metabolic syndrome and microvascular complications in patients with type 1 diabetes. *J Clin Endocrinol Metab.* (2009) 94:3530–4. doi: 10.1210/jc.2009-0960
8. Fourlanos S, Narendran P, Byrnes GB, Colman PG, Harrison LC. Insulin resistance is a risk factor for progression to type 1 diabetes. *Diabetologia.* (2004) 47:1661–7. doi: 10.1007/s00125-004-1507-3
9. Franck M, Paquot N, Scheen AJ. Influence of body weight on the natural history of and the therapeutic approaches to type 1 diabetes. *Rev Med Liege.* (2012) 67:461–7.
10. De Block CE, De Leeuw IH, Van Gaal LF. Impact of overweight on chronic microvascular complications in type 1 diabetic patients. *Diabetes Care.* (2005) 28:1649–55. doi: 10.2337/diacare.28.7.1649
11. Pories WJ, Swanson MS, MacDonald KG, Long S, Morris PG, Brown BM, et al. Who would have thought it? An operation proves to be the most effective therapy for adult-onset diabetes mellitus. *Ann Surg.* (1995) 222:339–50. doi: 10.1097/00000658-199509000-00011
12. Buchwald H, Estok R, Fahrbach K, Banel D, Jensen MD, Pories WJ, et al. Weight and type 2 diabetes after bariatric surgery: systematic review and meta-analysis. *Am J Med.* (2009) 122:e5. doi: 10.1016/j.amjmed.2008.09.041
13. Batterham RL, Cummings DE. Mechanisms of diabetes improvement following bariatric/metabolic surgery. *Diabetes Care.* (2016) 39:893–901. doi: 10.2337/dc16-0145
14. Vasas P, Por F. Surgical options for reducing body weight. *Orv Hetil.* (2014) 155:971–7. doi: 10.1556/OH.2014.29844
15. Czupryniak L, Wiszniewski M, SzymaÅski D, PawÅowski M, Loba J, Strzelczyk J. Long-term results of gastric bypass surgery in morbidly obese type 1 diabetes patients. *Obes Surg.* (2010) 20:506–8. doi: 10.1007/s11695-010-0074-6

16. Mendez CE, Tanenberg RJ, Pories W. Outcomes of Roux-en-Y gastric bypass surgery for severely obese patients with type 1 diabetes: a case series report. *Diabetes Metab Syndr Obes.* (2010) 3:281–3. doi: 10.2147/DMSO.S9981
17. Fuertes-Zamorano N, Sanchez-Pernaute A, Torres Garcia AJ, Rubio Herrera MA. Bariatric surgery in type 1 diabetes mellitus; long-term experience in two cases. *Nutr Hosp.* (2013) 28:1333–6. doi: 10.3305/nh.2013.28.4.6605
18. Chuang J, Zeller MH, Inge T, Crimmins N. Bariatric surgery for severe obesity in two adolescents with type 1 diabetes. *Pediatrics.* (2013) 132:e1031–4. doi: 10.1542/peds.2012-3640
19. Tang A, Milner KL, Tonks K, Campbell LV, Greenfield JR. Comment on Brethauer et al. Bariatric surgery improves the metabolic profile of morbidly obese patients with type 1 diabetes. *Diabetes Care.* (2014) 37:e248–9. doi: 10.2337/dc14-0578
20. Brethauer SA, Aminian A, Rosenthal RJ, Kirwan JP, Kashyap SR, Schauer PR. Bariatric surgery improves the metabolic profile of morbidly obese patients with type 1 diabetes. *Diabetes Care.* (2014) 37:e51–2. doi: 10.2337/dc13-1736
21. Lannoo M, Dillemans B, Van Nieuwenhove Y, Fieuws S, Mathieu C, Gillard P, et al. Bariatric surgery induces weight loss but does not improve glycemic control in patients with type 1 diabetes. *Diabetes Care.* (2014) 37:e173–4. doi: 10.2337/dc14-0583
22. Landau Z, Kowen-Sandbank G, Jakubowicz D, Raziel A, Sakran N, Zaslavsky-Paltiel I, et al. Bariatric surgery in patients with type 1 diabetes: special considerations are warranted. *Ther Adv Endocrinol Metab.* (2019) 10:2042018818822207. doi: 10.1177/2042018818822207
23. Vilarrasa N, Rubio MA, Miñambres I, Flores L, Caixàs A, Ciudin A, et al. Long-term outcomes in patients with morbid obesity and type 1 diabetes undergoing bariatric surgery. *Obes Surg.* (2017) 27:856–63. doi: 10.1007/s11695-016-2390-y
24. Raab H, Weiner RA, Frenken M, Rett K, Weiner S. Obesity and metabolic surgery in type 1 diabetes mellitus. *Nutr Hosp.* (2013) 28:31–4. doi: 10.3305/nh.2013.28.sup2.6711
25. Robert M, Belanger P, Hould FS, Marceau S, Tchernof A, Biertho L. Should metabolic surgery be offered in morbidly obese patients with type I diabetes? *Surg Obes Relat Dis.* (2015) 11:798–805. doi: 10.1016/j.soard.2014.12.016
26. Blanco J, Jiménez A, Casamitjana R, Flores L, Lacy A, Conget I, et al. Relevance of beta-cell function for improved glycemic control after gastric bypass surgery. *Surg Obes Relat Dis.* (2014) 10:9–13. doi: 10.1016/j.soard.2013.07.020
27. Reyes Garcia R, Romero Munoz M, Galbis Verdu H. Bariatric surgery in type 1 diabetes. *Endocrinol Nutr.* (2013) 60:46–7. doi: 10.1016/j.endoen.2013.01.003
28. Rottenstreich A, Keidar A, Yuval JB, Abu-Gazala M, Khalaileh A, Elazary R. Outcome of bariatric surgery in patients with type 1 diabetes mellitus: our experience and review of the literature. *Surg Endosc.* (2016) 30:5428–33. doi: 10.1007/s00464-016-4901-2
29. Middelbeek RJ, James-Todd T, Cavallerano JD, Schlossman DK, Patti ME, Brown FM. Gastric bypass surgery in severely obese women with type 1 diabetes: anthropometric and cardiometabolic effects at 1 and 5 years postsurgery. *Diabetes Care.* (2015) 38:e104–5. doi: 10.2337/dc15-0396
30. Maraka S, Kudva YC, Kellogg TA, Collazo-Clavell ML, Mundi MS. Bariatric surgery and diabetes: implications of type 1 vs. insulin-requiring type 2. *Obesity (Silver Spring).* (2015) 23:552–57. doi: 10.1002/oby.20992
31. Faucher P, Poitou C, Carette C, Tezenas du Montcel S, Barsamian C, Touati E, et al. Bariatric surgery in obese patients with type 1 diabetes: effects on weight loss and metabolic control. *Obes Surg.* (2016) 26:2370–8. doi: 10.1007/s11695-016-2106-3
32. Al Sabah S, Al Haddad E, Muzaffar TH, Almulla A. Laparoscopic sleeve gastrectomy for the management of type 1 diabetes mellitus. *Obes Surg.* (2017) 27:3187–93. doi: 10.1007/s11695-017-2777-4
33. Moreno-Fernandez J, Chico A, Working Group of Diabetes and Technology of the Spanish Diabetes Association, Spain. Bariatric surgery results in patients with type 1 diabetes mellitus on continuous subcutaneous insulin infusion therapy. *Endocrinol Nutr.* (2016) 63:571–2. doi: 10.1016/j.endoen.2016.09.014
34. Chow A, Switzer NJ, Dang J, Shi X, de Gara C, Birch DW, et al. A systematic review and meta-analysis of outcomes for type 1 diabetes after bariatric surgery. *J Obes.* (2016) 2016:6170719. doi: 10.1155/2016/6170719
35. Ashrafian H, Harling L, Toma T, Athanasiou C, Nikiteas N, Efthimiou E, et al. Type 1 diabetes mellitus and bariatric surgery: a systematic review and meta-analysis. *Obes Surg.* (2015) 26:1697–704. doi: 10.1007/s11695-015-1999-6
36. Middelbeek RJ, James-Todd T, Patti ME, Brown FM. Short-term insulin requirements following gastric bypass surgery in severely obese women with type 1 diabetes. *Obes Surg.* (2014) 24:1442–6. doi: 10.1007/s11695-014-1228-8
37. Demaria EJ, Winegar DA, Pate VW, Hutcher NE, Ponce J, Pories WJ. Early postoperative outcomes of metabolic surgery to treat diabetes from sites participating in the ASMBS bariatric surgery center of excellence program as reported in the Bariatric outcomes longitudinal database. *Anna Surg.* (2010) 252:559–67. doi: 10.1097/SLA.0b013e3181f2aed0
38. Kirwan, J.P., Aminian A, Kashyap SR, Burguera B, Brethauer SA, Schauer PR. Bariatric surgery in obese patients with type 1 diabetes. *Diabetes Care.* (2016) 39:941–8. doi: 10.2337/dc15-2732
39. Aminian A, Kashyap SR, Burguera B, Punchai S, Sharma G, Froylich D, et al. The incidence and clinical features of diabetic ketoacidosis after bariatric and metabolic surgery. *Diabetes Care.* (2016) 39:e50–3. doi: 10.2337/dc15-2647
40. Dowsett, J., Humphreys R, Krones R. Normal blood glucose and high blood ketones in a critically unwell patient with T1DM post-bariatric surgery: a case of euglycemic diabetic ketoacidosis. *Obes Surg.* (2019) 29:347–49. doi: 10.1007/s11695-018-3548-6
41. Raveendran AV, Chacko EC, Pappachan JM. Non-pharmacological treatment options in the management of diabetes mellitus. *Eur Endocrinol.* (2018) 14:31–9. doi: 10.17925/EE.2018.14.2.31
42. Han SH, White S, Patel K, Dutson E, Gracia C, Mehran A. Acute gastric remnant dilation after laparoscopic Roux-en-Y gastric bypass operation in long-standing type I diabetic patient: case report and literature review. *Surg Obes Relat Dis.* (2006) 2:664–6. doi: 10.1016/j.soard.2006.08.005
43. Gletsu-Miller N, Wright BN. Mineral malnutrition following bariatric surgery. *Adv Nutr.* (2013) 4:506–17. doi: 10.3945/an.113.004341
44. Brolin RE, Leung M. Survey of vitamin and mineral supplementation after gastric bypass and biliopancreatic diversion for morbid obesity. *Obes Surg.* (1999) 9:150–4. doi: 10.1381/096089299765553395
45. Halverson JD. Micronutrient deficiencies after gastric bypass for morbid obesity. *Am Surg.* (1986) 52:594–8.
46. Decker GA, Swain JM, Crowell MD, Scolapio JS. Gastrointestinal and nutritional complications after bariatric surgery. *Am J Gastroenterol.* (2007) 102:2571–80. doi: 10.1111/j.1572-0241.2007.01421.x
47. Rhode BM, Arseneau P, Cooper BA, Katz M, Gilfix BM, MacLean LD. Vitamin B-12 deficiency after gastric surgery for obesity. *Am J Clin Nutr.* (1996) 63:103–9. doi: 10.1093/ajcn/63.1.103
48. Brolin RE, Gorman JH, Petschenik AJ, Bradley LJ, Kenler HA, Cody RP. Are vitamin B12 and folate deficiency clinically important after roux-en-Y gastric bypass? *J Gastrointest Surg.* (1998) 2:436–42. doi: 10.1016/S1091-255X(98)80034-6
49. Updegraff TA, Neufeld NJ. Protein, iron, and folate status of patients prior to and following surgery for morbid obesity. *J Am Diet Assoc.* (1981) 78:135–40.
50. Alvarez-Leite JI. Nutrient deficiencies secondary to bariatric surgery. *Curr Opin Clin Nutr Metab Care.* (2004) 7:569–75. doi: 10.1097/00075197-200409000-00010
51. Brolin RE, LaMarca LB, Kenler HA, Cody RP. Malabsorptive gastric bypass in patients with superobesity. *J Gastrointest Surg.* (2002) 6:195–205. doi: 10.1016/S1091-255X(01)00022-1
52. Guney E, Kisakol G, Ozgen G, Yilmaz C, Yilmaz R, Kabalak T. Effect of weight loss on bone metabolism: comparison of vertical banded gastroplasty and medical intervention. *Obes Surg.* (2003) 13:383–8. doi: 10.1381/096089203765887705
53. Goldner WS, O'Dorisio TM, Dillon JS, Mason EE. Severe metabolic bone disease as a long-term complication of obesity surgery. *Obes Surg.* (2002) 12:685–92. doi: 10.1381/096089202321019693
54. Hamoui N, Kim K, Anthone G, Crookes PF. The significance of elevated levels of parathyroid hormone in patients with morbid obesity before and after bariatric surgery. *Arch Surg.* (2003) 138:891–7. doi: 10.1001/archsurg.138.8.891
55. Arterburn DE, Courcoulas AP. Bariatric surgery for obesity metabolic conditions in adults. *BMJ.* (2014) 349:g3961. doi: 10.1136/bmj.g3961

56. King WC, Chen JY, Mitchell JE, Kalarchian MA, Steffen KJ, Engel SG, et al. Prevalence of alcohol use disorders before after bariatric surgery. *JAMA.* (2012) 307:2516–25. doi: 10.1001/jama.2012.6147
57. Hagedorn JC, Encarnacion B, Brat GA, Morton JM. Does gastric bypass alter alcohol metabolism? *Surg Obes Relat Dis.* (2007) 3:543–8. doi: 10.1016/j.soard.2007.07.003
58. Klockhoff H, Naslund I, Jones AW. Faster absorption of ethanol and higher peak concentration in women after gastric bypass surgery. *Br J Clin Pharmacol.* (2002) 54:587–91. doi: 10.1046/j.1365-2125.2002.01698.x
59. Adams TD, Gress RE, Smith SC, Halverson RC, Simper SC, Rosamond WD, et al. Long-term mortality after gastric bypass surgery. *N Engl J Med.* (2007) 357:753–61. doi: 10.1056/NEJMoa066603
60. Adams TD, Davidson LE, Litwin SE, Kolotkin RL, LaMonte MJ, Pendleton RC, et al. Health benefits of gastric bypass surgery after 6 years. *JAMA.* (2012) 308:1122–31. doi: 10.1001/2012.jama.11164
61. Tindle HA, Omalu B, Courcoulas A, Marcus M, Hammers J, Kuller LH. Risk of suicide after long-term follow-up from bariatric surgery. *Am J Med.* (2010) 123:1036–42. doi: 10.1016/j.amjmed.2010.06.016
62. Peterhänsel C, Petroff D, Klinitzke G, Kersting A, Wagner B. Risk of completed suicide after bariatric surgery: a systematic review. *Obes. Rev.* (2013) 14:369–82. doi: 10.1111/obr.12014
63. Lagerros YT, Brandt L, Hedberg J, Sundbom M, Bodén S. Suicide, self-harm, and depression after gastric bypass surgery: a nationwide cohort study. *Ann Surg.* (2017) 265:235–43. doi: 10.1097/SLA.0000000000001884
64. Lim RBC, Zhang MWB, Ho RCM. Prevalence of all-cause mortality and suicide among bariatric surgery cohorts: a meta-analysis. *Int J Environ Res Public Health.* (2018) 15:1519. doi: 10.3390/ijerph15071519
65. Pérez-Pevida B, Escalada J, Miras AD, Frühbeck G. Mechanisms underlying type 2 diabetes remission after metabolic surgery. *Front Endocrinol (Lausanne).* (2019) 10:641. doi: 10.3389/fendo.2019.00641
66. Ferrannini E, Mingrone G. Impact of different bariatric surgical procedures on insulin action and beta-cell function in type 2 diabetes. *Diabetes Care.* (2009) 32:514–20. doi: 10.2337/dc08-1762
67. le Roux CW, Aylwin SJ, Batterham RL, Borg CM, Coyle F, Prasad V, et al. Gut hormone profiles following bariatric surgery favor an anorectic state, facilitate weight loss, and improve metabolic parameters. *Ann Surg.* (2006) 243:108–14. doi: 10.1097/01.sla.0000183349.16877.84
68. Jorgensen NB, Jacobsen SH, Dirksen C, Bojsen-Møller KN, Naver L, Hvolris L, et al. Acute and long-term effects of Roux-en-Y gastric bypass on glucose metabolism in subjects with type 2 diabetes and normal glucose tolerance. *Am J Physiol Endocrinol Metab.* (2012) 303:E122–31. doi: 10.1152/ajpendo.00073.2012
69. Romero F, Nicolau J, Flores L, Casamitjana R, Ibarzabal A, Lacy A, et al. Comparable early changes in gastrointestinal hormones after sleeve gastrectomy and Roux-en-Y gastric bypass surgery for morbidly obese type 2 diabetic subjects. *Surg Endosc.* (2012) 26:2231–39. doi: 10.1007/s00464-012-2166-y
70. Korner J, Inabnet W, Febres G, Conwell IM, McMahon DJ, Salas R, et al. Prospective study of gut hormone and metabolic changes after adjustable gastric banding and Roux-en-Y gastric bypass. *Int J Obes.* (2009) 33:786–95. doi: 10.1038/ijo.2009.79
71. Jorgensen NB, Dirksen C, Bojsen-Moller KN, Jacobsen SH, Worm D, Hansen DL, et al. Exaggerated glucagon-like peptide 1 response is important for improved beta-cell function and glucose tolerance after Roux-en-Y gastric bypass in patients with type 2 diabetes. *Diabetes.* (2013) 62:3044–52. doi: 10.2337/db13-0022
72. Jimenez A, Casamitjana R, Flores L, Delgado S, Lacy A, Vidal J. GLP-1 and the long-term outcome of type 2 diabetes mellitus after Roux-en-Y gastric bypass surgery in morbidly obese subjects. *Ann Surg.* (2013) 257:894–99. doi: 10.1097/SLA.0b013e31826b8603
73. Scrocchi LA, Brown TJ, MacLusky N, Brubaker PL, Auerbach AB, Joyner AL, et al. Glucose intolerance but normal satiety in mice with a null mutation in the glucagon-like peptide receptor gene. *Nat Med.* (1996) 2:1254–58. doi: 10.1038/nm1196-1254
74. Yusta B, Baggio LL, Estall JE, Koehler JA, Holland DP, Li H, et al. GLP-1 receptor activation improves b-cell function and survival following induction of endoplasmic reticulum stress. *Cell Metab.* (2006) 4:391–406. doi: 10.1016/j.cmet.2006.10.001
75. Garibay D, McGavigan AK, Lee SA, Ficorilli JV, Cox AL, Michael MD, et al. Beta-cell glucagon-like peptide- 1 receptor contributes to improved glucose tolerance after vertical sleeve gastrectomy. *Endocrinology.* (2016) 157:3405–09. doi: 10.1210/en.2016-1302
76. Shah M, Law JH, Micheletto F, Sathananthan M, Dalla Man C, Cobelli C, et al. Contribution of endogenous glucagon-like peptide 1 to glucose metabolism after Rouxen-Y gastric bypass. *Diabetes.* (2014) 63:483–93. doi: 10.2337/db13-0954
77. Service GJ, Thompson GB, Service FJ, Andrews JC, Collazo-Clavell ML, Lloyd RV. Hyperinsulinemic hypoglycemia with nesidioblastosis after gastricbypass surgery. *N Engl J Med.* (2005) 353:249–54. doi: 10.1056/NEJMoa043690
78. Patti ME, McMahon G, Mun EC, Bitton A, Holst JJ, Goldsmith J, et al. Severe hypoglycaemia post-gastric bypass requiring partial pancreatectomy: evidence for inappropriate insulin secretion and pancreatic islet hyperplasia. *Diabetologia.* (2005) 48:2236–40. doi: 10.1007/s00125-005-1933-x
79. Salehi M, Gastaldelli A, D'Alessio DA. Blockade of glucagon-like peptide 1 receptor corrects postprandial hypoglycemia after gastric bypass. *Gastroenterology.* (2014) 146:669–80. doi: 10.1053/j.gastro.2013.11.044
80. Vidal J, de Hollanda A, Jimenez A. GLP-1 is not the key mediator of the health benefits of metabolic surgery. *Surg Obes Relat Dis.* (2016) 12:1225–29. doi: 10.1016/j.soard.2016.02.029
81. Mokadem M, Zechner JF, Margolskee RF, Drucker DJ, Aguirre V. Effects of Roux-en-Y gastric bypass on energy and glucose homeostasis are preserved in two mouse models of functional glucagon-like peptide-1 deficiency. *Mol Metab.* (2014) 3:191–201. doi: 10.1016/j.molmet.2013.11.010
82. Wilson-Perez HE, Chambers AP, Ryan KK, Li B, Sandoval DA, Stoffers D, et al. Vertical sleeve gastrectomy is effective in two genetic mouse models of glucagonlike peptide-1 receptor deficiency. *Diabetes.* (2013) 62:2380–85. doi: 10.2337/db12-1498
83. Goldfine AB, Mun EC, Devine E, Bernier R, Baz-Hecht M, Jones DB, et al. Patients with neuroglycopenia after gastric bypass surgery have exaggerated incretin and insulin secretory responses to a mixed meal. *J Clin Endocrinol Metab.* (2007) 92:4678–85. doi: 10.1210/jc.2007-0918
84. Korner J, Bessler M, Inabnet W, Taveras C, Holst JJ. Exaggerated glucagon-like peptide-1 and blunted glucose-dependent insulinotropic peptide secretion are associated with Roux-en-Y gastric bypass but not adjustable gastric banding. *Surg Obes Relat Dis.* (2007) 3:597–601. doi: 10.1016/j.soard.2007.08.004
85. Lee WJ, Chen CY, Chong K, Lee YC, Chen SC, Lee SD. Changes in postprandial gut hormones after metabolic surgery: a comparison of gastric bypass and sleeve gastrectomy. *Surg Obes Relat Dis.* (2011) 7:683–90. doi: 10.1016/j.soard.2011.07.009
86. Bojsen-Moller KN, Dirksen C, Jorgensen NB, Jacobsen SH, Serup AK, Albers PH, et al. Early enhancements of hepatic and later of peripheral insulin sensitivity combined with increased postprandial insulin secretion contribute to improved glycemic control after Roux-en-Y gastric bypass. *Diabetes.* (2014) 63:1725–37. doi: 10.2337/db13-1307
87. Camastra S, Gastaldelli A, Mari A, Bonuccelli S, Scartabelli G, Frascerra S, et al. Early and longer term effects of gastric bypass surgery on tissue-specific insulin sensitivity and beta cell function in morbidly obese patients with and without type 2 diabetes. *Diabetologia.* (2011) 54:2093–102. doi: 10.1007/s00125-011-2193-6
88. Isbell JM, Tamboli RA, Hansen EN, Saliba J, Dunn JP, Phillips SE, et al. The importance of caloric restriction in the early improvements in insulin sensitivity after Roux-en-Y gastric bypass surgery. *Diabetes Care.* (2010) 33:1438–42. doi: 10.2337/dc09-2107
89. Foo J, Krebs J, Hayes MT, Bell D, Macartney-Coxson D, Croft T, et al. Studies in insulin resistance following very low calorie diet and/or gastric bypass surgery. *Obes Surg.* (2011) 21:1914–20. doi: 10.1007/s11695-011-0527-6
90. Jackness C, Karmally W, Febres G, Conwell IM, Ahmed L, Bessler M, et al. Very low-calorie diet mimics the early beneficial effect of Roux-en-Y gastric bypass on insulin sensitivity and β-cell function in type 2 diabetic patients. *Diabetes.* (2013) 62:3027–32. doi: 10.2337/db12-1762
91. Gastaldelli A, Iaconelli A, Gaggini M, Magnone MC, Veneziani A, Rubino F, et al. Short-term effects of laparoscopic adjustable gastric banding vs. Roux-en-Y gastric bypass. *Diabetes Care.* (2016) 39:1925–31. doi: 10.2337/dc15-2823

92. Muscelli E, Mingrone G, Camastra S, Manco M, Pereira JA, Pareja JC, et al. Differential effect of weight loss on insulin resistance in surgically treated obese patients. *Am J Med.* (2005) 118:51–7. doi: 10.1016/j.amjmed.2004.08.017
93. Campos GM, Rabl C, Peeva S, Ciovica R, Rao M, Schwarz JM, et al. Improvement in peripheral glucose uptake after gastric bypass surgery is observed only after substantial weight loss has occurred and correlates with the magnitude of weight lost. *J Gastrointest Surg.* (2010) 14:15–23. doi: 10.1007/s11605-009-1060-y
94. Rowlands J, Heng J, Newsholme P, Carlessi R. Pleiotropic effects of GLP-1 and analogs on cell signaling, metabolism, and function. *Front Endocrinol.* (2018) 9:672. doi: 10.3389/fendo.2018.00672
95. Cabou C, Burcelin R. GLP-1, the gut-brain, brain-periphery axes. *Rev Diabetic Stud.* (2011) 8:418–31. doi: 10.1900/RDS.2011.8.418
96. Seo S, Ju S, Chung H, Lee D, Park S. Acute effects of glucagon-like peptide-1 on hypothalamic neuropeptide and AMP activated kinase expression in fasted rats. *Endocr J.* (2008) 55:867–74. doi: 10.1507/endocrj.K08E-091
97. Lockie SH, Heppner KM, Chaudhary N, Chabenne JR, Morgan DA, Veyrat-Durebex C, et al. Direct control of brown adipose tissue thermogenesis by central nervous system glucagon-like peptide-1 receptor signaling. *Diabetes.* (2012) 61:2753–62. doi: 10.2337/db11-1556
98. de Silva A, Salem V, Long CJ, Makwana A, Newbould RD, Rabiner A, et al. The gut hormones PYY 3-36 and GLP-1 7-36 amide reduce food intake and modulate brain activity in appetite centers in humans. *Cell Metab.* (2011) 14:700–6. doi: 10.1016/j.cmet.2011.09.010
99. Morinigo R, Moizé V, Musri M, Lacy AM, Navarro S, Marín JL, et al. Glucagon-like peptide-1, peptide YY, hunger, and satiety after gastric bypass surgery in morbidly obese subjects. *J Clin Endocrinol Metab.* (2006) 91:1735–40. doi: 10.1210/jc.2005-0904
100. Korner J, Bessler M, Cirilo LJ, Conwell IM, Daud A, Restuccia NL, et al. Effects of Roux-en-Y gastric bypass surgery on fasting and postprandial concentrations of plasma ghrelin, peptide YY, and insulin. *J Clin Endocrinol Metab.* (2005) 90:359–65. doi: 10.1210/jc.2004-1076
101. Madsbad S, Dirksen C, Holst JJ. Mechanisms of changes in glucose metabolism and bodyweight after bariatric surgery. *Lancet Diabet Endocrinol.* (2014) 2:152–64. doi: 10.1016/S2213-8587(13)70218-3
102. Pournaras DJ, le Roux CW. Are bile acids the new gut hormones? Lessons from weight loss surgery models. *Endocrinology.* (2013) 154:2255–56. doi: 10.1210/en.2013-1383
103. Patti ME, Houten SM, Bianco AC, Bernier R, Larsen PR, Holst JJ, et al. Serum bile acids are higher in humans with prior gastric bypass: potential contribution to improved glucose and lipid metabolism. *Obesity.* (2009) 17:1671–7. doi: 10.1038/oby.2009.102
104. Mencarelli A, Renga B, D'Amore C, Santorelli C, Graziosi L, Bruno A, et al. Dissociation of intestinal and hepatic activities of FXR and LXRα supports metabolic effects of terminal ileum interposition in rodents. *Diabetes.* (2013) 62:3384–93. doi: 10.2337/db13-0299
105. Gomez-Ambrosi J, Andrada P, Valenti V, Rotellar F, Silva C, Catalan V, et al. Dissociation of body mass index, excess weight loss and body fat percentage trajectories after 3 years of gastric bypass: relationship with metabolic outcomes. *Int J Obes.* (2017) 41:1379–87. doi: 10.1038/ijo.2017.134
106. Frikke-Schmidt H, O'Rourke RW, Lumeng CN, Sandoval DA, Seeley RJ. Does bariatric surgery improve adipose tissue function? *Obes Rev.* (2016) 17:795–809. doi: 10.1111/obr.12429
107. Faraj M, Havel PJ, Phelis S, Blank D, Sniderman AD, Cianflone K. Plasma acylation-stimulating protein, adiponectin, leptin, and ghrelin before and after weight loss induced by gastric bypass surgery in morbidly obese subjects. *J Clin Endocrinol Metab.* (2003) 88:1594–602. doi: 10.1210/jc.2002-021309
108. Liou AP, Paziuk M, Luevano JM Jr., Machineni S, Turnbaugh PJ, et al. Conserved shifts in the gut microbiota due to gastric bypass reduce host weight and adiposity. *Sci Transl Med.* (2013) 5:178ra141. doi: 10.1126/scitranslmed.3005687
109. Baud G, Daoudi M, Hubert T, Raverdy V, Pigeyre M, Hervieux E, et al. Bile diversion in Roux-en-Y gastric bypass modulates sodium-dependent glucose intestinal uptake. *Cell Metab.* (2016) 23:547–53. doi: 10.1016/j.cmet.2016.01.018
110. Harvey EJ, Arroyo K, Korner J, Inabnet WB. Hormone changes affecting energy homeostasis after metabolic surgery. *Mt Sinai J Med.* (2010) 77:446–65. doi: 10.1002/msj.20203
111. Cummings DE, Weigle DS, Frayo RS, Breen PA, Ma MK, Dellinger EP, et al. Plasma ghrelin levels after diet-induced weight loss or gastric bypass surgery. *N Engl J Med.* (2002) 346:1623–30. doi: 10.1056/NEJMoa012908
112. Sista F, Abruzzese V, Clementi M, Carandina S, Amicucci G. Effect of resected gastric volume on ghrelin and GLP-1 plasma levels: a prospective study. *J Gastrointest Surg.* (2016) 20:1931–41. doi: 10.1007/s11605-016-3292-y
113. Saeidi N, Meoli L, Nestoridi E, Gupta NK, Kvas S, Kucharczyk J, et al. Reprogramming of intestinal glucose metabolism and glycemic control in rats after gastric bypass. *Science.* (2013) 341:406–10. doi: 10.1126/science.1235103
114. Troy S, Soty M, Ribeiro L, Laval L, Migrenne S, Fioramonti X, et al. Intestinal gluconeogenesis is a key factor for early metabolic changes after gastric bypass but not after gastric lap-band in mice. *Cell Metab.* (2008) 8:201–11. doi: 10.1016/j.cmet.2008.08.008
115. Thorens B, Larsen PJ. Gut-derived signaling molecules and vagal afferents in the control of glucose and energy homeostasis. *Curr Opin Clin Nutr Metab Care.* (2004) 7:471–8. doi: 10.1097/01.mco.0000134368.91900.84
116. Pozzilli P, Guglielmi C, Caprio S, Buzzetti R. Obesity, autoimmunity, and double diabetes in youth. *Diabetes Care.* (2011) 34:S166–70. doi: 10.2337/dc11-s213
117. Dirksen C, Jacobsen SH, Bojsen-Møller KN, Jørgensen NB, Naver LS, Hvolris LE, et al. Reduction in cardiovascular risk factors and insulin dose, but no beta-cell regeneration 1 year after Roux-en-Y gastric bypass in an obese patient with type 1 diabetes: a case report. *Obes Res Clin Pract.* (2013) 7:e269–74. doi: 10.1016/j.orcp.2012.01.002
118. Madsbad S, Faber OK, Binder C, McNair P, Christiansen C, Transbøl I. Prevalence of residual beta-cell function in insulin-dependent diabetics in relation to age at onset and duration of diabetes. *Diabetes.* (1978) 27:262–4. doi: 10.2337/diab.27.1.S262
119. Levetan C. Distinctions between islet neogenesis and β-cell replication: Implications for reversal of type 1 and 2 diabetes. *J Diabetes.* (2010) 2:76–84. doi: 10.1111/j.1753-0407.2010.00074.x
120. Seisser. J. Latent (slowly progressing) autoimmune diabetes in adults. *Curr Diab Rep.* (2008) 8:94–100. doi: 10.1007/s11892-008-0018-x
121. Brophy S, Yderstraede K, Mauricio D, Hunter S, Hawa M, Pozzilli P, et al. Time to insulin initiation cannot be used in defining latent autoimmune diabetes in adults. *Diab Care.* (2008) 31:439–41. doi: 10.2337/dc07-1308
122. Hironaka JY, Kitahama S, Sato H, Inoue M, Takahashi T, Tamori Y. Sleeve gastrectomy induced remission of slowly progressive type 1 diabetes in a morbidly obese Japanese patient. *Intern Med.* (2019) 58:675–8. doi: 10.2169/internalmedicine.1217-18
123. Uno K, Seki Y, Kasama K, Wakamatsu K, Hashimoto K, Umezawa A, et al. Mid-term results of bariatric surgery in morbidly obese Japanese patients with slow progressive autoimmune diabetes. *Asian J Endosc Surg.* (2018) 11:238–43. doi: 10.1111/ases.12443
124. Lindqvist A, Spegel P, Ekelund M, Garcia Vaz E, Pierzynowski S, Gomesz MF, et al. Gastric bypass improves beta-cell function and increases β-cell mass in a porcine model. *Diabetes.* (2014) 63:1665–71. doi: 10.2337/db13-0969

9

Male Obesity Associated Gonadal Dysfunction and the Role of Bariatric Surgery

*Sana Sultan[1], Ameet G. Patel[2], Shamsi El-Hassani[3], Benjamin Whitelaw[1], Bianca M. Leca[1], Royce P. Vincent[4], Carel W. le Roux[5], Francesco Rubino[2], Simon J. B. Aywlin[1] and Georgios K. Dimitriadis[1]**

[1] Department of Endocrinology and Metabolic Medicine, King's College Hospital NHS Foundation Trust, London, United Kingdom, [2] Department of Minimal Access Surgery, King's College Hospital NHS Foundation Trust, London, United Kingdom, [3] Minimal Access and Bariatric Unit, Princess Royal University Hospital, King's College Hospital NHS Foundation Trust, Orpington, United Kingdom, [4] Department of Clinical Biochemistry, King's College Hospital NHS Foundation Trust, London, United Kingdom, [5] Diabetes Complication Research Centre, School of Medicine and Medical Science, UCD Conway Institute, University College Dublin, Belfield, Ireland

***Correspondence:**
Georgios K. Dimitriadis
g.dimitriadis@nhs.net

Obesity is an ever growing pandemic and a prevalent problem among men of reproductive age that can both cause and exacerbate male-factor infertility by means of endocrine abnormalities, associated comorbidities, and direct effects on the precision and throughput of spermatogenesis. Robust epidemiologic, clinical, genetic, epigenetic, and preclinical data support these findings. Clinical studies on the impact of medically induced weight loss on serum testosterone concentrations and spermatogenesis is promising but may show differential and unsustainable results. In contrast, literature has demonstrated that weight loss after bariatric surgery is correlated with an increase in serum testosterone concentrations that is superior than that obtained with only lifestyle modifications, supporting a further metabolic benefit from surgery that may be specific to the male reproductive system. The data on sperm and semen parameters is controversial to date. Emerging evidence in the burgeoning field of genetics and epigenetics has demonstrated that paternal obesity can affect offspring metabolic and reproductive phenotypes by means of epigenetic reprogramming of spermatogonial stem cells. Understanding the impact of this reprogramming is critical to a comprehensive view of the impact of obesity on subsequent generations. Furthermore, conveying the potential impact of these lifestyle changes on future progeny can serve as a powerful tool for obese men to modify their behavior. Healthcare professionals treating male infertility and obesity need to adapt their practice to assimilate these new findings to better counsel men about the importance of paternal preconception health and the impact of novel non-medical therapeutic interventions. Herein, we summarize the pathophysiology of obesity on the male reproductive system and emerging evidence regarding the potential role of bariatric surgery as treatment of male obesity-associated gonadal dysfunction.

Keywords: obesity, male reproductive system, male obesity related hypogonadism, bariatric surgery, metabolic surgery, male subfertility, oligospermia, erectile dysfunction

INTRODUCTION

Obesity is a multifactorial global pandemic, which affects virtually every system in the body and can have significant bio-psycho-social impacts on the patients. It is increasingly becoming a significant health issue, which now affects all age groups and is seen in the developed and developing world (1). In the year 2016, the World Health Organization (WHO) data showed that 39% of the world's population is overweight and 13% are obese (1).

Obesity results from complex interactions between metabolic, genetic, environmental, nutritional, and psychosocial factors. Excess body weight has been established as a clear risk for increased morbidity and mortality and is a known risk factor for several serious physical health conditions such as hypertension, type II diabetes mellitus (T2DM), dyslipidemia, cerebrovascular, and cardiovascular illness (2). In addition we now know that obesity also impacts both male and female sexual and reproductive function (2). Throughout history and pervading many civilizations the penis in an erect state has been a powerful symbol of male fertility, virility, and dominance. Therefore, the inability to achieve and/or maintain an erection can have profound negative physical and psychological effects on the patient as an individual and indirectly on the partner (3).

AETIOPATHOGENESIS OF MALE OBESITY RELATED HYPOGONADISM

Testosterone Deficiency

The male reproductive system is a multilevel complex physiological system that is controlled by various feedback mechanisms and signaling molecules, which are all in a delicate balance. Hypogonadism is defined as decreased or absent gonadal function and in males is characterized by reduced testosterone levels (4). There exists an expectation that testosterone levels will naturally decline with age and can lead to or strongly contribute to hypogonadism (5). Obesity and in particular, visceral adipose tissue expansion, represents a strong risk factor for the development of male hypogonadism and this state is referred to as male obesity secondary hypogonadism (MOSH) (6). The effects of MOSH will manifest themselves as testosterone deficiency, erectile dysfunction, changes in sperm, and semen parameters and overall sexual dysfunction (6). The current scientific literature shows established links between obesity and secondary hypogonadism where one cross sectional study has demonstrated an 8.7-fold increase in risk of secondary hypogonadism in patients with a BMI >30 kg/m^2 (7).

Furthermore, men with a BMI of 35–40 kg/m^2 can have up to 50% less free and total testosterone when compared to age matched peers with a normal BMI (8). There is overwhelming undisputed evidence of the link between obesity and male sexual and reproductive dysfunction however the exact mechanisms for this remains to be elucidated (7–9).

The Cohen hypothesis was the first suggested link between testosterone and obesity in the literature (10). This is based on the observation that testosterone and obesity have a circular relationship in which obesity acts as a strong independent risk factor to testosterone deficiency (10). Similarly suboptimal testosterone levels can in their own right exacerbate obesity leading to a vicious cycle, which can only be broken with substantial reduction in body mass (10). **Figure 1** shows this relationship and highlights other contributing causes.

Testosterone is known to be a hormone that has potent metabolic effects and it is now accepted that testosterone levels and subsequent effects are closely related to body mass although the exact mechanism remain to be elucidated (11). In suboptimal levels, testosterone will facilitate the differentiation of pluripotent stem cells into adipocytes, which will cause increased aromatization of testosterone into oestradiol (11). This will act via negative feedback mechanism to the hypothalamic – pituitary axis (HPA) to suppress further gonadal stimulation and testosterone release (11).

In addition to those mechanisms in Cohen's hypothesis, testosterone deficiency is known to play indirect metabolic roles preventing physiological compensatory mechanisms (11). This is explored in the hypogonadal—obesity—adipocytokine hypothesis, which expands this idea further (11). Testosterone is known to enhance the activity of lipoprotein lipase enzyme, which leads to a rise in triglyceride uptake into adipocytes (11). Furthermore, larger numbers of adipocytes lead to increases in insulin resistance, production of pro-inflammatory cytokines tumor necrosis factor-a. interleukin-1 and interleukin-6 (TNF-α, IL-1, and IL-6), and increases in leptin and oestradiol levels (11, 12).

Leptin is a hormone produced by adipocytes, and acts to regulate energy balance ensuring reduced fat storage (13). It

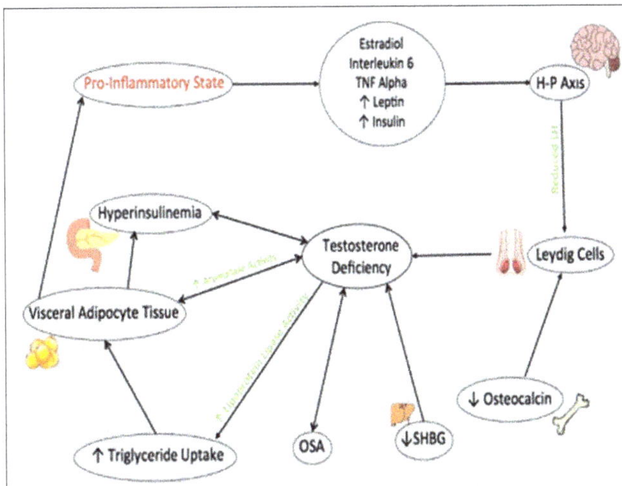

FIGURE 1 | The metabolic and reproductive effects of testosterone in relation to obesity. Factors related to obesity, such as OSA and reduced SHGB contribute to Testosterone deficiency. Reduced Osteocalcin output from Osteoblasts is also newly associated with contributing to testosterone deficiency. Testosterone deficiency increases activity of Lipoprotein Lipase and therefore triglyceride uptake which increases visceral adipose tissues. This further exacerbates htperinsulinemia and testosterone deficiency through the activities of Aromatase enzyme. Visceral adipose tissue increases production of cytokines and inflammatory mediators leading to a pro-inflammatory and contribute to hypothalamic-pituitary suppression leading to further testosterone deficiency.

also has other roles and acts at the hypothalamic- pituitary level to influence the reproductive system in both male and female patients (13). In normal conditions, Leptin potentiates the release of testosterone, by acting at the hypothalamic level, stimulating neurons to release gonadotrophin releasing hormone (GnRH), and subsequently luteinizing hormone (LH) from the pituitary gland (13). However, in obesity these neurons become resistant to the actions of Leptin (11, 13). In addition, receptors for Leptin have been found in testicular tissue and studies have shown that Leptin can directly inhibit gonadotrophic actions on Leydig cells thus further exacerbating testosterone deficiency and therefore obesity (11, 13).

The initial signals that activate the hypothalamic- pituitary-gonadal axis originate in the arcuate nucleus and periventricular nucleus of the hypothalamus (14). These neurons release neuropeptide Kisspeptin, which in turn stimulates the release of GnRH (14). Excess levels of oestradiol and pro-inflammatory cytokines act at the hypothalamic level to inhibit the neuronal release of Kisspeptin, which will lead to a profound reduction in GnRH signals leading to a sustained state of hypogonadotropic hypogonadism (12, 15).

Another hypothesis for male hypogonadism in obesity is the Gelding theory. Currently, within the scientific literature there has been more evidence supporting this theory as at least contributing to testosterone deficiency. Within the gastrointestinal system there exists on average 1.5 kg (100 trillion) of bacteria (16, 17). This tends to be largely gram-negative bacteria, which produce a pro-inflammatory lipopolysaccharide and endotoxin (16, 17). Under normal circumstances these proinflammatory substances are confined to the gastrointestinal tract (16, 17). However, a highly calorific and fatty diet has been shown to contribute to breakdown in the intestinal mucosa leading to passage of bacterial endotoxins into the general circulation, which further contributes to a pro-inflammatory state (16, 17). Exposure to lipopolysaccharide from the general circulation is hypothesized to cause impaired testicular function thereby contributing to testosterone deficiency. The exact mechanism of how this occurs remains unclear (16, 17).

Sex Hormone Binding Globulin (SHBG) is a glycoprotein produced by the liver. In the circulation, ~98% of testosterone is bound to albumin and SHBG (18, 19). Suboptimal SHBG levels can exacerbate testosterone deficiency through pro-inflammatory effects and increased deposition of lipids within macrophages and adipocytes. This will exacerbate the existing inflammatory state of obesity and propagate further weight gain (18). In addition, it is now accepted that suboptimal levels of SHBG and testosterone significantly contribute to insulin resistance and therefore a pre-diabetic state. The MRFIT and the Massachusetts Male Aging Study followed up 176 and 1,156 patients over 5 and 7–10 years, respectively (20, 21). Both showed results that are consistent with the wider literature, which is that low levels of testosterone and SHBG were strongly associated with the development of diabetes (20, 21). In obese patients there exists a state of hyperinsulinemia due to reduced insulin sensitivity in peripheral tissues (6). This leads to high levels of insulin, which have been shown to contribute to firstly central hypogonadism through the modulation of GnRH and therefore gonadotrophin output and secondly to peripheral hypogonadism through direct actions on Leydig cells (6, 22, 23).

Testosterone levels are also influenced by Obstructive Sleep Apnea (OSA), which is a common condition and often co-exists with obesity and excess body weight (24, 25). The underlying pathophysiological mechanism of OSA involves partial or complete upper airway obstruction, which results in intermittent hypoxia, sleep fragmentation, reduced deep, and rapid eye movement (REM) sleep and daytime somnolence (24, 25) OSA has been associated with pituitary-gonadal dysfunction in male patients, which is manifested as suboptimal testosterone levels, erectile dysfunction, and reduced libido (24, 25). Suboptimal testosterone levels found in OSA are due to reduced quality and quantity of sleep, which in turn worsens both obesity and OSA (24, 25).

Erectile Dysfunction

Testosterone deficiency also leads to difficulties in achieving and maintaining an erection. Healthy erectile function is dependent on interactions of erectile tissue, central, and peripheral nervous system, several endocrine, and psychological factors (3). Sexual stimulation results in activation of non-adrenergic, non-cholinergic, and parasympathetic cholinergic nerve fibers leading to the release of nitric oxide and acetylcholine, respectively (3). This will lead to increased cyclic guanosine monophosphate (GMP) and reduced intracellular calcium levels thus facilitating the relaxation of smooth muscles and vasodilatation causing increased blood flow to corpus cavernosum causing veno-occlusion of the subtunical venules (3). Disturbances in one or more of these mechanisms can contribute or lead to erectile dysfunction (3, 26).

Excess body weight has been strongly linked to erectile dysfunction and in fact current research has suggested high BMI as a significant risk factor for erectile dysfunction (27, 28). Obesity leads to a pro-inflammatory physiological state, which favors widespread arteriolar endothelial dysfunction and impaired activity of nitric oxide. In addition, it also leads to increased insulin and leptin resistance, which can exacerbate T2DM and resultant peripheral neuropathies (29). Obesity is also known to cause both central and peripheral hypogonadism and testosterone deficiency thus further exacerbating erectile dysfunction (29).

Current literature has shown that patients with a raised BMI have a 30% increased risk of erectile dysfunction than those of a normal BMI, and 96.5% of obese patients with metabolic syndrome report erectile dysfunction (30, 31). A multivariate analysis conducted by Bacon et al. showed an increased risk of erectile dysfunction at 19 and 33% in men with a BMI of 25–26.9 and 27–29.9kg/m^2, respectively (32, 33). The risk of erectile dysfunction is further compounded in patients with obesity due to the presence of other co-morbid conditions such as cardiovascular dysfunction and T2DM (29, 34). A meta-analysis investigating the prevalence of erectile dysfunction in T2DM showed that 52.5% of diabetic patients report erectile dysfunction giving prevalence odds of approximately 3.5 times more than healthy individuals (34).

Erectile dysfunction is essentially reflective of underlying vascular disease in those patients with obesity and some researchers have suggested that the presence of erectile dysfunction can be used as a prompt for further assessment of cardiovascular system (28).

Sperm and Semen Parameters

Obesity has a clear negative effect on male reproductive and sexual function, however the effect of obesity on sperm and semen parameters remains ambiguous. It is wholly accepted that obesity increases oxidative stress through a prolonged and sustained pro-inflammatory state, which is hypothesized to cause oxidative damage to the sperm. This is thought to lead to decreased motility, increased DNA damage, reduced acrosomal reactions, and therefore lower successful outcomes following *in vitro* Fertilization (IVF) (6, 35).

Some studies have suggested that elevated BMI results in a detrimental effect on sperm morphology, motility, and concentration however others have found no association (36–38). Belloc et al. investigated 10,665 semen samples and found that in morbidly obese patients (BMI >40 kg/m^2) there was reduced semen volume, concentration, total sperm count, and reduced motility (39). There were also significant increases found in azoospermia and cryptozoospermia from 1.9 and 4.7% to 9.1 and 15.2%, respectively (39). Similarly Sermondade et al. carried out a systemic review investigating the effect of BMI on sperm count. They found that compared to men of normal BMI, those in the obese or morbidly obese categories had an odds ratio of 1.28 (1.06–1.55) and 2.04 (1.59–2.62) for oligozospermia and azoospermia, respectively (40). In contrast, a cross sectional study by Rufus et al. carried out a comparison of semen quality in 206 men of varying BMI (41). The overall outcome of the study was that elevated BMI did not have a significant effect on semen quality (41).

It is clear that there is no consensus in the current literature regarding the effects of obesity and excess body weight on sperm and semen parameters. Further research is required into this area so that we may better understand the effects of obesity on male reproduction. This will inevitably allow the provision of more targeted and therefore more effective treatment for reproductive issues in male patients with obesity.

Effects of Paternal Obesity Through Future Generations

Intragenerational inheritance occurs when induced epigenetic changes in the gametes are passed on to the subsequent generation (42). This epigenetic inheritance can lead to changes to the phenotype of the offspring and beyond generations. Transmission of epigenetic signatures for the paternal gamete, includes any sperm epigenetic signatures altered throughout a man's life (or even that were induced *in utero*) from the father to the child only and termed intergenerational. Whereas, the inheritance of an altered epigenetic state beyond immediate offspring is termed transgenerational inheritance. According to epidemiological evidence, many types of environmental challenges imposed on the parent, such as hunger, specific diets, toxins, and trauma, have been found to influence the development of the offspring (43). Paternal age, subfertility, smoking, obesity, and exposure to a range of environmental influences, including air pollution, radiofrequency electromagnetic radiation and others, have also been implicated (44). The Dutch famine study showed that severe caloric restriction in parents during wartime starvation in World War II, resulted in significant cardiometabolic abnormalities in the *post-utero* life of their offsprings (45).

Obesity has been shown to directly drive transgenerational effects in successive generations. Preclinical studies with the use of animal models have found altered metabolic processing in offspring sired by obese fathers (46). Further studies using murine models have shown similar patterns of offspring metabolic perturbations but have also identified specific epigenetic alterations in the sperm (47). In humans, an intriguing recent study found alterations in DNA methylation at the insulin-like growth factor 2 gene in newborns sired by obese fathers (48). Taken together, data from experimental studies strongly suggest that obesity can affect sperm function, embryogenesis, and even offspring health; though, the same results have not been clearly demonstrated in humans (49, 50).

Donkin et al., demonstrated that the expression level of specific miRNAs, and small nuclear RNA (snRNA) fragments was altered in the spermatozoa of obese men. They speculated that this altered expression coordinately modulated the expression of genes involved in behavior and food intake and could participate in predisposing the offspring to obesity (50).

MANAGEMENT OF MALE OBESITY RELATED HYPOGONADISM

Non-surgical Interventions

Current management of obesity entails access to specialized secondary and tertiary care services that allow patients to engage with a multidisciplinary team to aid weight loss and maintenance. Lifestyle modifications such as caloric deficit diets and increased physical activity are the mainstay of non-surgical therapies. Recently, treatment with a Glucagon Like Peptide−1 (GLP-1) receptor agonist has shown beneficial effects with regards to weight loss but have also shown increased levels of gonadotrophins and subsequent increases in testosterone (50).

Several studies have demonstrated benefits with regards to improvement and recovery in the male reproductive system following significant and sustained weight loss. The European Male Aging Study (EMAS) has shown that changes in total body weight of ≥15% are correlated to changes in testosterone whereby gaining weight reduces testosterone levels and vice versa (51). Similarly the Massachusetts Male Aging Study established that a 4–5 kg/m^2 increase in BMI significantly contributes to a reduction in total testosterone level comparable to 10 years of aging (52). Hakonsen et al. also demonstrated similar results in a pilot cohort study of 43 men who were enrolled in a residential weight loss program. This study showed an average weight loss of 15%, which correlated to improvement in hormonal profile and an increase in total sperm count and semen volume (53). Mir et al. also showed that weight loss leads to significant reduction in DNA fragmentation index and therefore improved sperm morphology (37).

In a cross-sectional prospective cohort study, Bacon et al. demonstrate that physical activity is associated with 30% decreased risk of erectile dysfunction (31). Further studies have explored the relationship of weight to erectile function and have used the International Index of Erectile Function (IIEF) score. One such study demonstrated that lifestyle measures can cause a reduction in BMI from 36.9 to 31.2 kg/m^2 and improvement in IIEF score from 13.9 to 17, respectively (54).

Bariatric Surgery: Hormonal and Metabolic Effects

Intense and sustained lifestyle modifications can show adequate weight loss of up to 10% at 1 year with up to 5.3% maintained at 8 years (55). However, a subset of obese and morbidly obese patients will require surgical interventions in the form of bariatric surgery (55). Eligibility for surgical intervention in the treatment of obesity is globally variable; however, it is generally accepted that bariatric surgery could be an appropriate option for patients with a BMI >40 kg/m^2 or those with a BMI of 35–40 kg/m^2 with co-morbid conditions (55). There are different surgeries available however all seem to show favorable outcomes. In a systematic review by O'Brien et al., patients achieved 71, 60, and 49% excess weight loss with a biliopancreatic diversion with duodenal switch (BPD/DS), laparoscopic Roux en Y gastric bypass (RYGB) and laparoscopic adjustable gastric band (LAGB), respectively. (56, 57). Such drastic and sustained weight loss will have profound effects on alleviation of obesity and associated co-morbid conditions. **Table 1** shows relevant studies investigating the effect of bariatric surgery on hormonal and metabolic profile, erectile dysfunction, and semen and sperm parameters.

In addition to significant and sustained weight loss, several studies have also demonstrated improvement in total testosterone, SHBG levels, insulin resistance, and several other metabolic parameters (63, 72). Interestingly, the improvements in these parameters are not procedure specific (63, 72). Extensive and sustained weight loss leading to improvement in MOSH has consistently been reported in the literature. In a systematic review and meta-analysis of 45 articles, MOSH was present in 64% of patients preoperatively with resolution seen in 87% of patients post-operatively (73). Similarly, Pellitero et al. carried out an observational study of 33 men undergoing bariatric surgery and showed that 1 year post-operatively there was significant excess weight loss observed at 18.8% with an increase in total and free testosterone, SHBG and FSH and decrease in estradiol and prolactin (63).

Further studies have also demonstrated that decreases in visceral adipose tissue leads to increases in free testosterone and these effects are thought to be long lasting (6, 74). Visceral adipose tissue is known to contain higher levels of aromatase enzyme thereby contributing to excess conversion of testosterone to estradiol (6, 74). Therefore, it would make sense that reduction in visceral adipose tissue could disturb this mechanism and lead to a rise in testosterone levels and therefore overall improvement in MOSH (6).

It is now accepted that obesity and excess body weight creates a pro-inflammatory physiological state that directly causes or exacerbates several health conditions including MOSH. Studies have shown favorable outcomes in terms of reduction in pro-inflammatory mediators following bariatric surgery. This is seen in a study of 20 morbidly obese subjects undergoing adjustable gastric banding. One year post operatively they had significant reduction in BMI from 41.6 to 30.8 kg/m^2 and high sensitivity C Reactive Protein (hs-CRP) from 1.33 to 0.4 mg/dl, respectively (62). These results were replicated in a study of 47 patients (BMI >40 kg/m^2), and post operatively, subjects were found to have lost an average of 33% of their body weight, which was correlated with a reduction of hs-CRP from 0.83 to 0.18 mg/dl (56, 75).

Bariatric surgery clearly shows immediate and sustained reduction in BMI and therefore improvement in pathophysiological factors causing or contributing to hypogonadism. Pham et al. have also shown that these effects do persist long term (71). They carried out a randomized controlled trial of 32 male obese patients assigned to medical therapy or surgical treatment (76). Surgical patients showed an increase of 47.4% in free testosterone compared to medical patients at a 2.2% increase only. The increases in testosterone also correlated to decreased high sensitivity CRP, leptin, and overall BMI (76).

Experimental evidence has suggested potential links between the skeletal and reproductive system. Osteoblasts produce a hormone called Osteocalcin, which acts directly on the Leydig cells in the testes to produce testosterone (77). Samavat et al. have shown that reduction in BMI leads to increased levels in Osteocalcin, which also correlates to an increased level of testosterone (78). It is widely accepted that testosterone is a hormone, which exerts significant metabolic effects in both direct and indirect manners (78). This is clearly an area that is promising however requires further research to elucidate exact effects and how dependent they may be on other risk factors such as age or other comorbidities.

Bariatric Surgery: Erectile Dysfunction

There is agreement in the literature regarding the detrimental effects of obesity and excess body weight on erectile function. The impact of erectile dysfunction on the individual patient but also in a partnership is profound and can lead to significant negative effects on quality of life. This effect is ameliorated with reduction in BMI and improvements can be seen in biological and psychological factors contributing to reproductive and sexual function (58, 65). In a systematic review and meta-analysis assessing erectile function in patients with obesity pre- and post-operatively showed a 4.10 increase in the IIEF score demonstrating statistical significance (79). Furthermore, a study of 97 patients with obesity undergoing bariatric surgery showed improvement in sexual drive, erectile and ejaculatory function, and sexual satisfaction post operatively. These effects were directly correlated to percentage of excess body weight lost (64). In a prospective study by Arolfo et al. data was collected pre- and 12 months post-operatively on 44 male patients. Patients had significant improvement in IIEF 12 months after surgery (59).

Improvement in sexual function and specifically erectile function is clearly seen with bariatric surgery and correlated to

TABLE 1 | Effects of bariatric surgery on hormonal and metabolic profile, erectile dysfunction, semen and sperm parameters.

Level of evidence	References	Sample Size	Intervention	Outcome
Level Ib	Samavat et al. (58)	103	Gastric bypass	Post operative time point review: 9 months Weight loss achieved: Mean −36.2 ± 20.24 kg Outcome: significant increase in free and total testosterone, OCN and SHBG; decrease in Oestradiol
Level Ib	Arolfo et al. (59)	44	Roux-en-y gastric bypass; Sleeve gastrectomy	Post operative time point review: 9 months Weight loss achieved: Mean-39.75 ± 24 kg Outcome: Significant increase in total testosterone, SHBG and IIEF score; decrease in HbA1c, insulin, triglycerides, HDL cholesterol, and CRP
Level Ib	Legro et al. (60)	6	Roux-en-y gastric bypass	Post operative time point review: 1, 3, 6 months Weight loss achieved: Mean −55 ± 30 kg Outcome: improvement in testosterone level
Level Ib	Reis et al. (61)	20	Lifestyle modifications, Gastric bypass	Post operative time point review: 4 and 24 months Weight loss achieved: inaccessible Outcome: improvement in total and free testosterone and FSH and reduced prolactin levels
Level IIb	Liu et al. (62)	45	Roux-en-y gastric bypass	Post operative time point review: Weight loss achieved: inaccessible Outcome: increase in total testosterone with reduced visceral fat
Level IIIb	Calderon et al. (63)	35	Gastric bypass; Sleeve gastrectomy; Gastric Banding	Post operative time point review: 6 months or more (not specified) Weight loss achieved: −51.0 ± 20.7 kg for RYGB group and −31.1 ± 17.6 kg for the restrictive surgery group Outcome: increase in total testosterone and SHBG; decrease in fasting glucose and insulin
Level Ia	Glina et al. (64)	7 articles	Bariatric surgery—Review article	Outcome: improvement in IIEF score
Level IIb	Dallal et al. (65)	97	Gastric bypass	Post—operative time point review: 19 months Weight loss achieved: Mean 53 ± 29 kg Outcome: improvement in sexual drive, erectile function, ejaculatory function, and sexual satisfaction
Level IIb	Kun et al. (66)	39	Roux-en-y gastric bypass	Post operative time point review: 12 months Weight loss achieved: Unspecified Mean pre-op BMI: 41.2 ± 8.5 kg/m^2 and post-op 32.1 ± 7.3 kg/m^2 Outcome: improvement in cavernosal thickness and vasculopathy, endothelial function scores, and IIEF
Level Ia	Wei et al. (67)	6 articles	Gastric bypass—Review article	Outcome: increase in semen volume; no changes in semen concentration or motility
Level IIa	Carette et al. (68)	46	Gastric bypass; Sleeve gastrectomy	Post operative time point review: 6 and 12 months Weight loss achieved: inaccessible Outcome: increase sperm count likely due to resolution of hypogonadism and DNA fragmentation
Level IIb	Samavat et al. (69)	31	Roux-en-y gastric bypass; Medical management	Post operative time point review: 0 and 6 months Weight loss achieved: Mean −34.7 ± 16.7 kg Outcome: improvement in total sperm motility and number; Statistically significant increase in semen volume. Reduced Il- 8 levels and sperm DNA fragmentation
Level IV	Sermondade et al. (70)	3	Roux-en-y gastric bypass; Sleeve gastrectomy	Post operative time point review: not specified Weight loss achieved: Unspecified Case 1: −32.3 kg/m^2 Case 2: −23.1 kg/m^2 Case 3: −11.1 kg/m^2 Outcome: severe worsening of parameters in 2 patients; reversibility seen in 1 patient 2 years post-operatively

Levels of evidence based on Oxford Center for Evidence Based Medicine criteria (71).
OCN, Osteocalcin; SHBG, Serum Hormone Binding Globulin; IIEF, International Index of Erectile Function; HDL, High Density Lipoproteins; CRP, C-Reactive Protein; FSH, Follicle Stimulating Hormone.

improvements in hormonal profile. However, the positive effects seen on erectile function are thought to be due to more than just an improvement in hormonal and metabolic profiles. We know that erectile dysfunction in part results from issues with the integrity of blood vessels in penis. In fact, some researchers have also suggested that erectile dysfunction could be a manifestation of vascular disease and endothelial dysfunction (59). This theory was reinforced in a retrospective cohort study by Kun et al. in which 39 obese men were investigated and 46.2 and 53.8% had cavernosal vasculopathy and carotid vasculopathy, respectively (76). This reduced post bariatric surgery to 15.4 and 23.1% and subsequently led to an improvement in IIEF from 17.3 to 23.8 (80).

In reality, improvement in erectile function and in fact reversal of erectile dysfunction is likely due to a drastic and maintained reduction in excess weight leading to a more favorable hormonal and metabolic profile. Further amelioration of other co-morbidities and risk factors such as endothelial dysfunction clearly significantly contributes to better outcomes.

Bariatric Surgery: Sperm and Semen Parameters

The effects of bariatric surgery on hormonal profiles and erectile function in male patients with obesity are clearly favorable. However, the impact on semen and sperm parameters remains inconsistent within the current literature. Samavat et al. assessed morbidly obese patients 6 months after laparoscopic RYGB and found improvement in overall semen volume and viability (66). In addition, they found a decrease in serum Il-8 levels and sperm DNA fragmentation (66).

Similarly, a systematic review and meta-analysis of 6 articles showed that patients who had undergone gastric bypass surgery had an increase in semen volume (69).

Conversely, Lee et al. carried out a systematic review and meta-analysis of 28 cohort studies in which sperm parameters were reported in only three of those articles and showed no statistically significant difference pre- and post- bariatric surgery (67). Furthermore the BARIASPERM study, assessing 46 male patients with no prior history of infertility, showed that sperm count at 6 and 12 months post operatively was significantly reduced (81). Patients underwent either a gastric bypass surgery or a sleeve gastrectomy with both showing reduced total sperm count at −41.1 million and −91.1 million, respectively (81).

The reasons underlying these negative effects are likely multifactorial involving different underlying pathophysiological mechanisms. Rapid and sizeable excess body weight loss can lead to nutritional deficiencies such as iron, calcium, and vitamins. This occurs in varying severity depending on the surgical procedure and can have a negative effect on spermatogenesis leading to worsening parameters (68). In addition, weight loss of such proportion can lead to release of liposoluble toxic substances that can cause alterations in spermatogenesis (68). A case series by Sermondade et al. analyzed three patients and found worsening sperm parameters in all three patients however in one case this effect was reversed after 24 months (68). This further supports the theory above suggesting that over time stabilization of nutritional status and reduction in toxic metabolites may have eventually led to improved sperm parameters (58). It is clear that there is no consensus currently in the scientific literature on the effects of bariatric surgery on sperm and semen parameters. Further studies with larger populations are required to elucidate exact effects and suggest underlying pathophysiological mechanisms.

CONCLUSION

Obesity has become a global pandemic affecting both developed and developing nations. It has significant health consequences on the individual including issues relating to sexual and reproductive health. Bariatric surgery, as a metabolic treatment for obesity, is clearly very effective in terms of rapid and sustained reductions in BMI leading to restoration of reproductive and metabolic hormonal profile. Significant weight loss also alleviates the pro-inflammatory state that is associated with obesity and other co-morbid conditions and helps restore endothelial integrity thereby reducing erectile dysfunction and other cardiovascular risk burden. Bariatric surgery produces successful and encouraging outcomes in terms of the patient's overall health and well-being but more specifically seems to ameliorate hypogonadism and sexual dysfunction.

There remain several unanswered questions in relation to the effects of bariatric surgery on male fertility. The evidence of the effects of surgical interventions on sperm and semen parameters remains conflicting with no consensus reached in the current literature. It is clear from this review that most studies included are small and largely involve retrospective data analysis which is a clear area of improvement in future research and a limitation of this manuscript. Experimental medicine studies interrogating the elusive pathophysiology of obesity and male reproductive system can be invaluable in the optimisation of current and development of future tailored metabolic interventions to treat male obesity related reproductive dysfunction.

AUTHOR CONTRIBUTIONS

SS and GD wrote the manuscript. AP, SE-H, BW, RV, CR, FR, SA, and GD revised the final version of the manuscript. All authors contributed to the article and approved the submitted version.

REFERENCES

1. Obesity and overweight. Who.int (2019). Available online at: https://www.who.int/news-room/fact-sheets/detail/obesity-and-overweight (accessed December 9, 2019).
2. Khaodhiar L, McCowen K, Blackburn G. Obesity and its comorbid conditions. *Clin Cornerstone.* (1999) 2:17–31. doi: 10.1016/S1098-3597(99)90002-9
3. Yafi FA, Jenkins L, Albersen M, Corona G, Isidori AM, Goldfarb S, et al. Erectile dysfunction. *Nat Rev Dis Prim.* (2016) 2:16003. doi: 10.1038/nrdp.2016.3
4. De Lorenzo A, Noce A, Moriconi E, Rampello T, Marrone G, Di Daniele N, et al. MOSH Syndrome (male obesity secondary hypogonadism): clinical assessment and possible therapeutic approaches. *Nutrients.* (2018) 10:474. doi: 10.3390/nu10040474

5. Seyam O, Gandhi J, Joshi G, Smith N, Khan S. Obesity's role in secondary male hypogonadism: a review of pathophysiology and management issues. *SN Comprehensive Clin Med.* (2019) 1:408–18. doi: 10.1007/s42399-019-00056-7
6. Di Vincenzo A, Busetto L, Vettor R, Rossato M. Obesity, male reproductive function and bariatric surgery. *Front Endocrinol.* (2018) 9:769. doi: 10.3389/fendo.2018.00769
7. Tajar A, Forti G, O'Neill TW, Lee DM, Silman AJ, Finn JD, et al. Characteristics of secondary, primary, and compensated hypogonadism in aging men: evidence from the European male ageing study. *J Clin Endocrinol Metab.* (2010) 95:1810–8. doi: 10.1210/jc.2009-1796
8. Fui MN, Dupuis P, Grossmann M. Lowered testosterone in male obesity: mechanisms, morbidity and management. *Asian J Androl.* (2014) 16:223–31. doi: 10.4103/1008-682X.122365
9. Mihalca R, Fica S. The impact of obesity on the male reproductive axis. *J Med Life.* (2014) 7:296–300.
10. Cohen P. The hypogonadal–obesity cycle: role of aromatase in modulating the testosterone–estradiol shunt – a major factor in the genesis of morbid obesity. *Med Hypotheses.* (1999) 52:49–51. doi: 10.1054/mehy.1997.0624
11. Kelly D, Jones T. Testosterone: a metabolic hormone in health and disease. *J Endocrinol.* (2013) 217:R25–45. doi: 10.1530/JOE-12-0455
12. Schulster M, Bernie AM, Ramasamy R. The role of estradiol in male reproductive function. *Asian J Androl.* (2016) 18:435–40. doi: 10.4103/1008-682X.173932
13. Isidori A, Caprio M, Strollo F, Moretti C, Frajese G, Isidori A, et al. Leptin and androgens in male obesity: evidence for leptin contribution to reduced androgen levels1. *J Clin Endocrinol Metab.* (1999) 84:3673–80. doi: 10.1210/jcem.84.10.6082
14. Harter C, Kavanagh G, Smith J. The role of kisspeptin neurons in reproduction and metabolism. *J Endocrinol.* (2018) 238:R173–R183. doi: 10.1530/JOE-18-0108
15. George J, Millar R, Anderson R. Hypothesis: kisspeptin mediates male hypogonadism in obesity and type 2 diabetes. *Neuroendocrinology.* (2010) 91:302–7. doi: 10.1159/000299767
16. Tremellen K. Gut endotoxin leading to a decline IN gonadal function (GELDING) - a novel theory for the development of late onset hypogonadism in obese men. *Basic Clin Androl.* (2016) 26:7. doi: 10.1186/s12610-016-0034-7
17. Tremellen K, McPhee N, Pearce K, Benson S, Schedlowski M, Engler H. Endotoxin-initiated inflammation reduces testosterone production in men of reproductive age. *Am J Physiol Endocrinol Metab.* (2018) 314:E206–13. doi: 10.1152/ajpendo.00279.2017
18. Yamazaki H, Kushiyama A, Sakoda H, Fujishiro M, Yamamotoya, T, Nakatsu Y, et al. Protective effect of sex hormone-binding globulin against metabolic syndrome: *in vitro* evidence showing anti-inflammatory and lipolytic effects on adipocytes and macrophages. *Mediators Inflamm.* (2018) 2018:3062319. doi: 10.1155/2018/3062319
19. DeVan M, Bankson D, Abadie J. To what extent are free testosterone (FT) values reproducible between the two washingtons, and can calculated FT be used in lieu of expensive direct measurements?. *Am J Clin Pathol.* (2008) 129:459–63. doi: 10.1309/6PYTC60ALVQQ59RQ
20. Stellato R, Feldman H, Hamdy O, Horton E, McKinlay J. Testosterone, sex hormone-binding globulin, and the development of type 2 diabetes in middle-aged men: prospective results from the Massachusetts male aging study. *Diabetes Care.* (2000) 23:490–4. doi: 10.2337/diacare.23.4.490
21. Haffner S, Shaten J, Stem M, Smith G, Kuller L. Low levels of sex hormone-binding globulin and testosterone predict the development of non-insulin-dependent diabetes mellitus in men. *Am J Epidemiol.* (1996) 143:889–97. doi: 10.1093/oxfordjournals.aje.a008832
22. Benitez A, Diaz J. Effect of streptozotocin-diabetes and insulin treatment on regulation of leydig cell function in the rat. *Hormone Metab Res.* (1985) 17:5–7. doi: 10.1055/s-2007-1013433
23. Pitteloud N, Hardin M, Dwyer A, Valassi E, Yialamas M, Elahi D, et al. Increasing insulin resistance is associated with a decrease in leydig cell testosterone secretion in men. *J Clin Endocrinol Metab.* (2005) 90:2636–41. doi: 10.1210/jc.2004-2190
24. Kim SD, Cho KS. Obstructive sleep apnea and testosterone deficiency. *World J Mens Health.* (2019) 37:12–18. doi: 10.5534/wjmh.180017
25. Fernandez CJ, Chacko EC, Pappachan JM. Male obesity-related secondary hypogonadism - pathophysiology, clinical implications and management. *Eur Endocrinol.* (2019) 15:83–90. doi: 10.17925/EE.2019.15.2.83
26. Traish A, Feeley R, Guay A. Mechanisms of obesity and related pathologies: androgen deficiency and endothelial dysfunction may be the link between obesity and erectile dysfunction. *FEBS J.* (2009) 276:5755–67. doi: 10.1111/j.1742-4658.2009.07305.x
27. Feldman HA, Johannes CB, Derby CA, Kleinman KP, Mohr BA, Araujo AB. Erectile dysfunction and coronary risk factors: prospective results from the Massachusetts male aging study. *Prev Med.* (2000) 30:328–38. doi: 10.1006/pmed.2000.0643
28. Fung MM, Bettencourt R, Barrett-Connor H. Heart disease risk factors predict erectile dysfunction 25 years later. *J Am Coll Cardiol.* (2004). 43:1405–11. doi: 10.1016/j.jacc.2003.11.041
29. Miscio G, Guastamacchia G, Brunani A, Priano L, Baudo S, Mauro A. Obesity and peripheral neuropathy risk: a dangerous liaison. *J Peripher Nerv Syst.* (2005) 10:354–8. doi: 10.1111/j.1085-9489.2005.00047.x
30. Corona G, Mannucci E, Schulman C, Petrone L, Mansani R, Cilotti A, et al. Psychobiologic correlates of the metabolic syndrome and associated sexual dysfunction. *Eur Urol.* (2006) 50:595–604. doi: 10.1016/j.eururo.2006.02.053
31. Bacon C, Mittleman M, Kawachi I, Giovannucci E, Glasser D, Rimm E. Sexual function in men older than 50 years of age: results from the health professionals follow-up study. *Ann Intern Med.* (2003) 139:161–8. doi: 10.7326/0003-4819-139-3-200308050-00005
32. Bacon C, Mittleman M, Kawachi I, Giovannucci E, Glasser D, Rimm E. A prospective study of risk factors for erectile dysfunction. *J Urol.* (2006) 176:217–21. doi: 10.1016/S0022-5347(06)00589-1
33. Sanchez E, Pastuszak AW, Khera M. Erectile dysfunction, metabolic syndrome, and cardiovascular risks: facts and controversies. *Transl Androl Urol.* (2017) 6:28–36. doi: 10.21037/tau.2016.10.01
34. Kouidrat Y, Pizzol D, Cosco T, Thompson T, Carnaghi M, Bertoldo A, et al. High prevalence of erectile dysfunction in diabetes: a systematic review and meta-analysis of 145 studies. *Diabet Med.* (2017) 34:1185–92. doi: 10.1111/dme.13403
35. Marseglia L, Manti S, D'Angelo G, Nicotera A, Parisi E, Di Rosa G, et al. Oxidative stress in obesity: a critical component in human diseases. *Int J Mol Sci.* (2014) 16:378–400. doi: 10.3390/ijms16010378
36. Wang EY, Huang Y, Du QY, Yao GD, Sun YP. Body mass index effects sperm quality: a retrospective study in Northern China. *Asian J Androl.* (2017) 19:234–7. doi: 10.4103/1008-682X.169996
37. Håkonsen LB, Thulstrup AM, Aggerholm AS, Olsen J, Bonde JP, Andersen Y, et al. Does weight loss improve semen quality and reproductive hormones? Results from a cohort of severely obese men. *Reprod Health.* (2011) 8:24. doi: 10.1186/1742-4755-8-24
38. Palmer NO, Bakos HW, Fullston T, Lane M. Impact of obesity on male fertility, sperm function and molecular composition. *Spermatogenesis.* (2012) 2:253–63. doi: 10.4161/spmg.21362
39. Belloc S, Cohen-Bacrie M, Amar E, Izard V, Benkhalifa M, Dalléac A, et al. High body mass index has a deleterious effect on semen parameters except morphology: results from a large cohort study. *Fertil Steril.* (2014) 102:1268–73. doi: 10.1016/j.fertnstert.2014.07.1212
40. Sermondade N, Faure C, Fezeu L, Shayeb A, Bonde J, Jensen T, et al. BMI in relation to sperm count: an updated systematic review and collaborative meta-analysis. *Hum Reprod Update.* (2012) 19:221–31. doi: 10.1093/humupd/dms050
41. Rufus O, James O, Michael A. Male obesity and semen quality: any association? *Int J Reprod Biomed.* (2018) 16:285–90. doi: 10.29252/ijrm.16.4.285
42. Bohacek J, Mansuy IM. Epigenetic inheritance of disease and disease risk. *Neuropsychopharmacology.* (2013) 38:220–36. doi: 10.1038/npp.2012.110

43. Nilsson EE, SkinnerMK. Environmentally induced epigenetic transgenerational inheritance of disease susceptibility. *Transl Res.* (2015) 165:12–7. doi: 10.1016/j.trsl.2014.02.003
44. Yuan TF, Li A, Sun X, Ouyang H, Campos C, Rocha NB, et al. Transgenerational inheritance of paternal neurobehavioral phenotypes: stress, addiction, ageing and metabolism. *Mol Neurobiol.* (2016) 53:6367–76. doi: 10.1007/s12035-015-9526-2
45. Smith CA. The effect of wartime starvation in Holland upon pregnancy and its product. *Am J Obstet Gynecol.* (1947) 53:599–608. doi: 10.1016/0002-9378(47)90277-9
46. de Castro Barbosa T, Ingerslev LR, Alm PS, Versteyhe S, Massart J, Rasmussen M, et al. High-fat diet reprograms the epigenome of rat spermatozoa and transgenerationally affects metabolism of the offspring. *Mol Metab.* (2016) 5:184–97. doi: 10.1016/j.molmet.2015.12.002
47. Fullston T, Ohlsson Teague EM, Palmer NO, DeBlasio MJ, Mitchell M, Corbett M, et al. Paternal obesity initiates metabolic disturbances in two generations of mice with incomplete penetrance to the F2 generation and alters the transcriptional profile of testis and sperm microRNA content. *FASEB J.* (2013) 27:4226–43. doi: 10.1096/fj.12-224048
48. Soubry A, Schildkraut JM, Murtha A, Wang F, Huang Z, Bernal A, et al. Paternal obesity is associated with IGF2 hypomethylation in newborns: results from a newborn epigenetics study (NEST) cohort. *BMC Med.* (2013) 11:29. doi: 10.1186/1741-7015-11-29
49. Craig JR, Jenkins TG, Carrell DT, Hotaling JM. Obesity, male infertility, and the sperm epigenome. *Fertil Steril.* (2017) 107:848–59. doi: 10.1016/j.fertnstert.2017.02.115
50. Donkin I, Versteyhe S, Ingerslev LR, Qian K, Mechta M, Nordkap L, et al. Obesity and bariatric surgery drive epigenetic variation of spermatozoa in humans. *Cell Metab.* (2016) 23:369–78. doi: 10.1016/j.cmet.2015.11.004
51. Jensterle M, Podbregar A, Goricar K, Gregoric N, Janez A. Effects of liraglutide on obesity-associated functional hypogonadism in men. *Endocr Connect.* (2019) 8:195–202. doi: 10.1530/EC-18-0514
52. Camacho E, Huhtaniemi I, O'Neill T, Finn J, Pye S, Lee D, et al. Age-associated changes in hypothalamic–pituitary–testicular function in middle-aged and older men are modified by weight change and lifestyle factors: longitudinal results from the European male ageing study. *Eur J Endocrinol.* (2013) 168:445–55. doi: 10.1530/EJE-12-0890
53. Travison T, Araujo A, Kupelian V, O'Donnell A, McKinlay J. The relative contributions of aging, health, and lifestyle factors to serum testosterone decline in men. *J Clin Endocrinol Metab.* (2007) 92:549–55. doi: 10.1210/jc.2006-1859
54. Mir J, Franken D, Andrabi S, Ashraf M, Rao K. Impact of weight loss on sperm DNA integrity in obese men. *Andrologia.* (2018) 50:e12957. doi: 10.1111/and.12957
55. Esposito K, Giugliano F, Di Palo C, Giugliano G, Marfella R, D'Andrea F, et al. Effect of lifestyle changes on erectile dysfunction in obese men. *JAMA.* (2004) 291:2978. doi: 10.1001/jama.291.24.2978
56. Wolfe BM, Kvach E, Eckel RH. Treatment of obesity: weight loss and bariatric surgery. *Circ Res.* (2016) 118:1844–55. doi: 10.1161/CIRCRESAHA.116.307591
57. O'Brien PE, Hindle A, Brennan L, Skinner S, Burton P, Smith A, et al. Long-term outcomes after bariatric surgery: a systematic review and meta-analysis of weight loss at 10 or more years for all bariatric procedures and a single-centre review of 20-year outcomes after adjustable gastric banding. *Obes Surg.* (2019) 29:3–14. doi: 10.1007/s11695-018-3525-0
58. Samavat J, Facchiano E, Cantini G, Di Franco A, Alpigiano G, Poli G, et al. Osteocalcin increase after bariatric surgery predicts androgen recovery in hypogonadal obese males. *Int J Obes.* (2013) 38:357–63. doi: 10.1038/ijo.2013.228
59. Arolfo S, Scozzari G, Di Benedetto G, Vergine V, Morino M. Surgically induced weight loss effects on sexual quality of life of obese men: a prospective evaluation. *Surg Endosc.* (2020). doi: 10.1007/s00464-019-07356-y. [Epub ahead of print].
60. Legro R, Kunselman A, Meadows J, Kesner J, Krieg E, Rogers A, et al. Time-related increase in urinary testosterone levels and stable semen analysis parameters after bariatric surgery in men. *Reprod BioMed Online.* (2015) 30:150–6. doi: 10.1016/j.rbmo.2014.10.014
61. Reis L, Zani E, Saad R, Chaim E, de Oliveira L, Fregonesi A. Bariatric surgery does not interfere with sperm quality—a preliminary long-term study. *Reprod Sci.* (2012) 19:1057–62. doi: 10.1177/1933719112440747
62. Liu F, Tu Y, Zhang P, Bao Y, Han J, Jia W. Decreased visceral fat area correlates with improved total testosterone levels after Roux-en-Y gastric bypass in obese Chinese males with type 2 diabetes: a 12-month follow-up. *Surg Obes Relat Dis.* (2018) 14:462–8. doi: 10.1016/j.soard.2017.11.009
63. Calderón B, Galdón A, Calañas A, Peromingo R, Galindo J, García-Moreno F, et al. Effects of bariatric surgery on male obesity-associated secondary hypogonadism: comparison of laparoscopic gastric bypass with restrictive procedures. *Obes Surg.* (2014) 24:1686–92. doi: 10.1007/s11695-014-1233-y
64. Glina F, de Freitas Barboza J, Nunes V, Glina S, Bernardo W. What is the impact of bariatric surgery on erectile function? A systematic review and meta-analysis. *Sex Med Rev.* (2017) 5:393–402. doi: 10.1016/j.sxmr.2017.03.008
65. Dallal R, Chernoff A, O'Leary M, Smith J, Braverman J, Quebbemann B. Sexual dysfunction is common in the morbidly obese male and improves after gastric bypass surgery. *J Am Coll Surgeons.* (2008) 207:859–64. doi: 10.1016/j.jamcollsurg.2008.08.006
66. Kun L, Pin Z, Jianzhong D, Xiaodong H, Haoyong Y, Yuqian B, et al. Significant improvement of erectile function after roux-en-Y gastric bypass surgery in obese chinese men with erectile dysfunction. *Obes Surg.* (2014) 25:838–44. doi: 10.1007/s11695-014-1465-x
67. Wei Y, Chen Q, Qian W. Effect of bariatric surgery on semen parameters: a systematic review and meta-analysis. *Med Sci Monit Basic Res.* (2018) 24:188–97. doi: 10.12659/MSMBR.910862
68. Carette C, Levy R, Eustache F, Baron G, Coupaye M, Msika S, et al. Changes in total sperm count after gastric bypass and sleeve gastrectomy: the BARIASPERM prospective study. *Surg Obes Relat Dis.* (2019) 15:1271–9. doi: 10.1016/j.soard.2019.04.019
69. Samavat J, Cantini G, Lotti, F, Di Franco A, Tamburrino L, Degl'Innocenti S, et al. Massive weight loss obtained by bariatric surgery affects semen quality in morbid male obesity: a preliminary prospective double-armed study. *Obes Surg.* (2018) 28:69–76. doi: 10.1007/s11695-017-2802-7
70. Sermondade N, Massin N, Boitrelle F, Pfeffer J, Eustache F, Sifer C, et al. Sperm parameters and male fertility after bariatric surgery: three case series. *Reprod BioMed Online.* (2012) 24:206–10. doi: 10.1016/j.rbmo.2011.10.014
71. Osland E, Yunus R, Khan S, Memon B, Memon M. Weight loss outcomes in laparoscopic vertical sleeve gastrectomy (LVSG) versus laparoscopic roux-en-Y gastric bypass (LRYGB) procedures. *Surg Laparosc Endosc Percutan Tech.* (2017) 27:e121. doi: 10.1097/SLE.0000000000000486
72. Howick J. Oxford centre for evidence-based medicine - levels of evidence (March 2009) - CEBM. *CEBM.* (2009). Available online at: https://www.cebm.net/2009/06/oxford-centre-evidence-based-medicine-levels-evidence-march-2009/ (accessed on January 31, 2020)
73. Pellitero S, Olaizola I, Alastrue A, Martínez E, Granada M, Balibrea J, et al. Hypogonadotropic hypogonadism in morbidly obese males is reversed after bariatric surgery. *Obes Surg.* (2012) 22:1835–42. doi: 10.1007/s11695-012-0734-9
74. Escobar-Morreale H, Santacruz E, Luque-Ramírez M, Botella Carretero J. Prevalence of 'obesity-associated gonadal dysfunction' in severely obese men and women and its resolution after bariatric surgery: a systematic review and meta-analysis. *Hum Reprod Update.* (2017) 23:390–408. doi: 10.1093/humupd/dmx012
75. Laimer M, Ebenbichler C, Kaser S, Sandhofer A, Weiss H, Nehoda H, et al. Markers of chronic inflammation and obesity: a prospective study on the reversibility of this association in middle-aged women undergoing weight loss by surgical intervention. *Int J Obes.* (2002) 26:659–62. doi: 10.1038/sj.ijo.0801970
76. Saleh M, Bertolami M, Assef J, Taha M, de Freitas W, Petisco A, et al. Improvement of atherosclerotic markers in non-diabetic patients after bariatric surgery. *Obes Surg.* (2012) 22:1701–7. doi: 10.1007/s11695-012-0706-0
77. Pham N, Bena J, Bhatt D, Kennedy L, Schauer P, Kashyap S. Increased free testosterone levels in men with uncontrolled type 2 diabetes five

years after randomization to bariatric surgery. *Obes Surg.* (2017) 28:277–80. doi: 10.1007/s11695-017-2881-5

78. Oury F, Sumara G, Sumara O, Ferron M, Chang H, Smith C, et al. Endocrine regulation of male fertility by the skeleton. *Cell.* (2011) 144:796–809. doi: 10.1016/j.cell.2011.02.004
79. Xu J, Wu Q, Zhang Y, Pei C. Effect of bariatric surgery on male sexual function: a meta-analysis and systematic review. *Sex Med.* (2019) 7:270–81. doi: 10.1016/j.esxm.2019.06.003
80. Jackson G. Erectile dysfunction and cardiovascular disease. *Arab J Urol.* (2013) 11:212–16. doi: 10.1016/j.aju.2013.03.003
81. Lee Y, Dang J, Switzer N, Yu J, Tian C, Birch D, et al. Impact of bariatric surgery on male sex hormones and sperm quality: a systematic review and meta-analysis. *Obes Surg.* (2018) 29:334–46. doi: 10.1007/s11695-018-3557-5

10

The Impact of Post-Bariatric Abdominoplasty on Secondary Weight Regain after Roux-en-Y Gastric Bypass

Jorunn Sandvik [1,2,3*], *Torstein Hole* [1,4], *Christian Klöckner* [2,5], *Bård Kulseng* [2,3] *and Arne Wibe* [6,7]

[1] *Clinic of Medicine and Rehabilitation, Møre and Romsdal Hospital Trust, Alesund, Norway,* [2] *Department of Surgery, Center for Obesity, St. Olav Hospital, Trondheim University Hospital, Trondheim, Norway,* [3] *Obesity Research Group, Department of Clinical and Molecular Medicine, Norwegian University of Science and Technology, Trondheim, Norway,* [4] *Faculty of Medicine and Health Sciences, Norwegian University of Science and Technology, Trondheim, Norway,* [5] *Department of Psychology, NTNU - Norwegian University of Science and Technology, Trondheim, Norway,* [6] *Department of Clinical and Molecular Medicine, Norwegian University of Science and Technology, Trondheim, Norway,* [7] *Department of Surgery, St. Olav Hospital, Trondheim University Hospital, Trondheim, Norway*

***Correspondence:**
Jorunn Sandvik
jorunn.sandvik@stolav.no;
jorunn.sandvik@mimer.no

Roux-en-Y gastric bypass (RYGB), implies a considerable weight loss during the first two years after surgery. Excess skin due to rapid weight loss might affect self-esteem, decrease quality of life and be a hindrance to physical activity. Removing excess skin might reduce secondary weight regain. Among plastic surgeons, a BMI < 30 kg/m^2 is usually required to have abdominoplasty (AP). Many RYGB patients never reach this threshold even if they have a considerable weight loss and experience practical as well as emotional problems due to excess skin. The aim of this study was to investigate the role of abominoplasty on weight development until five years, among patients who did and did not achieve a nadir BMI < 30 kg/m^2 during the first two years after RYGB. Data on 645 patients from a single center RYGB-quality register from 2004 to 2013 with baseline and follow-up data were analyzed. Post-bariatric AP was publicly funded if medically needed. Weight regain (WR) from nadir weight to five years was analyzed as percentage WR of maximal weight loss. Nadir BMI was available in 633 (98.1%) patients, and BMI after five years in 553 (85.7%) patients. The 233 patients with nadir BMI < 30 kg/m^2 who underwent AP regained 17.8 ($\pm$16.1) % of their maximal weight loss at five years compared to 24.2 ($\pm$19.7) % in 185 patients not having AP ($p < 0.001$). The 27 patients with nadir BMI > 30 kg/m^2 within two years after RYGB who underwent AP regained 12.9 ($\pm$19.3) % compared to 31.4 ($\pm$24.7) % in 188 patients without AP ($p < 0.001$). This procedure was more common among women than men, as 224 (46.4%) women, and 36 (22.2%) men underwent AP. Abdominoplasty was associated with reduced secondary weight regain after RYGB in this study. Whether this is caused by increased bodily satisfaction and better physical function, or a biological response to reduction of adipose tissue remains unclear. If removing abdominal subcutaneous adipose tissue prevent secondary weight regain and increase the robustness of bariatric surgery, this should be offered as part of the standard treatment after bariatric surgery.

Keywords: post-bariatric abdominoplasty, bariatric surgery, gastric bypass (RYGB), post-bariatric weight regain, post-bariatric body contouring

INTRODUCTION

Surgical procedures for treatment of severe obesity and obesity-related comorbidities have been integrated as part of public as well as private health care during the last two decades. The term *bariatric surgery*, with focus on weight reduction, has to a certain extent been replaced by the term *metabolic surgery*, with focus on the improvement of type 2 diabetes mellitus (T2DM), cardiovascular disease, and other diseases where inflammation plays a role. Worldwide, more than half a million people have bariatric surgery every year, and most of them experience considerable weight loss during the first years after surgery (1, 2). Usually the nadir weight is achieved between 1 and 2 years after surgery; however, most patients experience a varying degree of weight regain (WR) within the following years (3). Secondary WR after bariatric surgery might be regarded as a failure of the surgical method or as a natural progression of the chronic disease of obesity.

Many factors may contribute to the secondary WR, and the patients' motivation for lifelong changes in diet and habits of physical activity has been regarded as the main factor for weight loss maintenance after bariatric surgery. However, the knowledge on the biological mechanism beyond voluntary control of secondary WR after bariatric surgery is increasing (4).

One of the factors that seem to be associated with the degree and durability of weight loss is post-bariatric body contouring procedures (5–7). For some patients, considerable weight loss after bariatric surgery implies burdensome excess skin mainly on abdomen, but also on thighs, arms, breast, back, and face. The excess skin might result in intertrigo, skin infections, and mobility problems, as well as a negative body image, depression, and social dysfunction (8, 9).

When body contouring procedures are performed, excess skin and the adjacent subcutaneous adipose tissue are resected. Improvements in quality of life and bodily function after body contouring surgery have been related to psychological factors and improved self-esteem (10). However, metabolic consequences of removing excess subcutaneous adipose tissue by body contouring procedures have to a lesser extent been explored.

During the last years, an increasing number of the biological functions of adipose tissue have been revealed. Contrary to former beliefs, the adipose tissue is a dynamic and metabolic active organ, secreting various hormones and cytokines involved in appetite regulation, energy metabolism, and inflammation (11, 12). It is therefore relevant to question if removing excess skin and subcutaneous tissue has a beneficial biological effect on reducing secondary WR after bariatric surgery.

Studies on the metabolic effect of removing subcutaneous tissue by liposuction or lipectomy in people with obesity who did not undergo bariatric surgery have shown a reduction in inflammation, improvement in lipid profile, normalization of glucose and insulin levels, and improvement in cardiac function (13–15). In contrast, a meta-analysis on abdominal lipectomy in non-bariatric women from 2015 did not reveal significant effects on metabolic syndrome or insulin sensitivity, and only a short-term effect on body fat and weight (16, 17).

Bariatric surgery is performed in most countries in the world and in health care systems with various financial models. The access to bariatric surgery is limited by capacity as well as financial coverage for the patients. Post-bariatric body contouring surgery is even less accessible, and it may not be covered by public health service or private health insurance (18).

Among 37,906 patients who underwent bariatric surgery in New York from 2004 to 2010, <6% underwent an abdominoplasty during the following years (19). This low utilization of post-bariatric abdominoplasty was mainly explained by financial reasons.

Abdominoplasty is the most common post-bariatric body contouring procedure, but excess skin on thighs, arms, and upper truncus may also be a problem in need of surgical treatment (20). Most plastic surgeons have an upper body mass index (BMI) threshold of 28 or 30 kg/m^2 to perform abdominoplasty, because of the assumed increased risk of complications with higher BMI (21). Because only half of the patients undergoing bariatric surgery reach this BMI threshold, patients in the upper BMI levels before bariatric surgery may struggle with excess skin after a massive weight loss without any treatment alternatives. For them, the physical, mental, and social impairment of excess skin after bariatric surgery may imply an increase in secondary WR. Hence, the role of excess subcutaneous fat in secondary WR needs to be investigated.

Secondary WR after initial successful post-bariatric weight loss has been calculated in different ways; measuring WR as percentage of maximal weight loss is best associated with changes in clinical outcomes after bariatric surgery (22).

The aim of this study was to explore the role of abdominoplasty on weight development from the time of maximum weight loss until 5 years after roux-en-Y gastric bypass (RYGB), in a population who had access to abdominoplasty 2 years after surgery if they reached a nadir BMI of <30 kg/m^2, and there was a medical indication for the procedure.

MATERIALS AND METHODS

This study is a retrospective analysis of prospectively collected data on 645 adult patients who underwent laparoscopic RYGB from 2004 to 2013 as a primary treatment for severe obesity at Ålesund Hospital, a public hospital in Western Norway. Roux-en-Y gastric bypass was a treatment option for patients aged 18–60 years, with BMI >40 kg/m^2 or >35 kg/m^2 with obesity-related comorbidity. Details on the surgical method have been published in a previous article (23).

All patients who underwent RYGB at the hospital from 2004 were registered in a local quality registry, and data on weight changes, selected laboratory tests, body contouring procedures, and other relevant events related to the RYGB procedure were registered at baseline and at follow-up visits 2, 6, 12, 18, 24, 36, 48, and 60 months after surgery. Nadir BMI was the lowest BMI measured at the planned visits at 12, 18, or 24 months. Patients followed up for 5 years or more by the end of 2018 were included in the study.

Patients who wanted abdominoplasty or other body contouring procedures were referred to the plastic surgeon for assessment 18 months after RYGB if they had a BMI of <30 kg/m^2. In general, the patients had to wait at least 2 years after RYGB before they could have abdominoplasty, and the weight had to be stable during 6 months before surgery.

The abdominoplasty was not performed at the same hospital as the RYGB, but at private or public hospitals in the same region. The abdominoplasty was publicly funded regardless of where the operation was performed, if there was a medical indication for surgical treatment. Reports from the plastic surgeon were in most cases sent to the study hospital, and the date of the procedures was added to the quality registry. If reported, the amount of removed tissue and surgical technique were also registered.

Weight regain from nadir weight to 5 years after RYGB was analyzed as percentage WR of maximal weight loss, and WR in kilograms.

Continuous variables are given as means ± standard deviation (SD) if normally distributed, and as median and interquartile range (IQR) if non-normally distributed. Categorical variables are reported in numbers and percentages. Independent *t*-tests were performed for normally distributed continuous variables, and non-parametric test for non-normally distributed variables. χ^2-tests were performed for categorical variables. Differences were considered significant at $P < 0.05$.

RESULTS

From a total of 645 patients, 483 (75%) women, and 162 (25%) men, information on nadir BMI was available in 633 patients (98.1%), and BMI 5 years after RYGB was available in 553 patients (85.7%). Four patients had died within 5 years after RYGB, and 15 (patients 2.3%) had moved out of the region before 5 years. Details on comorbidities at baseline and T2DM after 5 years are given in **Table 1**.

Within 2 years after RYGB, a nadir BMI of 30 kg/m^2 or less was achieved by 418 patients (66.5%), as 331 (68.5%) of the women and 87 (53.7%) of the men reached this threshold ($P <$ 0.001). There was no difference in age among patients with nadir BMI greater than or less than 30 kg/m^2, with mean age of 40 (±9.7) years.

When comparing the patients with nadir BMI greater than or less than 30 kg/m^2, the patients who achieved BMI 30 kg/m^2 or less had a mean preoperative BMI of 42.0 (±3.6) kg/m^2, compared to 47.4 (±5.4) kg/m^2 in the patients who did not achieve a nadir BMI of less than this limit. Mean nadir BMI in the lower BMI group was 26.0 (±2.2) kg/m^2, compared to 33.4 (±2.8) kg/m^2, and mean BMI at 5 years was 29.0 (±3.5) kg/m^2 compared to 36.9 (±4.4) kg/m^2. The differences were significant at all points ($P < 0.001$) (**Figure 1**).

The mean percentage of total weight loss (%TWL) at nadir and after 5 years was 38.2% (±6.3%) and 30.5% (±9.0%) for the patients with nadir BMI of <30 kg/m^2, compared to 29.4% (±7.1%) and 21.3% (±9.6%) for the patients with nadir BMI of >30 kg/m^2 ($P < 0.001$).

Secondary WR measured as percentage of maximal weight loss from nadir to 5 years was 28.9% (±24.8%) in patients with nadir BMI of >30 kg/m^2 and 20.4% (± 18.0%) in all of the patients with nadir BMI below 30 kg/m^2 ($P < 0.001$).

Among the 418 patients who achieved BMI ≤ 30 kg/m^2, there were 233 patients (55.7%) who underwent abdominoplasty. The procedure was more common among women than men, as 202 (61.0%) of the women and 31 (35.6%) of the men with BMI ≤30 kg/m^2 underwent abdominoplasty ($P < 0.001$). The patients who had abdominoplasty were 39 (±8.8) years compared to 40.6 (±10.7) years in the patients who did not (ns). The median (IQR) time from RYGB to abdominoplasty was 31.0 (25.5–37) months.

In patients with nadir BMI of 30 kg/m^2 or less, preoperative BMI, nadir BMI, and BMI at 5 years were 42.4 (±3.7) kg/m^2, 25.6 (±2.0) kg/m^2, and 28.5 (±3.2) kg/m in the abdominoplasty

TABLE 1 | Comorbidities at baseline and T2DM status 5 years after RYGB in patients who achieved nadir BMI greater than or less than 30 kg/m^2, with and without abdominoplasty.

	Nadir BMI<30 kg/m^2 *n* = 418		*P*	Nadir BMI>30 kg/m^2 *n* = 210		*P*
	With AP *n* = 233	Without AP *n* = 185		With AP *n* = 27	Without AP *n* = 183	
T2DM at baseline	67 (16%)			38 (18.1%)		
	28 (12.0%)	39 (21.2%)	$P = 0.01$	3 (11.55)	34 (18.5%)	$P = 0.379$
T2DM at 5 years	13 (3.1%)			10 (4.8%)		
	5 (2.1%)	8(4.3%)	$P = 0.203$	0	10 (5.5%)	n.a.
Hypertension, baseline	105 (25.1%)			62(29.5%)		
	45 (19.3%)	60 (32.6%)	$P = 0.002$	3 (11.5%)	59 (32.2%)	$P = 0.031$
Sleep apnea baseline	95 (22.7%)			59 (28.4%)		
	45(19.4%)	50(27.2%)	$P = 0.062$	9 (33.3%)	51(27.9%)	$P = 0.557$
Hyperlipidemia baseline	52 (12.4%)			29 (13.8%)		
	18 (7.7%)	34 (18.4%)	$P = 0.001$	2 (7.4%)	27 (14.6%)	$P = 0.325$

AP, abdominoplasty; T2DM, type 2 diabetes mellitus.

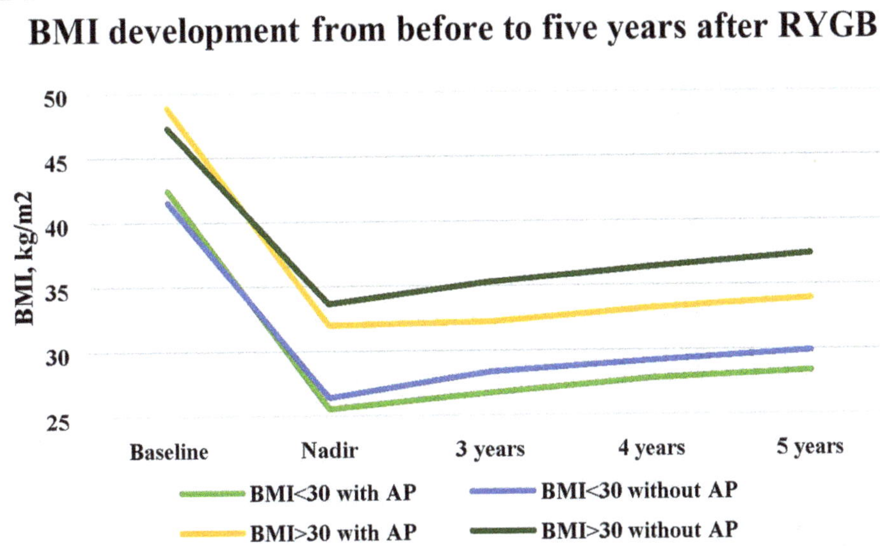

FIGURE 1 | Changes in mean BMI from baseline to 5 years after RYGB in patients with and without abdominoplasty and Nadir BMI above or below 30 kg/m^2.

group, and 41.6 (±3.5) kg/m^2, 26.4 (±2.3) kg/m^2, and 30.1 (±3.7) kg/m^2 among those who did not have abdominoplasty ($P < 0.001$ at all points) (**Table 2**).

From nadir to 5 years, the patients who achieved a nadir BMI of 30 kg/m^2 or less and underwent abdominoplasty in this period regained 17.8% (±16.1%) of their maximal weight loss compared to 24.2% (±19.7%) in patients who did not have abdominoplasty ($P < 0.001$) (**Figure 2**). When WR was measured in kilograms, the patients who had abdominoplasty had an increase of 8.4 (±7.3) kg, compared to 10.7 (±8.6) kg in the patients who did not have abdominoplasty ($P < 0.05$).

Abdominoplasty was mainly performed in the patients who achieved BMI of <30 kg/m^2 during the first 2 years after RYGB. However, from the 215 patients with a nadir BMI of >30 kg/m^2 during the first 2 years after RYGB, there were 27 (12.5%) patients, 22 women and 5 men, who had abdominoplasty at a median 35.5 (30.5–54.7) months after RYGB (**Table 2**). The secondary WR in this group was 6.1 (± 8.5) kg compared to 11.9 (±9.1) kg ($P <$ 0.001), or measured as WR in percentage of maximal weight loss 12.9% (±19.3%) compared to 31.4% (±24.7%) in the patients with nadir BMI of >30 kg/m^2 who did not undergo abdominoplasty ($P < 0.001$) (**Figure 2**). Men and women who underwent abdominoplasty had similar weight development (**Figure 3**).

When it comes to other body contouring procedures, 2 men and 48 women had breast corrections (reduction, lift, or augmentation). Also, 2 men and 43 women had excess skin on thighs removed, and 1 man and 29 women had plastic surgery on upper arms in the follow-up period. These procedures were performed at a later stage after RYGB and are not analyzed in relation to secondary WR in this study. Of all patients, 198 (30.7%) had one body contouring procedure, 52 (8.1%) had two procedures, and 25 (3.9%) had more than two procedures.

The reports from the plastic surgeons contained information on the amount of tissue removed at the abdominoplasty in 145 (55.8%) of 260 cases, the mean weight being 1.76 (±0.97) kg. As this information was not available for all patients who had abdominoplasty, individual values on excised tissue have not been implemented in the analyses of secondary WR in this study. However, a correlation between weight of excised tissue and secondary WR was not found in the subgroup with available data ($P = 0.737$).

DISCUSSION

In the present study, less secondary WR was found in the patients who underwent abdominoplasty after RYGB, and the difference was highest in the group with nadir BMI of >30 kg/m^2 within the first 2 years after RYGB. The number of patients in this group was low, and there was no information on BMI at time of abdominoplasty.

More women than men had abdominoplasty, as there were more women who achieved a BMI of <30 kg/m^2 within the first 2 years after RYGB. Moreover, the interest for body contouring surgery after bariatric surgery were higher among women than men, as has been found in other studies (24–26).

An assumed higher risk of post-operative complications has been the reason for limiting abdominoplasty after major weight loss to patients with BMI of <30 kg/m^2 (27). However, there are studies that did not find any difference in complications among patients with BMI greater than or less than 30 kg/m^2 undergoing post-bariatric body contorting surgery (28). In the present study, the abdominoplasties were mainly performed as day surgery in private hospitals without facilities for postoperative observation in a surgical ward. Furthermore, patients with higher surgical risk due to comorbidities or higher BMI had less access to

TABLE 2 | Patients' characteristics and weight changes.

	Nadir BMI <30 kg/m² *n* = 418		*P*	Nadir BMI >30 kg/m² *n* = 210		*P*
	With AP *n* = 233	**Without AP** *n* = 185		**With AP** *n* = 27	**Without AP** *n* = 183	
Age (±SD), years	39.2 (± 8.8)	40.6 (±10.7)	P = 0.125	36.6 (±8.2)	40.5 (±9.9)	P = 0.61
Female/male ratio	202/31	129/56	P < 0.001	22/5	118/65	P = 0.100
Baseline BMI (±SD) kg/m², *N*	42.4 (±3.7) 233	41.6 (±3.5) 185	P = 0.01	48.9 (±6.0) 27	47.3 (±5.3) 183	P = 0.172
Nadir BMI (±SD) kg/m², *n*	25.6 (±2.0) 233	26.4 (±2.3) 185	P < 0.001	32.0 (±2.0) 27	33.6 (±2.9) 183	P < 0.001
BMI 3 years after RYGB (±SD) kg/m², *n*	26.7 (±2.5) 220	28.4 (±3.2) 164	P < 0.001	32.2 (±2.7) 22	35.3 (±3.6) 141	P < 0.001
BMI 4 years after RYGB (±SD) kg/m², *n*	27.8 (±2.9) 212	29.2 (±3.4) 145	P < 0.001	33.2 (±2.7) 22	36.4 (±3.9) 145	P < 0.001
BMI 5 years after RYGB (±SD) kg/m², *n*	28.5 (±3.2) 212	30.1 (±3.7) 156	P < 0.001	33.9 (±3.2) 24	37.4 (±4.3) 152	P < 0.001
% TWL at nadir %, *n*	39.8 (±5.7) 233	36.3 (±6.4) 184	P < 0.001	33.8 (±7.2) 26	28.8 (±6.9) 183	P < 0.001
% TWL after 3 years %, *n*	36.5 (±7.3) 220	31.3 (±7.6) 164	P < 0.001	33.7 (±8.7) 22	24.3 (±8.1) 141	P < 0.001
% TWL after 4 years %, *n*	34.1 (±7.9) 212	29.1 (±8.0) 145	P < 0.001	31.0 (±8.0) 22	22.2 (±8.3) 145	P < 0.001
% TWL after 5 years %, *n*	32.7 (±8.1) 212	27.6 (±9.1) 156	P < 0.001	30.0 (±8.9) 24	20.0 (±9.0) 152	P < 0.001
% EWL at nadir %, *n*	97.6 (±11.9) 233	92.0 (±14.7) 185	P < 0.001	69.7 (±8.3) 26	61.1 (±10.9) 183	P < 0.001
% EWL after 3 years %, *n*	89.2 (±15.3) 220	79.4 (±18.9) 164	P < 0.001	68.1 (±11.9) 22	51.6 (±14.1) 141	P < 0.001
% EWL after 4 years %, *n*	83.4 (±17.4) 212	74.3 (±19.9) 145	P < 0.001	63.5 (±12.0) 22	46.9 (±15.1) 145	P < 0.001
% EWL after 5 years %, *n***	80.2 (±18.9) 212	69.5 (±21.6) 156	P < 0.001	60.9 (±14.2) 24	42.6 (±17.5) 152	P < 0.001
WR from nadir to 5 years after RYGB (SD) kg, *n***	8.4 (±7.3) 212	10.7 (±8.6) 156	P < 0.05	6.1 (±8.5) 24	11.9 (±9.1) 152	P < 0.001
% WR from nadir to 5 years after RYGB of maximal weight loss, %, *n*	17.8 (±16.1) 212	24.2 (±19.7) 156	P = 0.001	12.9 (±19.2) 24	31.4 (±24.7) 152	P < 0.001

*AP, abdominoplasty; **WR, weight regain.*

treatment due to limited capacity in the public hospitals in the region.

A study by de Vries et al. including 126 patients who underwent post-bariatric body contouring surgery found that there might be an association between body contouring surgery and weight loss maintenance after 3 and 4 years, but body contouring surgery was not associated with maintenance of achieved improvement of comorbidities (29). Two other cohort studies have reported less WR if body contouring procedures were performed after RYGB; the weight developments described in these studies were on the same level as in the present study (6, 7).

When it comes to the metabolic and biochemical modifications occurring after abdominoplasty in patients with BMI between 30 and 35 kg/m² who had not undergone bariatric surgery, a study by Cuomo et al. revealed an increase in adiponectin levels and a significant decrease in BMI at 1 year after abdominoplasty, leading the authors to suggest abdominoplasty or liposuction as a method for improvement of insulin sensitivity in people with moderate obesity (13). Several studies have indicated a significant reduction in cardiovascular risk score after large volume liposuction or abdominoplasty, at a level comparable to bariatric surgery (14). These findings might implicate that patients who have undergone bariatric

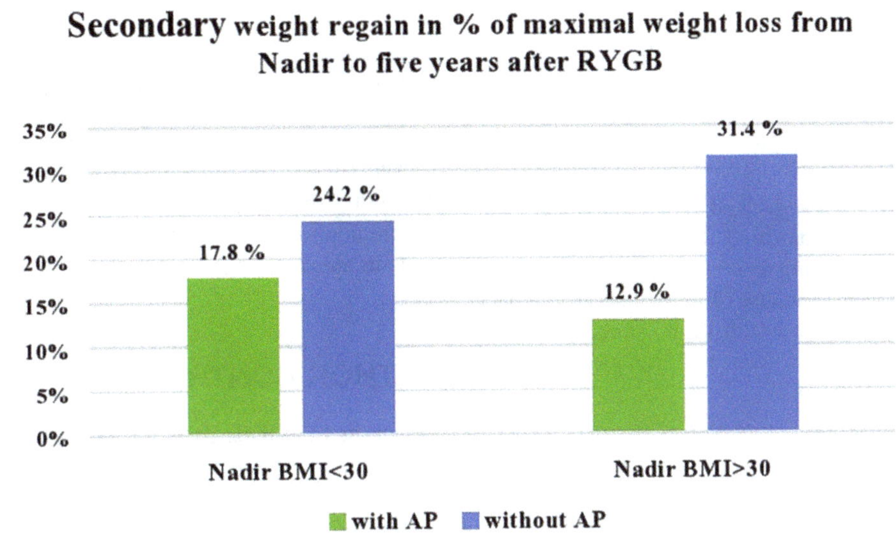

FIGURE 2 | Secondary weight regain from nadir to 5 years after Roux-en-Y gastric bypass in percent of maximal weight loss from surgery to nadir weight. The number of patients who underwent abdominoplasty was 233 out of 418 patients with nadir BMI < 30 kg/m^2, and 27 out of 215 patients with BMI > 30 kg/m^2.

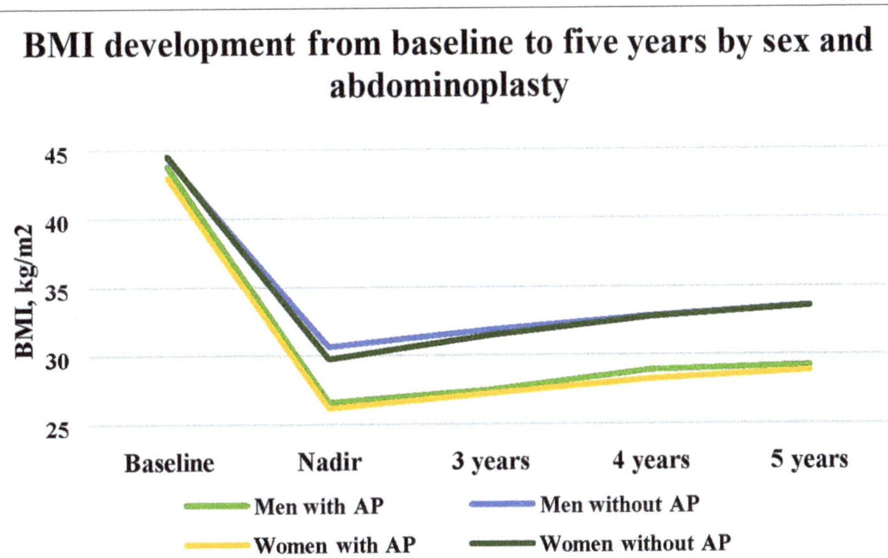

FIGURE 3 | Changes in mean BMI from baseline until 5 years after RYGB in men and women with and without abdominoplasty.

surgery have an additional beneficial metabolic effect of having abdominoplasty.

To our knowledge the role of body contouring procedures has not been emphasized when the favorable long-term effect of bariatric surgery on metabolic health and reduction in morbidity and mortality are presented. It is timely to ask if some of the effects attributed to bariatric surgery in fact are caused by removing adipose tissue in the period after the bariatric procedure.

More knowledge on the metabolic effects of plastic surgery in patients with obesity may lead to new treatment algorithms including abdominoplasty or liposuction as part of a multimodal program including non-surgical weight loss treatment, drugs, and plastic surgery, as well as bariatric surgery. As acceptance of obesity as a chronic relapsing disease worth treatment increases among patients as well as in the medical profession, more tools are needed to provide patients with the best treatment options in the various stages of the disease.

STRENGTHS AND LIMITATIONS

Compared to other studies that have found a beneficial effect of abdominoplasty on secondary WR after bariatric surgery, the present study had a higher number of patients and a higher percentage of patients undergoing abdominoplasty as the treatment was covered by public means. The data were collected prospectively, and the present cohort had a high rate of follow-up and an observation time of at least 5 years after RYGB.

A limitation in the present study is that data were collected in a clinical setting, and details related to technical aspects of the abdominoplasty were not registered. The reports from the plastic surgeons were not standardized, and information on the amount of tissue removed during abdominoplasty was available for only half of the patients. Because of limitations in the data available, changes in metabolic health or inflammation could not be documented by laboratory tests or clinical measurements before and after abdominoplasty.

CONCLUSION

Abdominoplasty was associated with reduced secondary WR after RYGB in this study, and particularly among the patients who did not achieve a nadir BMI of <30 kg/m^2 during the first 2 years after surgery. Whether this is caused by increased bodily satisfaction and better physical function or a biological response to reduction of adipose tissue remains unclear. If removing subcutaneous adipose tissue from abdomen prevents secondary WR and increases the robustness of bariatric surgery, this should be offered as part of the standard treatment after bariatric surgery.

The clinical relevance of the difference in secondary WR was not explored in this study, and the biological role of abdominoplasty on weight development after bariatric surgery remains an unanswered question.

AUTHOR CONTRIBUTIONS

JS collected the data. Analyses were performed by JS and CK. The conceptual framework was developed in discussion among all authors. JS wrote the first manuscript. All authors contributed to the final version of the manuscript.

REFERENCES

1. Angrisani L, Santonicola A, Iovino P, Vitiello A, Higa K, Himpens J, et al. IFSO worldwide survey 2016: primary, endoluminal, and revisional procedures. *Obes Surg.* (2018) 28:3783–94. doi: 10.1007/s11695-018-3450-2
2. Welbourn R, Hollyman M, Kinsman R, Dixon J, Liem R, Ottosson J, et al. Bariatric surgery worldwide: baseline demographic description and one-year outcomes from the fourth IFSO global registry report 2018. *Obes Surg.* (2018). doi: 10.1007/s11695-018-3593-1
3. Keith CJ Jr, Gullick AA, Feng K, Richman J, Stahl R, Grams J. Predictive factors of weight regain following laparoscopic Roux-en-Y gastric bypass. *Surg Endosc.* (2018) 32:2232–8. doi: 10.1007/s00464-017-5913-2
4. Karmali S, Brar B, Shi X, Sharma AM, de Gara C, Birch DW. Weight recidivism post-bariatric surgery: a systematic review. *Obes Surg.* (2013) 23:1922–33. doi: 10.1007/s11695-013-1070-4
5. Froylich D, Corcelles R, Daigle CR, Aminian A, Isakov R, Schauer PR, et al. Weight loss is higher among patients who undergo body contouring procedures after bariatric surgery. *Surg Obes Relat Dis.* (2016) 12:1731–6. doi: 10.1016/j.soard.2015.09.009
6. Balagué N, Combescure C, Huber O, Pittet-Cuénod B, Modarressi A. Plastic surgery improves long-term weight control after bariatric surgery. *Plast Reconstr Surg.* (2013) 132:826–33. doi: 10.1097/PRS.0b013e31829fe531
7. Smith OJ, Hachach-Haram N, Greenfield M, Bystrzonowski N, Pucci A, Batterham RL, et al. Body contouring surgery and the maintenance of weight-loss following Roux-En-Y gastric bypass: a retrospective study. *Aesthet Surg J.* (2018) 38:176–82. doi: 10.1093/asj/sjx170
8. Biorserud C, Olbers T, Fagevik Olsen M. Patients' experience of surplus skin after laparoscopic gastric bypass. *Obes Surg.* (2011) 21:273–7. doi: 10.1007/s11695-009-9849-z
9. Elander A, Biorserud C, Staalesen T, Ockell J, Fagevik Olsen M. Aspects of excess skin in obesity, after weight loss, after body contouring surgery and in a reference population. *Surg Obes Relat Dis.* (2019) 15:305–11. doi: 10.1016/j.soard.2018.10.032
10. Song P, Patel NB, Gunther S, Li CS, Liu Y, Lee CY, et al. Body image & quality of life: changes with gastric bypass and body contouring. *Ann Plast Surg.* (2016) 76(Suppl 3):S216–21. doi: 10.1097/SAP.0000000000000788
11. Fruhbeck G, Busetto L, Dicker D, Yumuk V, Goossens GH, Hebebrand J, et al. The ABCD of obesity: an EASO position statement on a diagnostic term with clinical and scientific implications. *Obes Facts.* (2019) 12:131–6. doi: 10.1159/000497124
12. Haczeyni F, Bell-Anderson KS, Farrell GC. Causes and mechanisms of adipocyte enlargement and adipose expansion. *Obes Rev.* (2018) 19:406–20. doi: 10.1111/obr.12646
13. Cuomo R, Russo F, Sisti A, Nisi G, Grimaldi L, Brandi C, et al. Abdominoplasty in mildly obese patients (BMI 30-35 kg/m^2): metabolic, biochemical and complication analysis at one year. *In Vivo.* (2015) 29:757–61.
14. Rocic P. Comparison of cardiovascular benefits of bariatric surgery and abdominal lipectomy. *Curr Hypertens Rep.* (2019) 21:37. doi: 10.1007/s11906-019-0945-8
15. Sailon AM, Wasserburg JR, Kling RR, Pasick CM, Taub PJ. Influence of large-volume liposuction on metabolic and cardiovascular health: a systematic review. *Ann Plast Surg.* (2017) 79:623–30. doi: 10.1097/SAP.0000000000001195
16. Seretis K, Goulis DG, Koliakos G, Demiri E. The effects of abdominal lipectomy in metabolic syndrome components and insulin sensitivity in females: a systematic review and meta-analysis. *Metabolism.* (2015) 64:1640–9. doi: 10.1016/j.metabol.2015.09.015
17. Seretis K, Goulis DG, Koliakos G, Demiri E. Short- and long-term effects of abdominal lipectomy on weight and fat mass in females: a systematic review. *Obes Surg.* (2015) 25:1950–8. doi: 10.1007/s11695-015-1797-1
18. Ngaage LM, Elegbede A, Pace L, Rosen C, Tannouri S, Rada EM, et al. Review of insurance coverage for abdominal contouring procedures in the postbariatric population. *Plast Reconstr Surg.* (2020) 145:545–54. doi: 10.1097/PRS.0000000000006513
19. Altieri MS, Yang J, Park J, Novikov D, Kang L, Spaniolas K, et al. Utilization of body contouring procedures following weight loss surgery: a study of 37,806 patients. *Obes Surg.* (2017) 27:2981–7. doi: 10.1007/s11695-017-2732-4
20. Lotfi P, Engdahl R. Concepts and techniques in postbariatric body contouring: a primer for the internist. *Am J Med.* (2019) 132:1017–26. doi: 10.1016/j.amjmed.2019.02.048
21. van der Beek ES, van der Molen AM, van Ramshorst B. Complications after body contouring surgery in post-bariatric patients: the importance of a stable weight close to normal. *Obes Facts.* (2011) 4:61–6. doi: 10.1159/000324567
22. King WC, Hinerman AS, Belle SH, Wahed AS, Courcoulas AP. Comparison of the performance of common measures of weight regain after bariatric

surgery for association with clinical outcomes. *JAMA.* (2018) 320:1560–9. doi: 10.1001/jama.2018.14433

23. Sandvik J, Hole T, Klockner CA, Kulseng BE, Wibe A. High-frequency of computer tomography and surgery for abdominal pain after Roux-en-Y gastric bypass. *Obes Surg.* (2018) 28:2609–16. doi: 10.1007/s11695-018-3223-y
24. Gusenoff JA, Messing S, O'Malley W, Langstein HN. Temporal and demographic factors influencing the desire for plastic surgery after gastric bypass surgery. *Plast Reconstr Surg.* (2008) 121:2120–6. doi: 10.1097/PRS.0b013e31817081a3
25. Cai A, Maringa L, Hauck T, Boos AM, Schmitz M, Arkudas A, et al. Body contouring surgery improves physical activity in patients after massive weight loss-a retrospective study. *Obes Surg.* (2020) 30:146–53. doi: 10.1007/s11695-019-04145-3
26. Monpellier VM, Antoniou EE, Mulkens S, Janssen IMC, van der Molen ABM, Jansen ATM. Body image dissatisfaction and depression in postbariatric patients is associated with less weight loss and a desire for body contouring surgery. *Surg Obes Relat Dis.* (2018) 14:1507–15. doi: 10.1016/j.soard.2018.04.016
27. Soldin M, Mughal M, Al-Hadithy N. National commissioning guidelines: body contouring surgery after massive weight loss. *J Plast Reconstr Aesthet Surg.* (2014) 67:1076–81. doi: 10.1016/j.bjps.2014.04.031
28. Hunecke P, Toll M, Mann O, Izbicki JR, Blessmann M, Grupp K. Clinical outcome of patients undergoing abdominoplasty after massive weight loss. *Surg Obes Relat Dis.* (2019) 15:1362–6. doi: 10.1016/j.soard.2019.06.001
29. de Vries CEE, Kalff MC, van Praag EM, Florisson JMG, Ritt M, van Veen RN, et al. The influence of body contouring surgery on weight control and comorbidities in patients after bariatric surgery. *Obes Surg.* (2020) 30:924–30. doi: 10.1007/s11695-019-04298-1

11

Comparison of Short and Long-Term Outcomes of Metabolic and Bariatric Surgery in Adolescents and Adults

Fatima Cody Stanford[1,2,3], *Tasnim Mushannen*[1,4], *Priscilla Cortez*[1,5], *Karen J. Campoverde Reyes*[1,6], *Hang Lee*[7], *Denise W. Gee*[3], *Janey S. Pratt*[8], *Paul A. Boepple*[2,3], *Miriam A. Bredella*[9], *Madhusmita Misra*[1,2] *and Vibha Singhal*[1,2,3]*

[1] *Neuroendocrine Unit, Massachusetts General Hospital and Harvard Medical School, Boston, MA, United States,* [2] *Pediatric Endocrinology, Massachusetts General Hospital and Harvard Medical School, Boston, MA, United States,* [3] *MGH Weight Center, Massachusetts General Hospital, Boston, MA, United States,* [4] *Weill Cornell Medicine, Education City, Al Rayyan, Qatar,* [5] *Department of Biology, College of Science, University of Arizona, Tucson, AZ, United States,* [6] *Liver Research Center, Beth Israel Deaconess Medical Center, Boston, MA, United States,* [7] *Departments of Biostatistics and Harvard Medical School, Boston, MA, United States,* [8] *Department of Surgery and Pediatric Surgery and Stanford University School of Medicine, Stanford, CA, United States,* [9] *Department of Radiology, Massachusetts General Hospital and Harvard Medical School, Boston, MA, United States*

***Correspondence:**
Vibha Singhal
vsinghal1@mgh.harvard.edu

Objective: We sought to compare the short and long-term outcomes of MBS in adolescents vs. adults who have undergone a Roux-en-Y gastric bypass (RYGB) or Sleeve gastrectomy (SG).

Design: Retrospective cohort study.

Setting: Single tertiary care academic referral center.

Participants: One hundred fifty adolescent (≤21-years) and adult (>21-years) subjects with severe obesity between 15 and 70 years of age who underwent RYGB or SG.

Outcomes: Metabolic parameters, weight and height measures were obtained pre-and post-surgery (at 3 and 6 months, and then annually for 4 years).

Results: Median pre-surgical body mass index (BMI) was higher in adolescents (n = 76) vs. adults (n = 74): 50 (45–57) vs. 44 (40–51) kg/m^2 ($p < 0.0001$). However, obesity related complications were greater in adults vs. adolescents: 66 vs. 21% had hypertension, 68 vs. 28% had dyslipidemia, and 42 vs. 21% had type 2 diabetes mellitus (all $p < 0.010$). % BMI reduction and % weight loss (WL) were greater in adolescents vs. adults at all time points ($p < 0.050$). %WL was higher in adolescents who underwent SG at each time point ($p < 0.050$), and trended higher among adolescents who underwent RYGB ($p = 0.060$), compared to adults with the respective procedure. Follow-up data showed greater resolution of type 2 diabetes and hypertension in adolescents than adults (87.5 vs. 54.8%; $p = 0.04$, and 68.7 vs. 35.4%; $p = 0.040$).

Conclusion: Adolescents compared to adults had greater reductions in BMI and weight, even at 4 years, and greater resolution of type 2 diabetes and hypertension. Earlier intervention in the treatment of severe obesity with MBS may lead to better outcomes.

Keywords: obesity surgery, weight loss, obesity complications, adolescent, adult, bariatric surgery

INTRODUCTION

Obesity, defined as a body mass index (BMI) $\geq$ 30 kg/m^2 in adults and BMI $\geq$ 95th percentile in children and adolescents of the same age and sex, is a pandemic complex multifactorial chronic disease. Despite public health efforts to reduce obesity, its prevalence has increased to 40% in adults and 19% in youth in the United States (1–3). Obesity causes significant physical, mental, and psychosocial complications and is associated with complications like hypertension (HTN), dyslipidemia (DYS), non-alcoholic fatty liver disease (NAFLD), diabetes mellitus type 2 (T2D), obstructive sleep apnea (OSA), anxiety, and depression (4–8).

While lifestyle modifications are the cornerstones of weight management, these are usually not enough to treat obesity, especially severe obesity (BMI $\geq$ 40 kg/m^2) (9). Only one weight loss medication, orlistat, is FDA approved in children and contributes to ~3% total body weight loss, insufficient in severe obesity. Timely metabolic and bariatric surgery (MBS) results in prolonged weight loss in both adolescents and adults (5, 6, 10–14). Biochemical markers of DYS, T2D, and non-alcoholic steatohepatitis (NASH) improve or resolve in most adult and adolescent patients after MBS (6, 12, 14–16). A recent study showed greater resolution of T2D and HTN in adolescents as compared to adults after Roux-en-Y gastric bypass (RYGB) suggesting a benefit of early intervention (17). However, data comparing long-term outcomes following sleeve gastrectomy (SG), the most commonly performed MBS is not available (18). Moreover, data comparing outcomes of RYGB and SG across age are lacking.

Our study seeks to compare outcomes from both RYGB and SG in a cohort of patients across a wide age spectrum at a single center. Our objective was to ascertain weight outcomes and resolution of obesity associated complications in adults vs. adolescents who undergo MBS via RYGB or SG. We hypothesized that adolescents would have better outcomes secondary to earlier intervention and overall lower disease burden at the time of intervention.

METHODS

We conducted a retrospective review of adults (> 21 years) and adolescents ($\leq$ 21 years) with obesity (BMI $\geq$ 30) who underwent RYGB or SG between 2001 and 2014 at a single institution. All consecutive adolescent (n = 76) and adult (n = 74) patients were included retrospectively from 2014. We collected demographics, weight, medications, complications pre-surgery and following surgery at 3, 6, and then yearly for 4 years. Since at our center at this time adolescents were recommended surgery only after completion of linear growth, we have used the single height measurement before surgery for all subsequent time points. We do not expect adults to change their height over time at this stage of life. The clinical and laboratory parameters included in this study were systolic and diastolic blood pressures, hemoglobin A1C (HbA1c), lipids (triglycerides, LDL, HDL, total cholesterol), liver enzymes [aspartate aminotransferase (AST), alanine-aminotransferase (ALT)], iron and vitamin studies [iron, ferritin, total iron binding capacity (TIBC), vitamin B12] and 25-hydroxy vitamin D (25-OHD) levels. Time to reach the lowest weight, the lowest weight (nadir weight), and percent of the total body weight lost (TBWL) were recorded. We extracted information from patient files regarding the specific obesity related diseases, i.e., HTN, T2D, DYS, NAFLD, OSA, and PCOS (based on predetermined criteria in **Supplementary Table 1**). Liver biopsies were taken at the time of surgery and analyzed for liver steatosis, NASH, and/or fibrosis.

Pre-surgery data were obtained from visits within 1 year of the date of surgery. Data from the visit closest to surgery were used. Post-surgery data were collected from visits specified by time point with the given timeframes: 3 months $\pm$ 1 month, 6 months $\pm$ 1 month, 1 year $\pm$ 3 months, 2 years $\pm$ 3 months, 3 years $\pm$ 6 months, 4 years $\pm$ 6 months.

Participants who were loss to follow-up did not differ from those in whom we had follow-up data for baseline weight, gender, type of surgery, and presence of comorbidities. We have listed the subjects with follow up weight data in the table with results. For or major comorbidity assessments; type 2 diabetes mellitus (T2D)—we had follow-up data on all 31 adults and 16 adolescents who had T2D at baseline. For HTN, we had follow-up data on 48 adults (1 missing) and all 16 adolescents who had hypertension before surgery. Similarly, for dyslipidemia, we had follow-up data on 49 adults (1 missing) and all 21 adolescents who initially had dyslipidemia.

We used JMP (v13; SAS Institute, Inc. Cary, NC, USA) for analyses. Normally distributed data were analyzed using a one-way Analysis of Variance (ANOVA), and non-parametrically distributed data were analyzed using the Wilcoxon rank-sum test. Data are reported as mean $\pm$ SD for parametric values or median (IQR) for non-parametric values. Pearson's Chi Square and Fisher's Exact Test were used to compare proportions. To control for confounders, we ran linear regression models for continuous outcomes (BMI, percent weight loss) and logistic regression for nominal variables like resolution of comorbidities. We controlled for baseline weight, type of surgery, gender, race, and baseline comorbidity depending on what was relevant for consideration as a confounder. We have elaborated the rationale of using the particular confounders further with the results.

Our institutional review board—The Partners Humans Research Committee (PHRC), affiliated to Massachusetts General Hospital and Harvard Medical School approved this study.

RESULTS

Baseline Characteristics

Baseline characteristics are shown in **Table 1**. Consistent with national trends regarding MBS, females comprised the majority in both age groups—adults and adolescents. Within both groups (adults and adolescents), the largest proportion of participants were Caucasian, followed by Hispanics, African Americans, and Asians. There was a wide distribution of ages between 15 and 70 years. Notably, the pre-surgery weight and BMI of adolescents was greater than those of adults. While both adolescents and adults were more likely to undergo RYGB vs. SG (given existing

TABLE 1 | Baseline demographics of the adult and adolescent groups.

	Adults ($n = 74$)	Adolescents ($n = 76$)	P
Age	46.5 (38.0–59.3)	18.0 (17.3–19.8)	**<0.010***
Sex (male/female)	31/43	13/63	**<0.010**
Height (in)	66.9 ± 4.2	65.9 ± 3.1	0.080
Weight (Kg)	127.3 (112.6–151.4)	140.9 (123.5–158.8)	**<0.010***
BMI (Kg/m2)	43.6 (40.0–51.3)	50.5 (45.3–56.7)	**<0.010***
RYGB (%)	59.5	77.6	**0.010**
SG (%)	40.5	22.4	
Race/Ethnicity (%)			
White	79.7	59.2	0.080
Hispanic	12.2	22.4	
African-American	2.7	7.9	
Asian	0	3.4	
>1 race	2.7	5.3	
Unknown	2.7	1.3	
Systolic BP (mm Hg)	129 (118–142)	126 (117–134)	0.220*
Diastolic BP (mm Hg)	77 (70.75–82)	75 (66–83.5)	0.560*
HDL (mg/dL)	41.5 (36.8–53.0)	39 (33.5–45.5)	0.100*
LDL (mg/dL)	108.6 ± 36.5	95.9 ± 4.0	**0.030**
Triglycerides (mg/dL)	146.5 (99.3–207.8)	102 (74.5–141.0)	**<0.001***
Cholesterol (mg/dL)	184.5 (159.3–205.5)	156.0 (140.0–179.0)	**<0.0001***
Hgb A1c (%)	6.2 (5.63–7.15)	5.6 (5.2–5.9)	**<0.0001***
ALT (IU/L)	26.0 (16.3–36.0)	23.0 (17.0–36.0)	0.760*
AST (IU/L)	23.0 (17.3–29.5)	22.0 (18.0–27.0)	0.640*
Alkaline phosphatase (IU/L)	74.0 (59.8–87.5)	82.5 (66.0–102.0)	**0.010***
TIBC (µg/dL)	321.6 ± 53.3	353.8 ± 61.9	**<0.010**
Iron (µg/dL)	67.0 (54.3–86.5)	54.5 (36.3–85.5)	**0.020***
Ferritin (ng/mL)	85.0 (39.0–168.8)	56.0 (34.5–81.0)	**0.020***
Vitamin B12 (pg/mL)	476.5 (349.3–673.5)	508.0 (396.0–620.0)	1.000*
Vitamin D (ng/ml)	25.5 (19.0–31.0)	23.0 (18.0–28.0)	0.210*

**Wilcoxon Test was used for non-normally distributed data.*
TIBC, Total iron binding capacity.
Bold value means statistically significant.

practice at that time), there was a higher prevalence of RYGB in adolescents.

Table 2 shows participants with pre-surgical obesity related conditions in adolescents and adults. As expected, more adults had HTN, T2D, and DYS than adolescents at the time of surgery. However, similar proportions of adolescents and adults (>80% in each) had NAFLD. More adolescents than adults had PCOS documented.

Weight Loss

Although adolescents on average had higher presurgical weight and BMI than adults, they lost a greater % of their weight than adults at every time point post-surgery (**Figure 1** and **Supplementary Table 1**). The peak difference in %WL was reached at 2 years, at which time adolescents had lost 1.51 times more weight than adults. The percent reduction in BMI was greater in adolescents vs. adults at all time points (Data not shown—similar to the percent weight loss data as a single height measurement at the presurgical visit was used for follow up). While BMI of adolescents was higher in the early postoperative period, the difference was no longer significant at 1 year and onwards. When we controlled for the type of surgery, adolescents had more %WL at most time points (except acutely at 3 months) (**Figure 1**). When we controlled for surgery type, race, and baseline weight, adolescents had more % WL at most time points (except acutely at 3 months and long-term at 4 years) (**Figure 1**). Inge and colleagues demonstrated similar %WL response at 5 years after RYGB, but their cohort did not include patients who underwent SG, (17) a procedure which has less %WL in the midterm and long-term based upon recent meta-analysis and systematic reviews (19). It is also important to note that our cohort likely differs from national data as our center is a tertiary referral center with patients with a high level of medical complexity.

Adolescents also showed greater %WL when they were stratified by surgical technique. At every year post-surgery, adolescents who underwent SG had greater %WL than adults ($p < 0.05$) (**Table 3**). These differences in %WL persisted after controlling for pre-surgical weight, race and gender. Specifically, after 4 years of SG, adolescents had lost 25–29% of their weight, while adults had lost 14–21% of their presurgical weight. However, %WL following RYGB did not differ in adolescents vs. adults at any time point. Adults who underwent RYGB vs. SG had greater %WL at all timepoints (even after controlling for baseline weight). This superiority of RYGB over SG was not observed in adolescents in our cohort.

Despite a dramatic response to surgery in both cohorts, a substantial proportion of patients continued to have obesity with a BMI $\geq$ 30 kg/m^2 (69.3% in adolescents vs. 62.2%, in adults; $p = 0.4$) and BMI $\geq$ 35 kg/m^2 (46.7% in adolescents vs. 35.1% in adults, $p = 0.15$) at nadir. At 4 years follow-up, 75.8% of adolescents vs. 81.6% of adults had a BMI $\geq$ 30 kg/m^2 ($p = 0.02$), and 60.6% of adolescents vs. 53.1%, of adults had a BMI $\geq$ 35 kg/m^2 ($p = 0.02$).

Resolutions and Improvements

Hypertension

Among participants pre-surgically diagnosed with HTN and who had follow-up data ($n = 64$; no data in 1 adult patient), almost two times as many adolescents vs. adults attained resolution of HTN and were off the medications at some time point over the course of four years ($p = 0.02$ unadjusted, $p = 0.05$ after adjusting for type of surgery) (**Figure 2**). Among all participants with follow-up data, regardless of a pre-surgical diagnosis of HTN and antihypertensive medication use, the proportion of participants with a blood pressure $\geq$ 140 mm systolic or $\geq$ 90 mm diastolic was similar between adults and adolescents at all time points post-surgery except at 1 year, at which time only 2.6% adolescents vs. 20.9% adults had documented blood pressures above 140/90 mm Hg ($p = 0.015$). Adolescents had either similar or better blood pressures than adults and were more likely to have resolution of HTN.

TABLE 2 | Distribution of pre-surgery weight related complications.

Adults ($n = 74$)	Adolescents ($n = 76$)	P
Hypertension ($n = 74$): 49/74 (66.22%)	Hypertension ($n = 76$): 16/76 (21.05%)	**<0.0001**
Dyslipidemia ($n = 74$): 50/74 (67.57%)	Dyslipidemia ($n = 76$): 21/76 (27.63%)	**<0.0001**
Type 2 Diabetes Mellitus ($n = 74$): 31/74 (41.89%)	Type 2 Diabetes Mellitus ($n = 76$): 16/76 (21.05%)	**0.005**
Obstructive Sleep Apnea ($n = 41$):	Obstructive Sleep Apnea ($n = 42$)	0.845
Y: 36/41 (87.80%)	Y: 35/42 (83.33%)	
N: 5/41 (12.20%)	N: 7/42 (16.67%)	
Non-alcoholic fatty liver disease ($n = 69$):	**Non-alcoholic fatty liver disease ($n = 74$)**	0.085
Y: 57/69 (82.61%)	Y: 68/74 (91.89%)	
N: 12/69 (17.39%)	N: 6/74 (8.11%)	
Steatosis ($n = 69$):	**Steatosis ($n = 74$):**	0.091
Y: 55/69 (79.71%)	Y: 67/74 (90.54%)	
N: 14/69 (20.29%)	N: 7/74 (9.46%)	
NASH ($n = 69$):	**NASH ($n = 71$):**	0.953
Y: 27/69 (39.13%)	Y: 26/71 (36.62%)	
N: 42/69 (60.87%)	N: 45/71 (63.38%)	
Fibrosis ($n = 65$):	**Fibrosis ($n = 71$):**	0.305
Y: 32/66 (48.48%)	Y: 27/71 (38.03%)	
N: 34/66 (51.52%)	N: 44/71 (61.97%)	

NASH, non-alcoholic steatohepatitis. Bold value means statistically significant.

Type 2 Diabetes Mellitus

87.5% adolescents ($n = 16$) vs. 54.8% adults ($n = 31$) had resolution of T2D ($p = 0.03$) over the course of 4 year follow up (**Figure 2**). Because the pre-surgical HbA1C and the type of surgery may affect the resolution of T2D, we consider them as confounder and controlled for these variables in our analyses. Adolescents had significantly lower HbA1C levels than adults at 3 months (5.39 vs. 5.83%; $p = 0.002$) and 4 years (5.29 vs. 6.27%; $p = 0.02$). A similar pattern was observed for changes in HbA1C values from baseline after controlling for the same variables, with greater reductions observed in adolescents than in adults at 3 months (−1.14 vs. −0.70%) and 4 years (−1.46 vs. −0.57%) ($p < 0.02$ for both).

Dyslipidemia

Adolescents did not differ from adults for the proportion that had resolution of dyslipidemia or change in absolute values of triglycerides, LDL, or total cholesterol at any time point post-surgery (**Figure 2**). However, after controlling for baseline HDL, surgery type, and gender, adults had higher HDL levels than adolescents in the early post-operative period at 3- and 6-months post-surgery (43.8 vs. 39.6 mg/dl, $p = 0.018$; 49.1 vs. 43.1 mg/dl, $p = 0.032$, respectively). However, subsequently, this difference was no longer observed, and HDL levels of adolescents rose to values similar to those observed in adults ($p > 0.3$). From 1 to 4 years, HDL values in adults ranged between 53 and 61 mg/dl while those of adolescents ranged between 55 and 58 mg/dl. By 1-year post-op, adolescents experienced substantially larger increases in HDL than adults.

Obstructive Sleep Apnea (OSA)

Assessments of resolution of OSA were not optimal. Approximately 95% of adults and 89% of adolescents who had OSA pre-surgically did not undergo a sleep study following surgery. However, the majority who did OSA had documented improvements of OSA noted in their medical records. There was no difference in the proportions of adolescents vs. adults with documented improvements of OSA at all time points except at 6 months, when 81.3% of adolescents vs. 45.0% of adults had documented improvement ($p = 0.04$). After 6 months, the proportion of adolescents with OSA improvement remained steady between 88 and 94%, while that in adults rose from 45% at 6 months to 75% at 4 years.

NAFLD and Liver Enzymes

Post-surgical assessments for NAFLD were rarely done as most patients did not undergo liver biopsies after surgery. Post-surgical information was only available in 24/76 (32%) of adolescents and 25/75 (33%) of adults; nevertheless, based on our predetermined definitions of NAFLD resolution (normalization of liver biopsy and/or liver enzymes if previously elevated), 16/24 (66.7%) of adolescents and 21/25 (84.0%) of adults attained resolution ($p = 0.16$).

ALT and AST levels in adolescents and adults were similar pre-surgically (23 vs. 26 U/L, $p = 0.76$; and 22 vs. 23 U/L, $p = 0.64$, respectively). At 3 months post-surgery, both ALT and AST levels were significantly higher in adolescents vs. adults (29.0 vs. 21.5 U/L, $p = 0.03$; and 26.0 vs. 22.5 U/L, $p = 0.03$, respectively). By 4 years post-surgery, ALT and AST levels were not different between adolescents and adults (23.0 vs. 19.7 U/L, $p = 0.43$; and 26.1 vs. 22.5 U/L, $p = 0.19$, respectively).

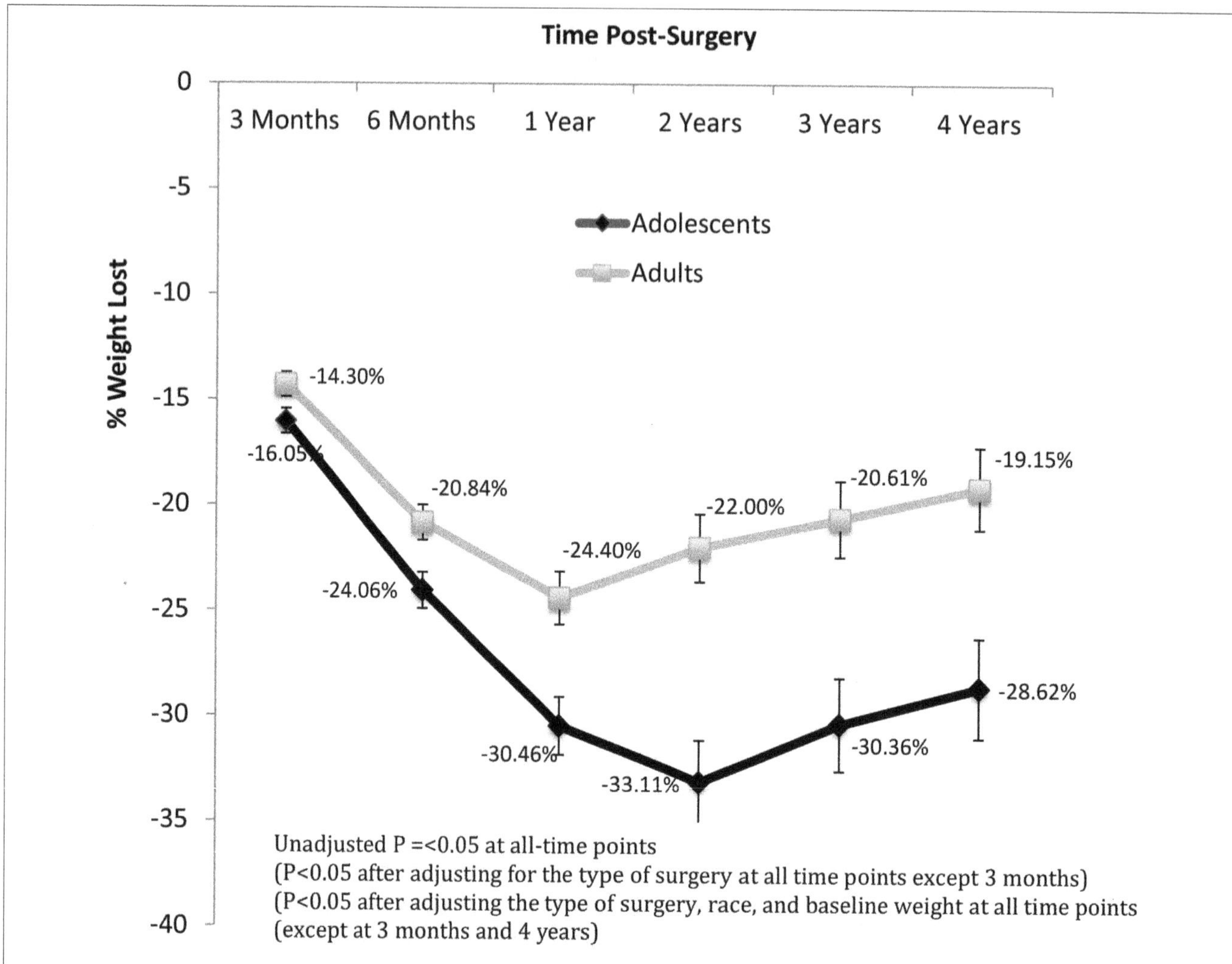

FIGURE 1 | Percent of total body weight loss post-surgery over time.

Vitamin and Mineral Deficiencies

25(OH)-D levels were similar in adolescents vs. adults pre-surgery (**Table 1**) and they were similar at the 4-year follow up (24 ± 12 vs. 29 ± 12 ng/dl; $p = 0.22$).

Ferritin and iron levels were higher in adults vs. adolescents pre-surgery (**Table 1**). At 4 years, ferritin and iron levels were similar in adolescents vs. adults [14.5 ng/mL (5.5–33.7) vs. 13 ng/mL (9.5–44.5); $p = 0.22$ and 60.5 μg/dl ± 29 vs. 75.1 μg/dl ± 43; $p = 0.44$, respectively].

Although adolescent and adult vitamin B12 levels were similar pre-surgically (**Table 1**), they were consistently lower in adolescents 4-years following surgery (485.4 ± 339 vs. 1027 ± 645, pg/mL respectively; $p = 0.003$).

DISCUSSION

Our study demonstrates that early intervention with MBS during adolescence leads to better weight loss outcomes and obesity related disease resolution compared to MBS performed in adulthood. To our knowledge, this is the first study to evaluate MBS outcomes after both RYGB and SG in adolescents and adults.

Literature comparing short and long-term outcomes of MBS (RYGB and SG) in adolescent and adult populations is scarce, and our data are promising as they demonstrate that outcomes are as better in adolescents compared to adults, especially for SG. The Swedish Obese Study (SOS) reviewed 5-year-follow-up data in adolescents vs. adults who underwent RYGB, and reported a mean reduction in BMI of 13.1 kg/m^2 in adolescents vs. 12.3 kg/m^2 in adults after 5 years of MBS (7). Khidir et al. showed a greater decrease in %WL after SG in adolescents vs. adults at 5-year follow-up (20). Similarly, Benedix et al. found that adolescents who underwent SG had better weight loss outcomes compared to adults. They described higher rates of resolution of HTN, T2D, and OSA in adolescents (21). However, these studies did not perform a head-to-head comparison of outcomes in different types of MBS, particularly RYGB vs. SG, the two most commonly performed MBS procedures in the adolescent and adult population. To our knowledge, this

TABLE 3 | Percent weight loss at different time points stratified by surgery type.

	Adults		Adolescents		*P*			
	RYGB (*n* = 44)	**SG (*n* = 30)**	**RYGB (*n* = 59)**	**SG (*n* = 17)**	**RYGB vs. SG (Adult)**	**RYGB vs. SG (Adol)**	**RYGB Adult vs. Adol**	**SG Adult vs. Adol**
3 Months	−15.9 ± 4.8 (*n* = 44)	−12.0 ± 4.8 (*n* = 30)	−16.0 ± 4.8 (*n* = 55)	−16.3 ± 5.3 (*n* = 17)	**0.0008**	0.843	0.939	**0.006**
6 Months	−23.1 ± 6.7 (*n* = 37)	−17.2 ± 7.8 (*n* = 23)	−24.4 ± 5.1 (*n* = 46)	−22.9 ± 4.9 (*n* = 12)	**0.002**	0.374	0.341	**0.027**
1 Year	−26.7 ± 10.5 (*n* = 36)	−21.1 ± 9.9 (*n* = 25)	−30.7 ± 8.9 (*n* = 43)	−29.2 ± 8.5 (*n* = 8)	**0.039**	0.670	0.071	**0.045**
2 Years	−30.2 (−36.2 to 20.5) (*n* = 31)	−19.3 (−26.7 to 12.5) (*n* = 25)	−33.8 (−40.6 to 26.9) (*n* =30)	−24.9 (−41.8 to 22.7) (*n* = 7)	**0.022***	0.473*	0.059*	**0.028**
3 Years	−26.5 ± 10.9 (*n* = 30)	−13.6 ± 12.3 (*n* = 25)	−31.0 ± 14.1 (*n* = 30)	−27.9 ± 13.2 (*n* = 7)	**0.0001**	0.601	0.172	**0.011**
4 Years	−24.7 ± 11.2 (*n* = 29)	−11.2 ± 12.3 (*n* = 20)	−32.3 (−36.6 to 22.5) (*n* = 26)	−24.4 (−27.4 to 19.1) (*n* = 7)	**0.0002**	0.243*	0.135*	**0.011***

**Wilcoxon Test used for non-normally distributed data. Bold value means statistically significant.*

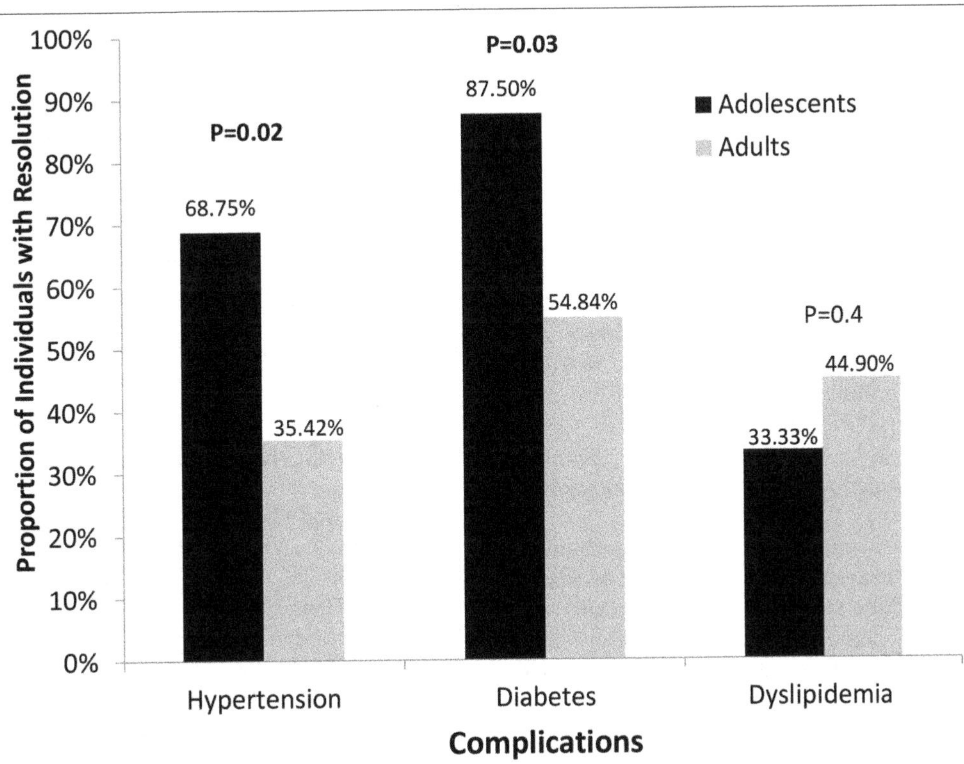

FIGURE 2 | Proportion of subjects with resolution of hypertension, diabetes, and dyslipidemia.

is one of the first studies to highlight the greater efficacy of MBS in adolescents compared to adults 4 years after SG or RYGB.

In our study, adolescents had better pre-surgery lipid, liver, glycemic, and hematological parameters, but their BMI was higher than adults. By the time of MBS, ~1/5 of adolescents had at least one obesity related complication, which over time increases their risk of mortality and adversely affects their quality of life (21). It is thus important to identify adolescents with moderate to severe obesity and escalate their obesity treatment according to the severity of their obesity.

Our data demonstrate that adolescents have greater weight loss than adults both acutely and at 4-year follow-up following MBS. Despite starting at a higher BMI than adults, the nadir BMI after MBS was not different between adults and adolescents suggesting that MBS has greater weight loss benefits at a younger age. Despite these positive results, almost 2/3 of the adolescents continued to have obesity at nadir weight and almost 50% had severe obesity. This is likely because adolescents often have delayed MBS intervention and have greater severity of obesity than adults at the time of MBS.

Studies have shown variation with regards to the ideal procedure in adults and adolescents (i.e., RYGB vs. SG). This study shows that regardless of the surgical technique utilized, adolescents have greater reductions in total body weight than adults over both the short and long-term. In our cohort, adults showed greater weight loss with RYGB than with SG at all time points. This superiority of RYGB was not seen in the adolescent group. Adolescents had a better response to SG than adults, which is consistent with previous studies (22, 23). This is encouraging and supportive of the current trend of more frequent SG, with its reduced complexity and lower post-surgical prevalence of micronutrient deficiencies than RYGB, particularly in adolescents (18).

Adolescents showed greater resolution of obesity related complications, especially HTN and T2D, than adults. These findings are supported by other studies which show that a longer duration of diabetes before MBS reduces the chances of resolution of T2D (24). Prolonged hyperglycemia and β-cell stress may lead to irreversible pancreatic damage and decrease the chances of improvement in glucose tolerance. Similar proportions of adolescents and adults had resolution of DYS, OSA and normalization of liver transaminases. After 6 months, adolescents had lower ALT levels than adults and maintained this at 4 years. Based on documentation in the medical records, adolescents had more rapid improvements of OSA, which suggests lower severity and greater reversibility of OSA in this age group. These data show that early MBS is equally or more beneficial in resolving obesity complications.

We did not find any difference between groups for vitamin D or iron levels. However, adolescents had lower levels of vitamin B12 after surgery than adults, suggesting lower compliance with supplement intake. This emphasizes the importance of follow-up and ongoing surveillance. While micronutrient deficiencies are a challenge, their long-term clinical impact in adolescents is unknown.

Limitations of the Study

As this was a retrospective study in one academic medical center, it might be challenging to extrapolate our results to other institutions. Despite this limitation, few centers in the US operate on both adult and pediatric patients with moderate to severe obesity, and this offers a unique opportunity to compare the two groups. There were limitations inherent to any retrospective study. Specifically, the number of participants who returned for follow up at the different timepoints was variable, and tests done at each time point were inconsistent.

We did not have enough follow up data to document resolutions of OSA and NAFLD in both adolescent and adult groups because only a small proportion had post-surgical polysomnography and liver biopsies and hence we only report documented improvements. Also, we were not able to obtain data on long term surgical complications due to inconsistent documentation. Moreover, despite having a diverse population, the predominant race was white, limiting the generalizability of these results to other racial and ethnic groups who may respond differently to MBS. Larger prospective studies that ensure racial diversity are necessary to confirm these findings.

CONCLUSION

Despite higher weight and BMI of adolescents at the time of MBS, adolescents had a greater percent total body weight loss and resolution of obesity co-morbidities (when present) than adults regardless of whether they underwent RYGB or SG. Our study results suggest that MBS surgical intervention at an early age portends better outcomes with regards to weight loss and obesity co-morbidity. As such, we encourage more utilization of MBS in adolescents with moderate to severe obesity as they are the age cohort most likely to glean benefits.

AUTHOR CONTRIBUTIONS

KC, TM, PC, and VS were responsible for acquisition of data and data analyses. FS, VS, and KC were responsible for interpreting the data. KC, TM, and PC were responsible for drafting the manuscript. FS and VS were responsible for the conception and design of the study and critical review of the paper. FS, MM, and VS were responsible for revising the article critically and adding important intellectual content. DG, PB, JP, MB, and HL were responsible for data collection and providing critical appraisal of the content. All authors have read and approved the final version of the paper and have made substantial contribution to the paper.

REFERENCES

1. Hales CM, Carroll MD, Fryar CD, Ogden CL. Prevalence of obesity among adults and youth: United States, 2015–2016. *NCHS Data Brief.* (2017) 1–8.
2. Pratt JSA, Browne A, Browne NT, Bruzoni M, Cohen M, Desai A, et al. ASMBS pediatric metabolic and bariatric surgery guidelines, 2018. *Surg Obes Relat Dis.* (2018) 14:882–901. doi: 10.1016/j.soard.2018.03.019
3. Skinner AC, Ravanbakht SN, Skelton JA, Perrin EM, Armstrong SC. Prevalence of obesity and severe obesity in US children, 1999-2016. *Pediatrics.* (2018) 141:e20173459. doi: 10.1542/peds.2017-3459
4. Escobar-Morreale HF, Botella-Carretero JI, Alvarez-Blasco F, Sancho J, San Millan JL. The polycystic ovary syndrome associated with morbid obesity may resolve after weight loss induced by bariatric surgery. *J Clin Endocrinol Metab.* (2005) 90:6364–9. doi: 10.1210/jc.2005-1490

5. Inge TH, Courcoulas AP, Jenkins TM, Michalsky MP, Helmrath MA, Brandt ML, et al. Weight loss and health status 3 years after bariatric surgery in adolescents. *N Engl J Med.* (2016) 374:113–23. doi: 10.1056/NEJMoa1506699
6. Inge TH, Jenkins TM, Xanthakos SA, Dixon JB, Daniels SR, Zeller MH, et al. Long-term outcomes of bariatric surgery in adolescents with severe obesity (FABS-5+): a prospective follow-up analysis. *Lancet Diabetes Endocrinol.* (2017) 5:165–73. doi: 10.1016/S2213-8587(16)30315-1
7. Olbers T, Beamish AJ, Gronowitz E, Flodmark CE, Dahlgren J, Bruze G, et al. Laparoscopic Roux-en-Y gastric bypass in adolescents with severe obesity (AMOS): a prospective, 5-year, Swedish nationwide study. *Lancet Diabetes Endocrinol.* (2017) 5:174–83. doi: 10.1016/S2213-8587(16)30424-7
8. Sawaya RA, Jaffe J, Friedenberg L, Friedenberg FK. Vitamin, mineral, and drug absorption following bariatric surgery. *Curr Drug Metab.* (2012) 13:1345–55. doi: 10.2174/138920012803341339
9. Savoye M, Shaw M, Dziura J, Tamborlane WV, Rose P, Guandalini C, et al. Effects of a weight management program on body composition and metabolic parameters in overweight children: a randomized controlled trial. *JAMA.* (2007) 297:2697–704. doi: 10.1001/jama.297.24.2697
10. Al-Sabah SK, Almazeedi SM, Dashti SA, Al-Mulla AY, Ali DA, Jumaa TH. The efficacy of laparoscopic sleeve gastrectomy in treating adolescent obesity. *Obes Surg.* (2015) 25:50–4. doi: 10.1007/s11695-014-1340-9
11. Douketis JD, Macie C, Thabane L, Williamson DF. Systematic review of long-term weight loss studies in obese adults: clinical significance and applicability to clinical practice. *Int J Obes.* (2005) 29:1153–67. doi: 10.1038/sj.ijo.0802982
12. Ikramuddin S, Korner J, Lee WJ, Connett JE, Inabnet WB, Billington CJ, et al. Roux-en-Y gastric bypass vs intensive medical management for the control of type 2 diabetes, hypertension, and hyperlipidemia: the diabetes surgery study randomized clinical trial. *JAMA.* (2013) 309:2240–9. doi: 10.1001/jama.2013.5835
13. Lennerz BS, Wabitsch M, Lippert H, Wolff S, Knoll C, Weiner R, et al. Bariatric surgery in adolescents and young adults–safety and effectiveness in a cohort of 345 patients. *Int J Obes.* (2014) 38:334–40. doi: 10.1038/ijo.2013.182
14. Maffazioli GD, Stanford FC, Campoverde Reyes KJ, Stanley TL, Singhal V, Corey KE, et al. Comparing outcomes of two types of bariatric surgery in an adolescent obese population: roux-en-y gastric bypass vs. sleeve gastrectomy. *Front Pediatr.* (2016) 4:78. doi: 10.3389/fped.2016.00078
15. Barker KB, Palekar NA, Bowers SP, Goldberg JE, Pulcini JP, Harrison SA. Non-alcoholic steatohepatitis: effect of roux-en-y gastric bypass surgery. *Am J Gastroenterol.* (2006) 101:368–73. doi: 10.1111/j.1572-0241.2006.00419.x
16. Mummadi RR, Kasturi KS, Chennareddygari S, Sood GK. Effect of bariatric surgery on nonalcoholic fatty liver disease: systematic review and meta-analysis. *Clin Gastroenterol Hepatol.* (2008) 6:1396–402. doi: 10.1016/j.cgh.2008.08.012
17. Inge TH, Courcoulas AP, Jenkins TM, Michalsky MP, Brandt ML, Xanthakos SA, et al. Five-year outcomes of gastric bypass in adolescents as compared with adults. *N Engl J Med.* (2019) 380:2136–45. doi: 10.1056/NEJMoa1813909
18. Griggs CL, Perez NP Jr, Goldstone RN, Kelleher CM, Chang DC, Stanford FC, et al. National trends in the use of metabolic and bariatric surgery among pediatric patients with severe obesity. *JAMA Pediatr.* (2018) 172:1191–2. doi: 10.1001/jamapediatrics.2018.3030
19. Shoar S, Saber AA. Long-term and midterm outcomes of laparoscopic sleeve gastrectomy versus Roux-en-Y gastric bypass: a systematic review and meta-analysis of comparative studies. *Surg Obes Relat Dis.* (2017) 13:170–80. doi: 10.1016/j.soard.2016.08.011
20. Khidir N, El-Matbouly MA, Sargsyan D, Al-Kuwari M, Bashah M, Gagner M. Five-year outcomes of laparoscopic sleeve gastrectomy: a comparison between adults and adolescents. *Obes Surg.* (2018) 28:2040–5. doi: 10.1007/s11695-018-3139-6
21. Benedix F, Krause T, Adolf D, Wolff S, Lippert H, Manger T, et al. Perioperative course, weight loss and resolution of comorbidities after primary sleeve gastrectomy for morbid obesity: are there differences between adolescents and adults? *Obes. Surg.* (2017) 27:2388–97. doi: 10.1007/s11695-017-2640-7
22. Stanford FC, Alfaris N, Gomez G, Ricks ET, Shukla AP, Corey KE, et al. The utility of weight loss medications after bariatric surgery for weight regain or inadequate weight loss: a multi-center study. *Multicenter Study.* (2017) 13:491–500. doi: 10.1016/j.soard.2016.10.018
23. Toth AT, Gomez G, Shukla AP, Pratt JS, Cena H, Biino G, et al. Weight loss medications in young adults after bariatric surgery for weight regain or inadequate weight loss: a multi-center study. *Children.* (2018) 5:116. doi: 10.3390/children5090116
24. Steven S, Carey PE, Small PK, Taylor R. Reversal of Type 2 diabetes after bariatric surgery is determined by the degree of achieved weight loss in both short- and long-duration diabetes. *Diabet Med.* (2015) 32:47–53. doi: 10.1111/dme.12567

12

The Effect of Metabolic Surgery on the Complications of Diabetes: What Are the Unanswered Questions?

Karl J. Neff[1*†] *and Carel W. Le Roux*[1,2†]

[1] *Diabetes Complications Research Centre, Conway Institute, University College Dublin, Dublin, Ireland,* [2] *Metabolic Medicine, Imperial College London, London, United Kingdom*

***Correspondence:**
Karl J. Neff
karl.neff@hse.ie

† *These authors have contributed equally to this work*

It is now established that metabolic surgery (also known as bariatric surgery or obesity surgery) is an effective treatment for type 2 diabetes. Data from several randomized controlled trials have shown that surgery, when used as an adjunct to best medical therapy, is superior to medical therapy alone in achieving glycaemic and metabolic treatment targets in diabetes care. This has resulting in metabolic surgery being recommended as a treatment option for obesity-associated type 2 diabetes in national and international diabetes care guidelines. While the superior glycaemic effect of surgery is clear, the effect of surgery on the complications of diabetes is not fully understood. There are observational and epidemiological data that indicate a preventative effect in cohorts who do not have complications at baseline, as well as a positive effect on those with established diabetic kidney disease. However, there is a dearth of randomized controlled studies that specifically examine the effect of surgery on the complications of diabetes. Therefore, we should remain cautious in some cases, especially in those with retinopathy or neuropathy, as there is potential for deterioration of disease post-operatively. Further study is needed on this important topic. A lot is known, but there remain several unanswered questions. This article summarizes what we know about the effect of metabolic surgery on the complications of diabetes, poses some unanswered questions, and suggests how we could answer them.

Keywords: metabolic surgery, diabetes, kidney disease, nephropathy, retinopathy, neuropathy

INTRODUCTION

Metabolic surgery (also referred to as bariatric surgery or obesity surgery) is now recommended as a mainstream treatment for type 2 diabetes in people who have both obesity and type 2 diabetes (1). This recommendation, supported by multiple international diabetes organizations including the American Diabetes Association and the International Diabetes Federation, is based on data from randomized controlled trials comparing surgical intervention to best medical therapy (2). In these trials, metabolic surgery has been proven to improve glycaemic control, in the short- and medium-term, to a greater extent than medical therapy alone (2). Surgery is particularly recommended for people with both obesity and type 2 diabetes in whom dietary and medical therapy has been unsuccessful in achieving diabetes treatment targets.

In many cases, the effect of surgery on type 2 diabetes can be so great as to induce remission of disease and normalization of glycaemia. It should be noted that this effect is often transient (3, 4). Therefore, surgery should not be offered as a "cure"' for diabetes, but rather as an effective treatment for type 2 diabetes. Approximately 50% of those who have metabolic surgery and achieve remission of their diabetes will have recurrence of diabetes within the subsequent 10 years (3). However, despite the recurrence of diabetes, these patients usually achieve much better glycaemic and metabolic control than they did before surgery, and so the beneficial glycaemic and metabolic effect of surgery, as compared to medical therapy alone, is retained (3).

However, it should be noted that surgical treatment of diabetes and obesity has associated complications (1, 2). The specific surgical complications are procedure dependent, but all surgical recipients will be at risk of hospitalization for treatment of complications of surgery, and will remain at high risk of micronutrient malnutrition, with the potential for associated anemia or neuropathy, for life (1). Surgery is not for everyone. An expert multidisciplinary assessment is needed for all surgical candidates to ensure that they are suitable and ready for surgery. Given the highly specialist nature of this work, surgery should only be performed in high volume centers by specialist surgeons who work within expert multidisciplinary teams (1).

The improved glycaemic control achieved with surgery could be expected to reduce the burden of microvascular complications in people with diabetes. However, there are not many randomized controlled trials specifically examining the effect of metabolic surgery on microvascular outcomes. There are experimental models, observational data, and one randomized controlled trial, that support the hypothesis that surgery could have a role in managing not only diabetes, but also its complications. However, many unanswered questions remain.

DIABETIC KIDNEY DISEASE

Diabetic Kidney Disease: What We Know

Type 2 diabetes and obesity often co-exist, and both can contribute to the development of renal dysfunction and disease (5–7). Obesity is associated with proteinuric renal disease even in the absence of diabetes (8). In cohorts with both diseases, there appears to be an additive effect. Having both obesity and diabetes increases the risk of developing renal disease, and a diagnosis of obesity is a key risk factor in the progression of diabetic kidney disease (DKD) (7, 9). Therefore, populations with both obesity and type 2 diabetes should be considered at elevated risk for the development of DKD. Given this pathological synergy, it seems sensible to suggest that in cohorts with both obesity and type 2 diabetes, treatment approaches should be simultaneously targeted at both diseases in order to prevent or treat any associated DKD.

In diabetic kidney disease (DKD), the first clinical manifestation is albuminuria. Metabolic surgery reduces the risk of developing albuminuria in the first instance (10–14). Surgery also results in reduced proteinuria, including albuminuria, even in cases of established disease (15, 16). This effect of surgery is seen within the first 12 months post-operatively, and lasts for at least five years (16–19). This effect is reported in cohorts with and without type 2 diabetes, and can lead to remission of established microalbuminuria in both cohorts (16, 18). A single randomized controlled trial has shown that Roux-en-Y gastric bypass is superior to best medical treatment in causing remission of albuminuria over 2 years, and thus inducing remission of early diabetic kidney disease (JAMA Surg; in press).

While the data for the effect of surgery on both preventing and remediating proteinuria are generally based on measured protein excretion, including 24 h urine collections, almost all of the data on the effect of metabolic surgery on renal function are based on estimated glomerular filtration rate (eGFR) rather than measured glomerular filtration rate (mGFR). It should be noted that in the context of significant weight loss, serum creatinine concentrations usually decrease, resulting in an apparent increase in eGFR (17, 20). Calculators for eGFR have not been validated for use in the context of significant and rapid weight loss, as occurs after metabolic surgery. Therefore, eGFR in this population should be interpreted with caution.

In general, there is no deleterious effect of surgery on eGFR in those with preserved renal function at the time of surgery (19). This seems to be the case for populations both with and without type 2 diabetes at baseline. There are data to suggest a potent renoprotective effect of surgery in people with type 2 diabetes and early DKD. In case-control data comparing metabolic surgery and medical therapy in people with type 2 diabetes, and albuminuria with preserved renal function, surgery was associated with stabilization of eGFR and remission of albuminuria over a 10 year follow-up period, as compared with a steady decline in renal function in the medical group (21).

While there are very few data on the effect of metabolic surgery on people with an eGFR of <60 ml/min/1.73 m^2 (stage 3–5 chronic kidney disease), the available data indicate potential benefit (17, 19, 22). When using eGFR, there seems to be a stablisation in renal function in recipients of metabolic surgery that can last up to 9 years post-operatively (19, 22–24). Notwithstanding the limitations of eGFR in this cohort, the renal data are reassuring. The maximal weight loss typically occurs within 2 years of surgery. After this point, weight loss stabilizes, and the eGFR calculators are presumably more robust (although this is not proven to be the case).

In clinical practice, metabolic surgery is offered to selected patients on dialysis who require transplantation, but who are excluded from transplant lists solely on the basis of their weight. While this cohort is understandably at high risk of peri-operative and post-operative morbidity and mortality, the benefits of surgery can exceed in the risks in some cases. For selected cohorts, surgery can be risk-acceptable and effective, resulting in successful renal transplantation (25). In some series of patients with end-stage renal disease who have surgery, cases of recovery of renal function in dialysis-dependent patients have been reported (26, 27). In these cases, histological markers of renal disease improved after surgery in parallel with the improvements in renal function.

The mechanisms for the above-described improvement in renal function and prevention of renal disease are not fully understood. Metabolic surgery reduces weight, improves hypertension and ameliorates hyperglycaemia, which can explain some of the effect on eGFR (3, 14, 19, 22, 28, 29). However, other mechanisms, such as resolution of pro-inflammatory pathways, may also contribute to the improvement in markers of renal disease (30, 31). The interplay between obesity and diabetes is difficult to tease out in human studies, but in animal models of DKD the inflammatory effect of obesity seems to be only partially responsible for improvements in proteinuria (30). Therefore, it seems that several mechanisms work together to produce the renal benefits seen in recipients of metabolic surgery.

Glomerular hyperfiltration is a phenomenon seen in obesity related renal disease, with or without co-morbid type 2 diabetes. Hyperfiltration results in glomerular hypertrophy, and the increased rate of filtration is associated with oxidative stress and activation of pro-inflammatory pathways. In some cases, the end-point of chronic hyperftltration is focal segmental glomerulosclerosis, with an associated clinical presentation of proteinuric renal disease termed obesity related glomerulopathy, which is similar in clinical presentation to diabetic kidney disease, but which can occur in the absence of diabetes or hyperglycaemia (8). This condition can result in end stage renal failure.

Obesity related glomerulopathy is a result of a confluence of pro-inflammatory pathways, ectopic lipid accumulation within the kidney, and podocyte dysfunction in the context of insulin resistance and oxidative stress (8). As it can occur in the absence of diabetes and hypertension, it is a clear demonstration of the importance of multiple non-glucocentric mechanisms that are involved in the onset and progression of diabetic kidney disease in those with type 2 diabetes and obesity (8). As is the case in diabetic kidney disease, metabolic and bariatric surgery can ameliorate obesity related glomerulopathy by remediating inflammation and reducing hyperfiltration (8).

Unanswered Questions in Diabetic Kidney Disease

GFR Accuracy—Do the Estimates Measure Up?

An essential question to answer is whether the estimated GFR calculators can be relied upon after metabolic surgery. Measured GFR before and after surgery appears stable when corrected for body surface area (17, 20, 32–36). However, in these studies there were very few participants with diabetes, and follow-up was less then 24 months in almost all cases.

This is problematic as we are basing our current ideas around the use of metabolic surgery in DKD on the effect of eGFR [usually estimated with the Modification of Diet in Renal Disease (MDRD) formula] in long-term epidemiological and cohort studies. The MDRD formula has been shown to be inaccurate in cohorts with type 2 diabetes and obesity (37, 38). Part of the problem is the presumption of a body surface area of 1.73 m^2, which is an underestimate in many people with obesity (38). However, even in longitudinal studies of measured GFR, concerns around eGFR calculators exist with respect to their validity in people with type 2 diabetes (39).

This issue is compounded by the changes in muscle mass that occurs after metabolic surgery (40). Serum creatinine is primarily derived from muscle mass, and so calculators based on serum creatinine may be prone to error if we compare eGFR before and after significant weight loss. The loss of muscle mass only appears to be significant in the first year after surgery, with apparent stabilization of muscle mass from the end of the first post-operative year (40). While the studies of measured GFR completed in the first year post operatively have been reassuring, very few participants were followed beyond the weight loss phase (17, 20–22). Therefore, it is unknown if the current creatinine based calculators for eGFR are valid in people with type 2 diabetes following metabolic surgery.

Calculators for eGFR other than MDRD can be used, although none appear to be as accurate as we would like (33). This is especially true in the weight loss phase in the first year after bariatric or metabolic surgery (33, 34, 37). Of the currently available calculators, CKD-EPI is the most accurate (33). CKD-EPI can underestimate GFR in people with obesity before surgery, and overestimate it in the post-operative phase, but the use of Cystatin C as a marker of filtration can enhance the accuracy of CKD-EPI (33, 34). However, Cystatin C is not widely available for use, and remains outside of standard clinical practice at present. While the estimated values may not be entirely accurate in any of the calculators, the trends over time do parallel, and so whatever calculator is used at the onset, should be consistently used over time to detect any significant changes in eGFR (22).

Given the above, in our opinion, it seems that that new studies are needed. These should be validation studies of eGFR calculators in populations with type 2 diabetes and obesity. Two cohorts are needed in these studies; a post-operative population who had metabolic surgery over 2 years before entry into the study, and a cohort matched for age, weight, and relevant comorbidities and medication use. It should be noted that given the dynamic physiological changes associated with surgery, eGFR calculation may not be able to achieve acceptably accurate results. Direct measurement of GFR is the only way to really gauge the effect of metabolic and bariatric surgery on renal function and disease. While the complexity of the measurement process means that measured GFR remains inaccessible for standard clinical care, the use of simplified direct measurement of GFR may prove to be the future of renal surveillance in this cohort.

Is Metabolic Surgery Better Than Medical Management for Treating People With DKD and an eGFR of <60 ml/min/1.73 m²?

There is abundant evidence that metabolic surgery is more effective than medical therapy alone in treating type 2 diabetes. There is also evidence that it can treat hypertension more effectively than with medication alone, although this evidence base is not as well-developed (3, 41). Given that these two major risk factors are well-treated by metabolic surgery, it seems logical to presume that surgery would be more effective than medical therapy in treating established DKD.

However, it remains the case that we still do not have any randomized controlled data from trials specifically powered to detect treatment effect differences between surgery and medical therapy in DKD with an eGFR <60 ml/min/1.73 kg/m^2. This is particularly important in the longer-term in people with renal impairment at baseline. While glycaemic control and blood pressure improve shortly after surgery, and remain improved in the medium to long-term, there is an increased risk of nephrolithiasis in surgical recipients (42). Oxalate nephropathy may develop after metabolic surgery, predisposing to nephrolithiasis and chronic renal disease (43). This risk appears to be procedure dependent, but is not well-quantified. However, it may be that in people with eGFRs of <60 ml/min/1.73 kg/m^2 the risk/benefit balance is not that strongly in favor of surgical treatment.

On balance, it seems likely that the potential renal benefits would exceed the risks. However, this needs to be specifically studied. Randomized controlled trials of surgery and best medical therapy are needed in people with established DKD and eGFR of <60 ml/min/1.73 m^2. These studies should incorporate a treat-to-target protocol, so that the medical arms achieve equivalent glycaemic and blood pressure targets. Best medical therapy should include renin-angiotensin-aldosterone system inhibitor or blockade, and sodium glucose co-transporter 2 inhibitor therapy. They should also include longer-term follow-up and measurement of urinary markers of nephrolithiasis.

DIABETIC RETINOPATHY

Diabetic Retinopathy: What We Know

There is little evidence to inform us on the effect of metabolic surgery on diabetic retinopathy. From the existing data, it seems that most people who do not have retinopathy pre-operatively, do not go on to develop it post-operatively (44–46). For those with pre-existing retinopathy, most either remain stable, or improve, in disease severity (44–46). However, some do deteriorate and develop more severe, and potentially sight-threatening, disease (44, 45, 47).

The existing longitudinal data on microvascular outcomes suggest that in most people surgery prevents the development or progression of diabetic retinopathy (11, 13, 14, 29). While none of these studies were specifically powered to examine the effect of surgery on retinopathy, these long-term real-world data are reassuring as they show that surgery is associated with significant reductions in the risk of developing retinopathy without a strong signal for significant deterioration of disease at population level (11, 13, 29).

This makes physiological sense, as surgery is proven to be more effective that medical therapy alone in helping people with type 2 diabetes meet glycaemic treatment targets (28, 48, 49). Hyperglycaemia is the major risk factor for the development and progression of retinopathy (50). Therefore, ameliorating hyperglycaemia with surgery would be expected to be protective against retinopathy.

However, while the long-term effect may be expected to be protective, the immediate post-operative period should be considered to be a time when the individual is at elevated risk of disease progression. This is due to the rapid improvement in glycaemic control seen after surgery. Rapid improvement in hyperglycaemia has long been associated with progression of retinopathy (51). Metabolic surgery results in an improvement in hyperglycaemia in the immediate post-operative period, with significant changes in HbA1c within months of treatment (48). This rapid improvement should be expected to put the surgical recipient at risk of progression of disease.

The existing evidence base is almost exclusively limited to cohort studies and uncontrolled case series. The populations studied are heterogenous with varying degrees of pre-operative disease and post-operative follow-up. There are very few randomized controlled data available on retinopathy. In the STAMPEDE trial, where 150 participants were randomized to sleeve gastrectomy, Roux-en-Y gastric bypass, or best medical therapy, formal scoring of retinopathy was not published, but it was reported that there was no significant change in retinopathy disease severity in any of the treatment groups (28).

However, the concern about the immediate post-operative effect of surgery on retinopathy is borne out in some of the published case series documenting the effect of surgery on retinopathy (44, 45, 47). In these series, many cases of disease progression have been described. Given the design of these studies, we cannot be clear as to the major risk factors for progression of disease, but it does seem that pre-operative hyperglycaemia is likely to be a major risk factor. In one study, the authors noted a difference in pre-operative HbA1c of over 11 mmol/mol (1%) between those who had progression of disease post-operatively and those who did not (47). The mean change in HbA1c was comparable between groups, but pre-operative HbA1c concentrations were higher in those who had post-operative progression of retinopathy (47).

In some cases, progression of disease can be sight threatening. From the reported cases, it appears to be a combination of pre-operative HbA1c, magnitude of change in HbA1c concentration post-operatively, and presence of pre-existing retinal disease, that is most important in determining the risk of progression to sight-threatening disease following surgery (44, 47, 52). Therefore, while in general surgery could be expected to prevent the development or progression of retinopathy, caution must be taken in candidates for surgery who have pre-existing retinopathy, especially if they are significantly off glycaemic targets pre-operatively.

Unanswered Questions in Retinopathy

What Is the Effect of Metabolic Surgery on Retinopathy?

The case series and cohort data outlined above suggest a rate of post-operative deterioration in retinopathy of between 1 and 45%. (46, 47, 52–56). This wide range is likely explained by the heterogeneity of the cohorts, both in terms of clinical characteristics and size. Different grading systems were also used across studies, which critically limits comparison between study cohorts.

This illustrates the need for robust prospective large-scale cohort studies examining the effect of surgery on retinopathy specifically. Any such study should include people with type 2 diabetes, both those with and without retinopathy, who are followed up after surgery with a robust validated grading system to determine if there is any change before and after surgery. In order to control for background rates of progression of retinopathy, the surgical cohort should be matched with a control cohort. Adequate matching will require a cohort with similar glycaemic control at baseline, comparable retinal grading at baseline, and equivalent duration of diabetes.

Follow-up for any study of retinopathy needs to be up to 5 years at least, as there can be changes in retinal scores for up to 4 years post-operatively (47). Therefore, even in those who achieve treatment targets, or even remission of diabetes, after surgery, a risk of progression of disease may exist. In the absence of definitive evidence, caution is best, and so in current practice, retinal screening should continue in those who have had surgery for at least 4 years. A longer-term study would inform us to the need for such an approach.

Are There Risk Factors for Development or Progression of Retinopathy After Metabolic Surgery?

There are signals in the existing cohort studies that pre-operative HbA1c concentrations, and grading of pre-existing retinopathy, are both important risk factors for progression of disease post-operatively. However, this needs to be proven and defined. What are the risk factors that are important in predicting progression? And what are the thresholds that define high-risk from normal risk? A well-designed prospective case control study could answer these questions.

In most studies, higher pre-operative HbA1c concentrations are associated with a higher rate of post-operative progression of retinopathy (47, 52, 54). The HbA1c threshold at which retinal risk really accelerates is not known, but in the cohort study with the highest rate of deterioration in retinopathy after surgery (9 people out of 20), the mean pre-operative HbA1c was 81 mmol/mol (9.5%) (54). In one study, the authors defined an increased risk of higher grades of post-operative retinopathy with every 1 mmol/mol increase in pre-operative HbA1c (47). This needs to be verified in a larger study.

As well as baseline HbA1c, the rapid change in HbA1c concentrations that often occur after surgery may be associated with progression of retinopathy. In this case, the cohort data have shown conflicting results. In some cohorts, there is a clear trend for deterioration in those who achieve the greatest improvement in HbA1c (52). In others, there is no such trend (47). However, the differing design of the studies, and differences in baseline characteristics between cohorts, explain this conflict. Based on the evidence for retinal disease progression with rapid improvements in glycemic control in other settings, it seems very likely that rapid changes in glycaemic control will prove to be a risk factor for progression of retinopathy. However, this remains to be proven. Theoretically, this risk factor could be modified with anti-diabetes medical therapy prior to surgery, in an effort to reduce HbA1c pre-operatively, thus reducing the rapid slope of change immediately after surgery.

There is no clear threshold for risk of post-operative progression of retinopathy. While baseline hyperglycaemia is clearly important, rapid improvement of hyperglycaemia is also important (51). Given what we know so far a pre-operative HbA1c of over 75 mmol/mol (9%) and a change in HbA1c of over 11 mmol/mol (1%) before and after surgery, seems reasonable as markers of risk (47, 52, 54). However, further study is needed to clearly define these glycaemic risk thresholds.

Recent data have suggested there are many phenotypes of type 2 diabetes that could be mapped genetically, and potentially via proteomic or metabolomics profiles (57). It is known that likelihood of remission of type 2 diabetes can be partially predicted by pre-operative factors including HbA1c and C-peptide concentrations (58). Using these parameters with other biochemical, metabolic, and anthropometric factors in multivariate models may be able to predict those who will have a rapid glycaemic response to surgery (59).

The other likely risk marker of post-operative deterioration in retinopathy is pre-operative grade of disease. It seems that any grade of retinopathy, no matter how early, increases the likelihood of higher grades post-operatively (47, 52). Most people who do not have retinopathy pre-operatively remain disease free after surgery (44–46). In those who do have deterioration of disease, there is no clear relationship between grade for pre-operative disease and eventual post-operative grading. Cases of severe and potentially sight-threatening disease have been described in people with minimal retinal disease pre-operatively (44, 45, 47). These cases are confounded by other changes in characteristics, predominantly glycaemic change, over time, and so the importance of the grade of retinal disease itself as a risk factor remains unclear.

Therefore, a large long-term case control study is needed, where people who go on to have metabolic surgery are well-characterized at baseline and then followed over at least 5 years. The surgical cohort should be matched to a control cohort for all relevant risk factors. Given the likely confounding effect of improvement in glycaemic control, statistical input should be sought as how to delineate the glycaemic effects from the effect of pre-existing grade of retinal disease and other potential risk factors.

While awaiting the results of any future study on retinopathy, it is best to be cautious. Therefore, we recommend pre-operative retinal assessment for all patients with type 2 diabetes who go on to have bariatric or metabolic surgery. Reassessment should be scheduled post-operatively. If there is any retinopathy, then reassessment should occur within three to 6 months post-operatively. If pre-proliferative retinopathy, or any maculopathy, is detected, then specialist ophthalmology advice should be sought to determine if pre-operative treatment is needed.

DIABETIC NEUROPATHY

Diabetic Neuropathy: What We Know

There are even fewer data on the effect of metabolic surgery on diabetic neuropathy than there are on the effect of surgery on retinopathy. However, the data that do exist demonstrate that metabolic surgery is associated with a reduced risk of developing diabetic neuropathy (13, 14, 28, 29, 60). These data were all derived from subjective reporting of neuropathy, either by patients themselves or from healthcare providers. In a small study using nerve conduction studies, there was no change in electrophysiological markers of neuropathy before and after surgery (46).

It is reasonable to expect that neuropathy would be less likely to occur after surgery given the significant improvement in glycaemic control induced by metabolic surgery. Therefore, the available data agree with expectation. However, there are very few people included in these studies with pre-existing neuropathy or diabetic foot disease. There is some cause for concern that surgery may result in treatment-induced neuropathy given the rapid rate of improvement in glycaemic control (61, 62).

Unanswered Questions in Neuropathy and Diabetic Foot Disease

Metabolic surgery can result in neuropathy, even in the absence of diabetes (63). The etiology of neuropathy after surgery varies, but can be related to deficiencies in micronutrients such as vitamin B12. While there is no evidence that treatment induced neuropathy is a common phenomenon after metabolic surgery, cases of serious diabetic neuropathy and arthropathy have been described in the context of rapid improvements in glycaemic control and weight (61, 62). Therefore, it will be necessary to study the effect of metabolic surgery on neuropathy, especially in people with pre-operative disease, in order to quantify the risk of post-operative deterioration.

As well as quantifying the effect of surgery on neuropathy, prospective cohort studies are needed to delineate the important mechanisms that could be associated with post-operative neuropathy. There are multiple potential insults associated with surgery. The rapid improvement in glycaemic control may induce a treatment-induced neuritis. Micronutrient deficiencies can also produce neuropathy. Anecdotal evidence would suggest that those that present with late onset of neuropathy, often many years after surgery, are those who are not taking regular comprehensive micronutrient supplementation. Specifically, deficiencies in B vitamins may be critical factors in the development of neuropathy. Therefore, any such study must be designed to comprehensively gather all the relevant data to allow a full analysis of all potential risk factors.

Diabetic foot disease is a source of major morbidity in people with type 2 diabetes. Neuropathy is a major contributor to diabetic foot disease. Therefore, if there was a risk of deterioration in neuropathy post-operatively, this may worsen existing diabetic foot disease or increase the risk of developing diabetic foot disease. There are no studies on this topic, but given the risk of harm in people with active diabetic foot disease (ulceration or arthropathy), there is an urgent need to investigate the effect of surgery on nerve function, both in those without neuropathy at baseline, and those with active diabetic foot disease.

CARDIOVASCULAR DISEASE

Cardiovascular Disease: What We Know

Metabolic surgery significantly improves blood pressure and cholesterol concentrations in tandem with improved glycaemic control in type 2 diabetes. Therefore, is it not surprising to note that surgery is consistently associated with reduced rates of myocardial infarction and stroke (4, 14, 64). This reduces the cardiovascular mortality rate in these cohorts by ~50%.

While the observational and epidemiological evidence are very convincing, it is not conclusively proven that surgery would be more effective than medical therapy in reducing cardiovascular mortality. There are no randomized controlled trials of surgery and best medical care where cardiovascular morbidity or mortality are primary outcomes. These studies remain to be completed, and should be focused on those with increased cardiovascular risk in the first instance.

Unanswered Questions in Cardiovascular Disease

Can We Determine Who Is Likely to Benefit Most From Metabolic Surgery?

It may be that there are certain cohorts who would benefit more from surgery than others. Those with existing cardiovascular disease may not be good surgical candidates. However, if metabolic surgery was being considered in order to reduce cardiovascular risk, it would be useful to know who would be most likely to benefit from intervention.

As mentioned above, there are different clinical phenotypes of type 2 diabetes that can be mapped to genotypes (57). It may be that some of these phenotypes would be more likely than others to respond to surgery in terms of weight loss or improved glycaemic control. However, it may also be the case that there are certain genotypes that would respond better than others in terms of improvements in cardiovascular risk factors. Multivariate models including phenotypic, genotypic, and proteomic parameters may be able to predict those who will have a good response to surgery (59).

Therefore, large-scale population studies are needed. People who go on to have surgery should be characterized genotypically and phenotypically. Samples for proteomic and metabolomics profiles should be taken. Then, as the population ages, and cardiovascular disease becomes apparent, modeling for identifiable risk markers should be completed. This would need to be a longer-term project if completed prospectively, but use of existing bariatric registries could make such a project more feasible (presuming that they included the relevant data).

Do Patients With Obesity and Type 2 Diabetes Have a Greater Health Economic Benefit From Surgery With Respect to Cardiovascular Disease?

Metabolic surgery is associated with reduced cardiovascular morbidity and mortality, including reduced rates of hospital admission for cardiovascular disease and heart failure (4, 64, 65). It is clear that in general metabolic surgery is cost-saving not just cost-effective (66). However, this is when people both with and without diabetes are included. A large proportion of the cost-saving is due to prevention of chronic disease, including diabetes and cardiovascular disease, and therefore reduced costs of treatment.

It would be reasonable to expect that there would be a greater cost saving associated with type 2 diabetes given the reduced medication and insulin use that generally occurs post-operatively (28). However, the health economic data are not entirely clear. Some studies indicate a greater cost benefit in people with type 2 diabetes, but others do not find a cost benefit (67, 68). This is likely due to differences in analysis. The lack of cost benefit is due to a greater number of hospital presentations for both routine follow-up care and emergency care (68). However, this is only a cost issue in the first 2 years post-operatively (68). In longer-term follow up, cost savings may be greater.

In cardiovascular disease and diabetes, it may be that there is a major cost saving. In addition to preventing primary events, metabolic surgery can offer secondary prevention and reduce costs associated with coronary artery disease treatment (69). This is not fully defined, and therefore a cost-analysis of people with both diabetes and cardiovascular disease at baseline is needed. It may be that due to a reduced number of secondary events and reduced medication use, people with both type 2 diabetes and cardiovascular disease offer greater health economic benefit to a healthcare system.

CONCLUSIONS

Metabolic surgery is an effective treatment for type 2 diabetes, and given the data available to date, is effective at preventing the development of diabetic complications. However, there is a lack of specific randomized controlled studies on the effect of surgery on the complications of diabetes. These are urgently needed. While waiting for these data, we should exercise care in people with retinopathy, neuropathy and diabetic foot disease, as there is potential for deterioration of disease post-operatively.

As well as physiological and clinical effects, more study is needed on the health economic effects of surgery. It seems logical to assume that people with type 2 diabetes and complications such as diabetic kidney disease or cardiovascular disease would be likely to offer greater cost savings to healthcare systems. Further studies are needed to determine if this is the case.

AUTHOR CONTRIBUTIONS

KN and CL both contributed to the literature review and the drafting of this article.

REFERENCES

1. Rubino F, Nathan DM, Eckel RH, Schauer PR, Alberti KG, Zimmet PZ, et al. Metabolic surgery in the treatment algorithm for type 2 diabetes: a joint statement by international diabetes organizations. *Diabetes Care.* (2016) 39:861–77. doi: 10.2337/dc16-0236
2. Park CH, Nam SJ, Choi HS, Kim KO, Kim DH, Kim JW, et al. Comparative efficacy of bariatric surgery in the treatment of morbid obesity and diabetes mellitus: a systematic review and network meta-analysis. *Obes Surg.* (2019) 29:2180–90. doi: 10.1007/s11695-019-03831-6
3. Sjostrom L, Lindroos AK, Peltonen M, Torgerson J, Bouchard C, Carlsson B, et al. Lifestyle, diabetes, and cardiovascular risk factors 10 years after bariatric surgery. *N Engl J Med.* (2004) 351:2683–93. doi: 10.1056/NEJMoa035622
4. Sjostrom L, Peltonen M, Jacobson P, Sjostrom CD, Karason K, Wedel H, et al. Bariatric surgery and long-term cardiovascular events. *JAMA.* (2012) 307:56–65. doi: 10.1001/jama.2011.1914
5. Wang Y, Chen X, Song Y, Caballero B, Cheskin LJ. Association between obesity and kidney disease: a systematic review and meta-analysis. *Kidney Int.* (2008) 73:19–33. doi: 10.1038/sj.ki.5002586
6. Kramer H, Reboussin D, Bertoni AG, Marcovina S, Lipkin E, Greenway FL III, et al. Obesity and albuminuria among adults with type 2 diabetes: the look AHEAD (Action for Health in Diabetes) study. *Diabetes Care.* (2009) 32:851–3. doi: 10.2337/dc08-2059
7. Go AS, Chertow GM, Fan D, McCulloch CE, Hsu CY. Chronic kidney disease and the risks of death, cardiovascular events, and hospitalization. *N Engl J Med.* (2004) 351:1296–305. doi: 10.1056/NEJMoa041031
8. D'Agati VD, Chagnac A, de Vries AP, Levi M, Porrini E, Herman-Edelstein M, et al. Obesity-related glomerulopathy: clinical and pathologic characteristics and pathogenesis. *Nat Rev Nephrol.* (2016) 12:453–71. doi: 10.1038/nrneph.2016.75
9. Collins AJ, Foley RN, Chavers B, Gilbertson D, Herzog C, Johansen K, et al. United States renal data system 2011 annual data report: atlas of chronic kidney disease & end-stage renal disease in the united states. *Am J Kidney Dis.* (2012) 59(1 Suppl 1):A7–e1–420. doi: 10.1053/j.ajkd.2011.11.015
10. Carlsson LM, Romeo S, Jacobson P, Burza MA, Maglio C, Sjöholm K, et al. The incidence of albuminuria after bariatric surgery and usual care in Swedish Obese Subjects (SOS): a prospective controlled intervention trial. *Int J Obes.* (2015) 39:169–75. doi: 10.1038/ijo.2014.72
11. Carlsson LMS, Sjoholm K, Karlsson C, Jacobson P, Andersson-Assarsson JC, Svensson PA, et al. Long-term incidence of microvascular disease after bariatric surgery or usual care in patients with obesity, stratified by baseline glycaemic status: a post-hoc analysis of participants from the Swedish Obese Subjects study. *lancet Diabetes Endocrinol.* (2017) 5:271–9. doi: 10.1016/S2213-858730061-X
12. Coleman KJ, Haneuse S, Johnson E, Bogart A, Fisher D, O'Connor PJ, et al. Long-term microvascular disease outcomes in patients with type 2 diabetes after bariatric surgery: evidence for the legacy effect of surgery. *Diabetes Care.* (2016) 39:1400–7. doi: 10.2337/dc16-0194
13. O'Brien R, Johnson E, Haneuse S, Coleman KJ, O'Connor PJ, Fisher DP, et al. Microvascular outcomes in patients with diabetes after bariatric surgery versus usual care: a matched cohort study. *Ann Intern Med.* (2018) 169:300–10. doi: 10.7326/M17-2383
14. Sjostrom L, Peltonen M, Jacobson P, Ahlin S, Andersson-Assarsson J, Anveden A, et al. Association of bariatric surgery with long-term remission of type 2 diabetes and with microvascular and macrovascular complications. *JAMA.* (2014) 311:2297–304. doi: 10.1001/jama.2014.5988
15. Afshinnia F, Wilt TJ, Duval S, Esmaeili A, Ibrahim HN. Weight loss and proteinuria: systematic review of clinical trials and comparative cohorts. *Nephrol Dial Transplant.* (2010) 25:1173–83. doi: 10.1093/ndt/gfp640
16. *Agrawal V, Khan I, Rai B, Krause KR, Chengelis DL, Zalesin KC*, et al. The effect of weight loss after bariatric surgery on albuminuria. *Clin Nephrol.* (2008) 70:194–202. doi: 10.5414/CNP70194
17. Navarro-Diaz M, Serra A, Romero R, Bonet J, Bayes B, Homs M, et al. Effect of drastic weight loss after bariatric surgery on renal parameters in extremely obese patients: long-term follow-up. *J Am Soc Nephrol.* (2006) 17(12 Suppl 3):S213–7. doi: 10.1681/ASN.2006080917
18. Heneghan HM, Cetin D, Navaneethan SD, Orzech N, Brethauer SA, Schauer PR. Effects of bariatric surgery on diabetic nephropathy after 5 years of follow-up. *Surg Obes Relat Dis.* (2013) 9:7–14. doi: 10.1016/j.soard.2012.08.016
19. Navaneethan SD, Yehnert H, Moustarah F, Schreiber MJ, Schauer PR, Beddhu S. Weight loss interventions in chronic kidney disease: a systematic review and meta-analysis. *Clin J Am Soc Nephrol.* (2009) 4:1565–74. doi: 10.2215/CJN.02250409
20. Chagnac A, Weinstein T, Herman M, Hirsh J, Gafter U, Ori Y. The effects of weight loss on renal function in patients with severe obesity. *J Am Soc Nephrol.* (2003) 14:1480–6. doi: 10.1097/01.ASN.0000068462.38661.89
21. Iaconelli A, Panunzi S, De Gaetano A, Manco M, Guidone C, Leccesi L, et al. Effects of bilio-pancreatic diversion on diabetic complications: a 10-year follow-up. *Diabetes Care.* (2011) 34:561–7. doi: 10.2337/dc10-1761
22. Neff KJ, Baud G, Raverdy V, Caiazzo R, Verkindt H, Noel C, et al. renal function and remission of hypertension after bariatric surgery: a 5-year prospective cohort study. *Obes Surg.* (2017) 27:613–9. doi: 10.1007/s11695-016-2333-7
23. Imam TH, Fischer H, Jing B, Burchette R, Henry S, DeRose SF, et al. Estimated GFR before and after bariatric surgery in CKD. *Am J Kidney Dis.* (2017) 69:380–8. doi: 10.1053/j.ajkd.2016.09.020

24. Chang AR, Chen Y, Still C, Wood GC, Kirchner HL, Lewis M, et al. Bariatric surgery is associated with improvement in kidney outcomes. *Kidney Int.* (2016) 90:164–71. doi: 10.1016/j.kint.2016.02.039
25. Freeman CM, Woodle ES, Shi J, Alexander JW, Leggett PL, Shah SA, et al. Addressing morbid obesity as a barrier to renal transplantation with laparoscopic sleeve gastrectomy. *Am J Transpl.* (2015) 15:1360–8. doi: 10.1111/ajt.13116
26. Alexander JW, Goodman HR, Hawver LR, Cardi MA. Improvement and stabilization of chronic kidney disease after gastric bypass. *Surg Obe Relat Dis.* (2009) 5:237–41. doi: 10.1016/j.soard.2008.08.016
27. Huan Y, Tomaszewski JE, Cohen DL. Resolution of nephrotic syndrome after successful bariatric surgery in patient with biopsy-proven FSGS. *Clin Nephrol.* (2009) 71:69–73. doi: 10.5414/CNP71069
28. Schauer PR, Bhatt DL, Kirwan JP, Wolski K, Aminian A, Brethauer SA, et al. Bariatric surgery versus intensive medical therapy for diabetes - 5-year outcomes. *N Engl J Med.* (2017) 376:641–51. doi: 10.1056/NEJMoa1600869
29. Johnson BL, Blackhurst DW, Latham BB, Cull DL, Bour ES, Oliver TL, et al. Bariatric surgery is associated with a reduction in major macrovascular and microvascular complications in moderately to severely obese patients with type 2 diabetes mellitus. *J Am Coll Surg.* (2013) 216:545–56. doi: 10.1016/j.jamcollsurg.2012.12.019
30. Neff KJ, Elliott JA, Corteville C, Abegg K, Boza C, Lutz TA, et al. Effect of roux-en-y gastric bypass and diet-induced weight loss on diabetic kidney disease in the zucker diabetic fatty rat. *Surg O Relat Dis.* (2017) 13:21–7. doi: 10.1016/j.soard.2016.08.026
31. Fenske WK, Dubb S, Bueter M, Seyfried F, Patel K, Tam FW, et al. Effect of bariatric surgery-induced weight loss on renal and systemic inflammation and blood pressure: a 12-month prospective study. *Surg Obes Relat Dis.* (2013) 9:559–68. doi: 10.1016/j.soard.2012.03.009
32. Brochner-Mortensen J, Rickers H, Balslev I. Renal function and body composition before and after intestinal bypass operation in obese patients. *Scand J Clin Lab Invest.* (1980) 40:695–702. doi: 10.3109/00365518009095584
33. Friedman AN, Moe S, Fadel WF, Inman M, Mattar SG, Shihabi Z, et al. Predicting the glomerular filtration rate in bariatric surgery patients. *Am J Nephrol.* (2014) 39:8–15. doi: 10.1159/000357231
34. Lieske JC, Collazo-Clavell ML, Sarr MG, Rule AD, Bergstralh EJ, Kumar R. Gastric bypass surgery and measured and estimated GFR in women. *Am J Kidney Dis.* (2014) 64:663–5. doi: 10.1053/j.ajkd.2014.06.016
35. Saliba J, Kasim NR, Tamboli RA, Isbell JM, Marks P, Feurer ID, et al. Roux-en-Y gastric bypass reverses renal glomerular but not tubular abnormalities in excessively obese diabetics. *Surgery.* (2010) 147:282–7. doi: 10.1016/j.surg.2009.09.017
36. Serpa Neto A, Bianco Rossi FM, Dal Moro Amarante R, Alves Buriti N, Cunha Barbosa Saheb G, Rossi M. Effect of weight loss after Roux-en-Y gastric bypass, on renal function and blood pressure in morbidly obese patients. *J Nephrol.* (2009) 22:637–46. doi: 10.13712Fjournal.pone.0163907
37. Chudleigh RA, Dunseath G, Peter R, Harvey JN, Ollerton RL, Luzio S, et al. Influence of body weight on the performance of glomerular filtration rate estimators in subjects with type 2 diabetes. *Diabetes Care.* (2008) 31:47–9. doi: 10.2337/dc07-1335
38. Nair S, Mishra V, Hayden K, Lisboa PJ, Pandya B, Vinjamuri S, et al. The four-variable modification of diet in renal disease formula underestimates glomerular filtration rate in obese type 2 diabetic individuals with chronic kidney disease. *Diabetologia.* (2011) 54:1304–7. doi: 10.1007/s00125-011-2085-9
39. Gaspari F, Ruggenenti P, Porrini E, Motterlini N, Cannata A, Carrara F, et al. The GFR and GFR decline cannot be accurately estimated in type 2 diabetics. *Kidney Int.* (2013) 84:164–73. doi: 10.1038/ki.2013.47
40. Davidson LE, Yu W, Goodpaster BH, DeLany JP, Widen E, Lemos T, et al. Fat-free mass and skeletal muscle mass five years after bariatric surgery. *Obesity.* (2018) 26:1130–6. doi: 10.1002/oby.22190
41. Schiavon CA, Bersch-Ferreira AC, Santucci EV, Oliveira JD, Torreglosa CR, Bueno PT, et al. Effects of bariatric surgery in obese patients with hypertension: the GATEWAY randomized trial (Gastric bypass to treat obese patients with steady hypertension). *Circulation.* (2018) 137:1132–42. doi: 10.1161/CIRCULATIONAHA.117.032130
42. Lieske JC, Mehta RA, Milliner DS, Rule AD, Bergstralh EJ, Sarr MG. Kidney stones are common after bariatric surgery. *Kidney Int.* (2015) 87:839–45. doi: 10.1038/ki.2014.352
43. Nasr SH, D'Agati VD, Said SM, Stokes MB, Largoza MV, Radhakrishnan J, et al. Oxalate nephropathy complicating Roux-en-Y gastric Bypass: an underrecognized cause of irreversible renal failure. *Clini J Am Soc Nephrol.* (2008) 3:1676–83. doi: 10.2215/CJN.02940608
44. Cheung D, Switzer NJ, Ehmann D, Rudnisky C, Shi X, Karmali S. The impact of bariatric surgery on diabetic retinopathy: a systematic review and meta-analysis. *Obes Surg.* (2015) 25:1604–9. doi: 10.1007/s11695-014-1539-9
45. Merlotti C, Ceriani V, Morabito A, Pontiroli AE. Bariatric surgery and diabetic retinopathy: a systematic review and meta-analysis of controlled clinical studies. *Obes Rev.* (2017) 18:309–16. doi: 10.1111/obr.12490
46. Miras AD, Chuah LL, Khalil N, Nicotra A, Vusirikala A, Baqai N, et al. Type 2 diabetes mellitus and microvascular complications 1 year after Roux-en-Y gastric bypass: a case-control study. *Diabetologia.* (2015) 58:1443–7. doi: 10.1007/s00125-015-3595-7
47. Chen Y, Laybourne JP, Sandinha MT, de Alwis NMW, Avery P, Steel DH, et al. Does bariatric surgery prevent progression of diabetic retinopathy? *Eye.* (2017) 31:1131–9. doi: 10.1038/eye.2017.119
48. Buchwald H, Estok R, Fahrbach K, Banel D, Jensen MD, Pories WJ, et al. Weight and type 2 diabetes after bariatric surgery: systematic review and meta-analysis. *Am J Med.* (2009) 122:248–56.e5. doi: 10.1016/j.amjmed.2008.09.041
49. Mingrone G, Panunzi S, De Gaetano A, Guidone C, Iaconelli A, Nanni G, et al. Bariatric-metabolic surgery versus conventional medical treatment in obese patients with type 2 diabetes:5 year follow-up of an open-label, single-centre, randomised controlled trial. *Lancet.* (2015) 386:964–73. doi: 10.1016/S0140-6736(15)00075-6
50. UK Prospective Diabetes Study (UKPDS) Group. Intensive blood-glucose control with sulphonylureas or insulin compared with conventional treatment risk of complications in patients with type 2 diabetes (UKPDS 33) UK Prospective Diabetes Study (UKPDS) Group. *Lancet.* (1998) 352:837–53. doi: 10.1016/S0140-6736(98)07019-6
51. Diabetes C, Complications Trial Research G, Nathan DM, Genuth S, Lachin J, Cleary P, et al. The effect of intensive treatment of diabetes on the development and progression of long-term complications in insulin-dependent diabetes mellitus. *N Engl J Med.* (1993) 329:977–86. doi: 10.1056/NEJM199309303291401
52. Murphy R, Jiang Y, Booth M, Babor R, MacCormick A, Hammodat H, et al. Progression of diabetic retinopathy after bariatric surgery. *Diabet Med.* (2015) 32:1212–20. doi: 10.1111/dme.12727
53. Brynskov T, Laugesen CS, Svenningsen AL, Floyd AK, Sorensen TL. Monitoring of diabetic retinopathy in relation to bariatric surgery: a prospective observational study. *Obes Surg.* (2016) 26:1279–86. doi: 10.1007/s11695-015-1936-8
54. Kim YJ, Seo du R, Kim MJ, Lee SJ, Hur KY, Choi KS. Clinical course of diabetic retinopathy in korean type 2 diabetes after bariatric surgery: a pilot study. *Retina.* (2015) 35:935–43. doi: 10.1097/IAE.0000000000000412
55. Thomas RL, Prior SL, Barry JD, Luzio SD, Eyre N, Caplin S, et al. Does bariatric surgery adversely impact on diabetic retinopathy in persons with morbid obesity and type 2 diabetes? A pilot study. *J Diabetes Compl.* (2014) 28:191–5. doi: 10.1016/j.jdiacomp.2013.10.006
56. Varadhan L, Humphreys T, Walker AB, Cheruvu CV, Varughese GI. Bariatric surgery and diabetic retinopathy: a pilot analysis. *Obes Surg.* (2012) 22:515–6. doi: 10.1007/s11695-012-0600-9
57. Ahlqvist E, Storm P, Karajamaki A, Martinell M, Dorkhan M, Carlsson A, et al. Novel subgroups of adult-onset diabetes and their association with outcomes: a data-driven cluster analysis of six variables. *lancet Diabetes Endocrinol.* (2018) 6:361–9. doi: 10.1016/S2213-8587(18)30051-2
58. Dixon JB, Chuang LM, Chong K, Chen SC, Lambert GW, Straznicky NE, et al. Predicting the glycemic response to gastric bypass surgery in patients with type 2 diabetes. *Diabetes Care.* (2013) 36:20–6. doi: 10.2337/dc12-0779
59. Szczerbinski L, Taylor MA, Citko A, Gorska M, Larsen S, Hady HR, et al. Clusters of glycemic response to oral glucose tolerance tests explain multivariate metabolic and anthropometric outcomes of bariatric surgery in obese patients. *J Clin Med.* (2019) 8:1091. doi: 10.3390/jcm8081091
60. Muller-Stich BP, Fischer L, Kenngott HG, Gondan M, Senft J, Clemens G, et al. Gastric bypass leads to improvement of diabetic neuropathy

independent of glucose normalization–results of a prospective cohort study (DiaSurg 1 study). *Ann Surg.* (2013) 258:760–5. doi: 10.1097/SLA.0b013e3182a618b2

61. Murchison R, Gooday C, Dhatariya K. The development of a charcot foot after significant weight loss in people with diabetes: three cautionary tales. *J Am Podiatr Med Assoc.* (2014) 104:522–5. doi: 10.7547/0003-0538-104.5.522
62. Gibbons CH, Freeman R. Treatment-induced neuropathy of diabetes: an acute, iatrogenic complication of diabetes. *Brain.* (2015) 138(Pt 1):43–52. doi: 10.1093/brain/awu307
63. Aghili R, Malek M, Tanha K, Mottaghi A. The effect of bariatric surgery on peripheral polyneuropathy: a systematic review and meta-analysis. *Obes Surg.* (2019) 29:3010–20. doi: 10.1007/s11695-019-04004-1
64. Adams TD, Gress RE, Smith SC, Halverson RC, Simper SC, Rosamond WD, et al. Long-term mortality after gastric bypass surgery. *N Engl J Med.* (2007) 357:753–61. doi: 10.1056/NEJMoa066603
65. Aleassa EM, Khorgami Z, Kindel TL, Tu C, Tang WHW, Schauer PR, et al. Impact of bariatric surgery on heart failure mortality. *Surg Obes Relat Dis.* (2019) 15:1189–96. doi: 10.1016/j.soard.2019.03.021
66. Borisenko O, Lukyanov V, Ahmed AR. Cost-utility analysis of bariatric surgery. *Br J Surgery.* (2018) 105:1328–37. doi: 10.1002/bjs.10857
67. James R, Salton RI, Byrnes JM, Scuffham PA. Cost-utility analysis for bariatric surgery compared with usual care for the treatment of obesity in Australia. *Surg Obes Relat Dis.* (2017) 13:2012–20. doi: 10.1016/j.soard.2016.12.016
68. Banerjee S, Garrison LP Jr, Flum DR, Arterburn DE. Cost and health care utilization implications of bariatric surgery versus intensive lifestyle and medical intervention for type 2 diabetes. *Obesity.* (2017) 25:1499–508. doi: 10.1002/oby.21927
69. Baimas-George M, Hennings DL, Al-Qurayshi Z, Emad K, DuCoin C. No more broken hearts: weight loss after bariatric surgery returns patients' postoperative risk to baseline following coronary surgery. *Surg Obes Relat Dis.* (2017) 13:1010–5. doi: 10.1016/j.soard.2016.12.008

13

Bariatric Surgery Modulates Urinary Levels of MicroRNAs Involved in the Regulation of Renal Function

Abdullah Alkandari [1,2], Hutan Ashrafian [1,3], Thozhukat Sathyapalan [4], Ara Darzi [1,3], Elaine Holmes [1], Thanos Athanasiou [1], Stephen L. Atkin [5] and Nigel J. Gooderham [1]*

[1] Department of Surgery and Cancer, Imperial College London, London, United Kingdom, [2] Dasman Diabetes Institute, Kuwait City, Kuwait, [3] Institute of Global Health Innovation, Imperial College London, London, United Kingdom, [4] Department of Academic Endocrinology, Diabetes, and Metabolism, Hull York Medical School, Kingston upon Hull, United Kingdom, [5] Weill Cornell Medical College Qatar, Qatar Foundation, Doha, Qatar

***Correspondence:**
Abdullah Alkandari
abdullah.alkandari@dasmaninstitute.org

Background: Obesity and diabetes cause chronic kidney disease with a common pathophysiology that is characterized by the accumulation of collagen in the extracellular matrix. Recent evidence has implicated the epithelial-to-mesenchymal transition (EMT) as a key step in this pathology with regulation by microRNAs. Weight loss leads to improvements in renal function; therefore, this study hypothesized that bariatric-surgery aided weight loss would lead to changes in urinary microRNAs involved in the regulation of renal function.

Materials and methods: Twenty-four bariatric patients undergoing Roux-en-Y gastric bypass and sleeve gastrectomy donated urine pre-operatively and at 2–6 months and 1–2 years post-operatively. Urine samples were also obtained from 10 healthy weight and 7 morbidly obese non-surgical controls. Expression levels of kidney microRNAs were assessed in urine and the function of microRNAs was assessed through the *in vitro* transfection of HK-2 cells, a kidney proximal tubule cell line.

Results: Levels of miR 192, miR 200a, and miR 200b were upregulated in urine following bariatric surgery. This increase was consistent across surgical type and diabetes status and was maintained and enhanced with time. Bariatric surgery alters urinary miR 192 expression from levels seen in morbidly obese patients to levels seen in healthy weight control patients. In mechanistic studies, the transfection of miR 192 in HK-2 cells increased miR 200a expression and decreased ZEB2, a key transcriptional promoter of kidney fibrosis.

Conclusions: Bariatric surgery increased miR 192 and miR 200 urinary levels, key anti-fibrotic microRNAs that could contribute to a renal-protective mechanism and may be of value as urinary biomarkers following surgery. These findings suggest that urinary microRNAs may represent potential novel biomarkers for obesity-associated renal function.

Keywords: microRNA, nephropathy, bariatric/metabolic surgery, urinary, longitudinal, diabetes

INTRODUCTION

Whilst obesity contributes to diabetes and hypertension, both leading causes of progressive chronic kidney disease (CKD), data suggests that obesity is an independent risk factor for CKD (1). Diabetes and obesity related CKD appear to share the same initial pathophysiology (1). Increasing BMI leads to renal hyperfiltration and proteinuria that eventually culminates in hypofiltration and CKD. Diabetic nephropathy (DN) occurs in approximately one third of cases of diabetes (both type 1 and type 2) and is the most common cause of CKD and end stage renal failure (2). DN is mediated by transforming growth factor-β1 (TGF-β1) and TGF-β1 promoted fibrosis is induced by increasing the number of local fibroblasts, which are the effecter cells in the production and accumulation of the extracellular matrix. Epithelial-to-mesenchymal transition (EMT) is increasingly recognized as a key component in this process by promoting the transition of resident renal epithelial cells to a fibroblast phenotype (3). Recently, multiple studies have implicated microRNAs in this process. MicroRNAs are small, endogenous RNAs that regulate gene expression by silencing the translation of mRNA. The microRNAs miR 192 and the miR 200 family contribute to kidney fibrosis by suppressing EMT, targeting zinc E-box binding homeobox 1 and 2 (ZEB1 and ZEB2) that encode for transcriptional repressors for E-cadherin, essential for maintaining the epithelial phenotype (4–6). This leads to an increase in collagen deposition in the extracellular matrix and the thickening of the glomerular basement, a common feature of DN.

Weight loss in the clinically obese patient, including that achieved surgically, leads to an improvement in renal function (7–9). Bariatric or metabolic surgery encompasses several gastrointestinal surgical procedures that offer metabolic modulation to diminish metabolic dysfunction and induce substantial weight loss through the BRAVE physiological steps–bile flow alteration, reduction of gastric size, anatomical gut rearrangement, and altered flow of nutrients, vagal manipulation, and enteric gut hormone modulation (10). The two most common bariatric procedures worldwide are the Roux-en-Y gastric bypass (RYGB) and the sleeve gastrectomy (11). In a RYGB, a small gastric pouch (15–30mL) is created and separated from the larger stomach remnant. The jejunum is then incised from the duodenum and anastomized to the small stomach pouch forming a distinctive "Y" shape that gives this procedure its name (12). In a sleeve gastrectomy, a longitudinal gastric sleeve is created running from the esophagus to the small intestine that is separated from the larger excised stomach (13). In comparison to non-surgical strategies, bariatric surgery is more effective at achieving sustained weight loss, improved quality of life and increased life expectancy (14, 15). Several studies have shown that bariatric surgery also leads to remission or resolution of type 2 diabetes and improved glycaemic control (16–19). These improvements are observed early post-operatively, before substantial weight loss and to a greater extent than in patients who achieve similar weight loss non-surgically, and are therefore, thought to offer weight-independent metabolic effects (20, 21) in addition to weight-dependent metabolic actions. Hypothesizes for this phenomenon include the foregut, hindgut, and midgut theories (22), but the precise mechanisms behind improvement of diabetes following bariatric surgery are still not fully understood. Bariatric surgery also leads to improvements in cancer risk, sleep apnoea, and other obesity-associated disorders (23, 24). Thus, bariatric surgery may target and improve renal function through direct mechanisms of weight loss as well as through diabetes dependent mechanisms.

MicroRNAs have attracted a great amount of recent attention as potential novel biomarkers of disease due to their stability in biofluids and their facile detection through PCR and profiling platforms (25, 26). Circulating microRNAs are reported biomarkers for cancer, obesity, and diabetes (25, 27, 28), and distinct bariatric microRNA profiles have been characterized in circulation (28, 29). Urinary microRNAs are reported biomarkers for immunoglobulin A nephropathy and bladder cancer (30, 31). Currently the non-invasive diagnosis of CKD relies on urinary microalbuminuria and estimated glomerular filtration rate (eGFR). However, the sensitivity and specificity of these markers are poor, particularly in obese patients, and only manifest late in the disease process.

We hypothesized that bariatric surgery modulates the urinary levels of microRNAs involved in the regulation of renal function. Therefore, we aimed to study urinary expression of renal microRNAs in bariatric patients before and after surgery in comparison to non-surgical control subjects.

MATERIALS AND METHODS

Study Design

Urine samples were collected for 10 healthy weight controls, seven morbidly obese controls and 24 bariatric surgical patients in Hull and East Yorkshire Hospitals and Imperial College Healthcare NHS Trusts under ethics approvals 09/H1304/46 and 08/H0711/123. Informed written consent was provided by all participants enrolled in this study and all appropriate guidelines were followed when conducting the methods. For the bariatric cohort, urine samples were obtained pre-operatively and at two periods post-operatively–between 2 and 6 months and between 1 and 2 years (**Table 1**). Nine out of the 24 bariatric patients had diabetes pre-operatively. Bariatric surgery was performed laparoscopically. Twenty bariatric patients had a RYGB and four had a sleeve gastrectomy. All bariatric patients fulfilled NICE qualifying criteria for bariatric surgery (32). All subjects had normal serum urea, creatinine, and eGFRs at baseline.

Urinary RNA Extraction

RNA was extracted from 250 μl of urine using the *mir*Vana PARIS kit (Ambion, Paisley, UK) according to the manufacturer's instructions with the one modification; to normalize and for carrier purposes, 30 femtomoles of synthetic *C. elegans* miR-39 (Ambion) was spiked into the urine samples prior to the acid-phenol:chloroform phase. Cel. miR-39 was chosen as carrier as it lacks sequence homology with human miRNAs. RNA was eluted in 100 μl nuclease free water.

TABLE 1 | Study summary.

	Controls		Bariatric cohort		
	Healthy	**Morbidly obese**	**RYGB + Sleeve**	**RYGB**	**Sleeve**
n	10	7	24	20	4
Age[†]	39.1 (16.3)	54 (11.7)	45.7 (10.8)	45 (10.4)	49.1 (13.7)
Female (*n*)	8	3	16	14	2
Diabetes (*n*)	0	1	9	8	1

[†] *Values represent mean. Standard deviation in parenthesis.*

Cell Culture

The human kidney proximal tubule cell (PTC) line HK-2 was obtained from ATCC (LGC Standards, Teddington, UK) and maintained in DMEM/Ham's F12, supplemented with 10% v/v fetal bovine serum (FBS), 1% Penicillin/Streptomycin antibiotics (100 U/ml, 100 μg/ml, respectively), and 1% Insulin-Transferrin-Sodium Selenite (Sigma-Aldrich, Gillingham, UK) as previously described (6).

Transfections

Endogenous microRNA levels were manipulated in HK-2 cells through the transfection of microRNA miR 192 mimic, a gain-of-function experiment designed to determine the biological activity of miR 192. mIRIDIAN microRNA mimics and mimic controls were purchased from Dharmacon (Lafayette, CO, USA). The siPORT NeoFX transfection agent was used according to the manufacturer's instructions. HK-2 cells at approximately 80% confluence were trypsinized and seeded at 50,000 cells per well in complete media in 24 well cell culture plates and transfected with miR-192 mimic at 10, 20, and 50 nM concentrations for 48 h. Following SiPORT transfection RNA was extracted from HK-2 cells using the *mir*VANA PARIS kit according to manufacturer's instructions and eluted in 75 μl nuclease free water.

Quantitative PCR

MicroRNA was reverse transcribed into cDNA using the TaqMan MicroRNA Reverse Transcription kit (Applied Biosystems, Paisley, UK) and messenger RNA (mRNA) was reverse transcribed using the High Capacity Reverse Transcription kit (Applied Biosystems) according to manufacturer's instructions. Relative microRNAs and mRNA levels were determined by real time, quantitative PCR using TaqMan Fast Universal Master Mix (Applied Biosystems). Quantitative PCR was performed in triplicate on the Applied Biosystems 7,500 Fast System. All PCR and RT probes were obtained from Applied Biosystems. Urinary microRNA expression was first normalized to creatinine to correct for diuretic effect (Creatinine Assay, R & D Systems, Abingdon, UK) and then normalized to cel. miR-39. Cellular microRNA expression following HK-2 transfections was normalized to U6 small nuclear RNA and mRNA expression was normalized to GAPDH, a frequently used housekeeping gene. Relative expression was calculated using the $2^{-\Delta Ct}$ method (33).

Statistical Analysis

Urinary microRNA data is expressed as fold change relative to pre-operative levels or morbidly obese control levels. Data is represented as mean ± standard error of mean (SEM). Statistical significance was determined using ANOVA (with a post-test for linear trend) and paired/unpaired Student's *t*-test where appropriate. Significance was considered as $p < 0.05$. Statistical analysis was performed using GraphPad Prism 6.0 (Graphpad, La Jolla, CA, USA).

RESULTS

Bariatric Clinical Outcomes

Bariatric surgery induced substantial clinical improvements in all bariatric patients (**Figure 1**). Reduction in BMI was significant within 100 days of surgery and mean BMI decreased by almost 30% at 100 days or more after surgery. Mean levels of fasting blood glucose also decreased following bariatric surgery, decreasing from 7.5 mmol/L pre-operatively to 5.6 mmol/L 100 days or more following surgery, although this decrease was not statistically significant. eGFR following bariatric surgery was unchanged (mean 74–79 mL/min).

Bariatric Surgery Increases Urinary miR 192 Levels

We initially assessed the urinary expression of miR 192, a consistently abundant renal microRNA (34). In patients who had laparoscopic RYGB, levels of miR 192 significantly increased 1.3 and 2.9-fold (relative to pre-operative levels) at 2–6 months and 1–2 years, respectively, following surgery (**Figure 2A**). A similar increase was observed in sleeve gastrectomy patients. MiR 192 levels increased 1.3-fold at 2–6 months following sleeve procedures and 4.7-fold (significant relative to pre-operative levels) at 1–2 years post-operatively (**Figure 2B**). Increase in urinary miR 192 levels was consistent when patients were stratified by pre-operative diabetes status. In patients with diabetes urinary levels of miR 192 increased 1.5-fold at 2–6 months and significantly 3.6-fold at 1–2 years following bariatric surgery (**Figure 2C**). Patients without diabetes demonstrated a significant 2.8-fold increase in miR 192 levels at 1–2 years following surgery (**Figure 2D**).

When expressed as fold change relative to the morbidly obese control group, bariatric pre-operative miR 192 levels were lower (0.6-fold), potentially reflecting the higher BMI in patients undergoing bariatric surgery (**Figure 3A**). Bariatric miR 192 expression was slightly higher 2–6 months following surgery (0.8-fold relative to morbidly obese controls). However, 1–2 years following bariatric surgery, mean miR 192 level was nearly 2-fold higher relative to the morbidly obese cohort and was comparable to miR 192 levels in those with a healthy weight (BMI under 25, **Figure 3A**). Although comparative two-way fold changes were not significant, the linear trend with time was ($p = 0.0117$, one-way ANOVA). An inverse correlation between miR 192-fold change and change in BMI post-operatively was also significant ($p = 0.0342$, Pearson's correlation, **Figure 3B**). The data show that bariatric surgery shifts urinary miR 192 expressions from

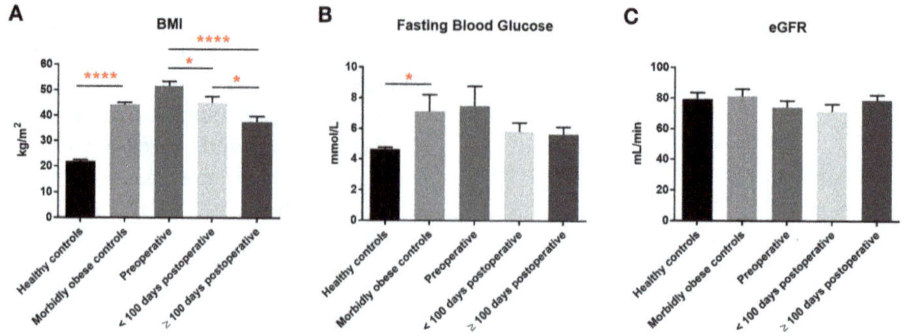

FIGURE 1 | Clinical measurements. Pre-operative, post-operative, and control levels of **(A)** BMI, **(B)** fasting blood glucose levels and **(C)** eGFR. Data represent mean ± SEM. $^{*}p < 0.05$, $^{****}p < 0.0001$ by Student's *t*-test.

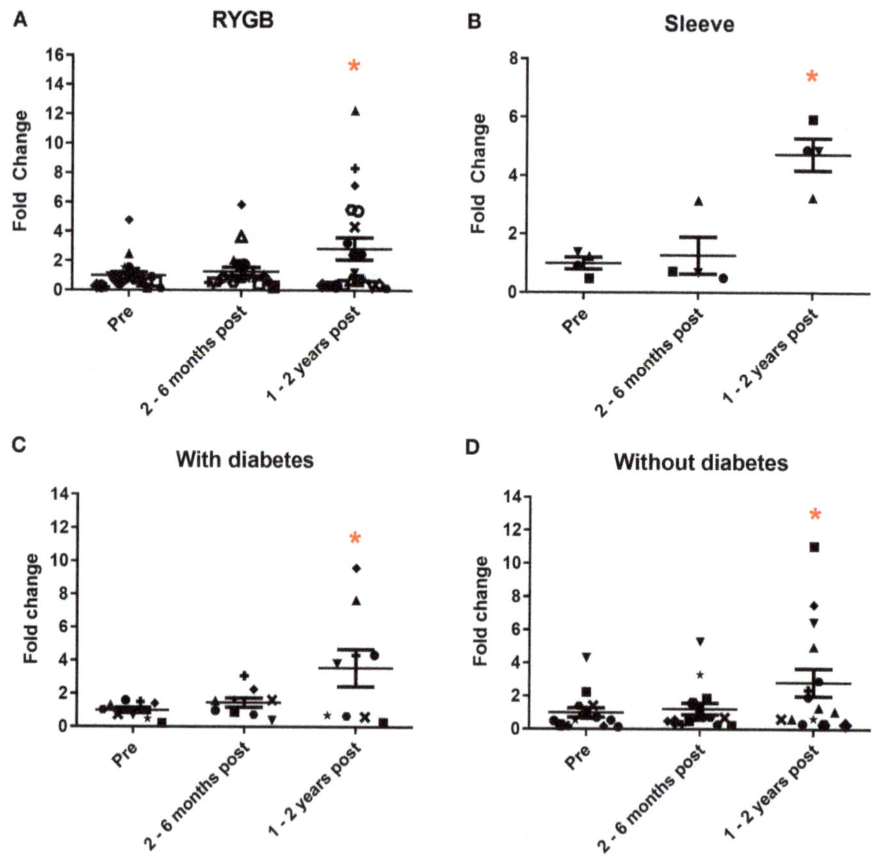

FIGURE 2 | Urinary miR 192 expression following bariatric surgery. **(A)** RYGB patients. **(B)** Sleeve gastrectomy patients. **(C)** Patients with diabetes. **(D)** Patients without diabetes. Data represents mean fold change ± SEM relative to mean preoperative expression. $n = 20$ for RYGB, $n = 4$ for sleeve, $n = 9$ for diabetes, and $n = 15$ for individuals without diabetes. Each patient is represented by a unique symbol. $^{*}p < 0.05$ vs. preoperative expression by paired *t*-test.

levels observed in a morbidly obese population to levels observed in a healthy weight population.

Of the 24 individuals who made up the bariatric cohort, 20 had increased urinary miR 192 expression post-operatively relative to their pre-operative levels, including 16 out of the 20 RYGB patients, eight out of nine patients with diabetes and all four sleeve gastrectomy patients. A timecourse of post-operative miR 192 expressions in RYGB and sleeve patients relative to their individual pre-operative miR 192 levels can be found in **Figure 3C**. A significant correlation was found between individual, personalized fold changed in miR 192 levels and days following surgery ($p = 0.0051$, Pearson's correlation). This illustrated a trend of a gradual, general increase in miR 192 levels in urine which is enhanced and sustained with

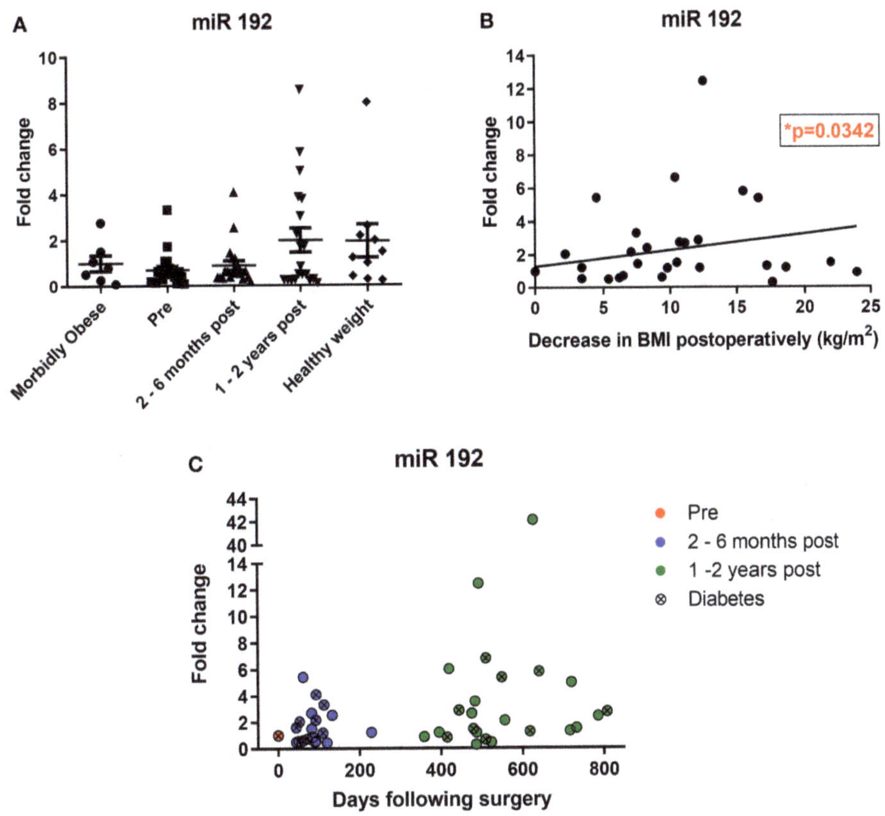

FIGURE 3 | Bariatric urinary miR 192 expression relative to a morbidly obese cohort. **(A)** Bariatric and healthy weight miR 192 expression relative to a morbidly obese control group. Data represents mean ± SEM relative to mean preoperative expression. Morbidly obese is a BMI $\geq$ 40 kg/m^2, healthy weight is a BMI < 25 kg/m^2. $n = 7$ for morbidly obese, n=10 healthy weight, $n = 24$ for preoperatively, 2–6 months and 1–2 years post-operatively. **(B)** Pearson correlation of miR 192-fold change against change in post-operative BMI. $n = 46$. **(C)** Timecourse of miR 192 expression following surgery. Data represented as fold change relative to individual preoperative expression for 24 bariatric patients.

time and consistent with migration toward the healthy weight control phenotype.

Bariatric Surgery Increases Urinary Levels of miR 200a and miR 200b

Urinary levels of miR 200a and miR 200b were also measured. Both are expressed in the kidney and change in their expression is associated with diabetic nephropathy (5, 6). MiR 200a urine levels increased 2.5-fold at 2–6 months and 3.4-fold at 1–2 years following surgery (**Figure 4A**), although neither increase achieved statistical significance. MiR 200b levels increased 5.8-fold at 2–6 months and strikingly 28.6-fold (significantly different from the pre-surgery levels) at 1–2 years post-operatively (**Figure 4B**). All but one patient demonstrated a post-operative increase of urinary miR 200a and all patients demonstrated an increase in urinary miR 200b relative to their individual pre-operative level. Significant correlations were observed between both miR 200a and miR 200b and days following bariatric surgery (**Figures 4C,D**, $p = 0.0071$ and 0.044, respectively, Pearson's correlation). There were also significant correlations between urinary levels of miR 192 and both miR 200a and miR 200b (**Supplementary Figure 1**, $p = 0.0364$ and $p < 0.0001$, respectively, Pearson's correlation).

Mechanistic Studies in the Human PTC Line, HK-2

To explore the mechanistic implications of altered microRNA expression following bariatric surgery, we used the human PTC HK-2 renal cell line to examine changes in phenotype. Transfection with all three concentrations of miR 192 mimic increased miR 192 expression 4,000, 16,000, and 18,000-fold, respectively, relative to cells transfected with a scrambled control (**Figure 5A**). Transfection of miR 192 increased levels of miR 200 at all concentrations, although the increase was only significant at 10 nM (**Figure 5B**). Expression levels of ZEB1 and Colα1 were unaltered for all three miR 192 mimic concentrations (**Figures 5C,E**). However, transfection with 50 nM miR 192 mimic concentration resulted in a significant 0.6-fold decrease in ZEB2 (**Figure 5D**).

DISCUSSION

There is a growing body of evidence that biofluid miRNA expression can be indicative of disease progression and prognosis (35–37). Urinary expression of microRNAs has also been proposed as useful in the diagnosis and prognosis of

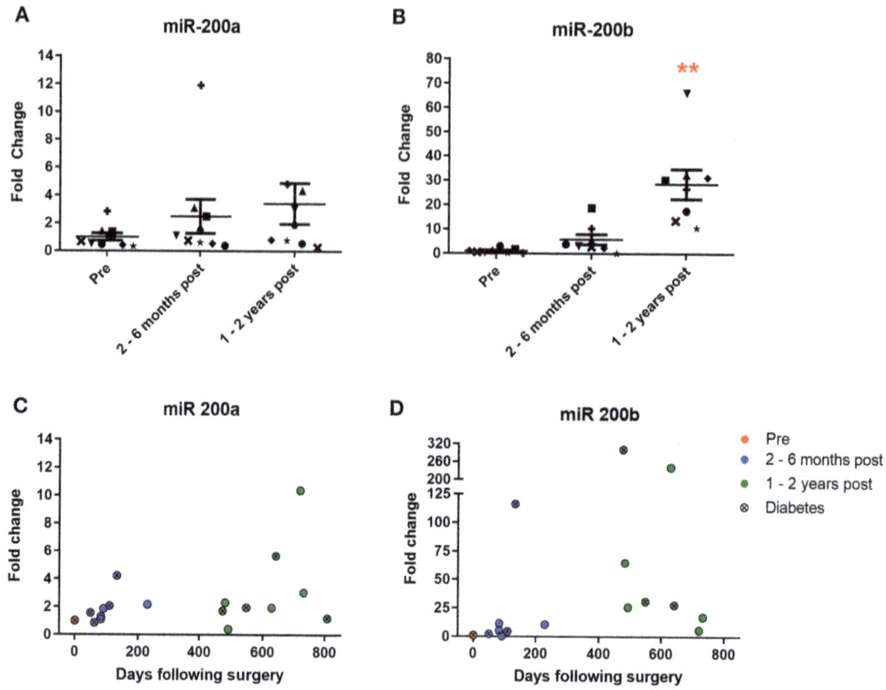

FIGURE 4 | Urinary expression of miR 200 following bariatric surgery. **(A)** miR-200a, $n = 9$ **(B)** miR-200b, $n = 8$. Data represents mean fold change ± SEM relative to mean preoperative expression. $^{**}p < 0.01$ vs. preoperative expression by paired *t*-test. Each patient is represented by a unique symbol. Timecourse of **(C)** miR 200a and **(D)** miR 200b expression following surgery. Data represented as fold change relative to individual preoperative expression.

renal disease (38). We therefore considered whether bariatric surgery modulates urinary levels of miRNAs that regulate kidney function.

Three kidney-expressed microRNAs, miR 192, miR 200a, and miR 200b, were shown to be upregulated in urine following bariatric surgery, an increase that was consistent across surgical type and diabetes status and was sustained and enhanced with time. Bariatric surgery shifts urinary miR 192 expression from levels seen in morbidly obese patients to levels comparable with those seen in a healthy cohort. In mechanistic studies, the transfection of miR 192 in a human kidney PTC cell line increased miR 200a and decreased ZEB2, a key transcriptional promoter of kidney fibrosis. These three microRNAs assessed in urine could potentially represent non-invasive, anti-fibrotic biomarkers for surgery-induced improvement in renal function.

The kidney-specific deletion of Dicer, a ribonuclease involved in microRNA biogenesis, leads to proteinuria, glomerular disease, and tubular injury in mice (39–41). This illustrates the important functional roles of microRNAs in kidney pathophysiology. MiR 192 is one of 5 microRNAs whose expression is higher in the kidney relative to other organs (34), and its levels are reduced in human renal biopsies from patients with advanced diabetic nephropathy, levels that correlate with tubulointerstitial fibrosis, and decreased GFR, reflecting miR 192's key anti-fibrotic role (6). *In vitro* incubation of PTCs with TGF-β1 decreases miR 192 expression and the overexpression of miR 192 suppresses ZEB1 and ZEB2, decreasing TGF-β1 mediated E-cadherin suppression (6). In diabetic apoE mice, miR 192 expression was downregulated in the kidney and treatment of PTCs with TGF-β1 results in a reduction of miR 192 (42). Renal levels of the miR 200 family are decreased in mouse models of renal scarring and by TGF-β1 in rat PTCs (43). Injection of miR 200b precursor antagonizes ZEB1/ZEB2 induction, decreases collagen synthesis, and ameliorates fibrosis (44). p53 tumor suppressor increases expression of miR 192 and miR 200, suppressing EMT (45). It has also been reported that miR 200 expression is a strong biomarker for epithelial vs. mesenchymal phenotype in cancer (46). MiR 200 overexpression results in mesenchymal to epithelial transition in mouse carcinomas and overexpressing miR 200 *in vitro* increases E-cadherin and represses EMT (4, 5). Here, miR 192 transfection of human PTCs led to an increase in miR 200a, indicating that miR 192 could act upstream to miR 200 in a hierarchical regulation pathway, suggesting miR 192 may be a master microRNA regulator in the kidney (**Figure 6**). Previously miR 192 has been shown to upregulate miR 200b/c expression in mesangial cells (47).

In contrast to their roles in PTCs, miR 192, and miR 200 appear to have pro-fibrotic effect in mesangial cells. TGF-β1 increases miR 192 in mouse mesangial cells and repression of ZEB1/ZEB2 expression by miR 192 leads to collagen synthesis (48). The inhibition of miR 192 in streptozotin-induced diabetic mice reduces proteinuria (49). In mesangial cells, miR 200 family represses ZEB1/ZEB2, promoting fibrosis (47). The pleiotropic, cell-specific roles miR 192 and miR 200 play in renal fibrosis reflect the complex physiology of the kidney. Indeed, the renal cortex and the medulla have different microRNA expression

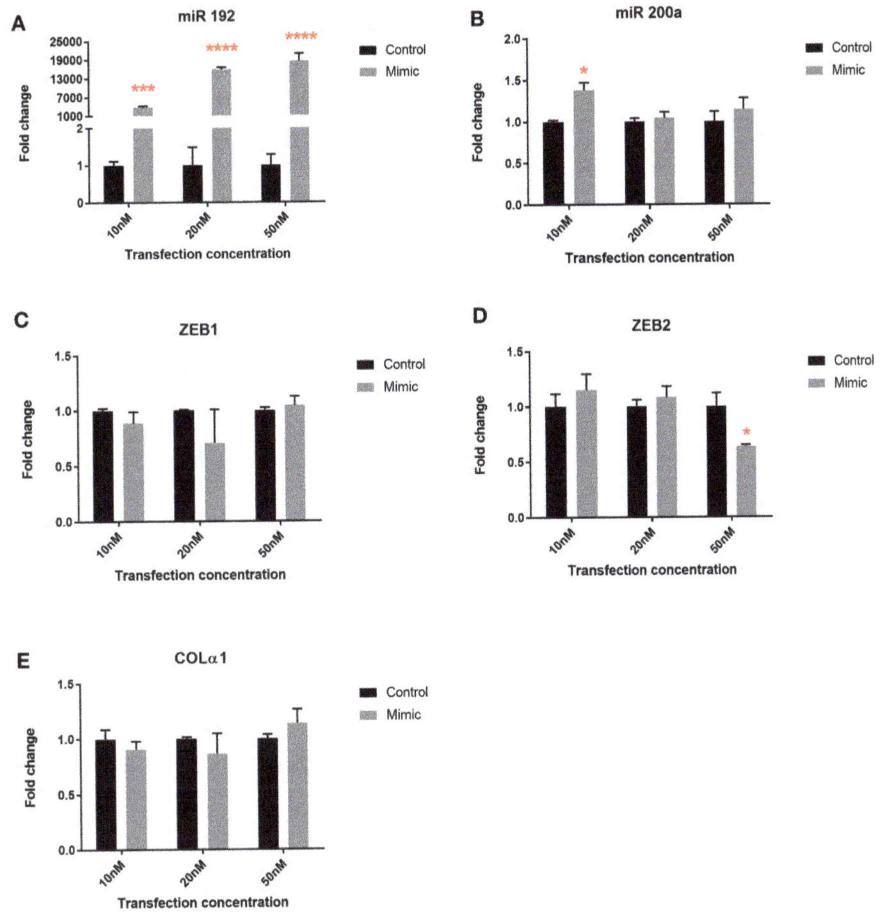

FIGURE 5 | miR 192 mimic transfection of HK2 cells illustrates its anti-fibrotic role. Expression of **(A)** miR 192 **(B)** miR 200a **(C)** ZEB1 **(D)** ZEB2 and **(E)** Colα1 following 48 h of 10, 20, and 50 nM miR 192 mimic transfection. Data represents mean ± SEM relative to transfection with a scrambled control. $^{*}p < 0.05$, $^{***}p < 0.001$, $^{****}p < 0.0001$, $n = 3$.

profiles (50). It is worth noting that proximal tubular cells are further along the urinary tract than mesangial cells of the glomerulas and that urinary levels of miR 192 and miR 200 are decreased in patients with bladder cancer, correlating with increased EMT (31).

In this study patients had normal renal function and therefore a change in renal function following surgery was not expected. However, other studies have reported improvements in renal function following bariatric procedures. Weight loss is associated with a reduction in proteinuria, including weight loss achieved surgically (7–9). Bariatric surgery improves renal function in patients with pre-existing glomerular hyperfiltration (9). Surgery also leads to reduced levels of albuminuria 1 year post-operatively, and levels continue to decrease up to 2 years and were maintained up to 5 years post-surgery (51, 52). Remission of microalbuminuria in individuals with diabetes can reach 60% 5 years following surgery. Surgery also has preventive effects, reducing the incidence of microalbuminuria by 80% and diabetic nephropathy by 60% compared to patients treated medically (52). Bariatric surgery can also lead to improvement and remission in patients with established CKD (53). The results presented here suggest miR 192 may mediate these renal improvements following bariatric surgery.

The early detection of DN is important in preventing progression to renal failure and there are considerable limitations of conventional markers of kidney function. Novel markers of DN have been reported, including proteins, peptides, and growth factors (54). Several studies have reported distinct microRNA profiles in urine, urinary sediments, and circulation in cases of kidney diseases. Urinary miR 29b, miR 29c, and miR 93 levels are correlated with proteinuria and renal scarring in patients with IgA nephropathy (55). Urinary microRNA profiles can also be used to differentiate various stages of diabetic nephropathy in individuals with type 1 diabetes (35). MicroRNA 145 is upregulated in the urinary exosomes of type 1 diabetes patients with microalbuminuria (56) and urinary microRNA levels, including levels of miR 192, can predict the development of microalbuminuria (57). In circulation, increased levels of miR 25, miR 27, miR 152, and miR 182 has been reported in patients with type 1 diabetes (58),

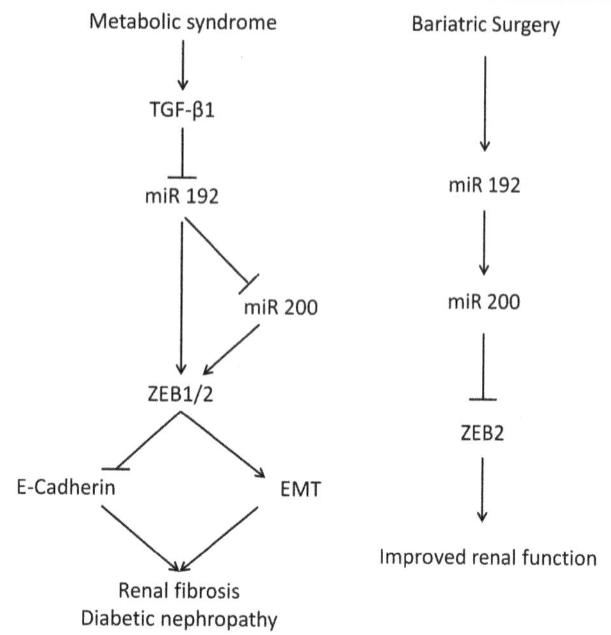

FIGURE 6 | The renal function of miR 192 and miR 200. **(Left)** Mechanism for glucose-mediated renal fibrosis in the proximal tubular cells. Diabetes increases TGF-β which inhibits miR 192/200, lifting the suppression on ZEB and EMT. **(Right)** Suggested mechanism following bariatric surgery.

and a recent report identified 10 elevated and two lowered microRNAs in patients with diabetes with DN relative to healthy controls (59). Circulating microRNAs can select diabetes patients with DN from those with good renal function, suggesting prognostic potential (59). This has led to interest in microRNAs as potential novel drug targets. The successful manipulation of miR 192 expression in the renal cortex of normal and diabetic mice (60) suggests the same may be possible in humans.

Other microRNAs have been reported to be involved in DN, including miR 21, miR 25, and miR 29 (61–63). The expression of more microRNAs needs to be assessed in bariatric urine samples and validated *in vitro*. However, there are limitations to using *in vitro* models of renal function, as EMT is more commonly observed in immortalized cell lines than *in vivo* renal fibrosis (64). The role of microRNAs in mediating the post-bariatric improvements in renal health needs to be confirmed in larger, prospective, multi-centre studies of bariatric patients including cohorts with varying degrees of kidney dysfunction.

In summary, bariatric surgery increased the urinary expression of the anti-fibrotic microRNAs miR 192 and miR 200 to levels found in the healthy controls. Several recent studies have assessed the suitability of urinary microRNAs as biomarkers, given the clinical ease of collecting and analyzing samples and the limitation of conventional markers of renal function. This study highlights the potential of urinary microRNAs as non-invasive biomarkers of health following bariatric surgery.

ETHICS STATEMENT

This study was carried out in accordance with the recommendations of East Yorkshire and North Lincolnshire Research Ethics Committee and the Charing Cross Research Ethics Committee under ethics approval 09/H1304/46 and 08/H0711/123, with written informed consent from all subjects. All subjects gave written informed consent in accordance with the Declaration of Helsinki. The protocol was approved by the East Yorkshire and North Lincolnshire Research Ethics Committee and the Charing Cross Research Ethics Committee.

AUTHOR CONTRIBUTIONS

AA, HA, TS, SA, and NG contributed to the conceptual design of this study. AA conducted the experiments and data analysis. AA, HA, and NG interpreted the data and wrote the article. AA, HA, TS, AD, EH, TA, SA, and NG critical evaluated and approved the final article.

ACKNOWLEDGMENTS

An abstract based on this work was presented at the 21st Pan Arab Conference on Diabetes in Cairo, Egypt and published in the conference proceedings (65).

REFERENCES

1. Maric-Bilkan C. Obesity and diabetic kidney disease. *Med Clin North Am.* (2013) 97:59–74. doi: 10.1016/j.mcna.2012.10.010
2. Molitch ME, DeFronzo RA, Franz MJ, Keane WF, Mogensen CE, Parving HH, et al. Nephropathy in diabetes. *Diabetes Care.* (2004) 27(Suppl 1):S79–83. doi: 10.2337/diacare.27.2007.S79
3. Bowen T, Jenkins RH, Fraser DJ. MicroRNAs, transforming growth factor beta-1, and tissue fibrosis. *J Pathol.* (2013) 229:274–85. doi: 10.1002/path.4119
4. Gregory PA, Bert AG, Paterson EL, Barry SC, Tsykin A, Farshid G, et al. The miR-200 family and miR-205 regulate epithelial to mesenchymal transition by targeting ZEB1 and SIP1. *Nat Cell Biol.* (2008) 10:593–601. doi: 10.1038/ncb1722

5. Korpal M, Lee ES, Hu G, Kang Y. The miR-200 family inhibits epithelial-mesenchymal transition and cancer cell migration by direct targeting of E-cadherin transcriptional repressors ZEB1 and ZEB2. *J Biol Chem.* (2008) 283:14910–4. doi: 10.1074/jbc.C800074200
6. Krupa A, Jenkins R, Luo DD, Lewis A, Phillips A, Fraser D. Loss of MicroRNA-192 promotes fibrogenesis in diabetic nephropathy. *J Am Soc Nephrol.* (2010) 21:438–47. doi: 10.1681/ASN.2009050530
7. Chagnac A, Weinstein T, Herman M, Hirsh J, Gafter U, Ori Y. The effects of weight loss on renal function in patients with severe obesity. *J Am Soc Nephrol.* (2003) 14:1480–6. doi: 10.1097/01.ASN.0000068462.38661.89
8. Morales E, Valero MA, Leon M, Hernandez E, Praga M. Beneficial effects of weight loss in overweight patients with chronic proteinuric nephropathies. *Am J Kidney Dis.* (2003) 41:319–27. doi: 10.1053/ajkd.2003.50039
9. Agnani S, Vachharajani VT, Gupta R, Atray NK, Vachharajani TJ. Does treating obesity stabilize chronic kidney disease? *BMC Nephrol.* (2005) 6:7. doi: 10.1186/1471-2369-6-7
10. Ashrafian H, Bueter M, Ahmed K, Suliman A, Bloom SR, Darzi A, et al. Metabolic surgery: an evolution through bariatric animal models. *Obes Rev.* (2010) 11:907–20. doi: 10.1111/j.1467-789X.2009.00701.x
11. Angrisani L, Santonicola A, Iovino P, Vitiello A, Zundel N, Buchwald H, et al. Bariatric surgery and endoluminal procedures: IFSO worldwide survey 2014. *Obes Surg.* (2017) 27:2279–89. doi: 10.1007/s11695-017-2666-x
12. Wittgrove AC, Clark GW, Tremblay LJ. Laparoscopic gastric bypass, Roux-en-Y: preliminary report of five cases. *Obes Surg.* (1994) 4:353–7. doi: 10.1381/096089294765558331
13. Marceau P, Biron S, Bourque RA, Potvin M, Hould FS, Simard S. Biliopancreatic diversion with a new type of gastrectomy. *Obes Surg.* (1993) 3:29–35. doi: 10.1381/096089293765559728
14. Salem L, Jensen CC, Flum DR. Are bariatric surgical outcomes worth their cost? A systematic review. *J Am Coll Surg.* (2005) 200:270–8. doi: 10.1016/j.jamcollsurg.2004.09.045
15. Sjostrom L, Narbro K, Sjostrom CD, Karason K, Larsson B, Wedel H, et al. Effects of bariatric surgery on mortality in Swedish obese subjects. *N Engl J Med.* (2007) 357:741–52. doi: 10.1056/NEJMoa066254
16. Pories WJ, Swanson MS, MacDonald KG, Long SB, Morris PG, Brown BM, et al. Who would have thought it? An operation proves to be the most effective therapy for adult-onset diabetes mellitus. *Ann Surg.* (1995) 222:339–50, discussion 350–332.
17. Buchwald H, Estok R, Fahrbach K, Banel D, Jensen MD, Pories WJ, et al. Weight and type 2 diabetes after bariatric surgery: systematic review and meta-analysis. *Am J Med.* (2009) 122:248–56 e245. doi: 10.1016/j.amjmed.2008.09.041
18. Mingrone G, Panunzi S, De Gaetano A, Guidone C, Iaconelli A, Leccesi L, et al. Bariatric surgery versus conventional medical therapy for type 2 diabetes. *N Engl J Med.* (2012) 366:1577–85. doi: 10.1056/NEJMoa1200111
19. Schauer PR, Kashyap SR, Wolski K, Brethauer SA, Kirwan JP, Pothier CE, et al. Bariatric surgery versus intensive medical therapy in obese patients with diabetes. *N Engl J Med.* (2012) 366:1567–76. doi: 10.1056/NEJMoa1200225
20. Laferrere B, Teixeira J, McGinty J, Tran H, Egger JR, Colarusso A, et al. Effect of weight loss by gastric bypass surgery versus hypocaloric diet on glucose and incretin levels in patients with type 2 diabetes. *J Clin Endocrinol Metab.* (2008) 93:2479–85. doi: 10.1210/jc.2007-2851
21. Fenske WK, Pournaras DJ, Aasheim ET, Miras AD, Scopinaro N, Scholtz S, et al. Can a protocol for glycaemic control improve type 2 diabetes outcomes after gastric bypass? *Obes Surg.* (2012) 22:90–6. doi: 10.1007/s11695-011-0543-6
22. Ashrafian H, Athanasiou T, Li JV, Bueter M, Ahmed K, Nagpal K, et al. Diabetes resolution and hyperinsulinaemia after metabolic Roux-en-Y gastric bypass. *Obes Rev.* (2011) 12:e257–272. doi: 10.1111/j.1467-789X.2010.00802.x
23. Ashrafian H, Ahmed K, Rowland SP, Patel VM, Gooderham NJ, Holmes E, et al. Metabolic surgery and cancer: protective effects of bariatric procedures. *Cancer.* (2010). doi: 10.1002/cncr.25738
24. Ashrafian H, le Roux CW, Rowland SP, Ali M, Cummin AR, Darzi A, et al. Metabolic surgery and obstructive sleep apnoea: the protective effects of bariatric procedures. *Thorax.* (2011) 67:442–9. doi: 10.1136/thx.2010.151225
25. Mitchell PS, Parkin RK, Kroh EM, Fritz BR, Wyman SK, Pogosova-Agadjanyan EL, et al. Circulating microRNAs as stable blood-based markers for cancer detection. *Proc Natl Acad Sci USA.* (2008) 105:10513–8. doi: 10.1073/pnas.0804549105
26. Sharkey JW, Antoine DJ, Park BK. Validation of the isolation and quantification of kidney enriched miRNAs for use as biomarkers. *Biomarkers.* (2012) 17:231–9. doi: 10.3109/1354750X.2012.657246
27. Guay C, Roggli E, Nesca V, Jacovetti C, Regazzi R. Diabetes mellitus, a microRNA-related disease? *Transl Res.* (2011) 157:253–64. doi: 10.1016/j.trsl.2011.01.009
28. Ortega FJ, Mercader JM, Catalan V, Moreno-Navarrete JM, Pueyo N, Sabater M, et al. Targeting the circulating microRNA signature of obesity. *Clin Chem.* (2013) 59:781–92. doi: 10.1373/clinchem.2012.195776
29. Alkandari A, Ashrafian H, Sathyapalan T, Sedman P, Darzi A, Holmes E, et al. Improved physiology and metabolic flux after Roux-en-Y gastric bypass is associated with temporal changes in the circulating microRNAome: a longitudinal study in humans. *BMC Obes.* (2018) 5:20. doi: 10.1186/s40608-018-0199-z
30. Wang G, Kwan BC, Lai FM, Chow KM, Kam-Tao Li P, Szeto CC. Expression of microRNAs in the urinary sediment of patients with IgA nephropathy. *Dis Markers.* (2010) 28:79–86. doi: 10.3233/DMA-2010-0687
31. Wang G, Chan ES, Kwan BC, Li PK, Yip SK, Szeto CC, et al. Expression of microRNAs in the urine of patients with bladder cancer. *Clin Genitourin Cancer.* (2012) 10:106–13. doi: 10.1016/j.clgc.2012.01.001
32. NICE. *Obesity: NICE Clinical Guideline 43.* London: National Institute for Health and Care Excellence (NICE) (2006). Available online at: http://www.nice.org.uk/CG43
33. Livak KJ, Schmittgen TD. Analysis of relative gene expression data using real-time quantitative PCR and the 2(-Delta Delta C(T)) Method. *Methods.* (2001) 25:402–8. doi: 10.1006/meth.2001.1262
34. Sun Y, Koo S, White N, Peralta E, Esau C, Dean NM, et al. Development of a micro-array to detect human and mouse microRNAs and characterization of expression in human organs. *Nucleic Acids Res.* (2004) 32:e188. doi: 10.1093/nar/gnh186
35. Argyropoulos C, Wang K, McClarty S, Huang D, Bernardo J, Ellis D, et al. Urinary microRNA profiling in the nephropathy of type 1 diabetes. *PLoS ONE.* (2013) 8:e54662. doi: 10.1371/journal.pone.0054662
36. Sathyapalan T, David R, Gooderham NJ, Atkin SL. Increased expression of circulating miRNA-93 in women with polycystic ovary syndrome may represent a novel, non-invasive biomarker for diagnosis. *Sci Rep.* (2015) 5:16890. doi: 10.1038/srep16890
37. Harling L, Lambert J, Ashrafian H, Darzi A, Gooderham NJ, Athanasiou T. Elevated serum microRNA 483-5p levels may predict patients at risk of post-operative atrial fibrillation. *Eur J Cardiothorac Surg.* (2017) 51:73–8. doi: 10.1093/ejcts/ezw245
38. Simpson K, Wonnacott A, Fraser DJ, Bowen T. MicroRNAs in diabetic nephropathy: from biomarkers to therapy. *Curr Diab Rep.* (2016) 16:35. doi: 10.1007/s11892-016-0724-8
39. Harvey SJ, Jarad G, Cunningham J, Goldberg S, Schermer B, Harfe BD, et al. Podocyte-specific deletion of dicer alters cytoskeletal dynamics and causes glomerular disease. *J Am Soc Nephrol.* (2008) 19:2150–8. doi: 10.1681/ASN.2008020233
40. Ho J, Ng KH, Rosen S, Dostal A, Gregory RI, Kreidberg JA. Podocyte-specific loss of functional microRNAs leads to rapid glomerular and tubular injury. *J Am Soc Nephrol.* (2008) 19:2069–75. doi: 10.1681/ASN.2008020162
41. Shi S, Yu L, Chiu C, Sun Y, Chen J, Khitrov G, et al. Podocyte-selective deletion of dicer induces proteinuria and glomerulosclerosis. *J Am Soc Nephrol.* (2008) 19:2159–69. doi: 10.1681/ASN.2008030312
42. Wang B, Herman-Edelstein M, Koh P, Burns W, Jandeleit-Dahm K, Watson A, et al. E-cadherin expression is regulated by miR-192/215 by a mechanism that is independent of the profibrotic effects of transforming growth factor-beta. *Diabetes.* (2010) 59:1794–802. doi: 10.2337/db09-1736
43. Wang B, Koh P, Winbanks C, Coughlan MT, McClelland A, Watson A, et al. miR-200a Prevents renal fibrogenesis through repression of TGF-beta2 expression. *Diabetes.* (2011) 60:280–7. doi: 10.2337/db10-0892
44. Oba S, Kumano S, Suzuki E, Nishimatsu H, Takahashi M, Takamori H, et al. miR-200b precursor can ameliorate renal tubulointerstitial fibrosis. *PLoS ONE.* (2010) 5:e13614. doi: 10.1371/journal.pone.0013614

45. Kim T, Veronese A, Pichiorri F, Lee TJ, Jeon YJ, Volinia S, et al. p53 regulates epithelial-mesenchymal transition through microRNAs targeting ZEB1 and ZEB2. *J Exp Med.* (2011) 208:875–83. doi: 10.1084/jem.20110235
46. Park SM, Gaur AB, Lengyel E, Peter ME. The miR-200 family determines the epithelial phenotype of cancer cells by targeting the E-cadherin repressors ZEB1 and ZEB2. *Genes Dev.* (2008) 22:894–907. doi: 10.1101/gad.1640608
47. Kato M, Arce L, Wang M, Putta S, Lanting L, Natarajan R. A microRNA circuit mediates transforming growth factor-beta1 autoregulation in renal glomerular mesangial cells. *Kidney Int.* (2011) 80:358–68. doi: 10.1038/ki.2011.43
48. Kato M, Zhang J, Wang M, Lanting L, Yuan H, Rossi JJ, et al. MicroRNA-192 in diabetic kidney glomeruli and its function in TGF-beta-induced collagen expression via inhibition of E-box repressors. *Proc Natl Acad Sci USA.* (2007) 104:3432–7. doi: 10.1073/pnas.0611192104
49. Putta S, Lanting L, Sun G, Lawson G, Kato M, Natarajan R. Inhibiting microRNA-192 ameliorates renal fibrosis in diabetic nephropathy. *J Am Soc Nephrol.* (2012) 23:458–69. doi: 10.1681/ASN.2011050485
50. Tian Z, Greene AS, Pietrusz JL, Matus IR, Liang M. MicroRNA-target pairs in the rat kidney identified by microRNA microarray, proteomic, and bioinformatic analysis. *Genome Res.* (2008) 18:404–11. doi: 10.1101/gr.6587008
51. Navarro-Diaz M, Serra A, Romero R, Bonet J, Bayes B, Homs M, et al. Effect of drastic weight loss after bariatric surgery on renal parameters in extremely obese patients: long-term follow-up. *J Am Soc Nephrol.* (2006) 17(12 Suppl 3):S213–7. doi: 10.1681/ASN.2006080917
52. Heneghan HM, Cetin D, Navaneethan SD, Orzech N, Brethauer SA, Schauer PR. Effects of bariatric surgery on diabetic nephropathy after 5 years of follow-up. *Surg Obes Relat Dis.* (2013) 9:7–14. doi: 10.1016/j.soard.2012.08.016
53. Alexander JW, Goodman HR, Hawver LR, Cardi MA. Improvement and stabilization of chronic kidney disease after gastric bypass. *Surg Obes Relat Dis.* (2009) 5:237–41. doi: 10.1016/j.soard.2008.08.016
54. Fassett RG, Venuthurupalli SK, Gobe GC, Coombes JS, Cooper MA, Hoy WE. Biomarkers in chronic kidney disease: a review. *Kidney Int.* (2011) 80:806–21. doi: 10.1038/ki.2011.198
55. Wang G, Kwan BC, Lai FM, Chow KM, Li PK, Szeto CC. Urinary miR-21, miR-29, and miR-93: novel biomarkers of fibrosis. *Am J Nephrol.* (2012) 36:412–8. doi: 10.1159/000343452
56. Barutta F, Tricarico M, Corbelli A, Annaratone L, Pinach S, Grimaldi S, et al. Urinary exosomal microRNAs in incipient diabetic nephropathy. *PLoS ONE.* (2013) 8:e73798. doi: 10.1371/journal.pone.0073798
57. Argyropoulos C, Wang K, Bernardo J, Ellis D, Orchard T, Galas D, et al. Urinary microRNA profiling predicts the development of microalbuminuria in patients with type 1 diabetes. *J Clin Med.* (2015) 4:1498–517. doi: 10.3390/jcm4071498
58. Nielsen LB, Wang C, Sorensen K, Bang-Berthelsen CH, Hansen L, Andersen ML, et al. Circulating levels of microRNA from children with newly diagnosed type 1 diabetes and healthy controls: evidence that miR-25 associates to residual beta-cell function and glycaemic control during disease progression. *Exp Diabetes Res.* (2012) 2012:896362. doi: 10.1155/2012/896362
59. Bijkerk R, Duijs JM, Khairoun M, Ter Horst CJ, van der Pol P, Mallat MJ, et al. Circulating microRNAs associate with diabetic nephropathy and systemic microvascular damage and normalize after simultaneous pancreas-kidney transplantation. *Am J Transplant.* (2015) 15:1081–90. doi: 10.1111/ajt.13072
60. Kato M, Natarajan R. Diabetic nephropathy–emerging epigenetic mechanisms. *Nat Rev Nephrol.* (2014) 10:517–30. doi: 10.1038/nrneph.2014.116
61. Fu Y, Zhang Y, Wang Z, Wang L, Wei X, Zhang B, et al. Regulation of NADPH oxidase activity is associated with miRNA-25-mediated NOX4 expression in experimental diabetic nephropathy. *Am J Nephrol.* (2010) 32:581–9. doi: 10.1159/000322105
62. Dey N, Das F, Mariappan MM, Mandal CC, Ghosh-Choudhury N, Kasinath BS, et al. MicroRNA-21 orchestrates high glucose-induced signals to TOR complex 1, resulting in renal cell pathology in diabetes. *J Biol Chem.* (2011) 286:25586–603. doi: 10.1074/jbc.M110.208066
63. Wang B, Komers R, Carew R, Winbanks CE, Xu B, Herman-Edelstein M, et al. Suppression of microRNA-29 expression by TGF-beta1 promotes collagen expression and renal fibrosis. *J Am Soc Nephrol.* (2012) 23:252–65. doi: 10.1681/ASN.2011010055
64. Kriz W, Kaissling B, Le Hir M. Epithelial-mesenchymal transition (EMT) in kidney fibrosis: fact or fantasy? *J Clin Invest.* (2011) 121:468–74. doi: 10.1172/JCI44595
65. Alkandari A, Ashrafian H, Sathyapalan T, Efthimiou E, Darzi A, Holmes E, et al. Urinary microRNAs as non-invasive biomarkers of surgery-induced improvement of renal function. In: *Abstracts of the 21st Pan Arab Conference on Diabetes PACD21, March 2017 and the 6th Middle East Congress on Clinical Nutrition, March 2017.* Cairo: Primary Care Diabetes (2017).

14

Metabolic and Endocrine Consequences of Bariatric Surgery

Isabel Cornejo-Pareja [1,2], Mercedes Clemente-Postigo [1,2] and Francisco J. Tinahones [1,2*]*

[1] Unidad de Gestión Clínica Endocrinología y Nutrición, Instituto de Investigación Biomédica de Málaga—IBIMA, Hospital Universitario Virgen de la Victoria, Universidad de Málaga, Málaga, Spain, [2] Centro de Investigación Biomédica en Red (CIBER) Fisiopatología de la Obesidad y Nutrición (CIBEROBN), Instituto de Salud Carlos III (ISCIII), Málaga, Spain

***Correspondence:**
Mercedes Clemente-Postigo
mer.cp@hotmail.com
Francisco J. Tinahones
fjtinahones@uma.es

Obesity is one of the most serious worldwide epidemics of the twenty-first century according to the World Health Organization. Frequently associated with a number of comorbidities, obesity threatens and compromises individual health and quality of life. Bariatric surgery (BS) has been demonstrated to be an effective treatment to achieve not only sustained weight loss but also significant metabolic improvement that goes beyond mere weight loss. The beneficial effects of BS on metabolic traits are so widely recognized that some authors have proposed BS as metabolic surgery that could be prescribed even for moderate obesity. However, most of the BS procedures imply malabsorption and/or gastric acid reduction which lead to nutrient deficiency and, consequently, further complications could be developed in the long term. In fact, BS not only affects metabolic homeostasis but also has pronounced effects on endocrine systems other than those exclusively involved in metabolic function. The somatotropic, corticotropic, and gonadal axes as well as bone health have also been shown to be affected by the various BS procedures. Accordingly, further consequences and complications of BS in the long term in systems other than metabolic system need to be addressed in large cohorts, taking into account each bariatric procedure before making generalized recommendations for BS. In this review, current data regarding these issues are summarized, paying special attention to the somatotropic, corticotropic, gonadal axes, and bone post-operative health.

Keywords: bariatric surgery, somatotropic axis, corticotropic axis, gonadal axis, bone metabolism

INTRODUCTION

Obesity is a chronic, progressive, and multifactorial disease involving genetic, metabolic, psychological, and endocrinology-related factors, among others. Obesity-associated comorbidities are numerous and are also related to higher mortality. Obesity is a risk factor for a number of other chronic illnesses related to metabolic syndrome including type 2 diabetes mellitus (T2DM), high blood pressure, dyslipidemia, cardiovascular diseases (CVD), respiratory disorders, joint diseases, psychosocial disorders, and even several types of cancer (including esophagus, colon, pancreas, prostate, and breast) (1).

The World Health Organization (WHO) has defined the term "obesity" as excessive fat accumulation that is harmful to health. Considered the twenty-first century epidemic, obesity is the main health problem in developed countries, reducing life expectancy and presenting a challenge for the global economy. This is a disease with exponential growth, and its rise and prevalence is also affecting the child population. In the last 40 years the proportion of the population that is obese has tripled. In 2016, 39% of adults aged 18 years and over were overweight and about 13% were obese. If nothing changes, the growing trend will continue and these numbers will increase in the coming years (2).

BARIATRIC SURGERY (BS): A TREATMENT FOR OBESITY

From the point of view of therapeutics, proper dietary re-education, together with lifestyle modification and physical exercise as well as psychological specialized support for obesity treatment are needed. However, studies such as Look AHEAD showed that weight loss and glycemic control is difficult to maintain in the long term, even with intensive lifestyle intervention (3). Thus, bariatric surgery (BS) is the most effective therapy in the long term for severely obese patients (grade II) with associated metabolic diseases and for morbidly and super morbidly obese patients (grades III-IV). In addition, there is increasing literature that supports the inclusion of BS for the treatment of T2DM and obese patients (1). In this context, a global approach developed by a multidisciplinary unit, which allows a personalized and comprehensive treatment for obese patients as well as the selection of those patients who can be benefit from surgical treatment is extremely relevant.

There are different effective surgical methods employed for obesity treatment and the majority of the most popular bariatric procedures such as Roux-en-Y gastric bypass (RYGB), sleeve gastrectomy (SG), mini-gastric bypass, and biliopancreatic diversion (BPD) are considered safe procedures that are efficient regarding obesity-associated comorbidities and weight loss (4). Nevertheless, there are some differences between bariatric procedures related to the magnitude of changes observed, complication rates or post-surgery morbidities in the short and long term (reintervention rates after surgery, gastroesophageal reflux disease). Due to these differences, an individualized treatment taking into account the characteristics of each patient is necessary (5–8).

After BS, many aspects are modified and imply a reduction in the risk of obesity-associated disorders as well as of all-cause mortality (9–11). Some of the beneficial effects of BS are improved physical function (12), sustained weight loss, reduction of comorbidities such as osteoarthritis and respiratory dysfunction (13), a more favorable metabolic profile, which implies an improvement in quality of life, and the resolution of cardiovascular risk factors (14–19) with lower triglyceride levels and higher HDL-C levels in most patients 1 year after surgery (20, 21).

Although there is extensive literature that claims beneficial health effects with BS, and the post-surgery mortality rate is <1%, these type of procedures are not exempt from long-term complications related to nutritional deficiencies. In general, mainly malabsorptive procedures, e.g., bypass procedures with duodenal exclusion of nutrients and a concomitant decrease in gastric acid, will have a higher risk of micronutrient and macronutrient deficiencies. Consequently, BS patients are at higher risk of developing nutrient deficiency-related disorders such as anemia, certain types of neuropathies or osteoporosis (22, 23).

EFFECTS OF BS ON GLYCEMIC PROFILE AND MECHANISMS INVOLVED IN T2DM RESOLUTION

A number of studies have explored metabolic changes after BS, and the efficiency of BS for the treatment of T2DM is well-established. BS therefore offers a safe and more effective alternative to achieve sustained glycemic control in diabetic obese patients in comparison with intensive medical treatment (24–26), which involves a decrease in chronic micro- and macroangiopathic complications (27).

The various surgical procedures usually employed in BS lead to partial or total T2DM remission of about 34–85.3% depending on the criteria applied to define T2DM remission, and 95% global success in glycemic control (28). When the different bariatric procedures are compared, biliopancreatic diversion (BPD) is the most effective for T2DM treatment, but this is a more complex procedure with higher surgical adverse event rates compared to other bariatric procedures (29). Risstad et al. reported better outcomes related to sustained weight loss, glycemic control and improvement in lipid profile after BPD than RYGB 5 years after surgery (14). Garrido-Sanchez et al. concluded that BPD takes less time to achieve insulin resistance improvement than SG (30).

RYGB is also a highly effective option for T2DM remission. Most patients who underwent RYGB did not require hypoglycemic drugs 1 year post-surgery, and it has been reported 84–90% and 29–50% T2DM remission one and 5 years after RYGB, respectively (31–35). However, T2DM remission rates in the literature vary. Yan et al. reported 56.81% (36.8–90.3%) T2DM remission in their meta-analysis (36), while Chang et al. found 95.15% (88.38–98.8%) T2DM remission (37).

Sleeve gastrectomy has gained popularity and appears to achieve glycemic control rates similar to RYGB but with fewer surgery-associated complications. The randomized controlled trial SMBOSS reported 60% T2DM remission rates after SG compared to 77% remission after RYGB 3 years after surgery (15). The STAMPEDE study compared the efficacy of intensive medical therapy alone or intensive medical therapy plus RYGB or plus SG (5-year follow-up) finding that, 28.6% of patients who underwent RYGB achieved HbA1c ≤6% in comparison with 23.4% of patients who underwent SG and 5.3% of patients who only received intensive medical therapy. The average improvement in HbA1c was 2.1% in surgery cohorts vs. 0.3% in intensive medical treatment cohorts (25). The SLEEVEPASS study showed that the effects of T2DM remitted completely or partially in 49% of patients who underwent SG and in 57% who underwent RYGB with no significant differences between procedures (16). However, it should be mentioned that the comparison between these two procedures based on the current literature is difficult due to study heterogeneity and because some of them are biased. Thus, their findings should be interpreted cautiously and further randomized controlled trials with a careful design are necessary (38).

Mechanisms for T2DM Remission After BS

Many explanations have been put forth for the metabolic improvements after BS. Early and pronounced improvement in hepatic insulin sensitivity after RYGB, which could be related to caloric restriction in the short-term post-operative period and the reduction in intrahepatic fat, has been reported. Moreover, an improvement in peripheral insulin sensitivity, which occurs later, and its relationship with the sustained weight loss has been described (39, 40).

Nevertheless, it is well-known that the metabolic improvements after BS take place in the days or weeks after surgery even before significant weight loss occurs (21, 41, 42). Therefore, mechanisms other than weight loss that cannot be explained solely by caloric restriction are likely triggered after BS and could account for the beneficial metabolic changes observed. This has promoted the use of the term "metabolic surgery" for this type of procedures (43).

Several hypotheses have been put forth to explain the early improvement in carbohydrate metabolism after BS, but the precise mechanisms for T2DM resolution are not yet completely understood (**Figure 1**). Among the factors which could be determining these improvements, in addition to caloric and excess nutrient restriction and the weight loss associated with food malabsorption, are changes in nutrient detection, improvements in pancreatic islet function, modulation of neural mechanisms and the secretion of gastrointestinal hormones implicated in energy and glucose homeostasis (e.g., glucagon-like peptide-1 (GLP1), peptide YY (PYY), cholecystokinin (CKK), ghrelin (44), glucagon (45, 46), obestatin levels (47), alteration in circulating adipokines (leptin decrease and adiponectin increase) (48, 49), bile acid secretion, or gut microbiota modulation (50). Most of the mechanisms proposed to explain the early metabolic improvements that occur independently from weight loss are related to the anatomic remodeling of the gastrointestinal tract, which highlights the relevance of the intestine in carbohydrate metabolism regulation after BS (51, 52).

Several hypotheses have been raised regarding the implication of the gastrointestinal system as a metabolically active organ:

- The "foregut hypothesis" is based on the exclusion of the duodenum and proximal jejunum from the nutrient traffic across the gastrointestinal tract, which may inhibit "anti-incretin" signal production such as gastric inhibitory polypeptide (GIP). The removal of this signaling would favor direct antidiabetic effects with a reduction in insulin resistance (53–55).
- The "hindgut hypothesis" posits that nutrients reach the distal jejunum quickly, ensuring optimal digestion and nutrient absorption as well as metabolic improvement and weight loss through stimulation of L cells in the distal ileum and proximal colon which secrete GLP-1, PYY, oxyntomodulin, and other hormones (56). This response leads to an improvement in insulin secretion by pancreatic β cells and a reduction in glucagon production and hence, to a better post-prandial response to glucose and lower insulin resistance. By contrast, various BS procedures have shown heterogeneous effects on circulating GIP levels, ranging from moderate to unnoticeable and sometimes even leading to a decrease (46, 57–60).
- Other possible mechanisms have been elucidated from the results of SG. Although it would initially be considered a purely restrictive bariatric procedure, evidence has highlighted that its effects cannot be explained by caloric restriction alone. SG also leads to complex hormonal changes such as diminished ghrelin levels, which enhance weight loss and improve post-prandial insulin response together with lower post-prandial glucose levels (61, 62), as well as higher post-prandial GLP-1 and PYY responses induced by a short intestinal transit after surgery (63).
- The modulation of bile acid circulation has been postulated as a feasible mechanism to explain some of the metabolic effects of BS. Bile acids could be involved in both weight loss and the improvement in glycemic control by the stimulation of intestinal L-cell secretion of GLP-1, PYY, and oxyntomodulin which favors insulin response and the feeling of satiety (64, 65). Human and animal studies support the key role of bile acids in glucose metabolism regulation by means of pathways activated by the interaction of bile acid with the nuclear and membrane receptors farnesoid X receptor (FXR) and Takeda G protein-coupled receptor 5 (TGR-5), which are present in a number of tissues and organs such as the gut, liver, pancreas, adipose tissue, and skeletal muscle. By means of these receptors, bile acids lead to an increase in insulin secretion by pancreatic β cells, improvements in glucose tolerance, enhancement of glucose uptake by adipose tissue, decrease in gluconeogenesis, increase in glycogen synthesis and promotion of hepatic glucose catabolism (20, 66–68).
- Another intestine-related effect of BS which could be involved in the BS metabolic effects is the modulation of gut microbiota. Gut microbiota composition has previously been associated with obesity, T2DM and other metabolic diseases (55). Thus, it has been proposed that the modulation of gut microbiota composition by BS might be, at least in part, responsible for the post-surgical metabolic improvements. In agreement with this hypothesis, significant changes in gut microbiota composition have been reported after BS (50), but results from different studies are heterogeneous and no clear conclusions have been drawn (69). RYGB has been associated with an increase in Proteobacteria (70–72), while others described a concomitant decrease in Firmicutes and Bacteroidetes (70, 71). However, other studies found different shifts in gut microbiota profile after BS. Kong et al. showed a decrease in bacteria belonging to Firmicutes phyla at 3 and 6 months after RYGB in obese women (most of them without T2DM) (72) and a recent study found that RYGB lead to a decrease in Bacteroidetes 1 year post-operatively in obese diabetic patients (73). More detailed information regarding changes in specific bacterium groups have been recently reviewed elsewhere, giving an idea of the heterogeneous results (69, 74). Independently of the specific changes in bacterium groups, an increased bacterial diversity (previously related to the healthy status) post-surgery was reported (72, 75). Few studies have analyzed

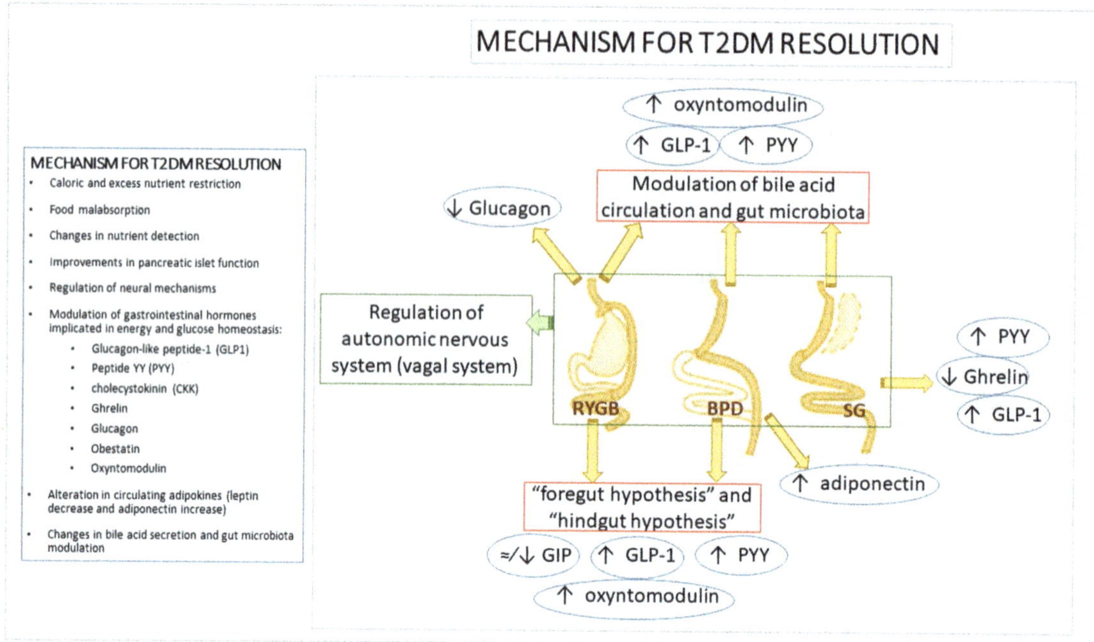

FIGURE 1 | Mechanism for T2DM resolution. Mechanisms and modifications of main gastrointestinal hormones involved in T2DM resolution after bariatric surgery. Several mechanisms have been proposed to explain the metabolic improvement after bariatric surgery. However, due to the fact that each bariatric procedure does not involve the same gastrointestinal tract modifications, it has been suggested that each procedure acts by means of different mechanisms to achieve T2DM resolution, including differential shifts in gastrointestinal hormones levels. It has been proposed that the exclusion of the duodenum and proximal jejunum in bariatric procedures such as RYGB or BPD would inhibit the "anti-incretin" signaling ("foregut hypothesis"). This kind of remodeling would also reduce the time that nutrients take to reach distal jejunum which could imply an early activation of incretin-secreting L-cells in the distal ileum and proximal colon ("hindgut hypothesis"). Incretins such as GLP-1, PYY, or oxyntomodulin improve pancreatic insulin secretion and reduce glucagon release. By contrast, the main gastrointestinal hormonal shift expected after SG is the decrease in the levels of the orexigenic hormone ghrelin due to the removal of the gastric fundus and therefore, of the ghrelin-producing mucosa. However, it has also been described an increase in GLP-1 and PYY levels after SG likely due to a shorter intestinal transit after surgery. Apart from changes in gastrointestinal hormone patterns, alterations in bile acid metabolism, gut microbiota composition, modification in gastrointestinal vagal signaling or changes in adipokines levels described after the different bariatric procedures, could be also involved in the bariatric metabolic improvement and T2DM resolution after surgery. BPD, biliopancreatic diversion; GIP, gastric inhibitory polypeptide; GLP-1, Glucagon-like Peptide 1; PYY, Peptide YY; RYGB, Roux-en-Y gastric bypass; SG, sleeve gastrectomy; T2DM, Type 2 diabetes mellitus.

other BS procedures than RYGB regarding their effects on gut microbiota composition (73, 76–78). Similar changes in gut microbiota composition were found after RYGB and vertical banded gastroplasty (VBG) (76). However, recent studies reported differences in post-surgical gut microbiota profile between RYGB and SG (73) and between RYGB and laparoscopic adjustable gastric banding (LAGB) (77). The different design and participant inclusion criteria (gender, presence of T2DM and other obesity comorbidities or follow-up after surgery) of the current studies could explain the discrepancies found. Moreover, the gut microbiota profile after BS can be also dependent on post-surgery analysis time, omeprazole intake and diet (73, 79). Despite firm conclusions regarding the specific intestinal bacterial switch have not yet been drawn, recent studies suggest that gut microbiota composition is related to the success of surgical intervention in terms of excess weight loss or T2DM remission (73, 80). In view of these results, it can be hypothesized that the inter-individual response to BS might be, at least in part, dependent on gut microbiota composition. Furthermore, several studies have reported that BS is related to the modulation of the mechanisms presumably involved in the gut microbiota-host metabolism crosstalk such as LPS translocation and inflammatory markers (41, 70, 81, 82), regulation of GI hormone secretion (77, 83), influence on AT function (72, 84), bile acid metabolism (79), or short-fatty acid (SCFA) production (77). All these evidence point out that there is a relationship between BS consequences and gut microbiota, although further homogeneous studies are necessary in order to get a comprehensive overview of the involvement of gut microbiota in the metabolic improvement at both the short- and long-term after BS and the precise mechanisms by which it can take place.

- Changes in the neuroendocrine system have also been suggested to be involved in the beneficial effects of BS. As summarized above, the principal hypotheses about beneficial neuroendocrine effects of BS include the modification of gastrointestinal hormone release with well-recognized effects on food intake and energy equilibrium. Most of these hormones not only communicate with the brain in an endocrine manner, but they also act in a paracrine fashion by interacting with specific receptors located on vagal afferent nervous fibers which innervate the gastrointestinal tract and are in close proximity to gastrointestinal endocrine cells (85, 86). In addition, vagal afferent endings also respond to mechanical stimuli such as distension (86, 87). The *nucleus tractus solitarius* (NTS; vagal afferent nucleus) senses afferent inputs to regulate energy balance, including hunger and satiety feelings by the activation of brain regions involved in food intake regulation, as well as by vagal efferent inputs that regulates splanchnic organs such as liver and endocrine pancreas (87–89). These pathways seem to be altered in obesity with vagal afferent over-activation likely due to a decreased sensitivity to stimuli of vagal afferents which requires higher stimuli to activate proper response to feeding which leads to hyperphagia (87). Accordingly, interventions aimed at both depletion or stimulation of vagal afferent fibers have been shown to improve weight loss and food intake control (90, 91). The fact that these opposite interventions as well as the existence of contradictory results regarding vagotomy suggests that the effect depend on the site where vagal afferents are intervened (92). Animal studies analyzing vagal afferent restructuring after BS support this hypothesis. Different vagal pathway reorganizations are induced after each bariatric procedure, but behavioral reduced food intake and increased satiety feelings are common after BS regardless the procedure (93). Both RYGB and SG involves the damage of gastric vagal afferent fibers but in different gastric regions (94). RYGB damages gastric branches close to their origin resulting in a decreased density of vagal afferents in the NTS, reduction of synapses and NTS microglia activation (95). It is noteworthy that other vagal afferent endings to the rest of the intestine and other splanchnic organs are preserved (96). By contrast, SG only damages terminal gastric vagal branches which oppositely results in increased density of vagal afferent in the NTS and the number of synapses, which has been suggested to be linked to higher sensitivity to nutrients and satiety feelings, and then to lower food intake (95). The fact that blocking of vagal afferent fibers in the band site abolishes AGB effects on food intake and satiety, highlights the role of vagal afferent pathways in mediating AGB effects likely by means of mechanoreception (97). Evidence from human studies dealing with the involvement of vagal system in BS effects are limited. Indirect evidence regarding how distension stimuli, and then mechanosensitivity by vagal afferent fibers, might be involved in the voluntary food intake reduction after RYGB and AGB has been reported (98, 99). Sundbom et al. used pancreatic polypeptide (PP) as marker for vagal efferent function after RYGB, finding a post-operatively decrease in ghrelin and PP associated with weight loss that authors attribute to vagal dysfunction (100). Accordingly, Tamboli et al. found an attenuation in PP response to ghrelin after RYGB (101). By contrast, Perathoner et al. did not find significant differences in satiety score, weight loss, motility or ghrelin and gastrin levels in RYGB patients with or without vagal nerve dissection (102). Although not having being directly related to vagal pathways, significant changes in neural response (specifically reduction of the activation of brain areas linked to the mesolimbic reward pathway) to food cues have been reported in morbidly obese patients undergone RYGB (103). Ten Kulve et al. suggested that the reduction in brain activation to food pictures and to the intake of palatable food in patients who underwent RYGB could be mediated by the post-operatively GLP1 increase, although precise mechanism linking GLP1 and brain activity response to food remains unknown (104). In view of these results, neural modifications that affect patient behavior regarding feeding habits could be induced by the different bariatric procedures. Nevertheless, the limited evidence in humans make difficult to confirm the relevance of these neural remodeling and whether are cause or consequence of BS effects.

BS also alters hormone levels other than incretins such as glucagon. Patients who underwent RYGB had decreased glucagon levels (105). This decrease was similar to the reduction due to general weight loss. However, other studies did not find a significant decrease in glucagon levels after other surgical procedures (106).

Obestatin levels have also been described to be implicated not only in food intake and gastric emptying but also to have beneficial effects on pancreatic β cells by reducing apoptosis and promoting proliferation, increasing insulin secretion and decreasing insulin resistance, which have a positive effect on systemic glucose homeostasis. It has been suggested that obestatin may play a role in T2DM remission (47).

Increased adiponectin levels after BS have also been described. Adiponectin is an anti-inflammatory hormone that improves insulin sensitivity, and its rise after BS has been correlated with higher T2DM remission rates in patients who underwent BPD (48, 49).

Despite the general overview that BS improves carbohydrate metabolism, there are also studies that have reported T2DM recurrence 5 years after surgery in 50–95% of patients who had achieved T2DM remission. This recurrence was associated with weight regain and a longer history of T2DM previous to the surgery (107, 108). Thus, more studies are necessary in order to provide clinical recommendations on the use of oral antidiabetic drugs in patients who have undergone BS with anatomical remodeling and the consequent physiological changes. Another relevant aspect that should be considered is neuroglycopenic hypoglycemia in BS patients, which could be related to the foregut hypothesis and low production of "anti-incretin" signals needed to counteract the dominant incretin action after surgery together with the hyperinsulinemia triggered by the increased incretin response in the distal intestine (55).

NON-METABOLIC BS-INDUCED ENDOCRINE ALTERATIONS

Aside from the well-known metabolic effects of BS, these surgical procedures also induce changes in other systems with further endocrine consequences (**Table 1**).

TABLE 1 | Endocrine consequences of bariatric surgery on somatotropic, corticotropic, and gonadal axes.

	Study	Surgery	Design	Follow-up	Sample size	Population	Primary outcome	Results
Somatotropic axis *General trend*: Somatotropic axis restoration	Mittempergher et al. (109)	BPD LAGB	Observational, prospective study	1 year	88 (34/54)	Obese patient (male/female)	GH IGF-1	Higher effects of mainly malabsorptive techniques than restrictive techniques.
	Camastra et al. (110)	RYGB	Observational, prospective study	6 months	23 (16/7)	Severely obese and non-obese controls.	GH	Significant increase in GH secretion.
	De marinis et al. (111)	BPD	Observational prospective study	16 and 24 months	30 (15/15)	Obese females and non-obese females.	IGF-1 GH peak after GHRH	Slower IGF-1 secretion in response to BS possibly attributed to underlying catabolic status, as GH response to GHRH severely increased.
	Mancini et al. (112)	RYGB	Observational prospective study	6 months	10	Non-diabetic premenopausal severely obese women	GH	Partial recovery of somatotropic axis.
	Britt Edén Engström et al. (113)	RYGB	Observational prospective study	6 and 12 months	63 (54/9)	Obese patients (female/male)	GH IGF-1	Increase in GH and IGF-1 levels.
	Savastano et al. (114)	LAGB	Observational prospective study	6 months	254 (104/36)	Moderately and severely obese patients (female/male)	GH IGF-1 GH peak after GHRH plus arginine (ARG) test	Higher weight loss and improvement of body composition profile in subjects who recovered GH response to stimulus and with normal IGF-1 levels after surgery.
	Di somma et al. (115)	LAGB	Observational prospective study	6 months	72	Severely obese females	GH peak after GHRH plus arginine test. IGF-1 IGFBP-3	Postoperative IGF-1 levels were the strongest determinant of body composition profile. So, recovered GH axis is related with higher success of surgery.

(Continued)

TABLE 1 | Continued

	Study	Surgery	Design	Follow-up	Sample size	Population	Primary outcome	Results
Corticotropic axis *General trend:* Short-term: cortisol increase immediately after BS (acute stress) Long-term: corticotropic axis activation (although there are controversial results)	Manco et al. (116)	BPD	Observational prospective study	2 years	10	Fertile non-diabetic obese women	CBG, Plasma cortisol suppression with dexamethasone suppression test	A significant decrease in circulating CBG levels and an increase in the free cortisol fraction in obese women. No difference was found in cortisol suppression after BS.
	Morrow et al. (117)	RYGB	Observational prospective study	2 and 5 months	24 (10/14)	Obese patients with presence or absence of night-eating syndrome undergoing BS	Fasting plasma cortisol	Decrease in fasting plasma cortisol in obese patients without night-eating syndrome after BS.
	Larsen et al. (118)	LAGB	Cross-sectional study		34 (16/18)	Obese women with and without binge syndrome	Salivary cortisol	Lower salivary cortisol levels during the day in obese women with binge syndrome than without binge disorder.
	Guldstrand et al. (119)	LAGB	Observational prospective study	~12 months ("After a stable body weight after BS")	8 (7/1)	Obese and non-diabetic patients (female/male)	Plasma cortisol	Reduction in cortisol levels in response to hypoglycemic clamp technique after BS-induced weight loss in comparison to the presurgical state characterized by exaggerated HPA axis activation.
	Ruíz-Tovar et al. (120)	SG	Observational prospective study	6 and 12 months	40	Morbidly obese patients	Serum cortisol, CRP	Cortisol levels decreased from 6 months after BS. CRP levels decreased significantly 12 months after BS.
	Valentine et al. (121)	BPD RYGB LAGB SG	Observational prospective study	6 and 12 months	24	Obese female participants	Salivary cortisol	A significant rise in morning salivary cortisol levels after BS, but no differences in nighttime salivary cortisol levels and the salivary cortisol awakening response.
	Hulme et al. (122)	RYGB LAGB SG	Observational prospective study	3 and 6 months	17 (14/3)	Obese patients (female/male)	Saliva Cortisol	No effect of BS on cortisol secretion daily patterns but morning cortisol showed a slightly non-significant increase.

(Continued)

TABLE 1 | Continued

		Study	Surgery	Design	Follow-up	Sample size	Population	Primary outcome	Results
Gonadal Axis General trends	*In women PCOS:* Improvement in gonadal function, menstrual irregularities and fertility. Androgen and hirsutism reduction.	Sarwer et al. (123)	RYGB LAGB	Observational prospective study	1 and 2 years	106	PCOS obese women	Total testosterone, estradiol, FSH, LH and SHGB levels	Significant improvements in general sexual quality, functioning and hormonal levels after BS.
		Jamal et al. (124)	RYGB	Observational prospective study	46.7 months	20	Obese female with ≥ 2 of 3 diagnostic criteria for PCOS	Hormonal levels (Testosterone, SHBG, LH, FSH, estradiol levels), menstrual cycles, hirsutism	An improvement in gonadal dysfunction in 82% of patients with a recovery in menstrual irregularities, 89% hirsutism resolution, and 50% achieve conception.
		Eid et al. (125)	RYGB	Observational prospective study	27.5 ± 16 months	24	PCOS obese women	Menstrual cycles, hirsutism, hormonal levels	Improvements in PCOS-associated symptoms including menstrual alteration resolution, and hirsutism. Successful conception was achieved by 5 patients.
		George and Azeez. (126)	SG	Retrospective analysis		132	PCOS Obese women	Clinical dates: menstrual cycles, hirsutism, hormonal levels and radiologic ovary pattern	Resolution of menstrual irregularities pattern in the majority of the cases, of hirsutism in 80% and of the radiologic pattern in PCOS in 81%.
		Skubleny et al. (127)	BPD RYGB LAGB SG	Meta-analysis	1-year	2130	PCOS Obese women	Hormonal levels and clinical sequelae of PCOS: menstrual cycles, hirsutism, and infertility.	PCOS significantly decrease from 45.6% pre-operatively to 6.8% 1 year post-operatively.
		Shekelle et al. (128)	BPD RYGB LAGB SG	Meta-analysis of cohort studies, case series and individual case reports.		57 articles analysis	Obese and reproductive age women	Fertility, contraception, pregnancy, weight management, and nutritional deficiencies.	Menstrual regularity was recovered in 71%; with an association between weight loss and ovulation recovery. Data suggest improvement fertility after BS with minimal nutritional deficiencies for mother and child and without higher complications in post-surgery pregnancies.

(Continued)

TABLE 1 | Continued

	Study	Surgery	Design	Follow-up	Sample size	Population	Primary outcome	Results
In MOSH men: MOSH is supposed to be a reversible situation in the majority of cases with normalization of serum testosterone levels, fertility improvement in male severe obesity, but there are discrepancies about spermatogenesis.	Reis et al. (129)	RYGB	Prospective randomized controlled trial	24 months	20 (10/10)	Obese men in 2 groups with life style modification and RYGB	IIEF test, serum estradiol, PRL, LH, FSH, free and total testosterone	Improvements in sexual functioning and hormonal levels (total testosterone, FSH and PRL).
	Mora et al. (130)	RYGB SG	Prospective observational case series study	1 year	39	Obese men	IIEF score, Testosterone, SHBG, estradiol, gonadotropins, inhibin B, PRL.	Improvement in sexual aspects (IIEF score and significant increment in testosterone level).
	Sarwer et al. (131)	RYGB	Prospective cohort study	4 years	32	Obese men	SHBG, IIEF, Testosterone	Increase total testosterone and SHBG levels 4 years post-operatively, but improvements in sexual dysfunction were not significant during the follow-up.
	Facchiano et al. (132)	BPD RYGB LAGB	Prospective study	6 months	20	Obese men	LH, FSH, Total and Free testosterone, SHBG, estradiol,	Increase in total testosterone, SHBG, LH and FSH levels with a relevant drop in estradiol levels.
	Luconi et al. (133)	BPD RYGB LAGB	Longitudinal study	6 and 12 months	24	Morbidly obese male	Free-testosterone, SHBG, LH, FSH	Increase in total and free testosterone levels as well as SHBG and gonadotropins (simultaneous increases in LH and FSH).
	Aarts et al. (134)	RYGB LAGB	Observational study	1-year	24 (13/11)	MOSH and eugonadal Obese men	Free-testosterone	Increase in free-testosterone in both MOSH and eugonadal groups.
	Samavat et al. (135)	BPD RYGB LAGB SG	Cohort study		55 (29/26)	Morbidly obese men (with MOSH and 26 without)	Total testosterone; Free testosterone; Gonadotropins. SHBG and estradiol levels.	Increase in androgen levels (total and free-testosterone) only in patients with hypogonadism. Decreased estradiol levels only in eugonadal patients. MOSH reversal that occurred early after surgery and was nearly complete.

BPD, Biliopancreatic diversion; SG, Sleeve gastrectomy; RYGB, Roux-en-Y gastric bypass; LAGB, Laparoscopic adjustable gastric band; IGF-1, Insulin-growth factor-1; GH, Growth hormone; GHRH, Growth hormone-releasing hormone; CBG, Corticosteroid-binding globulin; CRP, C-reactive protein; HPA axis, Hypothalamic-pituitary-adrenal axis; BS, bariatric surgery; PCOS, Polycystic ovary syndrome; MOSH, Obesity-associated secondary hypogonadism; IIEF, International Index of Erectile Function; PRL, Prolactin; LH, luteinizing hormone; FSH, Follicle-stimulating hormone; SHBG, Sex hormone binding globulin.

Somatotropic Axis: Growth Hormone (GH)/Insulin-Growth Factor-1 (IGF-1) After BS

GH is mainly regulated by two hypothalamic peptide hormones: GH-releasing hormone (GHRH) and somatostatin. However, other brain signaling pathways such as those related to sleep regulation are also involved in the regulation of GH secretion (136). Obesity is associated with an acquired functional reduction in GH secretion and in GH response to stimulus (e.g., insulin-induced hypoglycemia, arginine, arginine-GHRH, sleep, or exercise), which is reversible after significant weight loss (137, 138). Likewise, adiposity acts as a negative determinant for GH secretion frequency and width, and has been associated with an increase in GH removal, which implies a lower GH half-life (109). A combination of multiple somatotropic axis alterations might be responsible for the different grades of GH and IGF-1 deficiency in obese subjects. However, the physiological role of GH in obesity and the mechanisms that lead to the perturbations in its levels are not completely clear. Among the underlying neuroendocrine alterations of low plasma GH levels in obesity, hormonal GHRH, somatostatin, or ghrelin dysregulation have been proposed (136, 139). It should be also noted that gender is a relevant regulatory factor of GH secretion in healthy subjects (113).

Reports regarding serum IGF-1 levels in obesity have shown contradictory results with both normal (109, 140, 141) and decreased IGF-1 levels in obese subjects having been described (142). Recent studies have suggested that inflammatory mediators could play a relevant role in the decrease in IGF-1 bioactivity (143), which could be related to obesity which is characterized by a chronic low-grade inflammation. Obesity, specifically abdominal obesity, appears to be associated with a decrease in free IGF-1 levels. This finding is highly interesting since visceral fat mass plays a key role in the development of obesity-related diseases, and low IGF-1 levels have also been related to T2DM and CVD (144, 145).

Somatotropic axis alterations in obese subjects, similar to those in patients who have a GH deficit, are associated with a higher prevalence of cardiovascular risk factors and alterations in body composition (muscle mass and bone density reduction and rise in fat mass) (146–148). Concordantly, Di Somma et al. found that obese patients with severe somatotropic axis alterations showed an exacerbated cardio-metabolic risk with more serious sequelae compared to obese subjects without GH deficiency (114).

Several studies have reported a restoration of somatotropic axis alterations in severely obese patients after BS. A significantly increased secretion of GH after BPD has been described (110), as well as partial recovery of the somatotropic axis after RYGB (112). Mittempergher et al. determined that the GH increase after BS was higher after mainly malabsorptive procedures (2.7-fold increase) than after mainly restrictive procedures (1.4-fold increase) with parallel improvements in cardiovascular profile and BMI reduction. Therefore, in view of these results, malabsorptive procedures might be better recommended for patients with somatotropic deficiencies (109). However, further research is necessary in order to confirm these recommendations.

Britt Edén Engström et al. determined that GH secretion and IGF-1 levels, previously compromised in severe obese subjects, were augmented at 6 months in women and at 12 months in both women and men after RYGB. A concomitant BMI reduction was reported in men and women at 6 months, which was further improved at 12 months after surgery (113). Savastano et al. and Di Somma et al. reported significant correlations between body composition and GH response to stimulus (GHRH + arginine) before and after surgery in subjects who underwent LAGB, and also found higher success with surgical treatment (weight loss and improved body composition profile) in those subjects without somatotropic axis alterations as well as in patients who recovered GH response to stimulus after surgery (114, 115). BS-derived benefits can be influenced by presurgery GH response to stimuli and by previous IGF-1 levels adjusted for sex and age. Thus, these factors could be interesting markers of surgery success in weight loss and body composition improvement. Likewise, a somatotropic axis study may constitute a useful tool for obese patient follow-up after BS (115).

Although some discrepancies have been found in the literature (109, 149), IGF-1 secretion displays a slower response to BS, similar to that of non-surgical weight loss, and this can be related to an underlying catabolic status induced by BS (malabsorptive effects, pronounced restriction in caloric intake, etc.) (111, 113). Few studies have analyzed tissue response to GH in obesity. Some have described a more pronounced IGF-1 response in obese individuals compared to lean subjects (150, 151). Nevertheless, these findings were not confirmed by others (152). Britt Edén Engström et al. observed that most obese subjects showed high IGF-1 levels with regard to their GH status. Altogether, these findings may indicate that there is a specific tissue adaptation in obesity with higher GH sensitivity, especially to its anabolic effects (113). In view of these results, the acquired dysfunction in GH secretion secondary to obesity appears to be reversed after BS. The somatotropic axis status could constitute a useful tool for initial and post-surgery follow-up of BS patients as a marker of surgery success in terms of weight loss and body composition.

Hypothalamic-Pituitary-Adrenal (HPA) or Corticotropic Axis: Corticotropin-Releasing Hormone (CRH)/Corticotropin (ACTH)/Cortisol After BS

The HPA axis is a relevant pathway in the response to physiological stress which regulates cortisol secretion. Cortisol has a number of effects on the organism, including energy reserve mobilization to promote survival and to comply with metabolic requirements during stress. Cortisol is secreted by the suprarenal cortex after HPA axis activation in response to physiological or psychological stress and high cortisol levels are associated with intense emotional responses to stressful stimuli (153). However, cortisol metabolism is not only centrally regulated, but type 1 and 2 11-β- hydroxysteroid dehydrogenase enzymes also regulate cortisol in tissues (154, 155). Food intake also increases cortisol levels and an individual may feel a decrease in anxiety with eating (156). Thus, both high cortisol levels and distressed emotions, appear to be modulated by calorie-rich food intake. Once this neuroendocrine-behavioral response to chronic stress is initiated, it could become a habit that favors weight gain. The non-pathological HPA axis is characterized by a distinctive circadian profile that is disrupted when the HPA axis is deregulated (157, 158). The declining curve of daily cortisol secretion is usually less pronounced in chronic health disorders such as obesity (159, 160). During chronic stress, HPA axis adaptation results in a higher and more prolonged cumulative exposure to glucocorticoids, which are associated with negative effects including metabolic disorders and cardiovascular mortality (161–166). Emerging data suggest that metabolic syndrome patients could have a hyperactive HPA axis which would lead to "functional hypercortisolism." However, there are some controversial and heterogeneous findings in the studies analyzing this relationship (154, 155, 167). Moreover, there are disorders associated with HPA axis dysregulation that are more highly prevalent among obese subjects compared to the general population such as night-eating syndrome, binge eating disorder, sleep, and hormonal disorders as well as psychological symptoms (168–171). It is worth of mentioning that treatment for weight loss in obese subjects with these disorders is less successful than in obese individuals without these types of disorders (168, 172).

Very few studies have examined HPA axis regulation before and after BS in humans. The most commonly held idea is that weight loss tends to normalize cortisol levels and possible alterations in the HPA axis (173). Nevertheless, some studies suggest that long-term weight loss could be lessened when methods based on caloric restriction are employed, since caloric restriction could activate the HPA axis and increase circulating cortisol levels and these are associated with higher food intake and body weight (174–176). An increase in HPA axis tone during weight loss through food restriction can weaken behavioral modifications, which would make patient compliance to the prescribed diet and sustained weight loss in the long term difficult (177–179). Current evidence suggest that BS can affect HPA axis regulation, but controversial results have been found regarding the direction of this regulation (116, 119–121). Cortisol increases immediately after BS due to the acute stress caused by the surgery itself (180). However, the long-term effects of BS on cortisol have not yet been elucidated. Moreover, the few studies dealing with HPA axis after BS used different methodology for assessing HPA axis, which makes difficult to have clear conclusions regarding the effect of BS on HPA axis.

Morrow et al. studied HPA axis modulation in 24 severely obese participants (BMI = 40–70 Kg/m^2) without associated comorbidities who underwent RYGB. Participants were classified according to the presence or absence of night-eating syndrome. A decrease in fasting plasma cortisol levels 5 months after surgery was reported in patients without night-eating syndrome, but an increase was seen in the subgroup of patients who had night-eating syndrome. However, the two groups did not differ in weight loss or waist circumference (117). By contrast, Hulme et al. found that BS did not affect daily cortisol secretion patterns during the first 6 months after surgery, although morning cortisol showed a slightly non-significant post-operative increase (122).

Valentine et al. also found a significant rise in morning saliva cortisol levels 6 and 12 months after BS (54.2% after SG; 16.7% after LAGB; 12.5% after RYGB, and 8.3% after duodenal switch) in 24 obese women, but no differences were found in nighttime saliva cortisol levels or in salivary cortisol awakening response (121). High morning cortisol could be associated with an improvement in physiological health after BS that is expressed by the narrowing of the decreasing curve of diurnal cortisol secretion in contrast to plainer curve characteristics in chronic health disorders.

Larsen et al. analyzed salivary cortisol levels in obese women after LAGB and found that neuroendocrine regulation after BS differs in these patients depending on the presence or absence of binge eating disorder. Obese women with binge eating disorder had significantly lower salivary cortisol levels during the day than patients without binge disorder. It is of note that a normal weight control group was not included in this study (118).

Manco et al. described a significant decrease in circulating corticosteroid-binding globulin (CBG) levels and a concomitant increase in the metabolically free cortisol fraction in obese women 2 years after BPD (116). The increase in free cortisol fraction may contribute to adaptive enterocyte hyperplasia in the long term, favoring better functional morphology as cortisol is a regulator of crypt enterocyte proliferation (181). Likewise, hypophyseal response, and/or suprarenal sensitivity, assessed by intravenous dexamethasone infusion, differed between the patients who underwent BPD and the normal weight control group. Nevertheless, there were no differences in cortisol suppression induced by dexamethasone before and after BS (116).

Guldstrand et al. studied HPA axis changes after LAGB in 8 non-diabetic severely obese patients. For this purpose, cortisol levels were analyzed in response to hypoglycemic clamp technique and a reduction in counter-regulatory hormone (cortisol among them) response was observed during the sustained hypoglycemic state after BS-induced weight loss in comparison to the pre-surgical state characterized by exaggerated HPA axis activation (119).

Ruiz-Tovar et al. reported sustained high serum cortisol levels up to 6 months after BS in 40 morbidly obese patients who underwent laparoscopic SG. However, cortisol levels decreased and were directly associated with the CVD risk predictor triglyceride/HDL ratio from 6 months after BS (120).

In view of these studies, obesity-induced corticotropic axis activation is reduced after BS and a normalization in HPA circadian rhythms might be also occurring. This effect has not been described for caloric restriction, which could add value to the use of BS for obesity treatment. However, although current evidence suggest that BS can affect HPA axis regulation with improvement in axis physiological health, controversial results have been found regarding the direction of this regulation. Therefore, more studies on this issue are needed to homogenize criteria concerning which variables should be used to monitor corticotropic axis status.

Modifications in Gonadal Axis or Hypothalamic/Pituitary/Gonadal Axis: Gonadotropin-Releasing Hormone (GnRH)/Follicle-Stimulating Hormone (FSH), Luteinizing Hormone (LH)/Testosterone, and Estradiol After BS

The incidence of sexual dysfunction, reproductive disorders, and infertility increase with age. The relationship between sexual dysfunction and other medical conditions such as obesity (182), diabetes (183, 184), high blood pressure (185, 186), metabolic syndrome, CVD or smoking (187) is widely accepted.

It is also well-known that adipose tissue plays a relevant role in the metabolism of hormones, including sex hormones, secreted by different glands (188). Obesity-associated gonadal dysfunction is one of the most prevalent comorbidities in obese subjects who seek to lose weight (29% for women and 45% for men) (189). These disorders are particularly common in severely obese subjects who have undergone BS (190). Similar to other obesity comorbidities, the higher the BMI, the higher the risk of gonadal dysfunction (191–193). A number of recent studies have dealt with this issue. Sarwer et al. studied gonadal dysfunction prevalence in 250 obese patients (141 who were interested in BS and 109 in lifestyle changes) finding differences according to the preferred treatment for weight loss achievement. Among individuals interested in BS, 51.4% of women (according to the Female Sexual Function Index) and 36.4% of men (according to the International Index of Erectile Function) had sexual dysfunction. By contrast, 40.9% of women and 20% of men who sought lifestyle modifications had sexual dysfunction. These differences were mainly related to BMI discrepancies. Sexual dysfunction was associated with quality life and other psychosocial functions, particularly in women (192). Interestingly, the significant improvement found in sexual functioning occurred mainly in women (130, 187, 194).

It has been widely described that BS leads to an improvement in sex hormone and sexual hormone binding globulin (SHBG) levels in morbidly obese patients (132, 133, 193, 195), even higher than the effect attributable to weight loss alone (133). Thus, this supports the hypothesis that factors derived from excess adipose tissue may modulate the gonadal axis (196). An increase in SHBG and a modification in serum estradiol levels are detected after BS in men and women. This could be due to the effect on estrogen production from testosterone and steroid precursors mediated by aromatase (an enzyme whose higher activity has been associated with gonadal dysfunction pathology in obesity) in reduced adipose tissue after BS (197).

The main evidence found in this context are due to: (1) excess androgen in obese women, mainly associated with polycystic ovary syndrome (PCOS) (36%) and with idiopathic hyperandrogenism (198), and (2) androgen deficiency in obese men that is termed male obesity-associated secondary hypogonadism (MOSH). A recent meta-analysis highlights that PCOS and MOSH are among the most common comorbidities in severely obese patients who have undergone BS (36 and 64%, respectively) that are usually resolved after BS (96% of women with PCOS and 87% of men with MOSH), as highlighted by a recent meta-analysis (191).

This improvement in gonadal profile occurs in parallel with insulin resistance improvement and metabolic disorder resolution (191).

Sex-specific changes induced by BS have been reported as described below.

Modifications in the Gonadal Axis in Obese Women After BS

Excess adipose tissue in obese women may contribute to excess androgens by stimulating both ovary and hormonal secretion by the suprarenal glands as secondary effects of insulin resistance and compensatory hyperinsulinism. Specifically, abdominal adiposity may feed a vicious circle in which excess androgens favors body fat deposition and this visceral fat promotes ovary and adrenal-derived excess androgens in PCOS. However, for PCOS to develop in response to obesity and visceral fat accumulation, women must have a primary defect in steroidogenesis that promotes excess androgen secretion, predisposing to androgen excess disorders (199). In contrast, women without this primary defect in androgenic secretion do not develop excess androgens or PCOS, even in the case of extreme obesity or insulin resistance (198). Renowned authors in the field consider that obesity is one of the secondary phenotypes of PCOS, and in these cases, gonadal dysfunction improves and even resolves with weight loss (200). A recent meta-analysis has demonstrated that PCOS significantly decreased from 45.6% pre-operatively to 6.8% 1 year after surgery (127). A decrease in serum androgen levels (total testosterone) associated with a reduction in androsterone and sulfate dehydroepiandrosterone (DHEA) as well as with resolution of hirsutism and menstrual irregularities (53 and 96% of cases, respectively) has been reported. Improvements in estradiol, FSH and SHBG have also been described (191, 193, 201–203).

Studies dealing with fertility recovery in women with PCOS that have assessed fertility before and after BS are scarce. The existing studies suggest that female fertility improves after bariatric procedures and intensive weight loss. However, most of these are observational studies with high variability in age, in the bariatric procedure employed and without a control group. This makes reach a consensus about the role of BS in fertility management difficult. Accordingly, smarter studies with a precise design comparing the different bariatric procedures are required (204). Among the studies dealing with fertility, Eid et al. demonstrated that RYGB-induced weight loss was associated with improvements in PCOS-associated symptoms including menstrual alteration resolution in all the participants and hirsutism in half of the participants. In addition, successful conception was achieved by five patients who previous to surgery failed to conceive (125).

George and Azeez carried out a study that included 132 women with PCOS who underwent SG in whom resolution was achieved in the majority of the cases of menstrual irregularities, hirsutism (80%) and radiologic irregularities (81%) (126).

Jamal et al. also observed improved gonadal dysfunction in 82% of RYGB PCOS patients, with decreased menstrual irregularities and resolution of hirsutism in 29% of the patients, and 50% of patients who were unable to conceive prior to surgery were successful after surgery (124).

Balen et al. based on low-quality evidence, recommended BS use in obese PCOS women with a BMI>35 kg/m^2 and comorbidities such as gonadal dysfunction or BMI>40 kg/m^2 who had infertility problems despite programmed intensive and structured treatment (based on dietary-hygienic habit changes) with no response for at least 6 months. They also recommended to avoiding pregnancy in the rapid post-operative weight loss period for at least 6–12 months after BS and at later times, recommended that these women should be attended in a specialized multidisciplinary unit due to the risk of BS-associated nutritional deficiencies (205).

Although PCOS is the most frequent reproductive disorder in obese women (191), idiopathic hypogonadotropic hypogonadism has also been associated with higher obesity prevalence in the female population (206). Several studies have reported improvements in the gonadotropic axis as well as sexual functioning after BS in obese women that are not necessarily related to PCOS. Sarwer et al. reported that after BS, 106 women (80% RYGB and 20% LAGB patients) showed significant improvements in general sexual quality and functioning as well as sexual desire and satisfaction 1 year after surgery. These improvements were maintained up to 2 years after BS. These changes took place in parallel with psychosocial improvements, significant weight reduction of 32.7% and significant improvement in hormonal profile: decreased total testosterone, estradiol and DHEAS and increased FSH, LH and SHGB levels (123).

Bond et al. described that in 68% of obese women with sexual dysfunction (defined by the Female Sexual Function Index score), this condition resolved after BS. This improvement in sexual function was not dependent on type of surgery or amount of weight loss and appears to be an additional benefit for women undergoing BS (194).

As detailed above, weight loss after lifestyle modification, and particularly after BS, is associated with significant improvements in sexual functioning and resolution of both menstrual and ovulatory disorders that occur in nearly all patients. Thus, weight loss could also contribute to fertility restoration (191, 194, 201). However, Shekelle et al. pointed out in their review that most of the reports are observational studies and data should be interpreted cautiously (128). Moreover, except for PCOS, the definition of pre-operative reproductive disorders in obese female patients having undergone BS is not clearly defined. It is of interest to understanding whether results of these reports are referring to PCOS or to different and independent reproductive anomalies to confirm whether BS is also effective for the resolution of additional reproductive disorders.

Modifications in Gonadal Axis in Obese Men After BS

In obese men, excess adipose tissue appears to contribute to androgenic deficiency by means of pituitary gonadotropin inhibition. This suggests central production deterioration together with reduced gonadal sensitivity to LH and increased peripheral androgen degradation by their conversion to estrogens (207, 208). MOSH is characterized by reduced serum testosterone together with high relative estradiol levels and inappropriately low or normal levels of LH and FSH (209). Although serum LH levels and the pulse frequency are similar in obese and lean subjects, LH pulse width is noticeably reduced in obesity (210). Among mechanisms involved in MOSH pathogenesis, gonadotropin inhibition by excess peripheral estrogen production in adipose tissue has been reported. However, insulin resistance and the secretion of inflammatory mediators and adipokines may play a relevant role in MOSH physiopathology with an inhibitory action at the hypothalamic-pituitary level (196, 211, 212). Recent data suggest that not only hyperinsulinemia but also excess liver fat are among the main inhibitory influences on SHBG secretion in obese subjects, in a process in which pro-inflammatory cytokines derived from ectopic adipose tissue are likely implicated (213). Likewise, hypophyseal dysfunction induced by obstructive sleep apnea syndrome may also participate in MOSH development (214).

Thus, abdominal adiposity could favor a vicious cycle in MOSH development by inhibiting hypophyseal gonadotropin secretion (215–217) and simultaneously, the resulting androgen deficiency promotes body fat accumulation in parallel to a decrease in muscle and lean mass (218).

Substantial fat mass loss after intensive weight loss will likely tend to reduce aromatase activity and regulate estradiol/testosterone equilibrium, resulting in decreased estradiol production, and will favor LH increase which contributes to stimulating testosterone production and substrate availability for estradiol production. It is thought that the differences between obese subjects with normal gonadal function and those with hypogonadism might be determined by aromatase expression levels: MOSH would be induced when aromatase gene expression is elevated. By contrast, testosterone levels would remain within the normal range when aromatase expression levels are low (134). Similar to PCOS in obese women, MOSH is not a generalized condition in male obesity and underlying mechanisms are largely unknown.

An increase in serum androgen levels (for both total testosterone and the free testosterone index), which was even higher than the increase in SHBG levels in men has been reported (134, 191). Normalization of serum testosterone levels after BS is associated with improved fertility in severely obese men. Nevertheless, more specific fertility studies focused on spermatogenesis and androgen levels are needed given the discrepancies between the studies published to date (191). Some studies suggest a deterioration in seminal parameters (219, 220), while others have observed no effect (202, 221) or even beneficial effects on sperm quality (222). It has also been postulated that fat mass reduction associated with weight loss might reduce abdominal, thigh and scrotal fat depots. This leads to a decrease in testicular temperature and, consequently, facilitate spermiogenesis (207).

Chronic testosterone deficiency could reduce post-operative fat loss and enhance the catabolic effects of BS on muscle and bone. This would attenuate the positive effects of BS on insulin sensitivity. A number of recent studies dealing with the changes and benefits in gonadal dysfunction due to BS in obese men, are in agreement with BS-induced improvements in testosterone, SHBG and LH levels (129, 223, 224). Although diet and lifestyle changes and BS are associated with a significant increase in hormone levels, MOSH normalization (increased testosterone and gonadotropin levels together with decreased estradiol levels) was more effective with BS than with low-caloric diets. By contrast, results regarding FSH levels are more controversial (129, 193, 223).

Reis et al. found significant improvements in sexual functioning and levels of hormones such as total testosterone, FSH and prolactin in 10 RYGB patients (129).

Mora et al. observed a pronounced weight loss (77.18% of excess weight), metabolic profile improvement together with improvements in sexual aspects such as an improved score on the International Index of Erectile Function and a significant increase in testosterone levels 1 year after surgery (RYGB and SG in 46.2 and 53.4%, respectively) in a prospective study carried out in 39 obese men (130).

In agreement, Sarwer et al. reported a concomitant decrease in patient weight by nearly one third and increase in total testosterone and SHBG levels 4 years after surgery in their cohort of 32 men who underwent RYGB and who showed deficient sexual functioning prior to surgery. Despite this finding and although improvements in sexual dysfunction were seen in the short term after surgery, these changes were not significant during the follow-up (131).

Facchiano et al. reported an increase in total testosterone, SHBG, LH, and FSH levels with a relevant drop in the initially elevated estradiol levels at 6 months after BS (10 with RYGB, 8 with LAGB and 2 with BPD) in 20 obese men (132).

The findings of Luconi et al. confirmed the already known relationship between excess adiposity and hypogonadism in morbidly obese men. In the same line as previous studies, patients showed increased total and free testosterone levels as well as gonadotropins (simultaneous increases in LH and FSH). The increased testosterone and SHBG levels induced by BS were higher than those expected for the weight loss alone. Likewise, the increase in total testosterone may be related to an SHBG rise and peripheral aromatization reduction that contributes to the observed fall in estradiol levels. Moreover, the direct effect of weight loss on Leydig cell function should not be discarded in the improvement of gonadal profile (133).

Aarts et al. included 24 severely obese men (BMI = 35–59 Kg/m^2) in their study, 13 of them with MOSH and 11 eugonadal morbidly obese patients. One year after BS, an increase in free testosterone was observed in both MOSH and eugonadal groups. These levels were inversely related to weight loss. MOSH was a reversible situation in the majority of cases and this pre-operative condition was not adversely associated with BS efficiency in terms of weight, lipid and carbohydrate metabolism or with catabolic effects of surgery on muscle or bone mineral density (134).

Nevertheless, Samavat et al. in their study with morbidly obese BS patients (29 with hypogonadism and 26 eugonadal patients) observed that presurgery testosterone levels appear to moderate the BS effect on sex hormone recovery as an increase in androgen levels (total and free testosterone) only occurred in patients with hypogonadism. Preoperative estrogen levels were significantly lower in hypogonadal patients than in eugonadal patients. Moreover, estrogen levels only decreased after BS in eugonadal patients. Estradiol reduction in eugonadal patients was not related to testosterone level increment. As in the previous studies referenced above, Samavat et al. found a hypogonadism reversal that occurred early after surgery and was nearly complete. Taking into consideration these findings, the role of estradiol in obesity-related hypogonadism development might be limited (135).

All the revised studies, except for the study by Leenen et al. (225), reported a significant increase in total testosterone levels with weight loss and visceral fat reduction.

Few long-term studies have focused on the possible recurrence of gonadal dysfunction after weight regain. Rosenblatt et al. reported that patients who underwent RYGB from 6 to 16 years ago had high SHBG, total and free testosterone levels compared to non-surgical obese controls and these levels were comparable to those found in lean subjects. These findings agree with androgenic normalization in the long term. Nevertheless, the erectile function score was lower than in lean controls, which suggests incomplete functional restoration that may be related to weight gain and recurrent obesity comorbidities (226).

Recent research suggests reciprocal control between bone and testicles by means of osteocalcin (a peptide secreted by osteoblasts). It has been recently proposed that this peptide may be implicated in male fertility through direct stimulation of testosterone production by Leydig cells (227–231). Osteocalcin is decreased in obesity but it can also be produced by adipose tissue apart from bone production (232). Therefore, the inverse relationship between BMI and osteocalcin levels could indicate that only healthy adipose tissue may be involved in osteocalcin production (233). Weight loss induced by caloric restriction or BS is associated with the recovery of osteocalcin production. Samavat et al. analyzed 103 obese men, 76 patients who underwent RYGB and 27 controls who were waiting for surgery. The RYGB group showed an increase in osteocalcin, total testosterone and SHBG levels concomitant to a slight rise in gonadotropin levels, while estradiol levels fell likely due to a reduction in aromatase activity or expression. Osteocalcin levels were significantly associated with the restoration of testosterone levels in MOSH patients. Thus, osteocalcin may be an independent predictor for androgen restoration. It should be noted that no significant changes were seen in the non-surgical control group that had a slight weight loss. The osteocalcin levels increase might be explained by changes in leptin and adiponectin levels that regulate bone turnover in opposite ways. Likewise, insulin sensitivity improvement may enhance osteocalcin bone release (234). A recent report from Karsenty et al. supports the existence of a bone-testicle axis which is parallel to the pituitary-gonadal axis. In this way, osteocalcin and LH would act in parallel in both axes and osteocalcin would also be involved in human reproduction function (235).

In view of these results, BS is an effective method to treat gonadal dysfunction including recovery of fertility in comparison with lifestyle changes and diet-induced weight loss (200, 236, 237). Infertility or gonadal dysfunction could be used as criteria for indication for BS in obese patients with a BMI > 35 kg/m^2. The considerable resolution rate of PCOS and MOSH, the most representative gonadal dysfunction disorders in obese individuals, after BS consistently supports the causal relationship of both obesity and adipose tissue dysfunction with gonadal dysfunction in predisposed subjects. However, more long-term studies focusing on the persistence of gonadal dysfunction resolution after BS are required.

Modifications in Bone Metabolism After BS

It has been widely described that obese patients are at higher risk of vitamin D deficiency pre-operatively, although it is not clear whether this association is more closely related to obesity *per se* or to obesity-related diseases such as T2DM (238). Consequently, secondary hyperparathyroidism due to vitamin D deficiency has also been extensively reported in obesity (239). Paradoxically, obese patients are generally characterized by higher bone mineral density (BMD) and bone mineral content (BMC), and it has even been suggested that obesity could be protective against osteoporosis (240). Bone remodeling implies a continuous process of bone replacement (formation) and bone removal (resorption). When these two processes are unbalanced, net bone formation or bone loss, respectively, will occur (241). Bone remodeling not only promotes bone repair, but also helps to mechanical stress adaptation. Thus, mechanical bone loading determines bone strength, size, and mass. This has led to the suggestion that mechanical bone loading could be responsible for the protective role of obesity in bone health. Larger bone size (that can also be due to increased mechanical loading) and enhanced aromatase activity from adipose tissue have also been suggested factors favoring BMD in obesity (240–242).

The most common nutritional deficiencies after BS include folate, iron, vitamin B_{12}, calcium, vitamin D and zinc. Therefore, post-surgical changes in calcium and vitamin D can lead to bone loss resulting in higher fracture risk (243). In fact, it has generally been suggested that BS negatively affects bone health by diminishing BMD, enhancing bone resorption and impairing even further vitamin D levels and hyperparathyroidism (244). Most of the evidence comes from RYGB studies with fewer studies on other types of BS, but also finding negative effects from mainly restrictive procedures (245). One of the hypotheses posited to explain BMD and BMC after BS is mechanical unloading. A lower mechanical load due to weight loss can lead to less bone formation followed by a decrease in BMD. Concordantly, RYGB is associated with bone loss as reflected by BMD reduction at several sites 6 months (246), 1 year (247–251), and 2 years after surgery (22, 243, 252). Several studies have been carried out with longer follow-up periods up to 6 years finding a persistent bone loss (253–256). BPD has also been related to a higher incidence of metabolic bone disease 1–5 years after surgery (257) and Tsiftsis et al. reported decreased lumbar spine BMD 1 year after surgery (258). This BMD decrease could be site dependent since Marceau et al. found no changes in BMD in the hip but did find a decrease in the lumbar spine (259). Prospective studies comparing BMD at different sites between gastric bypass and SG, found that both procedures led to decreased BMD in the lumbar spine and femur. This decrease tended to be less pronounced after SG in most of the studies (260–262), but comparable in others (254, 263). Pluskiewicz et al. also reported a reduction in BMD in the lumbar spine, femoral neck and hip 6 months after SG (264). Results from LAGB are even more scarce. Decreased BMD and BMC have been reported 1 and 2 years after LAGB (265, 266). This negative effect seems to be smaller than that observed after RYGB (23). The effects of LAGB on BMC were compared to diet-induced weight loss and similar results were found (267). By contrast, Mach et al. did not find significant changes in BMC 1 year after LAGB (268).

BMD and BMC are determined by means of dual-energy X-ray absorptiometry (DXA), and technical limitations should be considered when data are interpreted. DXA are technically limited when applied to obese patients, particularly in severely obese subjects. Modifications in fat mass distribution due to drastic weight loss could influence measurement accuracy (22, 241, 269). Therefore, the controversial results regarding the effect of the different bariatric procedures on BMD and BMC could be due to technical issues.

In addition, it is unclear whether the reported BMD and BMC decrease after BS, is clinically relevant regarding osteoporosis incidence and fracture risk. As recently reviewed by Ben-Porat et al. different studies have found controversial results (245). In a study with a large sample size ($n = 2079$) in which most of the patients underwent LAGB, the risk for fracture was not increased 2 years after surgery (270). Nevertheless, when most of the population underwent RYGB, an increased fracture risk was observed in a retrospective study with a median follow-up of 7 years (271). These results were replicated after gastric bypass for a median follow-up time of 3.1 years (272). Studies that compared BS patients to obese and control patients, found higher fracture risk 4 years after surgery in the BS group than in the two control groups, significantly so with BPD. After 12 years there was also higher fracture risk after mainly malabsorptive procedures (273). A recent meta-analysis that included six studies concluded that BS is associated with increased fracture risk compared to control populations. However, the length of follow-up and the bariatric procedures were heterogeneous (274). Lack of long-term prospective studies does not help to elucidate the real effect of BS on osteoporosis development and fracture risk (245, 269).

The serum 25(OH)D form of vitamin D, calcium and parathyroid hormone (PTH) have also been measured to verify putative effects of BS on bone metabolism. As calcium is preferentially and actively absorbed in the proximal gut, and pancreatic secretion and bile acids are required for vitamin D absorption, bariatric procedures that bypass the duodenum and proximal jejunum could promote malabsorption of these micronutrients. Decreased stomach acid after SG and bypass of the proximal bowel would also reduce calcium absorption (22, 243). A meta-analysis analyzing 10 gastric bypass studies found, in addition to BMD reduction, a significant decrease in serum calcium levels (275). BPD was also associated with an increased prevalence of hypocalcemia (257). Gehrer et al. however, found no significant effect of RYGB or SG on serum calcium levels (276). Serum calcium levels are tightly regulated. While the intestine is responsible for calcium absorption from the diet, calcium reabsorption occurs in the kidneys. When these two mechanisms are insufficient to maintain serum calcium levels, calcium is released from the bones, which act as a calcium reservoir. Thus, despite normal calcium levels, low BMD could be present (22, 243). A more accurate way to evaluate calcium alteration after BS could be the direct determination of calcium absorption. Schafer et al. and Riedt et al. did this and found that gastric bypass led to a decline in calcium absorption 6 months after surgery (277, 278).

The tight regulation of serum calcium levels relies on PTH and the active form of Vitamin D (1,25$(OH)_2$D). PTH stimulates osteoclast differentiation and survival and calcium release from the bone matrix when serum calcium levels are low. Negative feedback avoids uncontrolled PTH-induced bone loss, by stimulating 1,25$(OH)_2$D synthesis. The active form of vitamin D inhibits PTH production and stimulates intestinal calcium absorption and FGF23 expression in bone (which leads to bone phosphorus loss) (241, 243). Although, it has been described as a pre-existing condition before BS, hyperparathyroidism has been reported after gastric bypass, LAGB, SG, and BPD (265, 275, 279–281). The prevalence of hyperparathyroidism increases with the time after BS, with higher prevalence after gastric bypass followed by RYGB, LAGB, and SG (281). Nevertheless, Tsiftsis et al. failed to find differences between pre-operative and post-operative PTH levels after BPD (258) and Guglielmi et al. found a decrease in PTH levels 6 months after SG (282). Likewise, hypovitaminosis D has been widely reported in obese patients prior to surgery. This status is sustained and even worsened after BS despite post-surgery vitamin D supplementation (283). It should be mentioned that BS patients usually receive vitamin D supplementation, but there is no consensus on the dose or duration of vitamin D supplementation. This should be taken into account for inter-study comparisons as this could be limiting conclusions regarding the magnitude of the effect of each BS procedure. Some studies compared 25(OH)D levels after different bariatric procedures in which patients were given the same vitamin D dose, and no differences were found between LAGB and RYGB on vitamin D deficiency incidence (284, 285). However, higher 25(OH)D levels were found after SG than RYGB after 2 years of follow-up (276, 286).

Vilarrasa et al. could not confirm these results when the administered doses of vitamin D were higher in the RYGB than in the SG group (254). This suggests that vitamin D supplementation should be adjusted depending on the bariatric procedure as 25(OH)D might be differentially affected depending on the technique. In addition, previous vitamin D deficiency and supplementation could be affecting post-surgical hypovitaminosis D. Furthermore, despite reaching normal 25(OH)D levels after BS, a higher incidence of bone diseases was reported after BPD which suggests that mechanisms other than PTH and vitamin D regulation could be affecting post-operative bone health (257).

Taking into account the limitation mentioned above regarding bone health assessment, bone turnover markers may also be an accurate approach to verify bone resorption and formation rates after BS. N-terminal propeptide of type 1 procollagen (P1NP) (cleaved from type 1 procollagen for collagen fiber assembling when incorporated into the bone matrix), bone-specific alkaline phosphatase (BAP) (a specific marker of bone formation osteoblast activity) and osteocalcin (a bone-specific protein produced by mature osteoblasts during bone matrix synthesis) are used as bone formation biomarkers. C-terminal and N-terminal telopeptides of type I collagen (CTX-1 and NTX-1, respectively; produced as a secondary product of collagen proteolytic cleavage during bone matrix degradation by osteoclasts) and tartrate-resistant acid phosphatase (TRACP; an enzyme highly expressed by osteoclasts) are considered bone resorption biomarkers (243, 287). SG and gastric bypass led to an increase in N-telopeptide but SG was also found to increase bone alkaline phosphatase (260). BPD also increased both bone formation and bone resorption markers. Despite this, BMD was reduced after surgery (258, 275). One year after LAGB, telopeptidases were reduced and correlated with bone loss (265). RYGB also decreased CTX 1 year after surgery (246). Crawford et al. recently analyzed the effect of weight loss through intensive medical therapy or by BS (RYGB or SG) on osteocalcin and CTX at 5 years. They found that surgical patients had increased levels of both CTX and osteocalcin, but no significant effect was seen with intensive medical therapy. A more noticeable effect was seen after RYGB than in SG (288).

Although some authors have questioned the mechanical unloading hypothesis (243), molecular mechanisms have been proposed to support this. Osteocytes act as mechanostat and comprise cellular response to environmental response to bone mechanical stress. Osteocytes sense mechanical bone deformation for mechanical loading and sclerostin production is inhibited. Sclerotin negatively regulates osteoblast differentiation and function and, conversely, sclerotin is upregulated under mechanical unloading. Thus, mechanical unloading could impair bone formation by impairing osteoblast function (241). Malnutrition, particularly after mainly malabsorptive techniques, has been also suggested as being responsible for bone metabolism deficiencies such as hypovitaminosis D or hyperparathyroidism as detailed above. But, further to mechanical stress and malnutrition, other hormonal mechanisms related to the well-described hormonal changes after the various bariatric procedures have been proposed (241). GLP-1, GIP, PYY, and ghrelin have been shown to act directly in bone (45, 46, 289). GIP inhibits osteoclast differentiation and its levels have been associated with bone formation markers (290, 291). Thus, the reported GIP decrease after BS procedures implies that proximal gut bypass could be associated with negative effects on bone. On the other hand, hormonal changes dependent on procedures involving stomach fundus removal such as SG, could also impair bone formation since ghrelin directly promotes osteoblast differentiation and proliferation (292), and its levels drop after this type of surgery. The relative function of GLP and PYY on bone metabolism and changes in their levels after BS do not correlate well, presupposing a harmful effect of BS on bone. PYY deficiency has been associated with low BMD (293), but its levels increase after RYGB, LAGB, SG, and BPD. Likewise, GLP-1 levels also rise after BS procedures such as BPD, but exogenous administration of GLP-1 and GLP-2 have been shown to improve BMD (294). Adipokines that decrease after BS, such as leptin, positively affect bone metabolism (295). On the other hand, adiponectin, which has been reported to raise after BS, has been negatively correlated with BMD (296). Moreover, adipose tissue is a source of estrogens which decrease bone resorption and enhance bone formation. Therefore, a weight loss-dependent estrogen decrease could also be associated with bone metabolism impairment after BS (223, 296).

All in all, there is sufficient evidence to assume that BS has an effect on bone metabolism. However, due to the fact that multiple mechanisms affected by BS could affect bone health in opposite ways, further research is needed to elucidate the net effect of each bariatric procedure on bone metabolism. Consensus on the best way to estimate bone health, taking into account technical limitations, should also be reached to obtain clear conclusions about what is really happening to bones in obese patients before and after surgery. Long-term prospective studies evaluating fracture risk and bone disease prevalence after BS, with large sample sizes and considering the type of post-surgery vitamin D and calcium supplementation, are further required to confirm BS effects on bone metabolism and to provide patients with accurate recommendations following each bariatric procedure.

CONCLUSION

Effects on metabolism and gastrointestinal hormones of BS are widely recognized, but the precise mechanisms are not yet completely understood. Moreover, it has been suggested that the different bariatric procedures are not equally effective in T2DM remission. However, heterogeneity regarding the criteria to define T2DM remission after BS makes difficult to state which surgical procedure is the most recommendable. Furthermore, other aspects than those exclusively metabolic should be taken into consideration since many other endocrine effects, but less explored up to date, are produced secondarily by the different bariatric procedures affecting corticotropic, somatotropic and gonadal axes as well as bone metabolism. Nevertheless, study design and criteria to evaluate the secondary consequences of BS are also heterogeneous which complicates the characterization of the precise effects of each bariatric procedure on these aspects. In addition, only few studies have evaluated BS consequences in the very long-term finding nutrient deficiency-related disorders, particularly after mainly malabsoprtive procedures which are at the same time considered as the most effective regarding T2DM resolution. Thus, although it is generally considered that benefits counteract by far the drawbacks of BS, further studies with homogeneous criteria and design, considering other bariatric consequences than merely metabolic effects, as well as the performance of a close long-term follow-up, are necessary in order to have a wider comprehensive overview of the consequences of each bariatric procedure. This would be useful for individualized surgical intervention recommendations depending on the different obesity co-morbidities previous to surgery of each patient as well as for preventing health-derived complications of BS.

AUTHOR CONTRIBUTIONS

IC-P, MC-P, and FT contributed to the manuscript design, to researching the literature and to the discussion, drafted and wrote the manuscript, and approved the final version.

FUNDING

IC-P was recipient of a post-doctoral grant (Río Hortega CM 17/00169) from the Instituto de Salud Carlos III (ISCIII; Madrid, Spain) and MC-P was recipient of a post-doctoral grant Juan de la Cierva Formación (FJCI-2017-32194) from the Ministerio de Ciencia, Innovación y Universidades (Spain). This study was supported by Centros de Investigación Biomédica En Red (CIBER, CB06/03/0018) of the ISCIII, Madrid (Spain), RIC-0539-2018 and PI-0092-2017 from Consejería de Salud (Junta de Andalucía), PI15/01114 and PI18/01160 from the ISCIII (Madrid, Spain) and co-funded by the Fondo Europeo de Desarrollo Regional (FEDER).

ACKNOWLEDGMENTS

The authors wish to thank FIMABIS and the help of Maria Repice for her language expertise in preparing this manuscript.

REFERENCES

1. Salas-Salvadó J, Rubio MA, Barbany M, Moreno B, de la SEEDO GC. Consenso SEEDO 2007 para la evaluación del sobrepeso y la obesidad y el establecimiento de criterios de intervención terapéutica. *Med Clin.* (2007) 28:184–96. doi: 10.1016/S0025-7753(07)72531-9
2. WHO. *Obesity and Overweight.* Available online at: https://www.who.int/news-room/fact-sheets/detail/obesity-and-overweight
3. Look AHEAD Research Group, Wing RR, Bolin P, Brancati FL, Bray GA, Clark JM, et al. Cardiovascular effects of intensive lifestyle intervention in type 2 diabetes. *N Engl J Med.* (2013) 369:145–54. doi: 10.1056/NEJMoa1212914
4. Daigle CR, Brethauer SA, Tu C, Petrick AT, Morton JM, Schauer PR, et al. Which postoperative complications matter most after bariatric surgery? Prioritizing quality improvement efforts to improve national outcomes. *Surg Obes Relat Dis.* (2018) 14:652–7. doi: 10.1016/j.soard.2018.01.008
5. Magouliotis DE, Tasiopoulou VS, Svokos KA, Svokos AA, Sioka E, Tzovaras G, et al. Banded vs. non-banded Roux-en-Y gastric bypass for morbid obesity: a systematic review and meta-analysis. *Clin Obes.* (2018) 8:424–33. doi: 10.1111/cob.12274
6. Tice JA, Karliner L, Walsh J, Petersen AJ, Feldman MD. Gastric banding or bypass? A systematic review comparing the two most popular bariatric procedures. *Am J Med.* (2008) 121:885–93. doi: 10.1016/j.amjmed.2008.05.036
7. Colquitt JL, Pickett K, Loveman E, Frampton GK. Surgery for weight loss in adults. *Cochrane Database Syst Rev.* (2014). 8:CD003641. doi: 10.1002/14651858.CD003641.pub4
8. Rachlin E, Galvani C. Metabolic surgery as a treatment option for type 2 diabetes mellitus: surgical view. *Curr Diab Rep.* (2018) 18:113. doi: 10.1007/s11892-018-1094-1
9. Schauer PR, Kashyap SR, Wolski K, Brethauer SA, Kirwan JP, Pothier CE, et al. Bariatric surgery versus intensive medical therapy in obese patients with diabetes. *N Engl J Med.* (2012) 366: 1567–76. doi: 10.1056/NEJMoa1200225
10. Sjöström L. Bariatric surgery and reduction in morbidity and mortality: experiences from the SOS study. *Int J Obes.* (2008) 32(Suppl. 7):S93–7. doi: 10.1038/ijo.2008.244

11. Sjöström L, Narbro K, Sjöström CD, Karason K, Larsson B, Wedel H, et al. Swedish obese subjects study. Effects of bariatric surgery on mortality in Swedish obese subjects. *N Engl J Med.* (2007) 357:741–52. doi: 10.1056/NEJMoa066254
12. Adil MT, Jain V, Rashid F, Al-Taan O, Whitelaw D, Jambulingam P. Meta-analysis of the effect of bariatric surgery on physical function. *Br J Surg.* (2018) 105:1107–18. doi: 10.1002/bjs.10880
13. Leonetti F, Capoccia D, Coccia F, Casella G, Baglio G, Paradiso F, et al. Obesity, type 2 diabetes mellitus, and other comorbidities: a prospective cohort study of laparoscopic sleeve gastrectomy vs medical treatment. *Arch Surg.* (2012) 147:694–700. doi: 10.1001/archsurg.2012.222
14. Risstad H, Søvik TT, Engström M, Aasheim ET, Fagerland MW, Olsén MF, et al. Five-year outcomes after laparoscopic gastric bypass and laparoscopic duodenal switch in patients with body mass index of 50 to 60: a randomized clinical trial. *JAMA Surg.* (2015) 150:352–61. doi: 10.1001/jamasurg.2014.3579
15. Peterli R, Wölnerhanssen BK, Vetter D, Nett P, Gass M, Borbély Y, et al. Laparoscopic sleeve gastrectomy versus Roux-Y-gastric bypass for morbid obesity-3-year outcomes of the prospective randomized Swiss Multicenter Bypass Or Sleeve Study (SM-BOSS). *Ann Surg.* (2017) 265:466–73. doi: 10.1097/SLA.0000000000001929
16. Salminen P, Helmiö M, Ovaska J, Juuti A, Leivonen M, Peromaa-Haavisto P, et al. Effect of laparoscopic sleeve gastrectomy vs laparoscopic Roux-en-Y gastric bypass on weight loss at 5 years among patients with morbid obesity: the SLEEVEPASS randomized clinical trial. *JAMA.* (2018) 319:241–54. doi: 10.1001/jama.2017.20313
17. Hofsø D, Nordstrand N, Johnson LK, Karlsen TI, Hager H, Jenssen T, et al. Obesity related cardiovascular risk factors after weight loss: a clinical trial comparing gastric bypass surgery and intensive lifestyle intervention. *Eur J Endocrinol.* (2010) 163:735–45. doi: 10.1530/EJE-10-0514
18. Adams TD, Pendleton RC, Strong MB, Kolotkin RL, Walker JM, Litwin SE, et al. Health outcomes of gastric bypass patients compared to nonsurgical, nonintervened severely obese. *Obesity.* (2010) 18:121–30. doi: 10.1038/oby.2009.178
19. Heo YS, Park JM, Kim YJ, Kim SM, Park DJ, Lee SK, et al. Bariatric surgery versus conventional therapy in obese Korea patients: a multicenter retrospective cohort study. *J Korean Surg Soc.* (2012) 83:335–42. doi: 10.4174/jkss.2012.83.6.335
20. Noel OF, Still CD, Argyropoulos G, Edwards M, Gerhard GS. Bile Acids, FXR, and metabolic effects of bariatric surgery. *J Obes.* (2016) 2016:4390254. doi: 10.1155/2016/4390254
21. Tinahones FJ, Queipo-Ortuño MI, Clemente-Postigo M, Fernnadez-Garcia D, Mingrone G, Cardona F. Postprandial hypertriglyceridemia predicts improvement in insulin resistance in obese patients after bariatric surgery. *Surg Obes Relat Dis.* (2013) 9:213–8. doi: 10.1016/j.soard.2011.08.022
22. Kim J, Brethauer S, ASMBS Clinical Issues Committee, American Society for Metabolic and Bariatric Surgery Clinical Issues Committee, Position Statement. Metabolic bone changes after bariatric surgery. *Surg Obes Relat Dis Off J Am Soc Bariatr Surg.* (2015) 11:406–11. doi: 10.1016/j.soard.2014.03.010.
23. Rodríguez-Carmona Y, López-Alavez FJ, González-Garay AG, Solís-Galicia C, Meléndez G, Serralde-Zúñiga AE. Bone mineral density after bariatric surgery. A systematic review. *Int J Surg Lond Engl.* (2014) 12:976–82. doi: 10.1016/j.ijsu.2014.08.002
24. Mingrone G, Panunzi S, De Gaetano A, Guidone C, Iaconelli A, Nanni G, et al. Bariatric-metabolic surgery versus conventional medical treatment in obese patients with type 2 diabetes: 5 year follow-up of anopen-label, singlecentre, randomised controlled trial. *Lancet.* (2015) 386:964–73. doi: 10.1016/S0140-6736(15)00075-6
25. Schauer PR, Bhatt DL, Kirwan JP, Wolski K, Aminian A, Brethauer SA, et al. STAMPEDE Investigators. Bariatric surgery versus intensive medical therapy for diabetes 5-year outcomes. *N Engl J Med.* (2017) 376:641–51. doi: 10.1056/NEJMoa1600869
26. Schauer PR, Bhatt DL, Kirwan JP, Wolski K, Brethauer SA, Navaneethan SD, et al. STAMPEDE Investigators. Bariatric surgery versus intensive medical therapy for diabetes—3-year outcomes. *N Engl J Med.* (2014) 370:2002–13. doi: 10.1056/NEJMoa1401329
27. Iaconelli A, Panunzi S, De Gaetano A, Manco M, Guidone C, Leccesi L, et al. Effects of bilio pancreatic diversion on diabetic complications: a 10 year follow up. *Diabetes Care.* (2011) 34:56–7. doi: 10.2337/dc10-1761
28. Singh AK, Singh R, Kota SK. Bariatric surgery and diabetes remission: who would have thought it? *Indian J Endocrinol Metab.* (2015) 19:563–76. doi: 10.4103/2230-8210.163113
29. Benotti P, Wood GC, Winegar DA, Petrick AT, Still CD, Argyropoulos G, et al. Risk factors associated with mortality after Roux-en-Y gastric bypass surgery. *Ann Surg.* (2014) 259:123–30. doi: 10.1097/SLA.0b013e31828a0ee4
30. Garrido-Sanchez L, Murri M, Rivas-Becerra J, Ocaña-Wilhelmi L, Cohen RV, Garcia-Fuentes E, et al. Bypass of the duodenum improves insulin resistance much more rapidly than sleeve gastrectomy. *Surg Obes Relat Dis.* (2012) 8:145–50. doi: 10.1016/j.soard.2011.03.010
31. Buchwald H, Avidor Y, Braunwald E, Jensen MD, Pories W, Fahrbach K, et al. Bariatric surgery: a systematic review and meta-analysis. *JAMA.* (2004) 292.1724–37. doi: 10.1001/jama.292.14.1724
32. PournarasDJ, AasheimET, Søvik TT, Andrews R, Mahon D, Welbourn R, et al. Effect of the definition of type II diabetes remission in the evaluation of bariatric surgery for metabolic disorders. *Br J Surg.* (2012) 99:100–3. doi: 10.1002/bjs.7704
33. Brethauer SA, Aminian A, Romero-Talam'as H, Batayyah E, Mackey J, Kennedy L, et al. Can diabetes be surgically cured? Long-term metabolic effects of bariatric surgery in obese patients with type 2 diabetes mellitus. *Ann Surg.* (2013) 258:628–36. Discussion 636–7. doi: 10.1097/SLA.0b013e3182a5034b
34. Buse JB, Caprio S, CefaluWT, Ceriello A, Del Prato S, Inzucchi SE, et al. How do we define cure of diabetes? *Diabetes Care.* (2009) 32:2133–5. doi: 10.2337/dc09-9036
35. Mingrone G, Panunzi S, De Gaetano A, Guidone C, Iaconelli A, Leccesi L, et al. Bariatric surgery versus conventional medical therapy for type 2 diabetes. *N Engl J Med.* (2012) 366:1577–85. doi: 10.1056/NEJMoa1200111
36. Yan Y, Sha Y, Yao G, Wang S, Kong F, Liu H, et al. Roux-en-Y Gastric bypass versus medical treatment for type 2 diabetes mellitus in obese patients: a systematic review and meta-analysis of randomized controlled trials. *Medicine.* (2016) 95:e3462. doi: 10.1097/MD.0000000000003462
37. Chang SH, Stoll CR, Song J, Varela JE, Eagon CJ, Colditz GA. The effectiveness and risks of bariatric surgery: an updated systematic review and meta-analysis, 2003-2012. *JAMA Surg.* (2014) 149: 275–87. doi: 10.1001/jamasurg.2013.3654
38. Wang F-G, Yan W-M, Yan M, Song M-M. Outcomes of Mini vs Roux-en-Y gastric bypass: a meta-analysis and systematic review, *Int J Surg.* (2018) 56:7–14. doi: 10.1016/j.ijsu.2018.05.009
39. Bojsen Møller KN, Dirksen C, Jørgensen NB, Jacobsen SH, Serup AK, Albers PH, et al. Early enhancements of hepatic and later of peripheral insulin sensitivity combined with increased postprandial insulin secretion contribute to improved glycemic control after Roux en Y gastric bypass. *Diabetes.* (2014) 63:1725–37. doi: 10.2337/db13-1307
40. Camastra S, Gastaldelli A, Mari A, Bonuccelli S, Scartabelli G, Frascerra S, et al. Early and longer term effects of gastric bypass surgery on tissue specific insulin sensitivity and beta cell function in morbidly obese patients with and without type 2 diabetes. *Diabetologia.* (2011) 54:2093–102. doi: 10.1007/s00125-011-2193-6
41. Clemente-Postigo M, Roca-Rodriguez Mdel M, Camargo A, Ocaña-Wilhelmi L, Cardona F, Tinahones FJ. Lipopolysaccharide and lipopolysaccharide-binding protein levels and their relationship to early metabolic improvement after bariatric surgery. *Surg Obes Relat Dis.* (2015) 11:933–9. doi: 10.1016/j.soard.2014.11.030
42. Murri M, García-Fuentes E, García-Almeida JM, Garrido-Sánchez L, Mayas MD, Bernal R, et al. Changes in oxidative stress and insulin resistance in morbidly obese patients after bariatric surgery. *Obes Surg.* (2010) 20:363–8. doi: 10.1007/s11695-009-0021-6
43. Ashrafian H, le Roux CW. Metabolic surgery and gut hormones– a review of bariatric entero-humoral modulation. *Physiol Behav.* (2009)97:620–31. doi: 10.1016/j.physbeh.2009.03.012
44. Santiago-Fernández C, García-Serrano S, Tome M, Valdes S, Ocaña-Wilhelmi L, Rodríguez-Cañete A, et al. Ghrelin levels could be involved in the improvement of insulin resistance after bariatric surgery. *Endocrinol Diabetes Nutr.* (2017) 64:355–62. doi: 10.1016/j.endien.2017.08.011

45. Meek CL, Lewis HB, Reimann F, Gribble FM, Park AJ. The effect of bariatric surgery on gastrointestinal and pancreatic peptide hormones. *Peptides.* (2016) 77:28–37. doi: 10.1016/j.peptides.2015.08.013
46. Jacobsen SH, Olesen SC, Dirksen C, Jørgensen NB, Bojsen-Møller KN, Kielgast U, et al. Changes in gastrointestinal hormone responses, insulin sensitivity, and beta-cell function within 2 weeks after gastric bypass in non-diabetic subjects. *Obes Surg.* (2012) 22:1084–96. doi: 10.1007/s11695-012-0621-4
47. Wang JL, Xu XH, Zhang XJ, Li WH. The role of obestatin in roux-en-Y gastric bypass-induced remission of type 2 diabetes mellitus. *Diabetes Metab Res Rev.* (2016) 32:470–7. doi: 10.1002/dmrr.2735
48. Adami GF, Gradaschi R, Andraghetti G, Scopinaro N, Cordera R. Serum leptin and adiponectin concentration in type 2 diabetes patients in the short and long term following Biliopancreatic diversion. *Obes Surg.* (2016) 26:2442–8. doi: 10.1007/s11695-016-2126-z
49. Malin SK, Bena J, Abood B, Pothier CE, Bhatt DL, Nissen S, et al. Attenuated improvements in adiponectin and fat loss characterize type 2 diabetes non-remission status after bariatric surgery. *Diabetes Obes Metab.* (2014) 16:1230–8. doi: 10.1111/dom.12376
50. Guo Y, Huang ZP, Liu CQ, Qi L, Sheng Y, Zou DJ. Modulation of the gut microbiome: a systematic review of the effect of bariatric surgery. *Eur J Endocrinol.* (2018) 178:43–56. doi: 10.1530/EJE-17-0403
51. Haluzík M, Kratochvílová H, Haluzíková D, Mráz M. Gut as an emerging organ for the treatment of diabetes: focus on mechanism of action of bariatric and endoscopic interventions. *J Endocrinol.* (2018) 237:R1–17. doi: 10.1530/JOE-17-0438
52. Jackness C, Karmally W, Febres G, Conwell IM, Ahmed L, Bessler M, et al. Very low-calorie diet mimics the early beneficial effect of Roux-en-Y gastric bypass on insulin sensitivity and beta-cell function in type 2 diabetic patients. *Diabetes.* (2013) 62:3027–32. doi: 10.2337/db12-1762
53. Rubino F, Forgione A, CummingsDE, Vix M, Gnuli D, Mingrone G, et al. The mechanism of diabetes control after gastrointestinal bypass surgery reveals a role of the proximal small intestine in the pathophysiology of type 2 diabetes. *Ann Surg.* (2006) 244:741–9. doi: 10.1097/01.sla.0000224726.61448.1b
54. Pournaras DJ, Glicksman C, Vincent RP, Kuganolipava S, Alaghband-Zadeh J, Mahon D, et al. The role of bile after Roux-en-Y gastric bypass in promoting weight loss and improving glycaemic control. *Endocrinology.* (2012) 153:3613–9. doi: 10.1210/en.2011-2145
55. Batterham RL, Cummings DE. Mechanisms of diabetes improvement following bariatric/metabolic surgery. *Diabetes Care.* (2016) 39:893–901. doi: 10.2337/dc16-0145
56. Jirapinyo P, Jin DX, Qazi T, Mishra N, Thompson CC. A meta-analysis of GLP-1 after Roux-en-Y gastric bypass: impact of surgical technique andmeasurement strategy. *Obes Surg.* (2018) 28:615–26. doi: 10.1007/s11695-017-2913-1
57. Svane MS, Bojsen-Møller KN, Nielsen S, Jørgensen NB, Dirksen C, Bendtsen, Fet al. Effects of endogenous GLP-1 and GIP on glucose tolerance after Roux-en-Y gastric bypass surgery. *Am J Physiol Endocrinol Metab.* (2016) 310:E505–14. doi: 10.1152/ajpendo.00471.2015
58. Mingrone G, Nolfe G, Gissey GC, Iaconelli A, Leccesi L, Guidone C, et al. Circadian rhythms of GIP and GLP1 in glucosetolerant and in type 2 diabetic patients after biliopancreatic diversion. *Diabetologia.* (2009) 52 873–81. doi: 10.1007/s00125-009-1288-9
59. Salinari S, Bertuzzi A, Asnaghi S, Guidone C, Manco M, Mingrone G. First-phase insulin secretion restoration and differential response to glucose load depending on the route of administration in type 2 diabetic subjects after bariatric surgery. *Diabetes Care.* (2009) 32:375–80. doi: 10.2337/dc08-1314
60. Oh TJ, Ahn CH, Cho YM. Contribution of the distal small intestine to metabolic improvement after bariatric/metabolic surgery: lessons from ileal transposition surgery. *J Diabetes Invest.* (2016) 7:94–101. doi: 10.1111/jdi.12444
61. Lo JC, Ljubicic S, Leibiger B, Kern M, Leibiger IB, Moede T, et al. Adipsin is an adipokine that improves β cell function in diabetes. *Cell.* (2014) 158:41–53. doi: 10.1016/j.cell.2014.06.005
62. Chronaiou A, Tsoli M, Kehagias I, Leotsinidis M, Kalfarentzos F, Alexandrides TK. Lower ghrelin levels and exaggerated postprandial peptide-YY, glucagon-like peptide-1, and insulin responses, after gastric fundus resection, in patients undergoing Roux-en-Y gastric bypass: a randomized clinical trial. *Obes Surg.* (2012) 22:1761–70. doi: 10.1007/s11695-012-0738-5
63. Still CD, Wood GC, Chu X, Erdman R, Manney CH, Benotti PN, et al. High allelic burden of four obesity SNPs is associated with poorer weight loss outcomes following gastric bypass surgery. *Obesity.* (2011):1676–83. doi: 10.1038/oby.2011.3
64. Flynn CR, Albaugh VL, Cai S, Cheung-Flynn J, Williams PE, Brucker RM, et al. Bile diversion to the distal small intestine has comparable metabolic benefits to bariatric surgery. *Nat Commun.* (2015) 6:7715. doi: 10.1038/ncomms8715
65. Shungin D, Winkler TW, Croteau-Chonka DC, Ferreira T, Locke AE, Mägi R, et al. New genetic loci link adipose and insulin biology to body fat distribution. *Nature.* (2015) 518:187–96. doi: 10.1038/nature14132
66. Kaska L, Sledzinski T, Chomiczewska A, Dettlaff-Pokora A, Swierczynski J. Improved glucose metabolism following bariatric surgery is associated with increased circulating bile acid concentrations and remodeling of the gut microbiome. *World J Gastroenterol.* (2016) 22:8698–719. doi: 10.3748/wjg.v22.i39.8698
67. Ryan KK, Tremaroli V, Clemmensen C, Kovatcheva-Datchary P, Myronovych A, Karns R, et al. FXR is a molecular target for the effects of vertical sleeve gastrectomy. *Nature.* (2014) 509:183–8. doi: 10.1038/nature13135
68. Schaap FG, Trauner M, Jansen PLM. Bile acid receptors as targets for drug development. *Nat Rev Gastroenterol Hepatol.* (2014) 11:55–67. doi: 10.1038/nrgastro.2013.151
69. Magouliotis DE, Tasiopoulou VS, Sioka E, Chatedaki C, Zacharoulis D. Impact of bariatric surgery on metabolic and gut microbiota profile: a systematic review and meta-analysis. *Obes Surg.* (2017) 27:1345–57. doi: 10.1007/s11695-017-2595-8
70. Graessler J, Qin Y, Zhong H, Zhang J, Licinio J, Wong M-L, et al. Metagenomic sequencing of the human gut microbiome before and after bariatric surgery in obese patients with type 2 diabetes: correlation with inflammatory and metabolic parameters. *Pharmacogenomics J.* (2013) 13:514–22. doi: 10.1038/tpj.2012.43
71. Zhang H, Di Baise JK, Zuccolo A, Kudrna D, Braidotti M, Yu Y, et al. Human gut microbiota in obesity and after gastric bypass. *Proc Natl Acad Sci USA.* (2009) 106:2365–70. doi: 10.1073/pnas.0812600106
72. Kong L-C, Tap J, Aron-Wisnewsky J, Pelloux V, Basdevant A, Bouillot J-L, et al. Gut microbiota after gastric bypass in human obesity: increased richness and associations of bacterial genera with adipose tissue genes. *Am J Clin Nutr.* (2013) 98:16–24. doi: 10.3945/ajcn.113.058743
73. Murphy R, Tsai P, Jüllig M, Liu A, Plank L, Booth M. Differential changes in gut microbiota after gastric bypass and sleeve gastrectomy bariatric surgery vary according to diabetes remission. *Obes Surg.* (2017) 27:917–25. doi: 10.1007/s11695-016-2399-2
74. Tabasi M, Ashrafian F, Khezerloo JK, Eshghjoo S, Behrouzi A, Javadinia SA, et al. Changes in gut microbiota and hormones after bariatric surgery: a bench-to-bedside review. *Obes Surg.* (2019) 29:1663–74. doi: 10.1007/s11695-019-03779-7
75. Palleja A, Kashani A, Allin KH, Nielsen T, Zhang C, Li Y, et al. Roux-en-Y gastric bypass surgery of morbidly obese patients induces swift and persistent changes of the individual gut microbiota. *Genome Med.* (2016) 8:67. doi: 10.1186/s13073-016-0312-1
76. Tremaroli V, Karlsson F, Werling M, Ståhlman M, Kovatcheva-Datchary P, Olbers T, et al. Roux-en-Y gastric bypass and vertical banded gastroplasty induce long-term changes on the human gut microbiome contributing to fat mass regulation. *Cell Metab.* (2015) 22:228–38. doi: 10.1016/j.cmet.2015.07.009
77. Ilhan ZE, DiBaise JK, Isern NG, Hoyt DW, Marcus AK, Kang D-W, et al. Distinctive microbiomes and metabolites linked with weight loss after gastric bypass, but not gastric banding. *ISME J.* (2017) 11:2047–58. doi: 10.1038/ismej.2017.71
78. Damms-Machado A, Mitra S, Schollenberger AE, Kramer KM, Meile T, Königsrainer A, et al. Effects of surgical and dietary weight loss therapy for obesity on gut microbiota composition and nutrient absorption. *Biomed Res Int.* (2015) 2015:806248. doi: 10.1155/2015/806248
79. Liu H, Hu C, Zhang X, Jia W. Role of gut microbiota, bile acids and their cross-talk in the effects of bariatric surgery on obesity and

type 2 diabetes. *J Diabetes Investig.* (2018) 9:13–20. doi: 10.1111/jdi.12687
80. Gutiérrez-Repiso C, Moreno-Indias I, de Hollanda A, Martín-Núñez GM, Vidal J, Tinahones FJ. Gut microbiota specific signatures are related to the successful rate of bariatric surgery. *Am J Transl Res.* (2019) 11:942–52. Available online at: http://www.ajtr.org/files/ajtr0085422.pdf
81. Furet J-P, Kong L-C, Tap J, Poitou C, Basdevant A, Bouillot J-L, et al. Differential adaptation of human gut microbiota to bariatric surgery-induced weight loss: links with metabolic and low-grade inflammation markers. *Diabetes.* (2010) 59:3049–57. doi: 10.2337/db10-0253
82. Clemente-Postigo M, Queipo-Ortuño MI, Murri M, Boto-Ordoñez M, Perez-Martinez P, Andres-Lacueva C, et al. Endotoxin increase after fat overload is related to postprandial hypertriglyceridemia in morbidly obese patients. *J Lipid Res.* (2012) 53:973–8. doi: 10.1194/jlr.P020909
83. Cani PD, Possemiers S, Van de Wiele T, Guiot Y, Everard A, Rottier O, et al. Changes in gut microbiota control inflammation in obese mice through a mechanism involving GLP-2-driven improvement of gut permeability. *Gut.* (2009) 58:1091–103. doi: 10.1136/gut.2008.165886
84. Clemente-Postigo M, Oliva-Olivera W, Coin-Aragüez L, Ramos-Molina B, Giraldez-Perez RM, Lhamyani S, et al. Metabolic endotoxemia promotes adipose dysfunction and inflammation in human obesity. *Am J Physiol Endocrinol Metab.* (2019) 316:E319–32. doi: 10.1152/ajpendo.00277.2018
85. Shin AC, Zheng H, Berthoud H-R. Vagal innervation of the hepatic portal vein and liver is not necessary for Roux-en-Y gastric bypass surgery-induced hypophagia, weight loss, and hypermetabolism. *Ann Surg.* (2012) 255:294–301. doi: 10.1097/SLA.0b013e31823e71b7
86. Kentish SJ, Page AJ. The role of gastrointestinal vagal afferent fibres in obesity. *J Physiol.* (2015) 593:775–86. doi: 10.1113/jphysiol.2014.278226
87. Blasi C. The role of the vagal nucleus tractus solitarius in the therapeutic effects of obesity surgery and other interventional therapies on type 2 diabetes. *Obes Surg.* (2016) 26:3045–57. doi: 10.1007/s11695-016-2419-2
88. Murphy KG, Bloom SR. Gut hormones and the regulation of energy homeostasis. *Nature.* (2006) 444:854–9. doi: 10.1038/nature05484
89. Badman MK, Flier JS. The gut and energy balance: visceral allies in the obesity wars. *Science.* (2005) 307:1909–14. doi: 10.1126/science.1109951
90. Kassir R, Barthelemy J-C, Roche F, Blanc P, Zufferey P, Galusca B, et al. Bariatric surgery associated with percutaneous auricular vagal stimulation: a new prospective treatment on weight loss. *Int J Surg Lond Engl.* (2015) 18:55–6. doi: 10.1016/j.ijsu.2015.04.033
91. Papasavas P, El Chaar M, Kothari SN, American Society for Metabolic and Bariatric Surgery Clinical Issues Committee. American Society for Metabolic and Bariatric Surgery position statement on vagal blocking therapy for obesity. *Surg Obes Relat Dis Off J Am Soc Bariatr Surg.* (2016) 12:460–1. doi: 10.1016/j.soard.2015.12.004
92. de Lartigue G, Diepenbroek C. Novel developments in vagal afferent nutrient sensing and its role in energy homeostasis. *Curr Opin Pharmacol.* (2016) 31:38–43. doi: 10.1016/j.coph.2016.08.007
93. Dixon JB, Lambert EA, Lambert GW. Neuroendocrine adaptations to bariatric surgery. *Mol Cell Endocrinol.* (2015) 418(Pt 2):143–52. doi: 10.1016/j.mce.2015.05.033
94. Stefanidis A, Oldfield BJ. Neuroendocrine mechanisms underlying bariatric surgery: insights from human studies and animal models. *J Neuroendocrinol.* (2017) 29:1–7. doi: 10.1111/jne.12534
95. Ballsmider LA, Vaughn AC, David M, Hajnal A, Di Lorenzo PM, Czaja K. Sleeve gastrectomy and Roux-en-Y gastric bypass alter the gut-brain communication. *Neural Plast.* (2015) 2015:601985. doi: 10.1155/2015/601985
96. Gautron L, Zechner JF, Aguirre V. Vagal innervation patterns following Roux-en-Y gastric bypass in the mouse. *Int J Obes 2005.* (2013) 37:1603–7. doi: 10.1038/ijo.2013.48
97. Stefanidis A, Forrest N, Brown WA, Dixon JB, O'Brien PB, Juliane Kampe null, et al. An investigation of the neural mechanisms underlying the efficacy of the adjustable gastric band. *Surg Obes Relat Dis Off J Am Soc Bariatr Surg.* (2016) 12:828–38. doi: 10.1016/j.soard.2015.11.020
98. Dixon AFR, Dixon JB, O'Brien PE. Laparoscopic adjustable gastric banding induces prolonged satiety: a randomized blind crossover study. *J Clin Endocrinol Metab.* (2005) 90:813–9. doi: 10.1210/jc.2004-1546
99. Björklund P, Laurenius A, Een E, Olbers T, Lönroth H, Fändriks L. Is the Roux limb a determinant for meal size after gastric bypass surgery? *Obes Surg.* (2010) 20:1408–14. doi: 10.1007/s11695-010-0192-1
100. Sundbom M, Holdstock C, Engström BE, Karlsson FA. Early changes in ghrelin following Roux-en-Y gastric bypass: influence of vagal nerve functionality? *Obes Surg.* (2007) 17:304–10. doi: 10.1007/s11695-007-9056-8
101. Tamboli RA, Antoun J, Sidani RM, Clements A, Harmata EE, Marks-Shulman P, et al. Metabolic responses to exogenous ghrelin in obesity and early after Roux-en-Y gastric bypass in humans. *Diabetes Obes Metab.* (2017) 19:1267–75. doi: 10.1111/dom.12952
102. Perathoner A, Weiss H, Santner W, Brandacher G, Laimer E, Höller E, et al. Vagal nerve dissection during pouch formation in laparoscopic Roux-Y-gastric bypass for technical simplification: does it matter? *Obes Surg.* (2009) 19:412–7. doi: 10.1007/s11695-008-9657-x
103. Ochner CN, Kwok Y, Conceição E, Pantazatos SP, Puma LM, Carnell S, et al. Selective reduction in neural responses to high calorie foods following gastric bypass surgery. *Ann Surg.* (2011) 253:502–7. doi: 10.1097/SLA.0b013e318203a289
104. Ten Kulve JS, Veltman DJ, Gerdes VEA, van Bloemendaal L, Barkhof F, Deacon CF, et al. Elevated postoperative endogenous GLP-1 levels mediate effects of Roux-en-Y gastric bypass on neural responsivity to food cues. *Diabetes Care.* (2017) 40:1522–9. doi: 10.2337/dc16-2113
105. Korner J, Inabnet W, Conwell IM, Taveras C, Daud A, Olivero-Rivera L, et al. Differential effects of gastric bypass and banding on circulating gut hormone and leptin levels. *Obesity.* (2006) 14:1553–61. doi: 10.1038/oby.2006.179
106. Kalinowski P, Paluszkiewicz R, Wróblewski T, Remiszewski P, Grodzicki M, Bartoszewicz Z, et al. Ghrelin, leptin, and glycemic control after sleeve gastrectomy versus Roux-en-Y gastric bypass-results of a randomized clinical trial. *Surg Obes Relat Dis Off J Am Soc Bariatr Surg.* (2017) 13:181–8. doi: 10.1016/j.soard.2016.08.025
107. DiGiorgi M, Rosen DJ, Choi JJ, Milone L, Schrope B, Olivero-Rivera L, et al. Re-emergence of diabetes after gastric bypass in patients with mid- to long-term follow-up. *Surg Obes Relat Dis.* (2010) 6:249–53. doi: 10.1016/j.soard.2009.09.019
108. Chikunguwo SM, Wolfe LG, Dodson P, Meador JG, Baugh N, Clore JN, et al. Analysis of factors associated with durable remission of diabetes after Roux-en-Y gastric bypass. *Surg Obes Relat Dis.* (2010) 6:254–9. doi: 10.1016/j.soard.2009.11.003
109. Mittempergher F, Pat G, Crea N, Di Betta E, Vilardi A, Chiesa D, et al. Preoperative prediction of Growth Hormone (GH)/Insulin-Like Growth Factor-1 (IGF-1) axis modification and postoperative changes in candidates for bariatric surgery. *Obes Surg.* (2013) 23:594–601. doi: 10.1007/s11695-012-0820-z
110. Camastra S, Manco M, Frascerra S, Iaconelli A, Mingrone G, Ferrannini F. Daylong pituitary hormones in morbid obesity: effects of bariatric surgery. *Int J Obes.* (2009) 33:166–72. doi: 10.1038/ijo.2008.226
111. De Marinis L, Bianchi A, Mancini A, Gentilella R, Perrelli M, Giampietro A, et al. Growth hormone secretion and leptin in morbid obesity before and after biliopancreatic diversion: relationships with insulin and body composition. *J Clin Endocrinol Metab.* (2004) 89:174–80. doi: 10.1210/jc.2002-021308
112. Mancini MC, Costa AP, deMelo M-E, Cercato C, Giannella-Neto D, Garrido AB Jr, et al. Effect of gastric bypass on spontaneous growth hormone and ghrelin release profiles. *Obesity.* (2006) 14:383–7. doi: 10.1038/oby.2006.51
113. Edén Engström B, Burman P, Holdstock C, Ohrvall M, Sundbom M, Karlsson FA. Effects of gastric bypass on the GH/IGF-I axis in severe obesity–and a comparison with GH deficiency. *Eur J Endocrinol.* (2006) 154:53–9. doi: 10.1530/eje.1.02069
114. Savastano S, Angrisani L, Di Somma C, Rota F, Savanelli MC, Cascella T, et al. Relationship between growth hormone/insulin-like growth factor-1 axis integrity and voluntary weight loss after gastric banding surgery for severe obesity. *Obes Surg.* (2010) 20:211–20. doi: 10.1007/s11695-009-9926-3
115. Di Somma C, Angrisani L, Rota F, Savanelli MC, Cascella T, Belfiore A, et al. GH and IGF-I deficiency are associated with reduced loss of fat mass after laparoscopic-adjustable silicone gastric banding. *Clin Endocrinol.* (2008) 69:393–9. doi: 10.1111/j.1365-2265.2008.03183.x
116. Manco M, Fernández-Real JM, Valera-Mora ME, Déchaud H, Nanni G, Tondolo V, et al. Massive weight loss decreases corticosteroid-binding

globulin levels and increases free cortisol in healthy obese patients: an adaptive phenomenon? *Diabetes Care.* (2007) 30:1494–500. doi: 10.2337/dc06-1353

117. Morrow J, Gluck M, Lorence M, Flancbaum L, Geliebter A. Night eating status and influence on body weight, body image, hunger, and cortisol pre- and post- Roux-en-Y Gastric Bypass (RYGB) surgery. *Eat Weight Disord.* (2008) 13:e96–9. doi: 10.1007/BF03327512
118. Larsen JK, van Ramshorst B, van Doornen LJ, Geenen R. Salivary cortisol and binge eating disorder in obese women after surgery for morbid obesity. *Int J Behav Med.* (2009) 16:311–5. doi: 10.1007/s12529-009-9036-6
119. Guldstrand M, Bo A, Wredling R, Backman L, Lins PE, Adamson U. Alteration of the counterregulatory responses to insulin-induced hypoglycemia and of cognitive function after massive weight reduction in severely obese subjects. *Metabolism.* (2003) 52:900–7. doi: 10.1016/S0026-0495(03)00103-3
120. Ruiz-Tovar J, Oller I, Galindo I, Llavero C, Arroyo A, Calero A, et al. Change in levels of C-reactive protein (CRP) and serum cortisol in morbidly obese patients after laparoscopic sleeve gastrectomy. *Obes Surg.* (2013) 23:764–9. doi: 10.1007/s11695-013-0865-7
121. Valentine AR, Raff H, Liu H, Ballesteros M, Rose JM, Jossart GH, et al. Salivary cortisol increases after bariatric surgery in women. *Hormone Metab Res.* (2011) 43:587–90. doi: 10.1055/s-0031-1279777
122. Hulme PA, McBride CL, Kupzyk KA, French JA. Pilot study on childhood sexual abuse, diurnal cortisol secretion, and weight loss in bariatric surgery patients. *J Child Sex Abus.* (2015) 24:385–400. doi: 10.1080/10538712.2015.1022293
123. Sarwer DB, Spitzer JC, Wadden TA, Mitchell JE, Lancaster K, Courcoulas A, et al. Changes in sexual functioning and sex hormone levels in women following bariatric surgery. *JAMA Surg.* (2014) 149:26–33. doi: 10.1001/jamasurg.2013.5022
124. Jamal M, Gunay Y, Capper A, Eid A, Heitshusen D, Samuel I. Roux-en-Y gastric bypass ameliorates polycystic ovary syndrome and dramatically improves conception rates: a 9-year analysis. *Surg Obes Relat Dis.* (2012) 8:440–4. doi: 10.1016/j.soard.2011.09.022
125. Eid GM, Cottam DR, Velcu LM, Mattar SG, Korytkowski MT, Gosman G, et al. Effective treatment of polycystic ovarian syndromewith Roux-en-Y gastric bypass. *Surg Obes Relat Dis.* (2005) 1:77–80. doi: 10.1016/j.soard.2005.02.008
126. George K, Azeez H. Resolution of gynaecological issues after bariatric surgery—a retrospective analysis. *Obes Surg.* (2013) 23:1043. doi: 10.1007/s11695-013-0986-z
127. Skubleny D, Switzer NJ, Gill RS, Dykstra M, Shi X, Sagle MA, et al. The impact of bariatric surgery on polycystic ovary syndrome: a systematic review and meta-analysis. *Obesity Surg.* (2016) 26:169–76. doi: 10.1007/s11695-015-1902-5
128. Shekelle PG, Newberry S, Maglione M, Li Z, Yermilov I, Hilton L, et al. Bariatric surgery in women of reproductive age: special concerns for pregnancy. *Evid Rep Technol Assess.* (2008) 1–51. Available online at: https://www.ncbi.nlm.nih.gov/books/NBK38559/
129. Reis LO, Favaro WJ, Barreiro GC, de Oliveira LC, Chaim EA, Fregonesi A, et al. Erectile dysfunction and hormonal imbalance in morbidly obese male is reversed after gastric bypass surgery: a prospective randomized controlled trial. *Int J Androl.* (2010) 33:736–44. doi: 10.1111/j.1365-2605.2009.01017.x
130. Mora M, Aranda GB, de Hollanda A, Flores L, Puig-Domingo M, Vidal J. Weight loss is a major contributor to improved sexual function after bariatric surgery. *Surg Endosc.* (2013) 27:3197–204. doi: 10.1007/s00464-013-2890-y
131. Sarwer DB, Spitzer JC, Wadden TA, Rosen RC, Mitchell JE, Lancaster K, et al. Sexual functioning and sex hormones in men who underwent bariatric surgery. *Surg Obes Relat Dis.* (2015) 11:643–51. doi: 10.1016/j.soard.2014.12.014
132. Facchiano E, Scaringi S, Veltri M, Samavat J, Maggi M, Forti G, et al. Age as a predictive factor of testosterone improvement in male patients after bariatric surgery: preliminary results of a monocentric prospective study. *Obes Surg.* (2013) 23:167–72. doi: 10.1007/s11695-012-0753-6
133. Luconi M, Samavat J, Seghieri G, Iannuzzi G, Lucchese M, Rotella C, et al. Determinants of testosterone recovery after bariatric surgery: is it only a matter of reduction of body mass index? *Fertil Steril.* (2013) 99:1872–9.e1. doi: 10.1016/j.fertnstert.2013.02.039
134. Aarts E, van Wageningen B, Loves S, Janssen I, Berends F, Sweep F, et al. Gonadal status and outcome of bariatric surgery in obese men. *Clin Endocrinol.* (2014) 81:378–86. doi: 10.1111/cen.12366
135. Samavat J, Facchiano E, Lucchese M, Forti G, Mannucci E, Maggi M, et al. Hypogonadism as an additional indication for bariatric surgery in male morbid obesity? *Eur J Endocrinol.* (2014) 171:555–60. doi: 10.1530/EJE-14-0596
136. Rasmussen MH. Obesity, growth hormone and weight loss. *Mol Cell Endocrinol.* (2010) 316:147–53. doi: 10.1016/j.mce.2009.08.017
137. Alvarez P, Isidro L, Leal-Cerro A, Casanueva FF, Dieguez, C Cordido F. Effect of withdrawal of somatostatin plus GH-releasing hormone stimulus of GH secretion in obesity. *Clin Endocrinol.* (2002) 56: 487–92. doi: 10.1046/j.1365-2265.2002.01487.x
138. Cordido F, Alvarez-Castro P, Isidro MI, Casanueva FF, Dieguez C. Comparison between insulin tolerance test, growth hormone releasing hormone (GHRH), GHRH plus acipimox and GHRH plus GH-releasing peptide-6 for the diagnosis of adult GH deficiency in normal subjects, obese and hypopituitary patients. *Eur J Endocrinol.* (2003) 149:117–22. doi: 10.1530/eje.0.1490117
139. Savastano S, Di Somma C, Barrea L, Colao A. The complex relationship between obesity and the somatropic axis: the long and winding road. *Growth Horm IGF Res.* (2014) 24:221–6. doi: 10.1016/j.ghir.2014.09.002
140. Park MJ, Kim HS, Kang JH, Kim DH, Chung CY. Serum levels of insulin-like growth factor (IGF)-I, free IGF-I, IGF binding (IGFBP)-1, IGFBP-3 and insulin in obese children. *J Pediatr Endocrinol Metab.* (1999) 12:139–44. doi: 10.1515/JPEM.1999.12.2.139
141. Ballerini MG, Ropelato MG, Domene HM, Pennisi P, Heinrich JJ, Jasper HG. Differential impact of simple childhood obesity on the components of the hormone-insulin-like growth factor (IGF)-IGF binding proteins axis. *J Pediatr Endocrinol Metab.* (2004) 17:749–57. doi: 10.1515/JPEM.2004.17.5.749
142. Attia N, Tamborlane WV, Heptulla R, Maggs D, Grozman A, Sherwin RS, et al. The metabolic syndrome and insulinlike growth factor I regulation in adult obesity. *J Clin Endocrinol Metab.* (1998) 83:1467–71. doi: 10.1210/jcem.83.5.4827
143. Street ME, Ziveri MA, Spaggiari C, Viani I, Volta C, Grzincich GL, et al. Inflammation is a modulator of the insulin-like growth factor (IGF)/IGF-binding protein system inducing reduced bioactivity of IGFs in cystic fibrosis. *Eur J Endocrinol.* (2006) 154:47–52. doi: 10.1530/eje.1.02064
144. Rasmussen MH, Juul A, Hilsted J. Effect of weight loss on free insulin-like growth factor-I in obese women with hyposomatotropism. *Obesity.* (2007) 15:879–86. doi: 10.1038/oby.2007.607
145. Johnsen SP, Hundborg HH, Sorensen HT, Schumacher H, Lichtinghagen R, Eschenfelder CC, et al. Insulin-like growth factor (IGF) I, -II, and IGF binding protein-3 and risk of ischemic stroke. *J Clin Endocrinol Metab.* (2005) 90: 5937–41. doi: 10.1210/jc.2004-2088
146. Maccario M, Grottoli S, Procopio M, Oleandri SE, Rossetto E, Gauna C, et al. The GH/IGF-I axis in obesity: influence of neuro-endocrine and metabolic factors. *Int J. Obes Relat Metab Disord.* (2000) 24:S96–9. doi: 10.1038/sj.ijo.0801289
147. Berryman DE, Gla CA, List EO, Johannsson G. The GH/IGF-1 axis in obesity: pathophysiology and therapeutic considerations, *Nat Rev Endocrinol.* (2013) 9:346–56. doi: 10.1038/nrendo.2013.64
148. Savastano S, Di Somma C, Belfiore A, Guida B, Orio F Jr, Rota F, et al. Growth hormone status in morbidly obese subjects and correlation with body composition. *J Endocrinol Invest.* (2006) 29:536–43. doi: 10.1007/BF03344144
149. Galli G, Pinchera A, Piaggi P, Fierabracci P, Giannetti M, Querci G, et al. Serum insulin-like growth factor-1 concentrations are reduced in severely obese women and raise after weight loss induced by laparoscopic adjustable gastric banding. *Obes Surg.* (2012) 22:1276–80. doi: 10.1007/s11695-012-0669-1
150. Maccario M, Tassone F, Gauna C, Oleandri SE, Aimaretti G, Procopio M, et al. Effects of short-term administration of low-dose rhGH on IGF-I levels

in obesity and Cushing's syndrome: indirect evaluation of the sensitivity to GH. *Eur J Endocrinol.* (2001) 144:251–6. doi: 10.1530/eje.0.1440251

151. Gianotti L, Pivetti S, Lanfranco F, Tassone F, Vittori E, Rossetto R, et al. Concomitant impairment of growth hormone secretion and peripheral sensitivity in obese patients with obstructive sleep apnoea syndrome. *J Clin Endocrinol Metab.* (2002) 87:5052–7. doi: 10.1210/jc.2001-011441
152. Buijs MM, Romijn JA, Burggraaf J, De Kam MI, Cohen AF, Frolich M, et al. Growth hormone blunts protein oxidation and promotes protein turnover to a similar extent in abdominally obese and normal-weight women. *J Clin Endocrinol Metab.* (2002) 87:5668–74. doi: 10.1210/jc.2002-020927
153. Biondi M, Picardi A. Psychological stress and neuroendocrine function in humans: the last two decades of research. *Psychother Psychosom.* (1999) 68:114–50. doi: 10.1159/000012323
154. Anagnostis P, Athyros VG, Tziomalos K, Karagiannis A, Mikhailidis DP. Clinical review: the pathogenetic role of cortisol in the metabolic syndrome: a hypothesis. *J Clin Endocrinol Metab.* (2009) 94:2692–701. doi: 10.1210/jc.2009-0370
155. Constantinopoulos P, Michalaki M, Kottorou A, Habeos I, Psyrogiannis A, Kalfarentzos F, et al. Cortisol in tissue and systemic level as a contributing factor to the development of metabolic syndrome in severely obese patients. *Eur J Endocrinol.* (2015) 172:69–78. doi: 10.1530/EJE-14-0626
156. Rosmond R, Holm G, Bjorntorp P. Food-induced cortisol secretion in relation to anthropometric, metabolic and haemodynamic variables in men. *Int J Obes Relat Metab Disord.* (2000) 24:416–22. doi: 10.1038/sj.ijo.0801173
157. Clow A. Cortisol as a biomarker of stress. *J Holist Healthc.* (2004) 1:10–14.
158. De Kloet ER. Hormones and the stressed brain. *Ann N YAcad Sci.* (2004) 1018:1–15. doi: 10.1196/annals.1296.001
159. Kumari M, Chandola T, Brunner E, Kivimaki M. A nonlinear relationship of generalized and central obesity with diurnal cortisol secretion in the Whitehall II study. *J Clin Endocr Metab.* (2010) 95:4415–23. doi: 10.1210/jc.2009-2105
160. Lasikiewicz N, Hendrickx H, Talbot D, Dye L. Exploration of basal diurnal salivary cortisol profiles in middle-aged adults: associations with sleep quality and metabolic parameters. *Psychoneuroendocrinology.* (2008) 33:143–51. doi: 10.1016/j.psyneuen.2007.10.013
161. De Kloet ER, Joels M, Holsboer F, Joëls M. Stress and the brain: from adaptation to disease. *Nat Rev Neurosci.* (2005) 6:463–75. doi: 10.1038/nrn1683
162. Kumari M, Shipley M, Stafford M, Kivimaki M. Association of diurnal patterns in salivary cortisol with all-cause and cardiovascular mortality: findings from the Whitehall II study. *J Clin Endocrinol Metab.* (2011) 96:1478–85. doi: 10.1210/jc.2010-2137
163. McEwen BS. The neurobiology of stress: from serendipity to clinical relevance. *Brain Res.* (2000) 886:172–89. doi: 10.1016/S0006-8993(00)02950-4
164. Dallman MF, Akana SF, Strack AM, Hanson ES, Sebastian RJ. The neural network that regulates energy balance is responsive to glucocorticoids and insulin and also regulates HPA axis responsivity at a site proximal to CRF neurons. *Ann N Y Acad Sci.* (1995) 771:730–42. doi: 10.1111/j.1749-6632.1995.tb44724.x
165. Jayo JM, Shively CA, Kaplan JR, Manuck SB. Effects of exercise and stress on body fat distribution in male cynomolgus monkeys. *Int J Obes Relat Metab Disord.* (1993) 17:597–604.
166. BjÖrntorp P, Rosmond R. Neuroendocrine abnormalities in visceral obesity. *Int J Obes Relat Metab Disord.* (2000) 24(Suppl. 2):S80–5. doi: 10.1038/sj.ijo.0801285
167. Reinehr T, Kulle A, Wolters B, Knop C, Lass N, Welzel M, et al. Relationships between 24-hour urinary free cortisol concentrations and metabolic syndrome in obese children. *J Clin Endocrinol Metab.* (2014) 99:2391–9. doi: 10.1210/jc.2013-4398
168. Geliebter A. Night-eating syndrome in obesity. *Nutrition.* (2001) 17:483–4. doi: 10.1016/S0899-9007(01)00550-0
169. Coutinho WF, Moreira RO, Spagnol C, Appolinario JC. Does binge eating disorder alter cortisol secretion in obese women? *Eat Behav.* (2007) 8:59–64. doi: 10.1016/j.eatbeh.2006.01.002
170. Monteleone P, Luisi M, De Filippis G, Colurcio B, Genazzani AR, Maj M. Circulating levels of neuroactive steroids in patients with binge eating disorder: a comparison with nonobese healthy controls and nonbinge eating obese subjects. *Int J Eat Disord.* (2003) 34:432–40. doi: 10.1002/eat.10199
171. Gluck ME, Geliebter A, Hung J, Yahav E. Cortisol, hunger, and desire to binge eat following a cold stress test in obese women with binge eating disorder. *Psychosom Med.* (2004) 66:876–81. doi: 10.1097/01.psy.0000143637.63508.47
172. Yanovski SZ. Binge eating disorder: current knowledge and future directions. *Obes Res.* (1993) 1:306–24. doi: 10.1002/j.1550-8528.1993.tb00626.x
173. Reinher T, Andler W. Cortisol and its relation to insulin resistance before and after weight loss in obese children. *Horm Res.* (2004) 62:107–12. doi: 10.1159/000079841
174. Flak JN, Jankord R, Solomon MB, Krause EG, Herman JP. Opposing effects of chronic stress and weight restriction on cardiovascular, neuroendocrine and metabolic function. *Physiol Behav.* (2011) 104:228–34. doi: 10.1016/j.physbeh.2011.03.002
175. Pankevich DE, Teegarden SL, Hedin AD, Jensen CL, Bale TL. Caloric restriction experience reprograms stress and orexigenic pathways and promotes binge eating. *J Neurosci.* (2010) 30:16399–407. doi: 10.1523/JNEUROSCI.1955-10.2010
176. Ulrich-Lai YM, Ryan KK. Neuroendocrine circuits governing energy balance and stress regulation: functional overlap and therapeutic implications. *Cell Metab.* (2014) 19:910–25. doi: 10.1016/j.cmet.2014.01.020
177. Witbracht MG, Laugero KD, Van Loan MD, Adams SH, Keim NL. Performance on the Iowa Gambling Task is related to magnitude of weight loss and salivary cortisol in a diet-induced weight loss intervention in overweight women. *Physiol Behav.* (2012) 106:291–7. doi: 10.1016/j.physbeh.2011.04.035
178. Tomiyama AJ, Mann T, Vinas D, Hunger JM, Dejager J, Taylor SE. Low calorie dieting increases cortisol. *Psychosom Med.* (2010) 72:357–64. doi: 10.1097/PSY.0b013e3181d9523c
179. Goodwin GM, Fairburn CG, Keenan JC, Cowen PJ. The effects of dieting and weight loss upon the stimulation of thyrotropin (TSH) by thyrotropin-releasing hormone (TRH) and suppression of cortisol secretion by dexamethasone in men and women. *J Affect Disord.* (1988) 14:137–44. doi: 10.1016/0165-0327(88)90056-0
180. Nguyen NT, Goldman CD, Ho HS, Gosselin RC, Singh A, Wolfe BM. Systemic stress response after laparoscopic and open gastric bypass. *J Am Coll Surg.* (2002) 194:557–66. doi: 10.1016/S1072-7515(02)01132-8
181. Quaroni A, Tian JQ, Goke M, Podolsky DK. Glucocorticoids have pleiotropic effects on small intestinal crypt cells. *Am J Physiol.* (1999) 277:G1027–40. doi: 10.1152/ajpgi.1999.277.5.G1027
182. Pasquali R. Obesity, fat distribution and infertility. *Maturitas.* (2006) 54:363–71. doi: 10.1016/j.maturitas.2006.04.018
183. Rosen RC, Wing RR, Schneider S, Wadden TA, Foster GD, West DS, et al. Erectile dysfunction in type 2 diabetic men: relationship to exercise fitness and cardiovascular risk factors in the Look AHEAD trial. *J Sex Med.* (2009) 6:1414–22. doi: 10.1111/j.1743-6109.2008.01209.x
184. De Berardis G, Franciosi M, Belfiglio M, Di Nardo B, Greenfield S, Kaplan SH, et al. Erectile dysfunction and quality of life in type 2 diabetic patients: a serious problem too often overlooked. *Diabetes Care.* (2002) 25:284–91. doi: 10.2337/diacare.25.2.284
185. Duncan LE, Lewis C, Jenkins P, Pearson TA. Does hypertension and its pharmacotherapy affect the quality of sexual function in women? *Am J Hypertens.* (2000) 13:640–7. doi: 10.1016/S0895-7061(99)00288-5
186. Grimm RH Jr, Grandits GA, Prineas RJ, McDonald RH, Lewis CE, Flack JM, et al. Long-term effects on sexual function of five antihypertensive drugs and nutritional hygienic treatment in hypertensive men and women. Treatment of Mild Hypertension Study (TOMHS). *Hypertension.* (1997) 29:8–14. doi: 10.1161/01.HYP.29.1.8
187. Dallal RM, Chernoff A, O'Leary MP, Smith JA, Braverman JD, Quebbemann BB. Sexual dysfunction is common in the morbidly obese male and improves after gastric bypass surgery. *J Am Coll Surg.* (2008) 207:859–64. doi: 10.1016/j.jamcollsurg.2008.08.006
188. Kirschner MA, Samojlik E. Sex hormone metabolism in upper and lower body obesity. *Int J Obes.* (1991) 15:101–8.
189. Moore RH, Sarwer DB, Lavenberg J, Lane IB, Evans JL, Volger S, et al. Relationship between sexual function and quality of life in persons seeking weight reduction. *Obesity.* (2013) 21:1966–74. doi: 10.1002/oby.20398

190. Steffen KJ, King WC, White GE, Subak LL, Mitchell JE, Courcoulas AP, et al. Sexual functioning of men and women with severe obesity before bariatric surgery. *Surg Obes Relat Dis.* (2017) 13:334–43. doi: 10.1016/j.soard.2016.09.022
191. Escobar-Morreale HF, Santacruz E, Luque-Ramírez M, Botella Carretero JI. Prevalence of "obesity-associated gonadal dysfunction" in severely obese men and women and its resolution after bariatric surgery: a systematic review and meta-analysis. *Hum Reprod Update.* (2017) 23:390–408. doi: 10.1093/humupd/dmx012
192. Sarwer DB, Spitzer JC, Wadden TA, Rosen RC, Mitchell JE, Lancaster K, et al. Sexual functioning and sex hormones in persons with extreme obesity and seeking surgical and nonsurgical weight loss. *Surg Obes Relat Dis.* (2013) 9:997–1007. doi: 10.1016/j.soard.2013.07.003
193. Corona G, Rastrelli G, Monami M, Saad F, Luconi M, Lucchese M, et al. Body weight loss reverts obesity-associated hypogonadotropic hypogonadism: a systematic review and meta-analysis. *Eur J Endocrinol.* (2013) 168:829–43. doi: 10.1530/EJE-12-0955
194. Bond DS, Wing RR, Vithiananthan S, Sax HC, Roye GD, Ryder BA, et al. Significant resolution of female sexual dysfunction after bariatric surgery. *Surg Obes Relat Dis.* (2011) 7:1–7. doi: 10.1016/j.soard.2010.05.015
195. Pellitero S, Olaizola I, Alastrue A, Martínez E, Granada ML, Balibrea JM, et al. Hypogonadotropic hypogonadism in morbidly obese males is reversed after bariatric surgery. *Obes Surg.* (2012) 22:1835–42. doi: 10.1007/s11695-012-0734-9
196. Saboor Aftab SA, Kumar S, Barber TM. The role of obesity and type 2 diabetes mellitus in the development of male obesity-associated secondary hypogonadism. *Clin Endocrinol.* (2013) 78:330–7. doi: 10.1111/cen.12092
197. Nelson LR, Bulun SE. Estrogen production and action. *J Am Acad Dermatol.* (2001) 45:S116–24. doi: 10.1067/mjd.2001.117432
198. Escobar-Morreale HF, Botella-Carretero JI, Alvarez-Blasco F, Sancho J, San Millan JL.The polycystic ovary syndrome associated with morbid obesity may resolve after weight loss induced by bariatric surgery. *J Clin Endocrinol Metab.* (2005) 90:6364–9. doi: 10.1210/jc.2005-1490
199. Escobar-Morreale HF, San Millan JL. Abdominal adiposity and the polycystic ovary syndrome. *Trends Endocrinol Metab.* (2007) 18:266–72. doi: 10.1016/j.tem.2007.07.003
200. Pasquali R, Diamanti-Kandarakis E, Gambineri A. Secondary polycystic ovary syndrome: theoretical and practical aspects. *Eur J Endocrinol.* (2016) 175:R157–69. doi: 10.1530/EJE-16-0374
201. Wing RR, Bond DS, Gendrano IN III, Wadden T, Bahnson J, Lewis CE, et al. Sexual Dysfunction Subgroup of the Look AHEAD Research Group. Effect of intensive lifestyle intervention on sexual dysfunction in women with type 2 diabetes: results from an ancillary Look AHEAD study. *Diabetes Care.* (2013) 36:2937–44. doi: 10.2337/dc13-0315
202. Reis LO, Zani EL, Saad RD, Chaim EA, de Oliveira LC, Fregonesi A. Bariatric surgery does not interfere with sperm quality–a preliminary long-term study. *Reprod Sci.* (2012) 19:1057–62. doi: 10.1177/1933719112440747
203. Kaukua J, Pekkarinen T, Sane T, Mustajoki P. Sex hormones and sexual function in obese men losing weight. *Obes Res.* (2003) 11:689–94. doi: 10.1038/oby.2003.98
204. Butterworth J, Deguara J, Borg CM. Bariatric surgery, polycystic ovary syndrome, and infertility. *J Obes.* (2016) 2016:1871594. doi: 10.1155/2016/1871594
205. Balen AH, Morley LC, Misso M, Franks S, Legro RS, Wijeyaratne CN, et al. The management of anovulatory infertility in women with polycystic ovary syndrome: an analysis of the evidence to support the development of global WHO guidance. *Hum Reprod Update.* (2016) 22:687–708. doi: 10.1093/humupd/dmw025
206. Bonomi M, Vezzoli V, Krausz C, Guizzardi F, Vezzani S, Simoni M, et al. Characteristics of a nationwide cohort of patients presenting with isolated hypogonadotropic hypogonadism (IHH). *Eur J Endocrinol.* (2018) 178:23–32. doi: 10.1530/EJE-17-0065
207. Rao SR, Kini S, Tamler R. Sex hormones and bariatric surgery in men. *Gend Med.* (2011) 8:300–11. doi: 10.1016/j.genm.2011.05.007
208. Tajar A, Forti G, O'Neill TW, Lee DM, Silman AJ, Finn JD, et al. Characteristics of secondary, primary, and compensated hypogonadism in aging men: evidence from the European Male Ageing Study. *J ClinEndocrinol Metab.* (2010) 95:1810–8. doi: 10.1210/jc.2009-1796
209. Hofstra J, Loves S, van Wageningen B, Ruinemans-Koerts J, Jansen I, de Boer H. High prevalence of hypogonadotropic hypogonadism in men referred for obesity treatment. *Neth J Med.* (2008) 66:103–109. Available online at: http://www.njmonline.nl/getpdf.php?id=637
210. Vermeulen A, Kaufman JM, Deslypere JP, Thomas G. Attenuated luteinizing hormone (LH) pulse amplitude but normal LH pulse frequency, and its relation to plasma androgens in hypogonadism of obese men. *J Clin Endocrinol Metab.* (1993) 76:1140–6. doi: 10.1210/jcem.76.5.8496304
211. Landry D, Cloutier F, Martin LJ. Implications of leptin in neuroendocrine regulation of male reproduction. *Reprod Biol.* (2013) 13:1–14. doi: 10.1016/j.repbio.2012.12.001
212. Bruning JC, Gautam D, Burks DJ, Gillette J, Schubert M, Orban PC, et al. Role of brain insulin receptor in control of body weight and reproduction. *Science.* (2000) 289:2122–5. doi: 10.1126/science.289.5487.2122
213. Simo R, Saez-Lopez C, Barbosa-Desongles A, Hernandez C, Selva DM. Novel insights in SHBG regulation and clinical implications. *Trends Endocrinol Metab.* (2015) 26:376–83. doi: 10.1016/j.tem.2015.05.001
214. Luboshitzky R, Aviv A, Hefetz A, Herer P, Shen-Orr Z, Lavie L, et al. Decreased pituitary-gonadal secretion in men with obstructive sleep apnea. *J Clin Endocrinol Metab.* (2002) 87:3394–8. doi: 10.1210/jc.87.7.3394
215. Michalakis K, Mintziori G, Kaprara A, Tarlatzis BC, Goulis DG. The complex interaction between obesity, metabolic syndrome and reproductive axis: a narrative review. *Metabolism.* (2013) 62:457–78. doi: 10.1016/j.metabol.2012.08.012
216. Burcelin R, Thorens B, Glauser M, Gaillard RC, Pralong FP. Gonadotropin-releasing hormone secretion from hypothalamic neurons: stimulation by insulin and potentiation by leptin. *Endocrinology.* (2003) 144:4484–91. doi: 10.1210/en.2003-0457
217. Dandona P, Dhindsa S. Update: hypogonadotropic hypogonadism in type 2 diabetes and obesity. *J Clin Endocrinol Metab.* (2011) 96: 2643–51. doi: 10.1210/jc.2010-2724
218. Escobar-Morreale HF, Alvarez-Blasco F, Botella-Carretero JI, Luque-Ramirez M. The striking similarities in the metabolic associations of female androgen excess and male androgen deficiency. *Hum Reprod.* (2014) 29:2083–91. doi: 10.1093/humrep/deu198
219. Lazaros L, Hatzi E, Markoula S, Takenaka A, Sofikitis N, Zikopoulos K, et al. Dramatic reduction in sperm parameters following bariatric surgery: report of two cases. *Andrologia.* (2012) 44:428–32. doi: 10.1111/j.1439-0272.2012.01300.x
220. Sermondade N, Massin N, Boitrelle F, Pfeffer J, Eustache F, Sifer C, et al. Sperm parameters and male fertility after bariatric surgery: three case series. *Reprod Biomed Online.* (2012) 24:206–10. doi: 10.1016/j.rbmo.2011.10.014
221. Legro RS, Kunselman AR, Meadows JW, Kesner JS, Krieg EF, Rogers AM, et al. Time-related increase in urinary testosterone levels and stable semen analysis parameters after bariatric surgery in men. *Reprod Biomed Online.* (2015) 30:150–6. doi: 10.1016/j.rbmo.2014.10.014
222. El Bardisi H, Majzoub A, Arafa M, AlMalki A, Al Said S, Khalafalla K, et al. Effect of bariatric surgery on semen parameters and sex hormone concentrations: a prospective study. *Reprod Biomed Online.* (2016) 33:606–11. doi: 10.1016/j.rbmo.2016.08.008
223. Hammoud A, Gibson M, Hunt SC, Adams TD, Carrell DT, Kolotkin RL, et al. Effect of Roux-en-Y gastric bypass surgery on the sex steroids and quality of life in obese men. *J Clin Endocrinol Metab.* (2009) 94:1329–32. doi: 10.1210/jc.2008-1598
224. Hammoud AO, Gibson M, Peterson CM, Meikle AW, Carrell DT. Impact of male obesity on infertility: a critical review of the current literature. *Fertil Steril.* (2008) 90:897–904. doi: 10.1016/j.fertnstert.2008.08.026
225. Leenen R, van der Kooy K, Seidell JC, Deurenberg P, Koppeschaar HP. Visceral fat accumulation in relation to sex hormones in obese men and women undergoing weight loss therapy. *J Clin Endocrinol Metab.* (1994) 78:1515–20. doi: 10.1210/jcem.78.6.8200956
226. Rosenblatt A, Faintuch J, Cecconello I. Sexual hormones and erectile function more than 6 years after bariatric surgery. *Surg Obes Relat Dis.* (2013) 9: 636–40. doi: 10.1016/j.soard.2012.06.010
227. Oury F, Sumara G, Sumara O, Ferron M, Chang H, Smith CE, et al. Endocrine regulation of male fertility by the skeleton. *Cell.* (2011) 144: 796–809. doi: 10.1016/j.cell.2011.02.004

228. Smith LB, Saunders PT. The skeleton: the new controller of male fertility? *Cell.* (2011) 144: 642–3. doi: 10.1016/j.cell.2011.02.028
229. Kirmani S, Atkinson EJ, Melton LJ III, Riggs BL, Amin S, Khosla S. Relationship of testosterone and osteocalcin levels during growth. *J Bone Miner Res.* (2011) 26:2212–6. doi: 10.1002/jbmr.421
230. Bolland MJ, Grey A, Horne AM, Reid IR. Testosterone levels following decreases in serum osteocalcin. *Calcif Tissue Int.* (2013) 93: 133–6. doi: 10.1007/s00223-013-9730-x
231. Hannemann A, Breer S, Wallaschofski H, Nauck M, Baumeister SE, Barvencik F, et al. Osteocalcin is associated with testosterone in the general population and selected patients with bone disorders. *Andrology.* (2013) 1:469–74. doi: 10.1111/j.2047-2927.2012.00044.x
232. Foresta C, Strapazzon G, De Toni L, Gianesello L, Calcagno A, Pilon C, et al. Evidence for osteocalcin production by adipose tissue and its role in human metabolism. *J Clin Endocrinol Metab.* (2010) 95: 3502–6. doi: 10.1210/jc.2009-2557
233. Kim SH, Lee JW, Im JA, Hwang HJ. Serum osteocalcin is related to abdominal obesity in Korean obese and overweight men. *Clin Chim Acta.* (2010) 411:2054–7. doi: 10.1016/j.cca.2010.08.046
234. Samavat J, Facchiano E, Cantini G, Di Franco A, Alpigiano G, Poli G, et al. Osteocalcin increase after bariatric surgery predicts androgen recovery in hypogonadal obese males. *Int J Obes.* (2014) 38:357–63. doi: 10.1038/ijo.2013.228
235. Oury F, Ferron M, Huizhen W, Confavreux C, Xu L, Lacombe J, et al. Osteocalcin regulates murine and human fertility through a pancreas-bone-testis axis. *J Clin Invest.* (2013) 123:2421–33. doi: 10.1172/JCI65952
236. Rastrelli G, Carter EL, Ahern T, Finn JD, Antonio L, O'Neill TW, et al. Development of and recovery from secondary hypogonadism in aging men: prospective results from the EMAS. *J Clin Endocrinol Metab.* (2015) 100:3172–82. doi: 10.1210/jc.2015-1571
237. Hoeger KM. Role of lifestyle modification in the management of polycystic ovary syndrome. *Best Pract Res Clin Endocrinol Metab.* (2006) 20:293–310. doi: 10.1016/j.beem.2006.03.008
238. Clemente-Postigo M, Muñoz-Garach A, Serrano M, Garrido-Sánchez L, Bernal-López MR, Fernández-García D, et al. Serum 25-hydroxyvitamin D and adipose tissue vitamin D receptor gene expression: relationship with obesity and type 2 diabetes. *J Clin Endocrinol Metab.* (2015) 100:E591–5. doi: 10.1210/jc.2014-3016
239. Hamoui N, Kim K, Anthone G, Crookes PF. The significance of elevated levels of parathyroid hormone in patients with morbid obesity before and after bariatric surgery. *Arch Surg Chic Ill. 1960.* (2003) 138:891–7. doi: 10.1001/archsurg.138.8.891
240. Gómez-Ambrosi J, Rodríguez A, Catalán V, Frühbeck G. The bone-adipose axis in obesity and weight loss. *Obes Surg.* (2008) 18:1134–43. doi: 10.1007/s11695-008-9548-1
241. Folli F, Sabowitz BN, Schwesinger W, Fanti P, Guardado-Mendoza R, Muscogiuri G. Bariatric surgery and bone disease: from clinical perspective to molecular insights. *Int J Obes. 2005.* (2012) 36:1373–9. doi: 10.1038/ijo.2012.115
242. Gómez JM, Vilarrasa N, Masdevall C, Pujol J, Solano E, Soler J, et al. Regulation of bone mineral density in morbidly obese women: a cross-sectional study in two cohorts before and after bypass surgery. *Obes Surg.* (2009) 19:345–50. doi: 10.1007/s11695-008-9529-4
243. Corbeels K, Verlinden L, Lannoo M, Simoens C, Matthys C, Verstuyf A, et al. Thin bones: Vitamin D and calcium handling after bariatric surgery. *Bone Rep.* (2018) 8:57–63. doi: 10.1016/j.bonr.2018.02.002
244. Stein EM, Silverberg SJ. Bone loss after bariatric surgery: causes, consequences, and management. *Lancet Diabetes Endocrinol.* (2014) 2:165–74. doi: 10.1016/S2213-8587(13)70183-9
245. Ben-Porat T, Elazary R, Sherf-Dagan S, Goldenshluger A, Brodie R, Mintz Y, et al. Bone Health following Bariatric Surgery: implications for management strategies to attenuate bone loss. *Adv Nutr Bethesda Md.* (2018) 9:114–27. doi: 10.1093/advances/nmx024
246. Schafer AL, Kazakia GJ, Vittinghoff E, Stewart L, Rogers SJ, Kim TY, et al. Effects of gastric bypass surgery on bone mass and microarchitecture occur early and particularly impact postmenopausal women. *J Bone Miner Res Off J Am Soc Bone Miner Res.* (2018) 33:975–86. doi: 10.1002/jbmr.3371
247. Casagrande DS, Repetto G, Mottin CC, Shah J, Pietrobon R, Worni M, et al. Changes in bone mineral density in women following 1-year gastric bypass surgery. *Obes Surg.* (2012) 22:1287–92. doi: 10.1007/s11695-012-0687-z
248. Carrasco F, Ruz M, Rojas P, Csendes A, Rebolledo A, Codoceo J, et al. Changes in bone mineral density, body composition and adiponectin levels in morbidly obese patients after bariatric surgery. *Obes Surg.* (2009) 19:41–6. doi: 10.1007/s11695-008-9638-0
249. Mahdy T, Atia S, Farid M, Adulatif A. Effect of Roux-en Y gastric bypass on bone metabolism in patients with morbid obesity: mansoura experiences. *Obes Surg.* (2008) 18:1526–31. doi: 10.1007/s11695-008-9653-1
250. Vilarrasa N, Gómez JM, Elio I, Gómez-Vaquero C, Masdevall C, Pujol J, et al. Evaluation of bone disease in morbidly obese women after gastric bypass and risk factors implicated in bone loss. *Obes Surg.* (2009) 19:860–6. doi: 10.1007/s11695-009-9843-5
251. Fleischer J, Stein EM, Bessler M, Della Badia M, Restuccia N, Olivero-Rivera L, et al. The decline in hip bone density after gastric bypass surgery is associated with extent of weight loss. *J Clin Endocrinol Metab.* (2008) 93:3735–40. doi: 10.1210/jc.2008-0481
252. Shanbhogue VV, Støving RK, Frederiksen KH, Hanson S, Brixen K, Gram J, et al. Bone structural changes after gastric bypass surgery evaluated by HR-pQCT: a two-year longitudinal study. *Eur J Endocrinol.* (2017) 176:685–93. doi: 10.1530/EJE-17-0014
253. Rousseau C, Jean S, Gamache P, Lebel S, Mac-Way F, Biertho L, et al. Change in fracture risk and fracture pattern after bariatric surgery: nested case-control study. *BMJ.* (2016) 354:i3794. doi: 10.1136/bmj.i3794
254. Vilarrasa N, de Gordejuela AGR, Gómez-Vaquero C, Pujol J, Elio I, San José P, et al. Effect of bariatric surgery on bone mineral density: comparison of gastric bypass and sleeve gastrectomy. *Obes Surg.* (2013) 23:2086–91. doi: 10.1007/s11695-013-1016-x
255. Elias E, Casselbrant A, Werling M, Abegg K, Vincent RP, Alaghband-Zadeh J, et al. Bone mineral density and expression of vitamin D receptor-dependent calcium uptake mechanisms in the proximal small intestine after bariatric surgery. *Br J Surg.* (2014) 101:1566–75. doi: 10.1002/bjs.9626
256. Raoof M, Näslund I, Rask E, Szabo E. Effect of gastric bypass on bone mineral density, parathyroid hormone and vitamin D: 5 years follow-up. *Obes Surg.* (2016) 26:1141–5. doi: 10.1007/s11695-016-2114-3
257. Compston JE, Vedi S, Gianetta E, Watson G, Civalleri D, Scopinaro N. Bone histomorphometry and vitamin D status after biliopancreatic bypass for obesity. *Gastroenterology.* (1984) 87:350–6. doi: 10.1016/0016-5085(84)90712-1
258. Tsiftsis DDA, Mylonas P, Mead N, Kalfarentzos F, Alexandrides TK. Bone mass decreases in morbidly obese women after long limb-biliopancreatic diversion and marked weight loss without secondary hyperparathyroidism. A physiological adaptation to weight loss? *Obes Surg.* (2009) 19:1497–503. doi: 10.1007/s11695-009-9938-z
259. Marceau P, Biron S, Lebel S, Marceau S, Hould FS, Simard S, et al. Does bone change after biliopancreatic diversion? *J Gastrointest Surg Off J Soc Surg Aliment Tract.* (2002) 6:690–8. doi: 10.1016/S1091-255X(01)00086-5
260. Nogués X, Goday A, Peña MJ, Benaiges D, de Ramón M, Crous X, et al. [Bone mass loss after sleeve gastrectomy: a prospective comparative study with gastric bypass]. *Cirugia Espanola.* (2010) 88:103–9. doi: 10.1016/S2173-5077(10)70015-6
261. Ivaska KK, Huovinen V, Soinio M, Hannukainen JC, Saunavaara V, Salminen P, et al. Changes in bone metabolism after bariatric surgery by gastric bypass or sleeve gastrectomy. *Bone.* (2017) 95:47–54. doi: 10.1016/j.bone.2016.11.001
262. Carrasco F, Basfi-Fer K, Rojas P, Valencia A, Csendes A, Codoceo J, et al. Changes in bone mineral density after sleeve gastrectomy or gastric bypass: relationships with variations in vitamin D, ghrelin, and adiponectin levels. *Obes Surg.* (2014) 24:877–84. doi: 10.1007/s11695-014-1179-0
263. Bredella MA, Greenblatt LB, Eajazi A, Torriani M, Yu EW. Effects of Roux-en-Y gastric bypass and sleeve gastrectomy on bone mineral density and marrow adipose tissue. *Bone.* (2017) 95:85–90. doi: 10.1016/j.bone.2016.11.014
264. Pluskiewicz W, BuŽga M, Holéczy P, Bortlík L, Šmajstrla V, Adamczyk P. Bone mineral changes in spine and proximal femur in individual obese

women after laparoscopic sleeve gastrectomy: a short-term study. *Obes Surg.* (2012) 22:1068–76. doi: 10.1007/s11695-012-0654-8
265. Pugnale N, Giusti V, Suter M, Zysset E, Héraïef E, Gaillard RC, et al. Bone metabolism and risk of secondary hyperparathyroidism 12 months after gastric banding in obese pre-menopausal women. *Int J Obes Relat Metab Disord J Int Assoc Study Obes.* (2003) 27:110–6. doi: 10.1038/sj.ijo.0802177
266. Giusti V, Gasteyger C, Suter M, Heraief E, Gaillard RC, Burckhardt P. Gastric banding induces negative bone remodelling in the absence of secondary hyperparathyroidism: potential role of serum C telopeptides for follow-up. *Int J Obes 2005.* (2005) 29:1429–35. doi: 10.1038/sj.ijo.0803040
267. Dixon JB, Strauss BJG, Laurie C, O'Brien PE. Changes in body composition with weight loss: obese subjects randomized to surgical and medical programs. *Obes Silver Spring Md.* (2007) 15:1187–98. doi: 10.1038/oby.2007.639
268. von Mach M-A, Stoeckli R, Bilz S, Kraenzlin M, Langer I, Keller U. Changes in bone mineral content after surgical treatment of morbid obesity. *Metabolism.* (2004) 53:918–21. doi: 10.1016/j.metabol.2004.01.015
269. Scibora LM, Ikramuddin S, Buchwald H, Petit MA. Examining the link between bariatric surgery, bone loss, and osteoporosis: a review of bone density studies. *Obes Surg.* (2012) 22:654–67. doi: 10.1007/s11695-012-0596-1
270. Lalmohamed A, de Vries F, Bazelier MT, Cooper A, van Staa T-P, Cooper C, et al. Risk of fracture after bariatric surgery in the United Kingdom: population based, retrospective cohort study. *BMJ.* (2012) 345:e5085. doi: 10.1136/bmj.e5085
271. Nakamura KM, Haglind EGC, Clowes JA, Achenbach SJ, Atkinson EJ, Melton LJ, et al. Fracture risk following bariatric surgery: a population-based study. *Osteoporos Int..* (2014) 25:151–8. doi: 10.1007/s00198-013-2463-x
272. Axelsson KF, Werling M, Eliasson B, Szabo E, Näslund I, Wedel H, et al. Fracture risk after gastric bypass surgery: a retrospective cohort study. *J Bone Miner Res.* (2018) 33:2122–31. doi: 10.1002/jbmr.3553
273. Lu C-W, Chang Y-K, Chang H-H, Kuo C-S, Huang C-T, Hsu C-C, et al. Fracture risk after bariatric surgery: a 12-year nationwide cohort study. *Medicine.* (2015) 94:e2087. doi: 10.1097/MD.0000000000002087
274. Zhang Q, Chen Y, Li J, Chen D, Cheng Z, Xu S, et al. A meta-analysis of the effects of bariatric surgery on fracture risk. *Obes Rev.* (2018) 19:728–36. doi: 10.1111/obr.12665
275. Liu C, Wu D, Zhang J-F, Xu D, Xu W-F, Chen Y, et al. Changes in bone metabolism in morbidly obese patients after bariatric surgery: a meta-analysis. *Obes Surg.* (2016) 26:91–7. doi: 10.1007/s11695-015-1724-5
276. Gehrer S, Kern B, Peters T, Christoffel-Courtin C, Peterli R. Fewer nutrient deficiencies after laparoscopic sleeve gastrectomy (LSG) than after laparoscopic Roux-Y-gastric bypass (LRYGB)-a prospective study. *Obes Surg.* (2010) 20:447–53. doi: 10.1007/s11695-009-0068-4
277. Schafer AL, Weaver CM, Black DM, Wheeler AL, Chang H, Szefc GV, et al. Intestinal calcium absorption decreases dramatically after gastric bypass surgery despite optimization of vitamin D status. *J Bone Miner Res.* (2015) 30:1377–85. doi: 10.1002/jbmr.2467
278. Riedt CS, Brolin RE, Sherrell RM, Field MP, Shapses SA. True fractional calcium absorption is decreased after Roux-en-Y gastric bypass surgery. *Obes Silver Spring Md.* (2006) 14:1940–8. doi: 10.1038/oby.2006.226
279. Youssef Y, Richards WO, Sekhar N, Kaiser J, Spagnoli A, Abumrad N, et al. Risk of secondary hyperparathyroidism after laparoscopic gastric bypass surgery in obese women. *Surg Endosc.* (2007) 21:1393–6. doi: 10.1007/s00464-007-9228-6
280. Tardio V, Blais J-P, Julien A-S, Douville P, Lebel S, Biertho L, et al. Serum parathyroid hormone and 25-hydroxyvitamin D concentrations before and after biliopancreatic diversion. *Obes Surg.* (2018) 28:1886–94. doi: 10.1007/s11695-017-3101-z
281. Wei J-H, Lee W-J, Chong K, Lee Y-C, Chen S-C, Huang P-H, et al. High incidence of secondary hyperparathyroidism in bariatric patients: comparing different procedures. *Obes Surg.* (2018) 28:798–804. doi: 10.1007/s11695-017-2932-y
282. Guglielmi V, Bellia A, Gentileschi P, Lombardo M, D'Adamo M, Lauro D, et al. Parathyroid hormone in surgery-induced weight loss: no glucometabolic effects but potential adaptive response to skeletal loading. *Endocrine.* (2018) 59:288–95. doi: 10.1007/s12020-017-1477-0
283. Chakhtoura MT, Nakhoul NN, Shawwa K, Mantzoros C, El Hajj Fuleihan GA. Hypovitaminosis D in bariatric surgery: a systematic review of observational studies. *Metabolism.* (2016) 65:574–85. doi: 10.1016/j.metabol.2015.12.004
284. DiGiorgi M, Daud A, Inabnet WB, Schrope B, Urban-Skuro M, Restuccia N, et al. Markers of bone and calcium metabolism following gastric bypass and laparoscopic adjustable gastric banding. *Obes Surg.* (2008) 18:1144–8. doi: 10.1007/s11695-007-9408-4
285. Fish E, Beverstein G, Olson D, Reinhardt S, Garren M, Gould J. Vitamin D status of morbidly obese bariatric surgery patients. *J Surg Res.* (2010) 164:198–202. doi: 10.1016/j.jss.2010.06.029
286. Lanzarini E, Nogués X, Goday A, Benaiges D, de Ramón M, Villatoro M, et al. High-dose vitamin D supplementation is necessary after bariatric surgery: a prospective 2-year follow-up study. *Obes Surg.* (2015) 25:1633–8. doi: 10.1007/s11695-015-1572-3
287. Shetty S, Kapoor N, Bondu JD, Thomas N, Paul TV. Bone turnover markers: emerging tool in the management of osteoporosis. *Indian J Endocrinol Metab.* (2016) 20:846–52. doi: 10.4103/2230-8210.192914
288. Crawford MR, Pham N, Khan L, Bena JF, Schauer PR, Kashyap SR. Increased bone turnover in type 2 diabetes patients randomized to bariatric surgery versus medical therapy at 5 years. *Endocr Pract.* (2018) 24:256–64. doi: 10.4158/EP-2017-0072
289. Rao RS, Kini S. GIP and bariatric surgery. *Obes Surg.* (2011) 21:244–52. doi: 10.1007/s11695-010-0305-x
290. Bollag RJ, Zhong Q, Phillips P, Min L, Zhong L, Cameron R, et al. Osteoblast-derived cells express functional glucose-dependent insulinotropic peptide receptors. *Endocrinology.* (2000) 141:1228–35. doi: 10.1210/en.141.3.1228
291. Zhong Q, Itokawa T, Sridhar S, Ding K-H, Xie D, Kang B, et al. Effects of glucose-dependent insulinotropic peptide on osteoclast function. *Am J Physiol Endocrinol Metab.* (2007) 292:E543–8. doi: 10.1152/ajpendo.00364.2006
292. Maccarinelli G, Sibilia V, Torsello A, Raimondo F, Pitto M, Giustina A, et al. Ghrelin regulates proliferation and differentiation of osteoblastic cells. *J Endocrinol.* (2005) 184:249–56. doi: 10.1677/joe.1.05837
293. Wong IP, Baldock PA, Herzog H. Gastrointestinal peptides and bone health. *Curr Opin Endocrinol Diabetes Obes.* (2010) 17:44–50. doi: 10.1097/MED.0b013e3283344a05
294. Nuche-Berenguer B, Moreno P, Esbrit P, Dapía S, Caeiro JR, Cancelas J, et al. Effect of GLP-1 treatment on bone turnover in normal, type 2 diabetic, and insulin-resistant states. *Calcif Tissue Int.* (2009) 84:453–61. doi: 10.1007/s00223-009-9220-3
295. Wucher H, Ciangura C, Poitou C, Czernichow S. Effects of weight loss on bone status after bariatric surgery: association between adipokines and bone markers. *Obes Surg.* (2008) 18:58–65. doi: 10.1007/s11695-007-9258-0
296. Hage MP, El-Hajj Fuleihan G. Bone and mineral metabolism in patients undergoing Roux-en-Y gastric bypass. *Osteoporos Int.* (2014) 25:423–39. doi: 10.1007/s00198-013-2480-9

15

Obesity-Related Epigenetic Changes after Bariatric Surgery

Andrea G. Izquierdo [1,2] *and Ana B. Crujeiras* [1,2*]

[1] Epigenomics in Endocrinology and Nutrition Group, Instituto de Investigacion Sanitaria (IDIS), Complejo Hospitalario Universitario de Santiago (CHUS/SERGAS), Santiago de Compostela, Spain, [2] CIBER Fisiopatologia de la Obesidad y Nutricion (CIBERobn), Madrid, Spain

***Correspondence:**
Ana B. Crujeiras
anabelencrujeiras@hotmail.com

Objective: In recent years, an increasing number of studies have begun focusing on epigenetics as a link between environmental factors and a greater predisposition to the development of obesity and its comorbidities. An important challenge in this field is the evaluation of the possibility of the reversal of obesity-related epigenetic marks by means of therapy to induce weight loss and if the beneficial effects of therapy in reducing obesity are mediated by epigenetic mechanisms. We aimed to offer an outline of the current results regarding to the impact of bariatric surgery on epigenetic regulation, as well as to show if the beneficial effect of this intervention could be mediated by epigenetic mechanisms.

Methods: A review of the scientific publications in PubMed was performed by using key words related to obesity, epigenetics and bariatric surgery to provide an update of recent findings in this area of research. The most relevant and recently published articles and abstracts were selected to frame this review.

Results: Previous studies have demonstrated the presence of differential DNA methylation after bariatric surgery and the differential expression of non-coding RNAs. Therefore, epigenetic regulation could mediate the benefit of bariatric surgery on body weight and the metabolic disturbances associated with excess body weight, such as insulin resistance, hypertension, and cardiovascular disease. This evidence is relatively new as epigenetic regulation was first evaluated in the obesity field only a few years ago. However, there is an urgent need to perform longitudinal studies to evaluate the capacity of epigenetic marks in the prediction of bariatric surgery response.

Conclusions: Bariatric surgery appears to be capable of partially reversing the obesity-related epigenome. The identification of potential epigenetic biomarkers predictive for the success of bariatric surgery may open new doors to personalized therapy for severe obesity.

Keywords: DNA methylation, epigenetic reprograming, metabolic balance, non-coding RNA (ncRNA), weight loss

INTRODUCTION

Obesity is currently a huge healthcare problem, worldwide, and is a risk factor for several diseases such as type 2 diabetes (T2D), cardiovascular disease and cancer (1). As the prevalence of obesity reaches pandemic proportions, this metabolic disease is estimated to become the biggest cause of mortality in the near future (2). In fact, it is extremely alarming, given that 2.3% of men and 5.0%

of women have a body mass index (BMI) ≥35 kg/m^2. The worldwide prevalence of morbid obesity was reported to be 0.64% in men and 1.6% in women (3).

Obesity is a multifaced chronic disease, the cause of which is a disbalance between energy consumed and the energy burned off. This disbalance is promoted by several factors such as unhealthy diet, sedentarism, and genotype (4). As consequence, surplus energy is stored in the adipocytes, and leading to an adipose tissue dysfunction characteristic of obesity, as well as other metabolic disorders, such as alterations in insulin sensitivity, blood pressure and the plasma lipid profile, which are risk factors that together define metabolic syndrome (5). Abdominal obesity is a powerfully risk factor of cardiovascular disease and T2D, independently of BMI (6).

Many of the aforementioned metabolic alterations occur as a result of an interplay between environmental, lifestyle and genetic factors (7). Metabolic diseases are strongly affected by physical inactivity and unhealthy dietary habits (8). Disappointingly, regardless of exhaustive genetic research on these disorders, the molecular mechanisms are scarcely elucidated. However, recently, it has been proposed that epigenetic mechanisms may be one factor underlying the development of the metabolic syndrome. Especially, there has been an growing interest in the potential role of epigenetics in the development of metabolic diseases, and in how lifestyle habits are associated with these changes (8).

In terms of weight-loss therapy, lifestyle changes such as those focusing on diet and exercise have poor long-term adherence, while pharmacological interventions are scarce.

Bariatric surgery is indicated when a patient shows a BMI higher than 40 kg/m^2 or higher than 30 kg/m^2 if obesity I coexisting with other comorbidities such as diabetes mellitus. The techniques of bariatric surgery are divided into restrictive and malabsortive or a combination of both. Among the most widely used techniques are the sleeve gastrectomy and the adjustable gastric band which are restrictive and the Roux-en Y gastric bypass (RYGB) which is a combined malabsorptive and restrictive procedure and it is the most used and most studied procedure. Other procedures such as the biliopancreeatic diversion are used with less frequency (9). Bariatric surgery is currently the most effective intervention (10), however, a significant number of patients are predisposed to recover the weight lost after surgery.

To underlying the mechanisms involved in this unsuccessful outcome and to find predictive biomarkers is a challenge for the obesity physicians (11). Additionally, the molecular mechanisms associated with the beneficial effect of bariatric surgery are still unclear. An important challenge in this field is to evaluate if it is possible to reverse the obesity-related epigenetic marks by means of therapy to induce weight loss and if the beneficial effects of therapy to reduce obesity are mediated by epigenetic mechanisms. Understanding the association between epigenetic mechanisms in obesity management could provide targets for personalized therapy.

In this review, we offer a snapshot of the current results in the epigenetics research field and bariatric surgery, as well as the impact of this intervention on epigenetic profiles in the counteraction of obesity and its comorbidities, and to predict the individual responses to this therapy.

MECHANISMS INVOLVED IN EPIGENETIC REGULATION

The genetic information is the same in all the types of cells present in an organism, although their functions and characteristics are different. The mechanisms responsible for this cellular differentiation that originate the different phenotypes are the epigenetic marks of the genomes. The concept of epigenetics was first defined by Conrad Waddington in the early 1940s. He defined epigenetics as "the branch of biology that studies the causal interactions between genes and their products that give rise to the phenotype" (12). In later years, this definition was elaborated upon and is nowadays commonly accepted as "the study of changes in genetic function that are mitotically and/or meiotically inheritable and that do not imply a change in the DNA sequence" (13). The genome of an organism is generally unchanging. In contrast, the epigenome can be altered by the effect of external environmental factors (including lifestyle, nutrient intake, stress, exposure to toxins, physical activity, medical history, etc.), allowing in a short-time to provide a dynamic response by the organism (14). Therefore, epigenetics may explain why many different cell types are generated during an organism development, in spite of containing the same genetic information (15). Hence, epigenetic investigations aim to understand how external factors regulate gene expression, and even phenotypic traits (16).

Epigenetic markers are chemical modifications mediated by DNA enzymes and their chromatin proteins that play a key role in the regulation of genomic functions. The main mechanisms that lead this epigenetic regulation are (**Figure 1**): DNA methylation, histone post-translational modification (PTM), and non-coding RNAs (ncRNAs) including microRNAs (miRNAs) and long non-coding RNAs (lncRNAs) (15). Among these mechanisms, DNA methylation is the most abundant in the organism and the most known.

DNA Methylation

Methylation corresponds to the biochemical addition of a methyl group to a molecule. In DNA from mammals, DNA methyltransferase enzymes (DNMTs) catalyzed this biochemical process and predominantly occurs in CG dinucleotides. The regions with a high density of CG dinucleotides, often found in genes in the promoter region, are referred to as CpG islands (17, 18).

DNA methylation can be evaluated in different genomic contexts: transcriptional start sites with or without CpG islands, in gene bodies, at regulatory elements and at repeat sequences (19). In general, CpG island methylation status has been correlated with transcription regulation, wherein methylated CpG islands in the promoter region are located upstream of switch off genes and unmethylated CpG islands are located upstream of switch on genes (20). While promoter methylation is associated with a decrease expression, it is known that

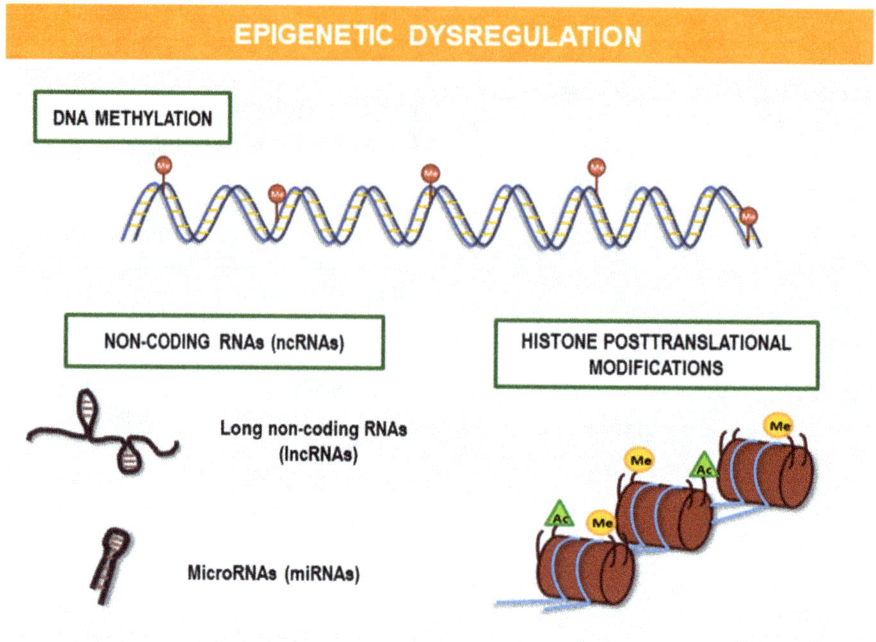

FIGURE 1 | Mechanisms of epigenetic regulation. The main mechanisms involved in epigenetic regulation are: DNA methylation, histone post-translational modifications (PTMs), and non-coding RNAs (ncRNAs) including microRNAs (miRNAs), and long non-coding RNAs (lncRNAs). These epigenetic modifications play a fundamental role in the development and regulation of gene expression throughout life. Recent studies demonstrate its relevance in clinical application as biomarkers or potential therapeutic targets for the early diagnosis and personalized treatment of diseases such as obesity and its comorbidities.

intragenic methylation (gene body, 5′UTR and 3′UTR) is related to increased gene expression (19).

As DNA methylation is modulated by environmental and lifestyle factors, this is an important mechanism underlying metabolic alterations (21). Different processes can be involved in the influence of lifestyle factors on the regulation of the epigenetic machinery (22). There is increasing evidence stating that lifestyle changes, including weight loss, can have an impact on DNA methylation and consequently in gene expression (23). Therefore, an important function of DNA methylation is to drive the gene expression (24). There are multiple types of epigenetic modification, and each type has a fundamental role in the development and regulation of gene expression throughout one's life course (18). In general, epigenetic marks are stable, although all levels of epigenetic modifications can be reverse. Specifically, DNA methylation can change from high levels to low levels of methylation and vice versa. This process can be promoted by different players, such as epigenetic drug intake [for example, the hypomethylating agent—5-aza-2′-deoxycytidine (5-aza-dC)] and healthy lifestyle habits (25). A dietary treatment with functional foods and exercise can modulate DNA methylation and as consequence, the gene expression leading to an improvement of a specific diseases phenotype (17, 26).

The assessment of DNA methylation has strong applicability to disease management (27). It is possible to identify biomarkers for obesity and other related diseases, which serve as predictors of an specific biological status for personalized medicine (28). Traditionally, DNA methylation studies were aimed on quantifying the methylation level of the target genes and determining the total level of 5-methyl-cytosine (5mC) (29). With the use of microarray hybridization technology, it is possible to measure the genome-wide DNA methylation. With the next-generation sequencing platforms genomic maps of DNA methylation can be built at a single-base resolution (30).

Greatest resolution and precision is obtained when DNA methylation is evaluated by bisulfite conversion and then sequenced (31). By means of the bisulfite treatment, DNA cytosines pass to uracil, but only when the cytosine is unmethylated. Thus, the sequencing assessment is able to distinguish methylated and unmethylated cytosines can be distinguished by sequencing (32).

Histone Post-translational Modification (PTM)

The post-translational modifications of histones play an important role in the control of gene expression, demonstrating their clinical relevance. Therefore, the number of investigations in this field has increased in recent years.

Histones are the main components of chromatin, a protein that together with DNA integrates chromosomes. Histones can be post-translationally altered by methylation, phosphorylation, acetylation or ubiquitination. These chemical processes are associated with the restructuring of chromatin, producing a more or less compacted state that activates (euchromatin) or inactivates (heterochromatin) the transcription of DNA (33). This modifications can occur at different sites simultaneously and the regulation between histone modifications can ensue within the same site, among different histone tails of in the same histone tail (15). Current studies have demonstrated the effect of histone modifications in adipogenesis (34, 35) and obesity (36, 37).

Non-coding RNAs (ncRNAs)

ncRNAs have arisen as relevant transcriptional factors in physiological and pathophysiological circumstances; therefore, gene silencing with their use can be employed as a therapeutic strategy. There are different types of ncRNAs in human genome as it was shown by whole-genome studies (38).

First, microRNAs (miRNA) are small, evolving, single-stranded and non-coding RNA molecules that represent 1–5% of the human genome and regulate at least 30% of the genes encoding proteins. Although little is currently known about biological functions, it is apparent that they are decisive players in the gene expression regulation that controls various cellular and metabolic pathways (39). MiRNAs are being increasingly described as having the capacity to impact alterations in the metabolism. The potential of miRNA as therapeutic targets, as well as disease markers to fight obesity has been highlighted (40, 41).

Additionally, long non-coding RNAs (lncRNAs) also represent a new emerging class of ncRNAs (17). For a long time, they were considered as the transcriptional "noise" of the genome; however, they have received considerable attention in recent years. LncRNAs are defined as RNA molecules with more than 200 nucleotides that present in large numbers in genome and they are involved in chromatin remodeling, as well as transcriptional and post-transcriptional regulation (42). Several lncRNAs have been identified for their role in the regulation of adipogenesis (white adipose tissue and brown adipose tissue) and energy metabolism (43). Therefore, their use as potential therapeutic targets to combat obesity is currently being considered.

EPIGENETICS IN OBESITY AND COMORBIDITIES

There is growing interest on epigenetics in the scientific community and its role in the development of chronic diseases such as obesity. The reason for this recent interest lies in the current knowledge that metabolic diseases are highly associated with epigenetic alterations. In fact, in the last two decades, scientists have generated a variety of valuable data and knowledge based on epigenetic and cellular metabolism studies (16). Recently, it has been claimed that epigenomes may represent the molecular bridge connecting gene regulation and environmental factors in defining the risk of obesity. Furthermore, it was hypothesized that epigenetic dysregulation could contribute to a rapid increase in the prevalence of obesity and its complications due to the heritability of acquired epigenetic marks (44).

Mostly of recent findings in the area of epigenetics and obesity research have been provided by human studies. These studies include those that investigate the relationship between total methylation, site-specific methylation or whole-genome methylation and obesity, as well as studies examining the impact of interventions on DNA methylation profiles and obesity (45).

DNA Methylation in Obesity

Differences in DNA methylation related to obesity or dietary interventions and weight loss use to be lower than 20%, even though this depend on the condition and tissue to be studied. A major limitation in many human studies is that epigenetic marks used to be measured in blood cells (as it is readily accessible for DNA analyses), instead of target tissues of metabolic disorders. Regardless of this, new studies have demonstrated the association between specific methylation sites in both blood and adipose tissue. According to this, Dick et al., demonstrated the association between DNA methylation levels and body mass index, the results in adipose tissue were reflected in whole blood (46). This warrants the use of DNA methylation profiling of blood cells for the detection of relevant epigenetic changes and offers a motivation for other appropriate studies (46, 47).

In line, our research group conducted a study using isolated DNA samples of subcutaneous adipose tissue and circulating leukocytes obtained from obese and non-obese patients (**Figure 2A**). This study provided new and valuable biomarkers for the DNA methylation of adipose tissue pathogenesis related to obesity, through peripheral blood analysis (48). There are several other examples regarding the objective of investigating whether the methylation signature of blood cell DNA is capable of reflecting the methylation status of adipose tissue. Specifically, it was determined in one study that the DNA methylation profile in peripheral blood mononuclear cells (PBMC) showed the methylation of white adipose tissue (WAT), with similar mean methylation of CpGs in the subcutaneous adipose and visceral adipose tissues (52). In another recent study, alterations in DNA methylation were identified in several tissues from obese patients, which influenced the pathogenesis of T2D (53).

Regarding the effect of DNA methylation in the promotion of obesity comorbidities, there is an abundance of evidence in the literature. For instance, an epigenetic analysis of the whole genome of the visceral adipose tissue of patients with morbid obesity was performed according to their sensitivity to insulin (49). The results obtained identified an methylome specific of insulin resistance in visceral adipose tissue, in which potential epigenetic biomarkers and new therapeutic targets for the alterations in insulin sensitivity associated with obesity were identified (**Figure 2B**) (49). In this line, a very recent study from the Methyl Epigenome Network Association (MENA) project evidenced that the methylation levels of 478 CpG sites in blood leukocytes are differentially methylation depending on the HOMA-IR cut off point of 3 units, being the methylation of these differentially methylated CpG sites good predictors of insulin resistance (54). Insulin resistance is the more relevant component of metabolic syndrome and related to this disorder, differential methylation was observed. Both global DNA methylation and the methylation levels of specific genes related to adipose tissue function and metabolism in visceral adipose tissue were found to be related to the metabolic syndrome etiology (55, 56). In blood leukocytes also a specific DNA methylation pattern was

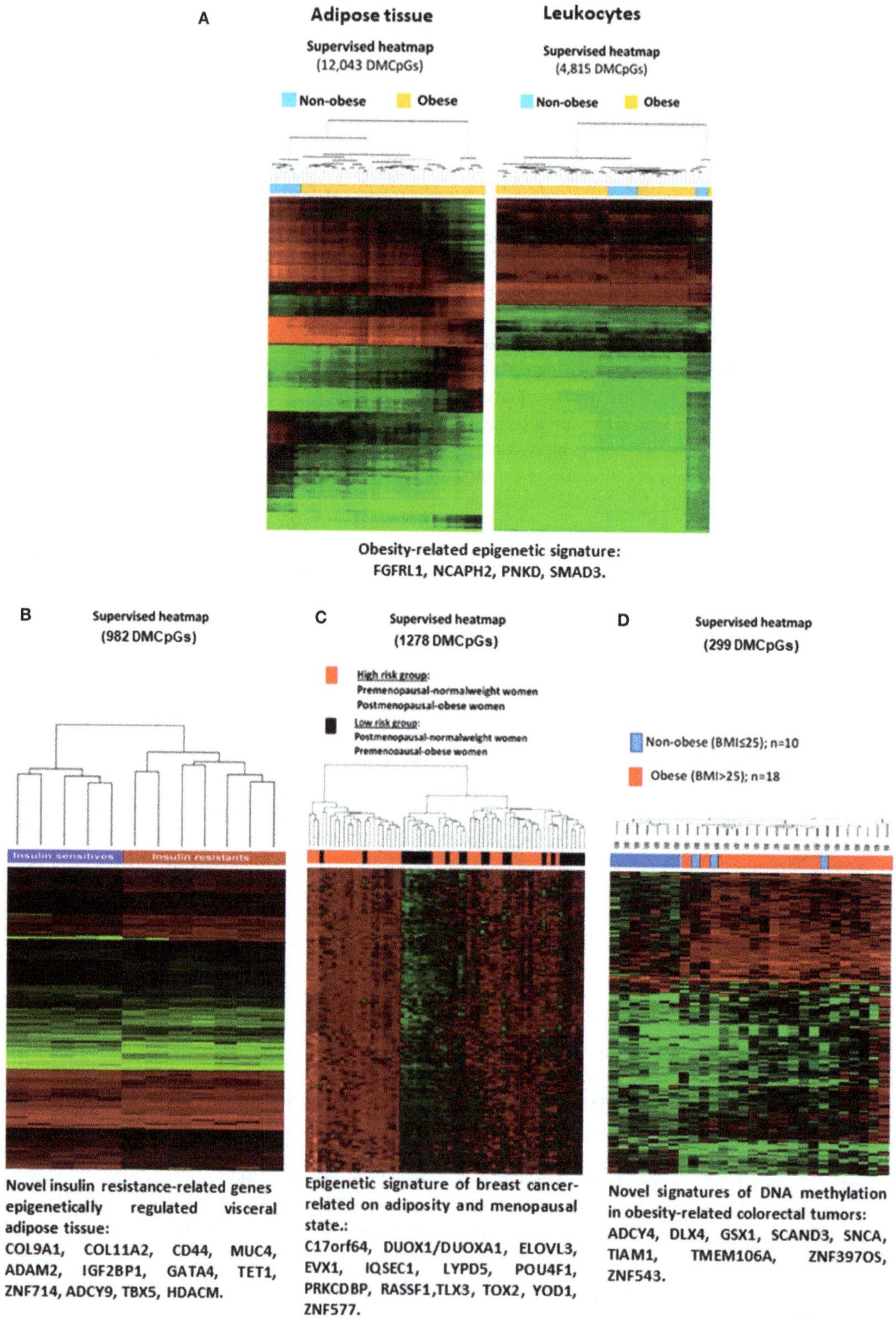

FIGURE 2 | Evidences of DNA methylation associated with obesity and codiseases. **(A)** Heatmap showing differences in the global methylation levels of the overall valid CpGs between the obese and non-obese subcutaneous adipose tissue samples (right panel) and leukocyte samples (left panel). Reprinted with permission from Crujeiras et al. (48). **(B)** Heatmap representing the differential DNA methylation in insulin-resistant and insulin sensitive patients. Reprinted with permission from Crujeiras et al. (49). **(C)** Supervised clustering of the CpGs found differentially methylated in breast tumor samples taking into account menopausal and adiposity status. Reprinted with permission from Crujeiras et al. (50). **(D)** Supervised clustering of the CpGs that were found to be differentially methylated in colorectal tumor samples from the obese and non-obese patients. Reprint with permission from Crujeiras et al. (51). DMCpGs, differentially methylation CpG sites.

found to be related to metabolic syndrome and the difference was consistent especially for ABCG1 gene (57).

Obesity is also related to the development and progression of non-alcoholic fatty liver disease (NAFLD). Moreover, epigenetics was proposed to be a relevant player in the onset of NAFLD. In this regards several differentially methylated regions (DMR) were found depending on the status of liver fibrosis. Importantly, these DMRs were associated with metabolic pathways and were reversed after weight loss (58).

Additionally, in the association between obesity and cancer, it was evidenced that epigenetic regulation, specially DNA methylation, may have a role. A specific methylome in post-menopausal breast cancer has been identified (**Figure 2C**) (50). Similarly, an analysis of the human colorectal cancer (CRC) methylome was associated with obesity (**Figure 2D**) (51). Some the BMI-associated CpG sites in blood leukocytes were also found to be related to hepatocellular carcinoma, evidencing the potential effect of obesity on hepatocellular carcinoma mediated by epigenetic mechanisms (59).

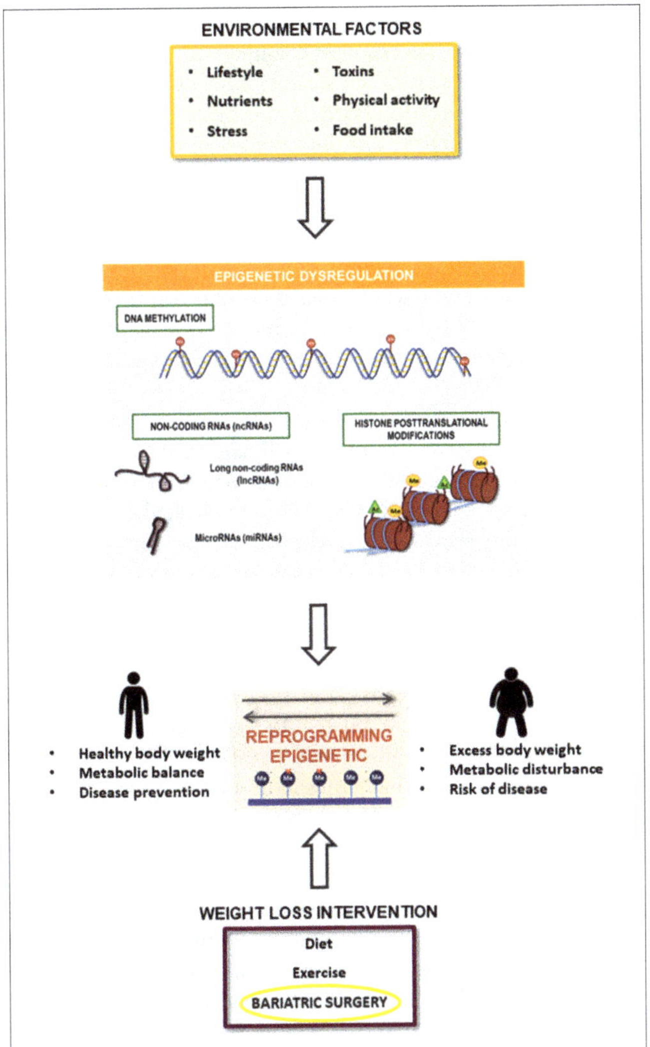

FIGURE 3 | Summary of the relationship between obesity development and bariatric surgery effect mediated by epigenetic mechanisms. Obesity is associated with a specific epigenetic dysregulation that is induced by several environmental factors such as toxics, dietary and physical activity habits and psychological events. On the other hand, bariatric surgery induces an improvement in obesity pathophysiology that could be mediated by the reversion of the obesity-related epigenetic dysregulation.

ncRNAs in Obesity

In terms of epigenetic regulation and obesity physiopathology, epigenetic mechanisms other than DNA methylation have also been evaluated. Studies have demonstrated the involvement of ncRNAs, such as miRNAs (60, 61) and lncRNAs (62) in body weight homeostasis and obesity co-morbidities. Emerging evidence suggests that microRNAs play a key role in the pathological development of obesity through their influence of adipocyte differentiation (63). In addition, interesting reports suggest that miRNAs may be regulated by diet and lifestyle factors. Slattery et al. showed some evidence of differences in miRNA expression associated with differences in food composition, even though this study did not find a relationship between miRNA expression and BMI (64). Also, miRNA may respond to various nutritional interventions (65). Moreover, miRNA expression profiles were correlated with subcutaneous adipose tissue and BMI (66). Other studies have aimed to identify the circulating miRNAs related to obesity that could be secreted from adipocytes and explore their possible role in the pathogenesis of metabolic disease (67, 68).

Several lncRNAs regulate adipogenesis (69), and they respond to metabolic transcription factors and hormones and nutrients (70). Three lncRNAs (lncRNA-p5549, lncRNA-p21015, and lncRNA-p19461) were found to be decreased in blood from obese individuals (71). From the identified lncRNAs, the lncRNA-p19461 expression level was found to be significantly increased in eight obese human individuals after a 12-week diet-induced weight-loss therapy, suggesting that circulating lncRNAs are altered in obesity and can be reversed after weight-loss treatment (71). LncRNAs, such as ASMER-1 and ASMER-2, have been proposed as key players in the insulin resistance associated with obesity (72) and as being involved in the potential mechanism in the link between obesity and cancer (73).In short, in recent years, numerous studies have been focusing on epigenetics as a link between environmental factors and a greater predisposition to the development of obesity and its comorbidities (17). This evidence proposes these epigenetic modifications as early prognostic markers for diseases such as obesity, allowing for the individuals stratification depending on the risk for developing a metabolic disorder, and the design of strategies for disease prevention and treatment in a personalized manner (26, 74). This has been demonstrated in studies focusing on epigenetics and precision medicine in obesity, and those on the epigenetic biomarkers of obesity and obesity-related diseases (75–77).

CHANGES IN EPIGENETIC MARKS AFTER BARIATRIC SURGERY

Bariatric surgery induces several beneficial effects on metabolism apart from weight loss. These beneficial effects lead to improvements in insulin sensitivity, resolving T2D (78). Additionally, after bariatric surgery, obese patients gain cardiovascular function (79). More relevantly, weight loss after bariatric surgery was found to be capable of decreasing the risk of hormone-related cancers in obese patients (80). These beneficial effects induced by weight loss and reduced calorie intake can be promoted by several pathways. It was recently demonstrated that bariatric surgery induces a new metabolic state that appears to be conserved in rodents and humans (81). After bariatric surgery, the chronic low-grade inflammation characteristic of obesity is resolved (82), and the release of incretin hormones is improved (83). Moreover, lipid oxidation and mitochondrial function improve after bariatric surgery (84). However, the molecular mechanism behind this is still unclear. As epigenetic regulation can be a relevant pathway in the expression modulation of the genes involved in the physiology and metabolism in human obesity (85), bariatric surgery could contribute to improvements in the metabolism by means of epigenetic regulation.

Several studies have evaluated the differences in DNA methylation levels after bariatric surgery (86, 87). Global DNA methylation data were inconsistent; however, RYGB surgery was able to modify the DNA methylation level of specific sites (86). For instance, in muscle tissue, it was observed obesity or weight loss induced by RYGB surgery is not associated with global cytosine methylation differences (88). Similarly, the methylation levels of long interspersed nuclear element 1 (LINE-1), a marker of global DNA methylation, did not change after RYGB bariatric surgery-induced weight loss (89, 90). In contrast, the methylation of specific genes underwent changes after weight loss-induced surgery. In muscle, significant changes were observed after RYGB in the DNA methylation profiles of PGC1A and PDK4, in addition to changes in the methylation at the CpG shores and exonic regions close to the transcription start sites. These changes after bariatric surgery were also associated with changes in the transcript levels, suggesting that these weight loss-induced epigenetic changes play a role in the regulation of metabolic gene transcription loss (88). A recent study demonstrated that weight loss induced by RYGB surgery is able to restored to normal levels the SORBS3 methylation and gene expression in the muscle (91). Alterations in the expression and methylation patterns of genes involved in insulin signaling as well as those related to specific non-alcoholic fatty liver disease (NAFLD) were also observed in liver biopsies after bariatric surgery (92). Adipose tissue, the key player in obesity biology, showed significant DNA methylation differences after RYGB bariatric surgery (93). These differences were observed in subcutaneous and omental adipose tissue and were correlated with differences in the transcript levels of differentially methylated genes, suggesting the role of adipose tissue DNA methylation in obesity and the possibility of its remodeling after surgery-induced weight loss (93).

Novel data were also observed when the epigenetic signature of obesity was evaluated in spermatozoa. DNA methylation of central control of appetite genes in sperm varied between obese and non-obese subjects and RYGB surgery-induced weight loss (94).

Apart from target tissue analysis, the methylation profile of specific genes was also evaluated in blood leukocytes before and after bariatric surgery. Although DNA methylation is tissue-specific, blood cells are easily accessible and useful tools for the performance of longitudinal epigenetic studies especially when the target tissue is inaccessible (17). After RYGB operation, the DNA methylation profile of obese individuals changed and resembled that of non-obese patients (95). The differentially methylated promoter was enriched in metabolic processes, demonstrating the potential association between the methylation pattern and beneficial effect of bariatric surgery on metabolic homeostasis. Moreover, the methylation of specific genes belonging to inflammatory pathways, such as SERPINE-1, IL-6, TNFA, IL-1B, and PKD4, was modulated after RYGB surgery (89, 96). A recent study demonstrated that the promoter methylation levels of the NFKB1 gene were significantly increased after surgery, and these changes were associated with changes in the circulating levels of inflammatory markers and blood pressure (97). Additionally, the methylation level of the genes involved in metabolic pathways also showed changes after bariatric surgery. The methylation levels of the stearoyl CoA desaturase-1 (SCD) gene promoter were decreased in morbidly obese individuals before bariatric surgery, and increased 6 months after RYGB, resembling those observed in individuals in the control group (98). SCD is an endoplasmic reticulum-bound enzyme that transforms different saturated fatty acids into monounsaturated fatty acids (99). In fact, this increase was associated with changes in the parameters related to insulin resistance, such as free fatty acid levels, homeostasis model assessment-estimated insulin resistance values, as well as the circulating levels of adiponectin (98).

DNA methylation is the most studied and abundant epigenetic mechanism. However, as mentioned above, other players in the epigenetic regulation exist such as ncRNA and chromatin remodeling. Several miRNAs have been implicated in the control of both insulin signaling and glucose metabolism at multiple levels and their expressions were associated with obesity (100). In line with this, Ortega et al. (101) evaluated the microRNAome in the adipose tissue obtained from morbidly obese patients before and after RYGB. This study demonstrated that 15 miRNAs were differentially expressed after surgery-induced weight loss and these miRNAs were related to cell cycle, development, lipid metabolism and inflammatory response (101). Similarly, after bariatric surgery, changes were observed in the adipocyte-derived exosomal microRNAs in association with improvements in insulin resistance (102). Other studies have evaluated the miRNA expression in serum or plasma. After RYGB, changes in the serum microRNA expression were observed compared to those before surgery, in association with insulin resistance parameters, demonstrating that microRNA expression could play an important and unique role in the effect of RYGB on the improvement of insulin secretion and insulin resistance, apart from the influence of decreased weight and body fat factors (103). A very recent study demonstrated that RYGB altered the circulating microRNAomes in a time-dependent manner, and the expression of 48 circulating microRNAs was significantly different. This study indicated that the circulating microRNAs differentially expressed after bariatric surgery are involved in pathways related to metabolic functions and their expression was correlated to BMI, body weight loss and fasting blood glucose levels (104).

LncRNAs constitute a novel class of RNAs that regulate gene expression; they are involved in the regulation of the expression of several genes belonging to relevant cellular functions. The exploration of their differential expression in relation to metabolism and endocrine regulation requires further investigation for the identification of potential therapeutic targets for obesity (62, 71). Few studies have explored the modulation of the expression of lncRNAs after bariatric surgery, and most of them were performed in animal models. In high-fat diet-induced diabetic mice, a total of 301 lncRNAs, including 232 that were upregulated and 69 that were downregulated, were differentially expressed in the duodenum between the duodenal-jejunal bypass and sham groups (105). These differentially expressed lncRNAs were related to pathways involved in inflammation and insulin secretion. It is suggested that the modulators of NONMMUG021726, the top-ranked gene, have the potential to be used as therapeutic targets or biomarkers for the prediction of bariatric surgery outcomes (105). NONMMUT023781 lncRNA expression was also identified as a potential target for glucose homeostasis after bariatric surgery in the jejune of high-fat diet-induced diabetic mice (106). This study demonstrated the differential expression of 827 jejunal lncRNAs in the duodenal-jejunal bypass group compared to the sham group (105). These dysregulated lncRNAs were related to neuromodulation-related pathways or biological processes, including serotonergic, glutamatergic, and dopaminergic synapses, suggesting the potential involvement of these lncRNA in the remission of T2D via the gut-brain axis (105).

Regarding other epigenetic mechanisms such as chromatin remodeling and histone modifications, no studies till date have focused on the effect of bariatric surgery. Further studies must evaluate the potential effect of bariatric surgery on these epigenetic mechanisms.

Transgenerational studies performed on the offspring of obese women before and after bariatric surgery provide potential evidence of the effect of bariatric surgery on epigenetic mechanisms. It was observed that children born before bariatric surgery show different methylome than children born after surgery, suggesting that the surgical intervention of mothers is able to modify the epigenetic mechanisms of the offspring. The identified genes differentially methylated between before bariatric surgery and after bariatric surgery siblings were related to insulin receptor signaling, type 2 diabetes signaling, and leptin signaling in obesity (107). A previous study demonstrated that the surgical treatment of severe maternal obesity resulted in sustained differences in the methylome and transcriptome of the genes involved in the inflammatory pathways in offspring born after the mothers underwent surgery, compared to their siblings conceived pre-surgery (108). On comparing the methylation profiles of siblings born before and after maternal bypass surgery, the CpG site-encoded genes involved in the glucoregulatory pathways were differentially methylated and potentially responsible for the improved cardiometabolic risk profile with greater insulin sensitivity in siblings conceived post-surgery (109). These studies demonstrate that the improvements in the obesity-related features of mothers following bariatric surgery are reflected in gene methylation and the expression levels of metabolic, immunologic, and inflammatory genes in their offspring. Thus, surgically induced reduction in body weight in a woman of reproductive age can reduce obesity in her children, potentially via epigenetic mechanisms (110).

Other issue that should be considered regarding to the association between the bariatric surgery effect on epigenetic mechanisms is that mediated by the microbiota composition. Bariatric surgery is able to modify the composition of microbiota and part of the beneficial effects of bariatric surgery could be mediated by the composition of microbiota after the surgical intervention and the changes correlate with changes in body composition and glucose homeostasis parameters (111). Importantly, the metabolites derived from microbiota can induce changes in DNA methylation and expression of non-coding-RNA. These changes in epigenetics machinery induced by microbial metabolites were proposed to have potential roles for preventing diseases development such as obesity (112). Further studies are needed to elucidate the crosstalk between microbiota metabolites and epigenetic machinery.

Taken together, the findings of all the aforementioned studies indicate that the beneficial effects induced by bariatric surgery on metabolism, immunity and inflammation can be mediated by epigenetic mechanisms, and also that these beneficial effects induce epigenetic mechanisms that determine descendant phenotype. Most of the studies were performed in small cohorts and therefore, the results have limited translation to the general population. However, the represent a very good start point for future studies in the field.

POSSIBLE THERAPEUTIC DIRECTION IN THE FUTURE

Relevant topics for discussion include the role of the epigenetic marks induced by bariatric surgery on the prognosis of obesity, as well as the susceptibility to the regain of weight loss. Bariatric surgery is able to induce long-term weight loss and resolves obesity co-morbidities with high efficacy. However, 1–2 years after surgery weight regain may occur (113). As mentioned above, epigenetic marks have been extensively proposed as biomarkers of the development and prognosis of several diseases, including obesity (17). However, few epigenetic studies till date have evaluated the association between the epigenetic marks induced by bariatric surgery and obesity-related prognoses. Only one very recent study focused on epigenomics and bariatric surgery efficacy. Even though it should be verified in an independent study, this work suggests that miR-448 and its target gene SIRT1 could serve as prognostic indicators for obese T2D patients after laparoscopic bariatric surgery (114). That study was performed using peripheral blood obtained from obese T2D patients. Patients were classified according to the clinical remission in response to bariatric surgery into the effective and ineffective groups. The time of efficacy evaluation was 3 months after surgery. Thus, the miR-448 expression was lower and mRNA and protein expression of SIRT1 was higher in the effective group than in the ineffective group after surgery (114). Regarding other epigenetic markers, patients who regained the weight loss induced by nutritional intervention exhibited differential DNA methylation patterns in the subcutaneous adipose tissue (115) or leukocytes (116) compared to patients who were able to maintain their weight loss over a short or long period. No relevant studies in this field have focused on bariatric surgery and obesity prognoses. Longitudinal studies must be conducted to explore the capacity of DNA methylation levels and other epigenetic marks in the prediction of the efficiency of bariatric surgery in the maintenance of weight loss and resolution of obesity co-morbidities, and provide potential therapeutic targets to guarantee the long-term success of bariatric surgery. On the other hand, changes in diet after bariatric surgery could be a relevant cause of changes in the epigenome. Longitudinal studies could also help to elucidate the effect of diet after bariatric surgery on epigenetics and its association with the success of the surgical intervention in counteraction obesity and its comorbidities.

CONCLUSIONS

Considering that obesity features are regulated by epigenetic mechanisms and that bariatric surgery appears to be capable of reversing the obesity-related epigenome, identification of potential epigenetic marks associated with the response to bariatric surgery may open new doors to the personalized therapy for severe obesity. This evidence is relatively new, as epigenetics regulation has been evaluated in the field of obesity only in the past few years, and few studies at present are involved in clarifying the role of epigenetic marks in obesity physiopathology and management. A limited number of studies have demonstrated differential DNA methylation after bariatric surgery and the differential expression of non-coding RNAs (miRNAs and lncRNAs). Epigenetic regulation appears to mediate the beneficial effect of bariatric surgery on body weight and the metabolic disturbances associated with excess body weight, such as insulin resistance, hypertension, cardiovascular disease. It is because bariatric surgery could be able to reprogram or reverse the epigenetic profile associated to obesity (**Figure 3**). However, regarding the prognosis of obesity after bariatric surgery, there is an urgent need to perform longitudinal studies to evaluate the capacity of epigenetic marks in the prediction of bariatric surgery response. Future interventional and long-term studies are required to further discover the mechanisms and predictive biomarkers of weight regain and inefficiency after bariatric surgery, focusing on epigenetic modifications, and the link between environment and cellular function.

AUTHOR CONTRIBUTIONS

AI and AC prepared the first draft of the manuscript. AI was involved in the literature search. AC critically revised and wrote the final version of the manuscript.

FUNDING

The study was supported by Centro de Investigación Biomedica en Red fisiopatología de la obesidad y nutricion (CIBERobn), an initiative of Instituto de Salud Carlos III (ISCIII) co-financed by the European Regional Development Fund (FEDER). AC is a Miguel Servet researcher (ISCIII; CP17/0008).

REFERENCES

1. Gadde KM, Martin CK, Berthoud HR, Heymsfield SB. Obesity: pathophysiology and management. *J Am Coll Cardiol.* (2018) 71:69–84. doi: 10.1016/j.jacc.2017.11.011
2. Upadhyay J, Farr O, Perakakis N, Ghaly W, Mantzoros C. Obesity as a disease. *Med Clin North Am.* (2018) 102:13–33. doi: 10.1016/j.mcna.2017.08.004
3. Collaboration NCDRF. Trends in adult body-mass index in 200 countries from 1975 to 2014: a pooled analysis of 1698 population-based measurement studies with 19.2 million participants. *Lancet.* (2016) 387:1377–96. doi: 10.1016/S0140-6736(16)30054-X
4. Marti A, Martinez-Gonzalez MA, Martinez JA. Interaction between genes and lifestyle factors on obesity. *Proc Nutr Soc.* (2008) 67:1–8. doi: 10.1017/S002966510800596X
5. Eckel RH, Grundy SM, Zimmet PZ. The metabolic syndrome. *Lancet.* (2005) 365:1415–28. doi: 10.1016/S0140-6736(05)66378-7
6. Casanueva FF, Moreno B, Rodriguez-Azeredo R, Massien C, Conthe P, Formiguera X, et al. Relationship of abdominal obesity with cardiovascular disease, diabetes and hyperlipidaemia in Spain. *Clin Endocrinol.* (2010) 73:35–40. doi: 10.1111/j.1365-2265.2009.03727.x
7. De Mello VD, Pulkkinen L, Lalli M, Kolehmainen M, Pihlajamaki J, Uusitupa M. DNA methylation in obesity and type 2 diabetes. *Ann Med.* (2014) 46:103–13. doi: 10.3109/07853890.2013.857259
8. Leech RM, Mcnaughton SA, Timperio A. The clustering of diet, physical activity and sedentary behavior in children and adolescents: a review. *Int J Behav Nutr Phys Act.* (2014) 11:4. doi: 10.1186/1479-5868-11-4
9. Elder KA, Wolfe BM. Bariatric surgery: a review of procedures and outcomes. *Gastroenterology.* (2007) 132:2253–71. doi: 10.1053/j.gastro.2007.03.057
10. Poirier P, Cornier MA, Mazzone T, Stiles S, Cummings S, Klein S, et al. Bariatric surgery and cardiovascular risk factors: a scientific statement from the American Heart Association. *Circulation.* (2011) 123:1683–701. doi: 10.1161/CIR.0b013e3182149099
11. Velapati SR, Shah M, Kuchkuntla AR, Abu-Dayyeh B, Grothe K, Hurt RT, et al. Weight regain after bariatric surgery: prevalence, etiology, and treatment. *Curr Nutr Rep.* (2018) 7:329–34. doi: 10.1007/s13668-018-0243-0
12. Waddington CH. Towards a theoretical biology. *Nature.* (1968) 218:525–7. doi: 10.1038/218525a0
13. Wu C, Morris JR. Genes, genetics, and epigenetics: a correspondence. *Science.* (2001) 293:1103–5. doi: 10.1126/science.293.5532.1103
14. Skinner MK, Manikkam M, Guerrero-Bosagna C. Epigenetic transgenerational actions of environmental factors in disease etiology. *Trends Endocrinol Metab.* (2010) 21:214–22. doi: 10.1016/j.tem.2009.12.007
15. Portela A, Esteller M. Epigenetic modifications and human disease. *Nat Biotechnol.* (2010) 28:1057–68. doi: 10.1038/nbt.1685
16. Xu W, Wang F, Yu Z, Xin F. Epigenetics and cellular metabolism. *Genet Epigenet.* (2016) 8:43–51. doi: 10.4137/GEG.S32160
17. Crujeiras AB, Diaz-Lagares A. DNA methylation in obesity and associated diseases. In: García-Giménez J, editor. *Epigenetic Biomarkers and Diagnostics* Madrid (2015). p. 313–29. doi: 10.1016/B978-0-12-801899-6.00016-4

18. Tollefsbol TO. An overview of medical epigenetics. In: Tollefsbol T, editor. *Medical Epigenetics* London (2016). p. 3–7. doi: 10.1016/B978-0-12-803239-8.00001-6
19. Jones PA. Functions of DNA methylation: islands, start sites, gene bodies and beyond. *Nat Rev Genet.* (2012) 13:484–92. doi: 10.1038/nrg3230
20. Kelly AD, Issa JJ. The promise of epigenetic therapy: reprogramming the cancer epigenome. *Curr Opin Genet Dev.* (2017) 42:68–77. doi: 10.1016/j.gde.2017.03.015
21. Coolen MW, Statham AL, Qu W, Campbell MJ, Henders AK, Montgomery GW, et al. Impact of the genome on the epigenome is manifested in DNA methylation patterns of imprinted regions in monozygotic and dizygotic twins. *PLoS ONE.* (2011) 6:e25590. doi: 10.1371/journal.pone.0025590
22. Ziech D, Franco R, Pappa A, Panayiotidis MI. Reactive oxygen species (ROS)–induced genetic and epigenetic alterations in human carcinogenesis. *Mutat Res.* (2011) 711:167–73. doi: 10.1016/j.mrfmmm.2011.02.015
23. Milagro FI, Gomez-Abellan P, Campion J, Martinez JA, Ordovas JM, Garaulet M. CLOCK, PER2 and BMAL1 DNA methylation: association with obesity and metabolic syndrome characteristics and monounsaturated fat intake. *Chronobiol Int.* (2012) 29:1180–94. doi: 10.3109/07420528.2012.719967
24. Yong WS, Hsu FM, Chen PY. Profiling genome-wide DNA methylation. *Epigenetics Chromatin.* (2016) 9:26. doi: 10.1186/s13072-016-0075-3
25. Estey EH. Epigenetics in clinical practice: the examples of azacitidine and decitabine in myelodysplasia and acute myeloid leukemia. *Leukemia.* (2013) 27:1803–12. doi: 10.1038/leu.2013.173
26. Milagro FI, Mansego ML, De Miguel C, Martinez JA. Dietary factors, epigenetic modifications and obesity outcomes: progresses and perspectives. *Mol Aspects Med.* (2013) 34:782–812. doi: 10.1016/j.mam.2012.06.010
27. Mikeska T, Craig JM. DNA methylation biomarkers: cancer and beyond. *Genes.* (2014) 5:821–64. doi: 10.3390/genes5030821
28. Agardh E, Lundstig A, Perfilyev A, Volkov P, Freiburghaus T, Lindholm E, et al. Genome-wide analysis of DNA methylation in subjects with type 1 diabetes identifies epigenetic modifications associated with proliferative diabetic retinopathy. *BMC Med.* (2015) 13:182. doi: 10.1186/s12916-015-0421-5
29. Lisanti S, Omar WA, Tomaszewski B, De Prins S, Jacobs G, Koppen G, et al. Comparison of methods for quantification of global DNA methylation in human cells and tissues. *PLoS ONE.* (2013) 8:e79044. doi: 10.1371/journal.pone.0079044
30. Laird PW. Principles and challenges of genomewide DNA methylation analysis. *Nat Rev Genet.* (2010) 11:191–203. doi: 10.1038/nrg2732
31. Cokus SJ, Feng S, Zhang X, Chen Z, Merriman B, Haudenschild CD, et al. Shotgun bisulphite sequencing of the Arabidopsis genome reveals DNA methylation patterning. *Nature.* (2008) 452:215–9. doi: 10.1038/nature06745
32. Hanna CW, Demond H, Kelsey G. Epigenetic regulation in development: is the mouse a good model for the human? *Hum Reprod Update.* (2018) 24:556–76. doi: 10.1093/humupd/dmy021
33. Egger G, Liang G, Aparicio A, Jones PA. Epigenetics in human disease and prospects for epigenetic therapy. *Nature.* (2004) 429:457–63. doi: 10.1038/nature02625
34. Steger DJ, Grant GR, Schupp M, Tomaru T, Lefterova MI, Schug J, et al. Propagation of adipogenic signals through an epigenomic transition state. *Genes Dev.* (2010) 24:1035–44. doi: 10.1101/gad.1907110
35. Okuno Y, Ohtake F, Igarashi K, Kanno J, Matsumoto T, Takada I, et al. Epigenetic regulation of adipogenesis by PHF2 histone demethylase. *Diabetes.* (2013) 62:1426–34. doi: 10.2337/db12-0628
36. Nie L, Shuai L, Zhu M, Liu P, Xie ZF, Jiang S, et al. The landscape of histone modifications in a high-fat Diet-Induced Obese (DIO) mouse model. *Mol Cell Proteomics.* (2017) 16:1324–34. doi: 10.1074/mcp.M117.067553
37. Abu-Farha M, Tiss A, Abubaker J, Khadir A, Al-Ghimlas F, Al-Khairi I, et al. Proteomics analysis of human obesity reveals the epigenetic factor HDAC4 as a potential target for obesity. *PLoS ONE.* (2013) 8:e75342. doi: 10.1371/journal.pone.0075342
38. Taft RJ, Pang KC, Mercer TR, Dinger M, Mattick JS. Non-coding RNAs: regulators of disease. *J Pathol.* (2010) 220:126–39. doi: 10.1002/path.2638
39. Macfarlane LA, Murphy PR. microRNA: biogenesis, function and role in cancer. *Curr Genomics.* (2010) 11:537–61. doi: 10.2174/138920210793175895
40. Peng Y, Yu S, Li H, Xiang H, Peng J, Jiang S. microRNAs: emerging roles in adipogenesis and obesity. *Cell Signal.* (2014) 26:1888–96. doi: 10.1016/j.cellsig.2014.05.006
41. Zaiou M, El Amri H, Bakillah A. The clinical potential of adipogenesis and obesity-related microRNAs. *Nutr Metab Cardiovasc Dis.* (2018) 28:91–111. doi: 10.1016/j.numecd.2017.10.015
42. Fang Y, Fullwood MJ. Roles, functions, and mechanisms of long non-coding RNAs in cancer. *Genom Proteom Bioinf.* (2016) 14:42–54. doi: 10.1016/j.gpb.2015.09.006
43. Wei S, Du M, Jiang Z, Hausman GJ, Zhang L, Dodson MV. Long non-coding RNAs in regulating adipogenesis: new RNAs shed lights on obesity. *Cell Mol Life Sci.* (2016) 73:2079–87. doi: 10.1007/s00018-016-2169-2
44. Bays H, Scinta W. Adiposopathy and epigenetics: an introduction to obesity as a transgenerational disease. *Curr Med Res Opin.* (2015) 31:2059–69. doi: 10.1185/03007995.2015.1087983
45. Casanello P, Krause BJ, Castro-Rodriguez JA, Uauy R. Epigenetics and obesity. *Rev Chil Pediatr.* (2016) 87:335–42. doi: 10.1016/j.rchipe.2016.08.009
46. Dick KJ, Nelson CP, Tsaprouni L, Sandling JK, Aissi D, Wahl S, et al. DNA methylation and body-mass index: a genome-wide analysis. *Lancet.* (2014) 383:1990–8. doi: 10.1016/S0140-6736(13)62674-4
47. Van Dijk SJ, Tellam RL, Morrison JL, Muhlhausler BS, Molloy PL. Recent developments on the role of epigenetics in obesity and metabolic disease. *Clin Epigenetics.* (2015) 7:66. doi: 10.1186/s13148-015-0101-5
48. Crujeiras AB, Diaz-Lagares A, Sandoval J, Milagro FI, Navas-Carretero S, Carreira MC, et al. DNA methylation map in circulating leukocytes mirrors subcutaneous adipose tissue methylation pattern: a genome-wide analysis from non-obese and obese patients. *Sci Rep.* (2017) 7:41903. doi: 10.1038/srep41903
49. Crujeiras AB, Diaz-Lagares A, Moreno-Navarrete JM, Sandoval J, Hervas D, Gomez A, et al. Genome-wide DNA methylation pattern in visceral adipose tissue differentiates insulin-resistant from insulin-sensitive obese subjects. *Transl Res.* (2016) 178:13–24 e15. doi: 10.1016/j.trsl.2016.07.002
50. Crujeiras AB, Diaz-Lagares A, Stefansson OA, Macias-Gonzalez M, Sandoval J, Cueva J, et al. Obesity and menopause modify the epigenomic profile of breast cancer. *Endocr Relat Cancer.* (2017b) 24:351–63. doi: 10.1530/ERC-16-0565
51. Crujeiras AB, Morcillo S, Diaz-Lagares A, Sandoval J, Castellano-Castillo D, Torres E, et al. Identification of an episignature of human colorectal cancer associated with obesity by genome-wide DNA methylation analysis. *Int J Obes.* (2018) 43:176–88. doi: 10.1038/s41366-018-0065-6
52. Arner P, Sahlqvist AS, Sinha I, Xu H, Yao X, Waterworth D, et al. The epigenetic signature of systemic insulin resistance in obese women. *Diabetologia.* (2016) 59:2393–405. doi: 10.1007/s00125-016-4074-5
53. Barajas-Olmos F, Centeno-Cruz F, Zerrweck C, Imaz-Rosshandler I, Martinez-Hernandez A, Cordova EJ, et al. Altered DNA methylation in liver and adipose tissues derived from individuals with obesity and type 2 diabetes. *BMC Med Genet.* (2018) 19:28. doi: 10.1186/s12881-018-0542-8
54. Arpon A, Milagro FI, Ramos-Lopez O, Mansego ML, Santos JL, Riezu-Boj JI, et al. Epigenome-wide association study in peripheral white blood cells involving insulin resistance. *Sci Rep.* (2019) 9:2445. doi: 10.1038/s41598-019-38980-2
55. Castellano-Castillo D, Moreno-Indias I, Fernandez-Garcia JC, Alcaide-Torres J, Moreno-Santos I, Ocana L, et al. Adipose tissue LPL methylation is associated with triglyceride concentrations in the metabolic syndrome. *Clin Chem.* (2018) 64:210–8. doi: 10.1373/clinchem.2017.277921
56. Castellano-Castillo D, Moreno-Indias I, Sanchez-Alcoholado L, Ramos-Molina B, Alcaide-Torres J, Morcillo S, et al. Altered adipose tissue DNA methylation status in metabolic syndrome: relationships between global DNA methylation and specific methylation at adipogenic, lipid metabolism and inflammatory candidate genes and metabolic variables. *J Clin Med.* (2019) 8:87. doi: 10.3390/jcm8010087
57. Akinyemiju T, Do AN, Patki A, Aslibekyan S, Zhi D, Hidalgo B, et al. Epigenome-wide association study of metabolic syndrome in African-American adults. *Clin Epigenetics.* (2018) 10:49. doi: 10.1186/s13148-018-0483-2
58. Hotta K, Kitamoto A, Kitamoto T, Ogawa Y, Honda Y, Kessoku T, et al. Identification of differentially methylated region (DMR) networks associated

with progression of non-alcoholic fatty liver disease. *Sci Rep*. (2018) 8:13567. doi: 10.1038/s41598-018-31886-5

59. Ramos-Lopez O, Riezu-Boj JI, Milagro FI, Alfredo Martinez J, Project M. Association of methylation signatures at hepatocellular carcinoma pathway genes with adiposity and insulin resistance phenotypes. *Nutr Cancer*. (2018) 20:1–12. doi: 10.1080/01635581.2018.1531136
60. Heneghan HM, Miller N, Kerin MJ. Role of microRNAs in obesity and the metabolic syndrome. *Obes Rev*. (2010) 11:354–61. doi: 10.1111/j.1467-789X.2009.00659.x
61. Dumortier O, Hinault C, Van Obberghen E. microRNAs and metabolism crosstalk in energy homeostasis. *Cell Metab*. (2013) 18:312–24. doi: 10.1016/j.cmet.2013.06.004
62. Giroud M, Scheideler M. Long non-coding RNAs in metabolic organs and energy homeostasis. *Int J Mol Sci*. (2017) 18:E2578. doi: 10.3390/ijms18122578
63. Lin Q, Gao Z, Alarcon RM, Ye J, Yun Z. A role of miR-27 in the regulation of adipogenesis. *FEBS J*. (2009) 276:2348–58. doi: 10.1111/j.1742-4658.2009.06967.x
64. Slattery ML, Herrick JS, Mullany LE, Stevens JR, Wolff RK. Diet and lifestyle factors associated with miRNA expression in colorectal tissue. *Pharmgenomics Pers Med*. (2017) 10:1–16. doi: 10.2147/PGPM.S117796
65. Palmer JD, Soule BP, Simone BA, Zaorsky NG, Jin L, Simone NL. microRNA expression altered by diet: can food be medicinal? *Ageing Res Rev*. (2014) 17:16–24. doi: 10.1016/j.arr.2014.04.005
66. Kloting N, Berthold S, Kovacs P, Schon MR, Fasshauer M, Ruschke K, et al. microRNA expression in human omental and subcutaneous adipose tissue. *PLoS ONE*. (2009) 4:e4699. doi: 10.1371/journal.pone.0004699
67. Wang YC, Li Y, Wang XY, Zhang D, Zhang H, Wu Q, et al. Circulating miR-130b mediates metabolic crosstalk between fat and muscle in overweight/obesity. *Diabetologia*. (2013) 56:2275–85. doi: 10.1007/s00125-013-2996-8
68. Doumatey AP, He WJ, Gaye A, Lei L, Zhou J, Gibbons GH, et al. Circulating MiR-374a-5p is a potential modulator of the inflammatory process in obesity. *Sci Rep*. (2018) 8:7680. doi: 10.1038/s41598-018-26065-5
69. Sun L, Goff LA, Trapnell C, Alexander R, Lo KA, Hacisuleyman E, et al. Long non-coding RNAs regulate adipogenesis. *Proc Natl Acad Sci USA*. (2013) 110:3387–92. doi: 10.1073/pnas.1222643110
70. Yang L, Li P, Yang W, Ruan X, Kiesewetter K, Zhu J, et al. Integrative transcriptome analyses of metabolic responses in mice define pivotal LncRNA metabolic regulators. *Cell Metab*. (2016) 24:627–39. doi: 10.1016/j.cmet.2016.08.019
71. Sun J, Ruan Y, Wang M, Chen R, Yu N, Sun L, et al. Differentially expressed circulating LncRNAs and mRNA identified by microarray analysis in obese patients. *Sci Rep*. (2016) 6:35421. doi: 10.1038/srep35421
72. Gao H, Kerr A, Jiao H, Hon CC, Ryden M, Dahlman I, et al. Long non-coding RNAs associated with metabolic traits in human white adipose tissue. *EBioMed*. (2018) 30:248–60. doi: 10.1016/j.ebiom.2018.03.010
73. Yau MY, Xu L, Huang CL, Wong CM. Long non-coding RNAs in obesity-induced cancer. *Noncoding RNA*. (2018) 4:E19. doi: 10.3390/ncrna4030019
74. Martinez JA, Milagro FI, Claycombe KJ, Schalinske KL. Epigenetics in adipose tissue, obesity, weight loss, and diabetes. *Adv Nutr*. (2014) 5:71–81. doi: 10.3945/an.113.004705
75. Fall T, Mendelson M, Speliotes EK. recent advances in human genetics and epigenetics of adiposity: pathway to precision medicine? *Gastroenterology*. (2017) 152:1695–706. doi: 10.1053/j.gastro.2017.01.054
76. Campanella G, Gunter MJ, Polidoro S, Krogh V, Palli D, Panico S, et al. Epigenome-wide association study of adiposity and future risk of obesity-related diseases. *Int J Obes*. (2018) 42:2022–35. doi: 10.1038/s41366-018-0064-7
77. Cheng Z, Zheng L, Almeida FA. Epigenetic reprogramming in metabolic disorders: nutritional factors and beyond. *J Nutr Biochem*. (2018) 54:1–10. doi: 10.1016/j.jnutbio.2017.10.004
78. Schauer PR, Mingrone G, Ikramuddin S, Wolfe B. Clinical outcomes of metabolic surgery: efficacy of glycemic control, weight loss, and remission of diabetes. *Diabetes Care*. (2016) 39:902–11. doi: 10.2337/dc16-0382
79. Benotti PN, Wood GC, Carey DJ, Mehra VC, Mirshahi T, Lent MR, et al. Gastric bypass surgery produces a durable reduction in cardiovascular disease risk factors and reduces the long-term risks of congestive heart failure. *J Am Heart Assoc*. (2017) 6:e005126. doi: 10.1161/JAHA.116.005126
80. Mackenzie H, Markar SR, Askari A, Faiz O, Hull M, Purkayastha S, et al. Obesity surgery and risk of cancer. *Br J Surg*. (2018) 105:1650–7. doi: 10.1002/bjs.10914
81. Ben-Zvi D, Meoli L, Abidi WM, Nestoridi E, Panciotti C, Castillo E, et al. Time-dependent molecular responses differ between gastric bypass and dieting but are conserved across species. *Cell Metab*. (2018) 28:310–23.e6. doi: 10.1016/j.cmet.2018.06.004
82. Zhang C, Zhang J, Liu Z, Zhou Z. More than an anti-diabetic bariatric surgery, metabolic surgery alleviates systemic and local inflammation in obesity. *Obes Surg*. (2018) 28:3658–68. doi: 10.1007/s11695-018-3400-z
83. Ma J, Vella A. What has bariatric surgery taught us about the role of the upper gastrointestinal tract in the regulation of postprandial glucose metabolism? *Front Endocrinol*. (2018) 9:324. doi: 10.3389/fendo.2018.00324
84. Fernstrom M, Bakkman L, Loogna P, Rooyackers O, Svensson M, Jakobsson T, et al. Improved muscle mitochondrial capacity following gastric bypass surgery in obese subjects. *Obes Surg*. (2016) 26:1391–7. doi: 10.1007/s11695-015-1932-z
85. Van Dijk SJ, Molloy PL, Varinli H, Morrison JL, Muhlhausler BS., Members of EpiSCOPE. Epigenetics and human obesity. *Int J Obes*. (2015) 39:85–97. doi: 10.1038/ijo.2014.34
86. Morcillo S, Macias-Gonzalez M, Tinahones FJ. The effect of metabolic and bariatric surgery on DNA methylation patterns. *Curr Atheroscler Rep*. (2017) 19:40. doi: 10.1007/s11883-017-0676-8
87. Sala P, De Miranda Torrinhas RSM, Fonseca DC, Ravacci GR, Waitzberg DL, Giannella-Neto D. Tissue-specific methylation profile in obese patients with type 2 diabetes before and after Roux-en-Y gastric bypass. *Diabetol Metab Syndr*. (2017) 9:15. doi: 10.1186/s13098-017-0214-4
88. Barres R, Kirchner H, Rasmussen M, Yan J, Kantor FR, Krook A, et al. Weight loss after gastric bypass surgery in human obesity remodels promoter methylation. *Cell Rep*. (2013) 3:1020–7. doi: 10.1016/j.celrep.2013.03.018
89. Nicoletti CF, Nonino CB, De Oliveira BA, Pinhel MA, Mansego ML, Milagro FI, et al. DNA methylation and hydroxymethylation levels in relation to two weight loss strategies: energy-restricted diet or bariatric surgery. *Obes Surg*. (2016) 26:603–11. doi: 10.1007/s11695-015-1802-8
90. Martin-Nunez GM, Cabrera-Mulero A, Alcaide-Torres J, Garcia-Fuentes E, Tinahones FJ, Morcillo S. No effect of different bariatric surgery procedures on LINE-1 DNA methylation in diabetic and non-diabetic morbidly obese patients. *Surg Obes Relat Dis*. (2017) 13:442–50. doi: 10.1016/j.soard.2016.10.014
91. Day SE, Garcia LA, Coletta RL, Campbell LE, Benjamin TR, De Filippis EA, et al. Alterations of sorbin and SH3 domain containing 3 (SORBS3) in human skeletal muscle following Roux-en-Y gastric bypass surgery. *Clin Epigenetics*. (2017) 9:96. doi: 10.1186/s13148-017-0396-5
92. Ahrens M, Ammerpohl O, Von Schonfels W, Kolarova J, Bens S, Itzel T, et al. DNA methylation analysis in non-alcoholic fatty liver disease suggests distinct disease-specific and remodeling signatures after bariatric surgery. *Cell Metab*. (2013) 18:296–302. doi: 10.1016/j.cmet.2013.07.004
93. Benton MC, Johnstone A, Eccles D, Harmon B, Hayes MT, Lea RA, et al. An analysis of DNA methylation in human adipose tissue reveals differential modification of obesity genes before and after gastric bypass and weight loss. *Genome Biol*. (2015) 16:8. doi: 10.1186/s13059-014-0569-x
94. Donkin I, Versteyhe S, Ingerslev LR, Qian K, Mechta M, Nordkap L, et al. Obesity and bariatric surgery drive epigenetic variation of spermatozoa in humans. *Cell Metab*. (2016) 23:369–78. doi: 10.1016/j.cmet.2015.11.004
95. Nilsson EK, Ernst B, Voisin S, Almen MS, Benedict C, Mwinyi J, et al. Roux-en Y gastric bypass surgery induces genome-wide promoter-specific changes in DNA methylation in whole blood of obese patients. *PLoS ONE*. (2015) 10:e0115186. doi: 10.1371/journal.pone.0115186
96. Kirchner H, Nylen C, Laber S, Barres R, Yan J, Krook A, et al. Altered promoter methylation of PDK4, IL1 B, IL6, and TNF after Roux-en Y gastric bypass. *Surg Obes Relat Dis*. (2014) 10:671–8. doi: 10.1016/j.soard.2013.12.019
97. Macias-Gonzalez M, Martin-Nunez GM, Garrido-Sanchez L, Garcia-Fuentes E, Tinahones FJ, Morcillo S. Decreased blood pressure is related to changes in NF-kB promoter methylation levels after bariatric

surgery. *Surg Obes Relat Dis.* (2018) 14:1327–34. doi: 10.1016/j.soard.2018.06.011

98. Morcillo S, Martin-Nunez GM, Garcia-Serrano S, Gutierrez-Repiso C, Rodriguez-Pacheco F, Valdes S, et al. Changes in SCD gene DNA methylation after bariatric surgery in morbidly obese patients are associated with free fatty acids. *Sci Rep.* (2017) 7:46292. doi: 10.1038/srep46292
99. Ntambi JM, Miyazaki M. Regulation of stearoyl-CoA desaturases and role in metabolism. *Prog Lipid Res.* (2004) 43:91–104. doi: 10.1016/S0163-7827(03)00039-0
100. Arner P, Kulyte A. microRNA regulatory networks in human adipose tissue and obesity. *Nat Rev Endocrinol.* (2015) 11:276–88. doi: 10.1038/nrendo.2015.25
101. Ortega FJ, Mercader JM, Moreno-Navarrete JM, Nonell L, Puigdecanet E, Rodriquez-Hermosa JI, et al. Surgery-induced weight loss is associated with the downregulation of genes targeted by microRNAs in adipose tissue. *J Clin Endocrinol Metab.* (2015) 100:E1467–76. doi: 10.1210/jc.2015-2357
102. Hubal MJ, Nadler EP, Ferrante SC, Barberio MD, Suh JH, Wang J, et al. Circulating adipocyte-derived exosomal microRNAs associated with decreased insulin resistance after gastric bypass. *Obesity.* (2017) 25:102–10. doi: 10.1002/oby.21709
103. Lirun K, Sewe M, Yong W. A pilot study: the effect of Roux-en-Y gastric bypass on the serum microRNAs of the type 2 diabetes patient. *Obes Surg.* (2015) 25:2386–92. doi: 10.1007/s11695-015-1711-x
104. Alkandari A, Ashrafian H, Sathyapalan T, Sedman P, Darzi A, Holmes E, et al. Improved physiology and metabolic flux after Roux-en-Y gastric bypass is associated with temporal changes in the circulating microRNAome: a longitudinal study in humans. *BMC Obes.* (2018) 5:20. doi: 10.1186/s40608-018-0199-z
105. Liang Y, Yu B, Wang Y, Qiao Z, Cao T, Zhang P. Duodenal long non-coding RNAs are associated with glycemic control after bariatric surgery in high-fat diet-induced diabetic mice. *Surg Obes Relat Dis.* (2017) 13:1212–26. doi: 10.1016/j.soard.2017.02.010
106. Liang Y, Yu B, Wang Y, Qiao Z, Cao T, Zhang P. Jejunal long non-coding RNAs are associated with glycemic control via gut-brain axis after bariatric surgery in diabetic mice. *Surg Obes Relat Dis.* (2018) 14:821–32. doi: 10.1016/j.soard.2018.03.006
107. Berglind D, Muller P, Willmer M, Sinha I, Tynelius P, Naslund E, et al. Differential methylation in inflammation and type 2 diabetes genes in siblings born before and after maternal bariatric surgery. *Obesity.* (2016) 24:250–61. doi: 10.1002/oby.21340
108. Guenard F, Tchernof A, Deshaies Y, Cianflone K, Kral JG, Marceau P, et al. Methylation and expression of immune and inflammatory genes in the offspring of bariatric bypass surgery patients. *J Obes.* (2013) 2013:492170. doi: 10.1155/2013/492170
109. Guenard F, Deshaies Y, Cianflone K, Kral JG, Marceau P, Vohl MC. Differential methylation in glucoregulatory genes of offspring born before vs. after maternal gastrointestinal bypass surgery. *Proc Natl Acad Sci USA.* (2013) 110:11439–44. doi: 10.1073/pnas.1216959110
110. Patti ME. Reducing maternal weight improves offspring metabolism and alters (or modulates) methylation. *Proc Natl Acad Sci USA.* (2013) 110:12859–60. doi: 10.1073/pnas.1309724110
111. Wang FG, Bai RX, Yan WM, Yan M, Dong LY, Song MM. Differential composition of gut microbiota among healthy volunteers, morbidly obese patients and post-bariatric surgery patients. *Exp Ther Med.* (2019) 17:2268–78. doi: 10.3892/etm.2019.7200
112. Cuevas-Sierra A, Ramos-Lopez O, Riezu-Boj JI, Milagro FI, Martinez JA. Diet, gut microbiota, and obesity: links with host genetics and epigenetics and potential applications. *Adv Nutr.* (2019) 10:S17–30.doi: 10.1093/advances/nmy078
113. Shantavasinkul PC, Omotosho P, Corsino L, Portenier D, Torquati A. Predictors of weight regain in patients who underwent Roux-en-Y gastric bypass surgery. *Surg Obes Relat Dis.* (2016) 12:1640–5. doi: 10.1016/j.soard.2016.08.028
114. Wang Y, Wang DS, Cheng YS, Jia BL, Yu G, Yin XQ, et al. Expression of microRNA-448 and SIRT1 and prognosis of obese type 2 diabetic mellitus patients after laparoscopic bariatric surgery. *Cell Physiol Biochem.* (2018) 45:935–50. doi: 10.1159/000487287
115. Bollepalli S, Kaye S, Heinonen S, Kaprio J, Rissanen A, Virtanen KA, et al. Subcutaneous adipose tissue gene expression and DNA methylation respond to both short- and long-term weight loss. *Int J Obes.* (2018) 42:412–23. doi: 10.1038/ijo.2017.245
116. Crujeiras AB, Campion J, Diaz-Lagares A, Milagro FI, Goyenechea E, Abete I, et al. Association of weight regain with specific methylation levels in the NPY and POMC promoters in leukocytes of obese men: a translational study. *Regul Pept.* (2013) 186:1–6. doi: 10.1016/j.regpep.2013.06.012

16

Diabetic and Elder Patients Experience Superior Cardiovascular Benefits after Gastric Bypass Induced Weight Loss

Pedro R. Pereira [1,2], *Marta Guimarães* [1,2,3], *Tiago Morais* [1,2], *Sofia S. Pereira* [1,2], *Mário Nora* [2,3] *and Mariana P. Monteiro* [1,2*]

[1] *Endocrine, Cardiovascular and Metabolic Research, Unit for Multidisciplinary Research in Biomedicine, University of Porto, Porto, Portugal,* [2] *Department of Anatomy, Abel Salazar Institute of Biomedical Sciences, University of Porto, Porto, Portugal,* [3] *Department of General Surgery, Centro Hospitalar de Entre o Douro e Vouga, Santa Maria da Feira, Portugal*

***Correspondence:**
Mariana P. Monteiro
mpmonteiro@icbas.up.pt

Background/Objetives: Obesity and obesity related co-morbidities are well-recognized risks for cardiovascular (CV) disease and mortality. Weight loss improves CV risk factors and the efficacy of bariatric surgery in decreasing CV mortality is now well-established. Our aim was to assess CV risk progression and occurrence of CV events in a cohort of patients that underwent Roux-en-Y gastric bypass (RYGB) for obesity treatment in a single academic public center.

Subjects and Methods: Ten year CV risk was estimated using the Framingham Equation at baseline and 2 years after RYGB surgery in our patients cohort ($n = 260$). In the subgroup with a follow-up time longer than 4 years after surgery ($n = 185$; mean 5.4 ± 0.1 years), CV risk adjusted for the time length after RYGB was similarly estimated and the occurrence of CV events for outcome adjudication was monitored during the same time period by reviewing the hospital patients' record, the electronic national health system patient register and our center outpatient clinic records.

Results: Ten year CV risk was significantly reduced 2 years after surgery when compared to baseline, with reductions of $1.65 \pm 0.25\%$ in the risk of CV disease. Patients with prior type 2 diabetes and aged 50 years or older experienced a significantly superior CV risk reduction, with diabetic patients experiencing a reduction of their 10–year CV disease risk of $3.58 \pm 1.11\%$ vs. a reduction of $1.31 \pm 0.20\%$ in non-diabetic patients and with the 10–year risk of CV disease dropping $3.41 \pm 0.75\%$ in patients older than 50 vs. a reduction of 0.99 ± 0.18 in patients up to 50 years. For the subgroup of patients with a longer follow-up time, baseline CV risk estimation predicted the occurrence of 6.08 ± 0.56 cardiovascular disease (CVD) events, 3.87 ± 0.39 coronary heart disease (CHD) events, 1.49 ± 0.22 myocardial infarctions (MI), 0.71 ± 0.09 strokes, 0. 28 ± 0.05 deaths from CHD and 0.35 ± 0.05 deaths from CVD. No CV events were adjudicated in this subgroup during follow-up.

Conclusions: RYGB significantly improves CV risk and prevents the occurrence of CV events. For similar weight loss, diabetic and elder patients experience a superior CV risk improvement and may have additional CV benefits after bariatric surgery.

Keywords: cardiovascular risk, cardiovascular outcome, obesity, bariatric/metabolic surgery, diabetes

INTRODUCTION

Obesity and obesity-related morbidities are well-established risks for cardiovascular (CV) disease and mortality (1). Obesity has direct effects on CV structure by increasing myocardial fat deposition and altering hemodynamic function (2). In addition, obesity triggers an increased sympathetic activity and a decreased systemic vascular resistance, which result in increased heart rate and cardiac output, generating cardiac overload and eventually leading to left ventricular hypertrophy, atria dilation (3), heart dysfunction and dysrhythmia (4). Moreover, obesity is the central feature of the metabolic syndrome, which includes other CV risk factors such as high blood pressure (BP), lipid abnormalities and altered glucose homeostasis or type 2 diabetes (T2D) (5). Indeed, obese individuals were shown to have at least twice the risk of developing heart failure compared to normal weight individuals (2, 6). Therefore, obesity is undeniably an independent predictor of CV disease (2, 6).

Weight loss allows the improvement of several CV risk factors and was demonstrated not only to decrease overall mortality, but also to specifically prevent CV related mortality (7–9). Bariatric surgery is the most effective means to achieve substantial and sustained weight loss in severely obese patients in whom previous conservative or medical interventions have repeatedly failed (10). Furthermore, there is now considerable evidence derived from prospective trials and meta-analyses that demonstrate the benefits of weight loss attained through bariatric surgery in improving CV risk factors, including reducing BP (11), improving dyslipidemia (12) and ameliorating glycemic control or even inducing clinical remission of T2D (13–15). Moreover, bariatric surgery not only proved to reduce CV risk scores, but also prevents the occurrence of CV events and reduces overall mortality (7, 16). In the Swedish Obesity Subjects Study (SOS study), post-bariatric patients when compared to non-operated weight matched controls, experienced 33% and 53% fewer total and fatal CV events, respectively (17).

Our aim was to evaluate the impact of weight loss attained through Roux-en-Y gastric bypass (RYGB) on CV outcomes by comparing the predicted vs. occurred CV event rate in a cohort of post-RYGB patients attended at a single academic public center.

METHODS

Subject Selection and Enrolment Criteria

Subjects enrolled in this study were attended at a single academic public center for Obesity Treatment. To be considered candidates for bariatric surgery patients had to meet the criteria of having a body mass index (BMI) over 40 kg/m^2 or over 35 kg/m^2 in the presence of obesity-related morbidities, provided previous non-invasive weight loss interventions had failed and there were no contraindications for the proposed surgical intervention. Participants were selected from our prospective database of post bariatric patients operated between 2005 and 2010 (N = 917) based on the following criteria: (1) availability of all clinical and analytical parameters required for CV risk calculation (N = 315) using the Framingham Heart Study (2008) score (as detailed in the section below), (2) having a minimum follow-up time of 2 years after surgery and (3) having a least of one observation in our center per year during the time of follow-up (N = 55 lost to follow-up), yielding the final subset of patients for data analysis (n = 260). To ensure homogeneity of clinical data acquisition and recording in our post-bariatric prospective register, all patients were attended by the same multidisciplinary team that includes endocrinologists, surgeons, psychologists, and nutritionists before and after the RYGB surgery.

Surgical Procedure

The RYGB procedure consisted in the creation of a neo-stomach with an approximate volume of 30 cm^3, which was anastomosed to a jejunum loop located 50–60 cm from the ligament of Treitz (gastro-jejunostomy), while the biliopancreatic flow was restored by an entero-enteric anastomosis performed 90 to 120 cm distal to the gastro-jejunostomy. Thereby, RYGB excludes from the gastrointestinal transit approximately 95% of the stomach, the entire duodenum and part of the jejunum.

CV Risk Calculation

To estimate CV risk (coronary, cerebrovascular, peripheral arterial disease and heart failure), the updated sex-specific multivariable risk factor algorithm derived from the Framingham Heart Study (2008) was used. This algorithm estimates an individual's overall risk for cardiovascular disease (CVD), as well as the isolated risk for coronary heart disease (CHD), myocardial infarction (MI), stroke, peripheral vascular disease, death from CHD, death from CVD and heart failure in a given period of time spanning from 4 to 10 years. To estimate the risk for each CV event, the Framingham equation uses fasting blood glucose, diagnosis of diabetes, blood pressure, total cholesterol, HDL cholesterol, presence of left ventricular hypertrophy (LVH), tobacco use and family history of CV events (18). Of note that the Framingham algorithm does not specifically include body weight nor BMI for CV risk calculation.

CV risk was estimated before (baseline T0) and 2 years after surgery (T2) in the entire patient cohort. In the subgroup with a follow-up time longer than 4 years after surgery (n = 185; mean 5.4 ± 0.01 years), CV risk adjusted for the time length after RYGB was similarly estimated. Occurrence of CV events was correspondingly monitored in this patient subgroup and for

TABLE 1 | Baseline patient demographics, anthropometric and biochemical features.

Age (years)	42.12 ± 0.62
Male:Female	22:238 91.6%:8.4%
BMI (Kg/m^2)	43.9 ± 0.4
Fasting glucose (mg/dL)	107 ± 2
HbA1c (%)[(1)]	5.0 ± 0.1
Systolic BP (mm Hg)	137 ± 1
Diastolic BP (mm Hg)	81 ± 1
Total Cholesterol (mg/dL)	195 ± 2
Triglycerides (mg/dL)	133 ± 4
HDL (mg/dL)	46 ± 1
LDL (mg/dL)	122 ± 2
Type 2 Diabetes (*n*, % of patients)	39 (14.9%)
Anti-diabetic drug (*n*, % of patients)	39 (14.9%)
Anti-hypertensive drug (*n*, % of patients)	63 (24.1%)
Anti-dyslipidemia drug (*n*, % of patients)	36 (13.8%)

[(1)] *HbA1c (%) value is for patient cohort (n = 260).*

TABLE 2 | Patient population distribution according to follow-up time and corresponding BMI and EBMIL.

Follow-up Time	N (%)	BMI (Kg/m^2)*	EBMIL (%)**
2 Years	260 (100)	29.91 ± 0.29	76.84 ± 1.33
4 Years	54 (20.8)	31.02 ± 0.65	71.31 ± 2.42
5 Years	44 (16.9)	30.97 ± 0.80	71.52 ± 3.30
6 Years	43 (16.6)	33.02 ± 0.68	54.49 ± 4.22
7 Years	44 (16.9)	31.72 ± 0.68	65.70 ± 3.18

**BMI, body mass index; **EBMIL, excess BMI loss.*

TABLE 3 | Patient anthropometric and biochemical features change from baseline at 2 years of follow-up.

	Baseline	2 y after surgery	Δ	*p*
BMI (Kg/m^2)	43.90 ± 0.39	29.92 ± 0.28	−13.98 ± 0.27	< 0.001
Fasting glucose (mg/dL)	107 ± 2	87 ± 1	−19 ± 2	< 0.001
Total Cholesterol (mg/dL)	195 ± 2	176 ± 2	−19 ± 2	< 0.001
Triglycerides (mg/dL)	133 ± 4	84 ± 2	−49 ± 4	< 0.001
LDL (mg/dL)	122 ± 2	102 ± 1	−20 ± 2	< 0.001
HDL (mg/dL)	46 ± 1	57 ± 1	11 ± 1	< 0.001
Systolic BP (mm Hg)	137 ± 1	134 ± 1	−3 ± 1	0.03
Diastolic BP (mm Hg)	81 ± 1	79 ± 1	−2 ± 1	0.04

the same time period. The means used for CV event adjudication included: (1) review of hospital patient records for the occurrence of CV events requiring in-hospital admission, (2) review of electronic national health system patient register depicting outpatient clinical records during routine appointments at the general practitioner and (3) review of our center outpatient clinic records. The protocol was reviewed and approved by the Institutional Ethical Review and Hospital Administration Boards in accordance with the recommendations of the Declaration of Helsinki and the European Data Protection Regulations.

Statistical Analysis

Results are presented as mean ± standard error of the mean (Mean ± SEM) unless otherwise specified. D'Agostino & Pearson omnibus test was used to determine the normality of the groups. Comparisons between three or more groups were performed with the Kruskal–Wallis test followed by the Dunn *post-hoc* test or with One-way ANOVA followed by a Holm-Sidak *post-hoc* test accordingly to the normality of the data. The difference between two independent experimental groups was evaluated using the unpaired Student *t*-test or Mann-Whitney U accordingly to the normality of the data. A $p < 0.05$ was considered statistically significant. All statistical analyzes were performed with the aid of the GraphPad Prism software version 7.00 for windows.

RESULTS

This post-RYGB patient cohort ($n = 260$) encompassed 91.6% females ($n = 238$) and 8.4% males ($n = 22$). At the time of surgery, subjects had a mean age of 42.12 ± 0.62 years and a mean BMI of 43.9 ± 0.4 kg/m^2, while 14.9% ($n = 39$) had been diagnosed with type 2 diabetes (T2D) prior undergoing bariatric surgery. Baseline patient demographics, anthropometric and biochemical features, irrespectively of specific drug treatment for any of these conditions are depicted on **Table 1**.

Patients had an average time after RYGB surgery of 4.41 ± 0.11 years, spanning from a minimum of 2 years to a maximum of 7 years, with the subsequent follow-up time distribution: 4 years 20.7% ($n = 54$), 5 years 17.3% ($n = 44$), 6 years 16.9% ($n = 43$) and 7 years 17.3% ($n = 44$). A maximum percentage of excess BMI loss [%EBMIL=100*($BMI_{Baseline}$-$BMI_{Follow-up}$)/($BMI_{Baseline}$-25)] of 76.84% ± 1.33% was achieved 2 years after surgery (**Table 2**). After RYGB surgery there was a significant improvement of several independent CV risk factors, including a decrease in BMI, fasting glucose, total cholesterol, LDL cholesterol, triglycerides, systolic, and diastolic blood pressure, along with an increase in HDL cholesterol (**Table 3**).

At baseline, the 10-year CV risk predicted by the Framingham Cardiovascular Risk Equation was 7.39 ± 0.48% for CVD, 4.67 ± 0.34% for CHD, 1.99 ± 0.20% for MI, 1.18 ± 0.11% for stroke, 0.58 ± 0.08% for death from CHD and 0.84 ± 0.10% for death from CVD (**Figure 1**). The 10-year CV risk recalculated 2 years after surgery decreased significantly predicting a risk of 5.74 ± 0.38% for CVD, 3.1 ± 0.22% for CHD, 1.09 ± 0.11% for MI, 1.27 ± 0.10% for stroke, 0.31 ± 0.04% for death from CHD and 0.59 ± 0.07% for death from CVD (**Figure 1**). Two years after RYGB surgery the 10-year CV risk reduction was statistically significant for most isolated CV events (−1.65 ± 0.25% for CVD, −1.57 ± 0.20% for CHD, −0.91 ± 0.13% for MI, −0.27 ± 0.06% for death

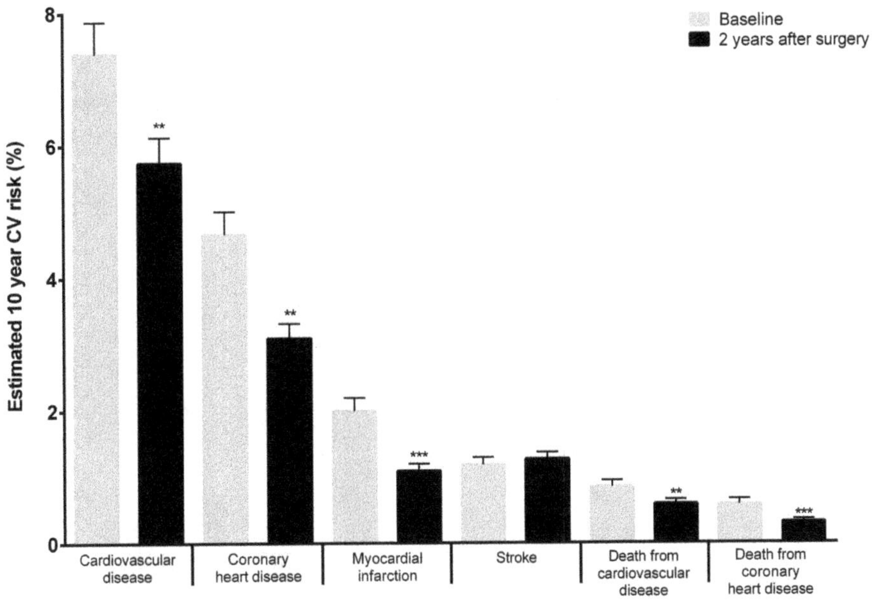

FIGURE 1 | Estimation of the 10-year risk of CV events applying the Framingham Heart Study (2008) score to patients' clinical and analytical features at baseline and 2 years after surgery. As an example, the Framingham Cardiovascular Risk equation predicted a baseline (pre-operative) 10-year risk for CVD events of 7.39 ± 0.49% and 2 years after surgery this risk was of 5.74 ± 0.38% (** $p < 0.01$; *** $p < 0.001$–baseline vs. 2 years after surgery).

from CHD and −0.26 ± 0.06% for death from CVD), with the sole exception of the risk for stroke that did not vary considerably since baseline (0.08 ± 0.08% for stroke; **Figure 1**).

Patients diagnosed with T2D prior to surgery had a significant decrease in 10-year risk for most CV events when compared to non-diabetic individuals, once excluded the risk for stroke (**Figure 2**). In addition, patient stratification according to age [<50 years (n = 182) and ≥ 50 years (n = 82)], showed that the elder group experienced a significant 10-year CV risk reduction when compared to the younger group (**Figure 3**); these differences prevailed even after excluding T2D patients from the analysis, as the condition was more frequent in the elder patient group (**Supplementary Data, Figure S1, Table S1**). Apart from fasting glucose levels that decreased significantly in T2D patients as compared to non-diabetic patients, the change from baseline of all other CV risk parameters that were evaluated experienced similar improvements, including BMI (**Table 4**). Similar findings were observed when the clinical profiles of younger and older patients before and after surgery were compared (**Table 5**).

For the subset of patients with more than 4 years of surgery the number of predicted CV events was calculated by adjusting the Framingham Equation to the follow-up time of each individual. Based on the CV risk estimation, 6.08 ± 0.56 CVD events, 3.87 ± 0.39 CHD events, 1.49 ± 0.22 MIs, 0.81 ± 0.09 strokes, 0.28 ± 0.05 deaths from CHD and 0.35 ± 0.05 deaths from CVD were predicted to occur in this subset of patients during the elapsed follow-up time (**Figure 4**).

No CV events were adjudicated during follow-up time.

DISCUSSION

Obesity is often associated with a high CV risk that weight loss can mitigate (8, 19). Bariatric surgery induces substantive and sustained weight reduction, in addition to improving several CV risk factors and decreasing CV events and mortality (17, 20, 21). RYGB is a bariatric surgery procedure widely performed for obesity treatment with a well-established effectiveness profile in inducing weight loss in addition to the ability to prevent or even to revert obesity related disorders, such as T2D and CV diseases (12, 22).

In this study we sought to evaluate the CV outcomes associated with weight loss achieved through RYGB surgery by comparing the predicted vs. occurred CV events in a cohort of patients attended in a single academic public center.

In this patient cohort, RYBG surgery induced a significant and sustained weight loss. The maximum weight reduction was achieved 2 years after surgery with a %EBMIL of 76.84%. At that same time point, the estimated 10-year CV risk also decreased significantly when compared to the estimated 10-year CV risk at baseline before the surgical procedure.

Moreover, CV risk reduction was significantly higher in patients with T2D diagnosed prior to surgery. In fact, the 10-year CV risk reductions with greater magnitude were observed for the risks of CHD, MI and CVD, outdoing the CV risk reductions experienced by non-diabetic patients. The sole exception was for the risk of stroke, which was not significantly altered after the intervention, corroborating earlier

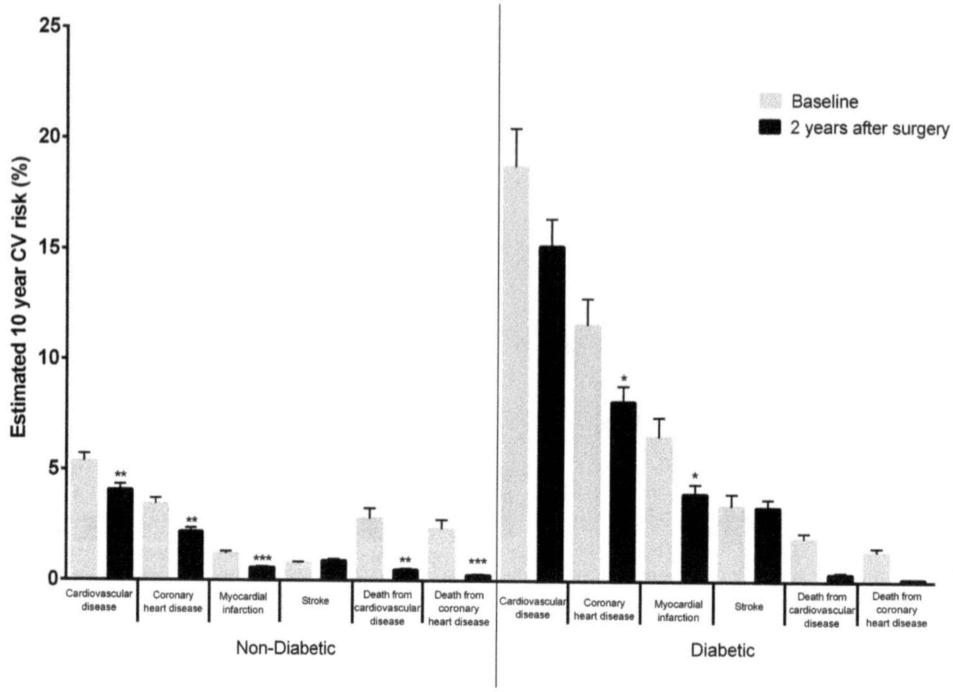

FIGURE 2 | Estimated 10-year CV risk applying the Framingham Heart Study (2008) score to patients' clinical and analytical data at baseline and 2 years after surgery in diabetic and non-diabetic patients. As an example, in non-diabetic patients, the Framingham Cardiovascular Risk equation predicted a pre-surgical 10-year risk of CVD events of 5.39 ± 0.34 and a 10-year risk for CVD events 2 years after surgery of 4.08 ± 0.28% while in diabetic patients, the Framingham Cardiovascular Risk equation predicted a pre-surgical 10-year risk of CVD events of 18.74 ± 1.72% and a 10-year risk for CV events 2 years after surgery of 15.16 ± 1.22% for CVD (*p < 0.05; **p < 0.01; ***p < 0.001–baseline vs. 2 years after surgery).

data from the SOS study, since weight loss after bariatric surgery has not shown to influence the incidence of stroke (23). Remarkably, this observation is quite consistent with other previous findings including those of large trials to assess the cardiovascular outcomes associated with glucose lowering drugs, such as the EMPA-REG trial, which has demonstrated that empaglifozin has several CV benefits in T2D patients and yet it failed to reduce the risk of stroke (24). Furthermore, weight loss elicited by bariatric surgery was proven to be particularly effective in decreasing the CV risk, as well as preventing CV events and mortality in individuals with high insulin and/or glucose levels at baseline (13, 23). Therefore, our data upholds the previous findings further supporting that T2D obese patients submitted to bariatric surgery may have additional CV benefits, besides the well-known glycemic improvement or even T2D clinical remission (17, 23). Subjects with diabetes are known for carrying a disproportionately higher risk of CV disease when compared to non-diabetic subjects. In fact, a significant proportion of T2D patients experience clinical remission of the disease after several bariatric surgical interventions, such as RYGB, along with a significant improvement of several independent CV risk factors, including blood glucose levels, blood pressure and lipid profile, which synergistically result in an overall decrease of the estimated CV risk (14). Moreover, the weight loss profile of patients with T2D diagnosed prior to RYGB surgery was no different from non-diabetic patients, reinforcing the effectiveness of this weight reducing intervention in T2D patients and the likely dissociation of the observed effects in what concerns body weight and CV risk factors.

Age is one of the most important determinants of CV health (25, 26). In earlier times, several national and international guidance's recommended that weight loss surgical interventions should be restricted to patients under 60 years old based on the concerns of age-related increased surgical risks (27). Nonetheless, as the amount of clinical evidence enlarged, it became recognizable that the surgical outcomes of bariatric surgery, including morbidity and mortality rates, in older patients were not significantly different than those observed in younger ones (28–31). Thus, the number of bariatric procedures performed in older patients has increased over the past decades (32, 33). Our data not only reinforces that weight loss achieved after RYGB in patients over 50 years old are not inferior to the observed in younger patients, but also suggests that the CV benefits in this patient group as compared to the younger ones are also more likely to be superior. This difference persists even after the exclusion of T2D patients from analysis, as the decrease in CV risk was still significantly higher in patients older than 50 years, further suggesting that age could be an additional factor to retrieve benefits from surgery.

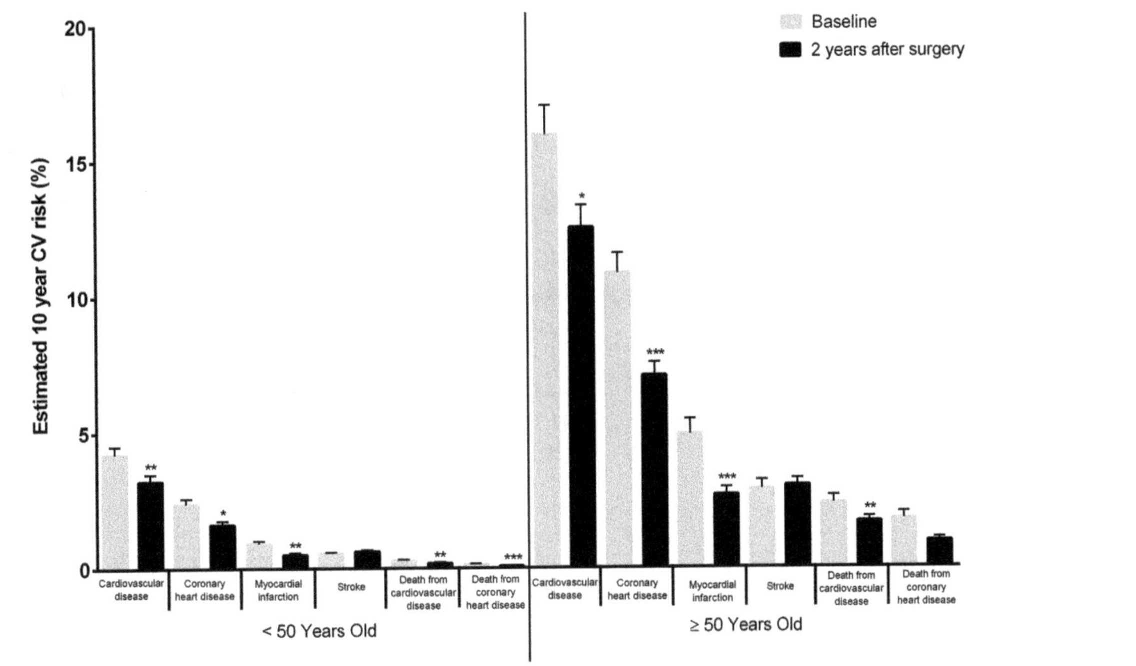

FIGURE 3 | Estimated 10-year CV risk in different age groups applying the Framingham Heart Study (2008) score to patients' clinical and analytical data prior to surgery and 2 years after surgery. As an example, the Framingham Cardiovascular Risk equation predicted a pre-surgical 10-year risk of CVD events of 4.23 ± 0.29% in patients younger than 50 while in patients with at least 50 years the same risk was of 15.97 ± 1.09%. Two years after surgery the 10-year risk of CVD had drop to 3.23 ± 0.25% for patients younger than 50 while for patients with at least 50 years it had drop to 12.55 ± 0.82% ($^{*}p < 0.05$; $^{**}p < 0.01$; $^{***}p < 0.001$–baseline vs. 2 years after surgery).

TABLE 4 | Comparison of clinical and biochemical features at baseline and 2 years after surgery according to the presence of type 2 diabetes prior to RYGB surgery.

	Non-Diabetic			**Diabetic**			**Change from baseline at 2 y**		
	Baseline	**2 y after surgery**	***p***	**Baseline**	**2 y after surgery**	***p***	**Non-Diabetic**	**Diabetic**	***p***
Age (years)	41.1 ± 0.7		48.2 ± 1.5						
Male/Female	18 8.1%		4 10.3%						
BMI (Kg/m2)	43.9 ± 0.4	29.8 ± 0.3	<0.001	43.8 ± 1.4	30.8 ± 0.9	<0.001	−14.2 ± 0.3	−12.9 ± 0.8	0.05
Fasting glucose (mg/dL)	102 ± 2	86 ± 1	<0.001	134 ± 8	95 ± 3	<0.001	−16 ± 2	−39 ± 7	< 0.001
Total Cholesterol (mg/dL)	195 ± 3	175 ± 2	<0.001	195 ± 7	181 ± 6	0.10	−19 ± 3	−14 ± 6	0.31
Triglycerides (mg/dL)	130 ± 4	83 ± 2	<0.001	148 ± 12	91 ± 5	<0.001	−47 ± 4	−56 ± 10	0.31
LDL (mg/dL)	122 ± 2	102 ± 2	<0.001	122 ± 5	106 ± 5	0.04	−21 ± 2	−15 ± 5	0.10
HDL (mg/dL)	46 ± 1	57 ± 1	<0.001	44 ± 2	56 ± 2	<0.001	11 ± 1	12 ± 2	0.65
Systolic BP (mm Hg)	137 ± 1	133 ± 1	0.03	141 ± 3	139 ± 3	0.64	−4 ± 1	−2 ± 4	0.66
Diastolic BP (mm Hg)	81 ± 1	79 ± 1	0.06	82 ± 2	81 ± 2	<0.001	−2 ± 1	−1 ± 2	0.32

The fact that our sample size is relatively small when compared to nationwide epidemiologic studies such as the SOS Study, is in no doubt the major limitation of this current study. However, given that our data refers to a single center population, with similar background demographic and clinical features, submitted to a single bariatric surgery technical procedure by the same multidisciplinary team and delivered the same standards of patient care, allowed the retrieval of robust data information for statistical analysis, and thus valid conclusions can be still be ascertained. Nevertheless, the fact that this was a retrospective review of patient records instead of a prospective study designed to assess CV outcomes with formal event adjudication, implies that the level of evidence retrieved from this study is not as high as it would be if derived from a clinical trial. Besides that, there was a 17.5% loss to follow-up rate of subjects that did not have a minimum of 4 years of follow-up after surgery or a minimum of one observation per year during the follow-up time, although, no significant differences in baseline characteristics between participants with long-term follow-up and drop outs were noticed.

TABLE 5 | Comparison of clinical and biochemical features at baseline and 2 years after surgery according to the patients age at the time of RYGB surgery.

	Age under 50 y			Age over 50 y			Change from baseline at 2 y		
	Baseline	**2 y after surgery**	***p***	**Baseline**	**2 y after surgery**	***p***	**Under 50 y**	**Over 50 y**	***p***
Age (years)	37.4 ± 0.5		55.1 ± 0.4						
Male/Female	15 7.9%		7 10.0%						
BMI (Kg/m2)	43.7 ± 0.4	29.7 ± 0.3	<0.001	44.5 ± 0.9	30.5 ± 0.6	<0.001	−14.0 ± 0.3	−14.1 ± 0.6	0.62
Type 2 diabetes (n. % of patients)	19 (10.0%)			20 (28.6%)					
Fasting glucose (mg/dL)	102 ± 2	86 ± 1	<0.001	121 ± 5	91 ± 2	<0.001	−16 ± 2	−30 ± 5	<0.001
Total Cholesterol (mg/dL)	192 ± 3	174 ± 2	<0.001	201 ± 4	181 ± 4	<0.001	−18 ± 3	−20 ± 5	0.99
Triglycerides (mg/dL)	131 ± 5	82 ± 2	<0.001	138 ± 7	90 ± 4	<0.001	−49 ± 4	−47 ± 7	0.87
LDL (mg/dL)	120 ± 3	101 ± 2	<0.001	128 ± 3	105 ± 3	<0.001	−19 ± 2	−23 ± 4	0.86
HDL (mg/dL)	46 ± 1	56 ± 1	<0.001	45 ± 1	58 ± 1	<0.001	10 ± 1	13 ± 2	0.37
Systolic BP (mm Hg)	136 ± 1	131 ± 1	0.01	142 ± 2	141 ± 2	0.75	−4 ± 1	−1 ± 3	0.30
Diastolic BP (mm Hg)	80 ± 1	78 ± 1	0.06	82 ± 2	81 ± 2	0.40	−2 ± 1	−1 ± 2	0.95

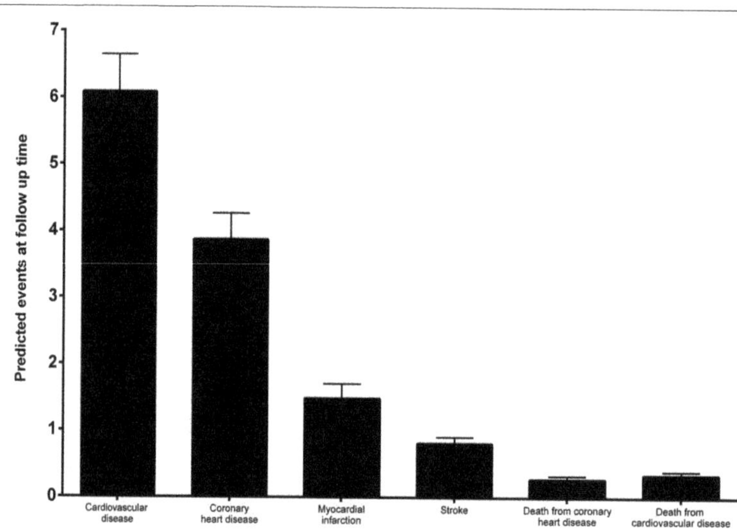

FIGURE 4 | Estimation of the predicted number of CV events during follow-up-time by applying the Framingham Heart Study (2008) score to baseline characteristics of patients with a minimum follow-up of 4 years.

Additionally, our data based on CV risk estimated before RYGB surgery predicted that 6 CVD events would have occurred during the elicited follow-up time if patients had not been intervened. However, there were no CV events adjudicated during the same time period. Overall, there was a significant difference between the estimated CV risk and the actual incidence of CV events observed, while RYGB surgery may have prevented 6 CV events in this patient population.

CONCLUSION

Weight loss attained trough RYGB surgery was associated with a substantial CV risk reduction and prevented the occurrence of CV events. In addition, diabetic and elder patients experience a superior CV risk reduction and may have additional CV benefits after bariatric surgery, despite depicting similar weight loss and risk factors improvement.

AUTHOR CONTRIBUTIONS

PP, TM, MG, SP, and MM planned and designed the study. PP, MG, and MN conducted data acquisition. TM performed the statistical analysis. PP, TM, and MM participated in analysis and interpretation of data. PP and MM wrote the manuscript; PP, TM, MG, SP, MN, and MM revised the manuscript. All authors approved the submitted version.

REFERENCES

1. Prospective Studies C, Whitlock G, Lewington S, Sherliker P, Clarke R, Emberson J, et al. Body-mass index and cause-specific mortality in 900 000 adults: collaborative analyses of 57 prospective studies. *Lancet* (2009) 373:1083–96. doi: 10.1016/S0140-6736(09)60318-4
2. Kenchaiah S, Evans JC, Levy D, Wilson PW, Benjamin EJ, Larson MG, et al. Obesity and the risk of heart failure. *N Engl J Med.* (2002) 347:305–13. doi: 10.1056/NEJMoa020245
3. Lavie CJ, Milani RV, Ventura HO. Obesity and cardiovascular disease: risk factor, paradox, and impact of weight loss. *J Am Coll Cardiol.* (2009) 53:1925–32. doi: 10.1016/j.jacc.2008.12.068
4. Lee GK, Cha YM. Cardiovascular benefits of bariatric surgery. *Trends Cardiovas. Med.* (2015) 26:280–9. doi: 10.1016/j.tcm.2015.07.006
5. Alberti KGMM, Eckel RH, Grundy SM, Zimmet PZ, Cleeman JI, Donato KA, et al. Harmonizing the metabolic syndrome. a joint interim statement of the international diabetes federation task force on epidemiology and prevention; national heart, lung, and blood institute; american heart association; world heart federation; international atherosclerosis society; and international association for the study of obesity. *Circulation* (2009) 120:1640–5. doi: 10.1161/circulationaha.109.192644
6. Hubert HB, Feinleib M, McNamara PM, Castelli WP. Obesity as an independent risk factor for cardiovascular disease: a 26-year follow-up of participants in the Framingham Heart Study. *Circulation* (1983) 67: 968–77.
7. Adams TD, Gress RE, Smith SC, Halverson RC, Simper SC, Rosamond WD, et al. Long-term mortality after gastric bypass surgery. *N Engl J Med.* (2007) 357:753–61. doi: 10.1056/NEJMoa066603
8. Ma C, Avenell A, Bolland M, Hudson J, Stewart F, Robertson C, et al. Effects of weight loss interventions for adults who are obese on mortality, cardiovascular disease, and cancer: systematic review and meta-analysis. *BMJ* (2017) 359:j4849. doi: 10.1136/bmj.j4849
9. Clifton PM, Keogh JB. Effects of different weight loss approaches on CVD risk. *Curr Atherosclerosis Rep.* (2018) 20:27. doi: 10.1007/s11883-018-0728-8
10. Gloy VL, Briel M, Bhatt DL, Kashyap SR, Schauer PR, Mingrone G, et al. Bariatric surgery versus non-surgical treatment for obesity: a systematic review and meta-analysis of randomised controlled trials. *BMJ* (2013) 347:f5934. doi: 10.1136/bmj.f5934
11. Livingston EH. Surgical volume impacts bariatric surgery mortality: a case for bariatric surgery centers of excellence. *Surgery* (2010) 147:751–3. doi: 10.1016/j.surg.2009.10.038
12. Sjostrom L, Lindroos AK, Peltonen M, Torgerson J, Bouchard C, Carlsson B, et al. Lifestyle, diabetes, and cardiovascular risk factors 10 years after bariatric surgery. *N Engl J Med.* (2004) 351:2683–93. doi: 10.1056/NEJMoa03562213
13. Ribaric G, Buchwald JN, McGlennon TW. Diabetes and weight in comparative studies of bariatric surgery vs conventional medical therapy: a systematic review and meta-analysis. *Obesity Surg.* (2014) 24:437–55. doi: 10.1007/s11695-013-1160-3
14. Nora M, Morais T, Almeida R, Guimaraes M, Monteiro MP. Should Roux-en-Y gastric bypass biliopancreatic limb length be tailored to achieve improved diabetes outcomes? *Medicine* (2017) 96:e8859. doi: 10.1097/md.0000000000008859
15. Beamish AJ, Olbers T, Kelly AS, Inge TH. Cardiovascular effects of bariatric surgery. *Nat Rev Cardiol.* (2016) 13:730–43. doi: 10.1038/nrcardio.2016.162
16. Kwok CS, Pradhan A, Khan MA, Anderson SG, Keavney BD, Myint PK, et al. Bariatric surgery and its impact on cardiovascular disease and mortality: a systematic review and meta-analysis. *Int J Cardiol.* (2014) 173:20–8. doi: 10.1016/j.ijcard.2014.02.026
17. Sjostrom L, Peltonen M, Jacobson P, Sjostrom CD, Karason K, Wedel H, et al. Bariatric surgery and long-term cardiovascular events. *JAMA* (2012) 307:56–65. doi: 10.1001/jama.2011.1914
18. D'Agostino RB, Sr., Vasan RS, Pencina MJ, Wolf PA, Cobain M, Massaro JM, et al. General cardiovascular risk profile for use in primary care: the Framingham heart study. *Circulation* (2008) 117:743–53. doi: 10.1161/circulationaha.107.699579
19. Vogel JA, Franklin BA, Zalesin KC, Trivax JE, Krause KR, Chengelis DL, et al. Reduction in predicted coronary heart disease risk after substantial weight reduction after bariatric surgery. *Am J Cardiol.* (2006) 99:222–6. doi: 10.1016/j.amjcard.2006.08.017
20. Chang SH, Stoll CR, Song J, Varela JE, Eagon CJ, Colditz GA. The effectiveness and risks of bariatric surgery: an updated systematic review and meta-analysis, 2003-2012. *JAMA Surg.* (2014) 149:275–87. doi: 10.1001/jamasurg.2013.3654
21. Sjostrom L, Narbro K, Sjostrom CD, Karason K, Larsson B, Wedel H, et al. Effects of bariatric surgery on mortality in Swedish obese subjects. *N Engl J Med.* (2007) 357:741–52. doi: 10.1056/NEJMoa066254
22. Mingrone G, Panunzi S, De Gaetano A, Guidone C, Iaconelli A, Nanni G, et al. Bariatric-metabolic surgery versus conventional medical treatment in obese patients with type 2 diabetes: 5 year follow-up of an open-label, single-centre, randomised controlled trial. *Lancet* (2015) 386:964–73. doi: 10.1016/S0140-6736(15)00075-6
23. Romeo S, Maglio C, Burza MA, Pirazzi C, Sjoholm K, Jacobson P, et al. Cardiovascular events after bariatric surgery in obese subjects with type 2 diabetes. *Diab Care* (2012) 35:2613–7. doi: 10.2337/dc12-0193
24. Zinman B, Wanner C, Lachin JM, Fitchett D, Bluhmki E, Hantel S, et al. Empagliflozin, cardiovascular outcomes, and mortality in type 2 diabetes. *N Engl J Med.* (2015) 373:2117–28. doi: 10.1056/NEJMoa1504720 25.
25. North BJ, Sinclair DA. The intersection between aging and cardiovascular disease. *Circulation Res.* (2012) 110:1097–108. doi: 10.1161/circresaha.111.246876
26. Finegold JA, Asaria P, Francis DP. Mortality from ischaemic heart disease by country, region, and age: statistics from World Health Organisation and United Nations. *Int J Cardiol.* (2013) 168:934–45. doi: 10.1016/j.ijcard.2012.10.046
27. Fried M, Yumuk V, Oppert JM, Scopinaro N, Torres A, Weiner R, et al. Interdisciplinary European guidelines on metabolic and bariatric surgery. *Obesity Surg.* (2014) 24:42–55. doi: 10.1007/s11695-013-1079-8
28. Giordano S, Victorzon M. Bariatric surgery in elderly patients: a systematic review. *Clin Interv Aging* (2015) 10:1627–35. doi: 10.2147/CIA.S70313
29. Dunkle-Blatter SE, St Jean MR, Whitehead C, Strodel W, III, Bennotti PN, Still C, et al. Outcomes among elderly bariatric patients at a high-volume center. *Surg Obesity Related Dis.* (2007) 3:163–9; discussion: 9–70. doi: 10.1016/j.soard.2006.12.004
30. Davidson LE, Adams TD, Kim J, Jones JL, Hashibe M, Taylor D, et al. Association of patient age at gastric bypass surgery with long-term all-cause and cause-specific mortality. *JAMA Surg.* (2016) 151:631–7. doi: 10.1001/jamasurg.2015.5501
31. Batsis JA, Miranda WR, Prasad C, Collazo-Clavell ML, Sarr MG, Somers VK, et al. Effect of bariatric surgery on cardiometabolic risk in elderly patients: a population-based study. *Geriatr Gerontol Int.* (2016) 16:618–24. doi: 10.1111/ggi.12527
32. Gonzalez-Heredia R, Patel N, Sanchez-Johnsen L, Masrur M, Murphey M, Chen J, et al. Does age influence bariatric surgery outcomes? *Bariatric Surg Pract Patient Care* (2015) 10:74–8. doi: 10.1089/bari.2015.0004
33. Gebhart A, Young MT, Nguyen NT. Bariatric surgery in the elderly: 2009-2013. *Surg Obesity Rel Dis.* (2015) 11:393–8. doi: 10.1016/j.soard.2014.04.014
34. Pereira PR. *O Impacto da Cirurgia Bariátrica no Risco Cardiovascular e na Prevalência de Eventos Cardiovasculares em Doentes Obesos.* Master's thesis, University of Porto—Portugal (2016).

17

Mechanisms Underlying Type 2 Diabetes Remission after Metabolic Surgery

Belén Pérez-Pevida [1,2*], ***Javier Escalada*** [2,3,4], ***Alexander D. Miras*** [1] ***and Gema Frühbeck*** [2,3,4*]

[1] Section of Investigative Medicine, Division of Diabetes, Endocrinology and Metabolism, Imperial College London, Hammersmith Campus, London, United Kingdom, [2] Department of Endocrinology and Nutrition, Clínica Universidad de Navarra, Pamplona, Spain, [3] Biomedical Research Networking Center for Physiopathology of Obesity and Nutrition (CIBEROBN), ISCIII, Pamplona, Spain, [4] Obesity and Adipobiology Group, Instituto de Investigación Sanitaria de Navarra (IdiSNA), Pamplona, Spain

***Correspondence:**
Belén Pérez-Pevida
bppevida@unav.es
Gema Frühbeck
gfruhbeck@unav.es

Type 2 diabetes prevalence is increasing dramatically worldwide. Metabolic surgery is the most effective treatment for selected patients with diabetes and/or obesity. When compared to intensive medical therapy and lifestyle intervention, metabolic surgery has shown superiority in achieving glycemic improvement, reducing number of medications and cardiovascular risk factors, which translates in long-term benefits on cardiovascular morbidity and mortality. The mechanisms underlying diabetes improvement after metabolic surgery have not yet been clearly understood but englobe a complex interaction among improvements in beta cell function and insulin secretion, insulin sensitivity, intestinal gluconeogenesis, changes in glucose utilization, and absorption by the gut and changes in the secretory pattern and morphology of adipose tissue. These are achieved through different mediators which include an enhancement in gut hormones release, especially, glucagon-like peptide 1, changes in bile acids circulation, gut microbiome, and glucose transporters expression. Therefore, this review aims to provide a comprehensive appraisal of what is known so far to better understand the mechanisms through which metabolic surgery improves glycemic control facilitating future research in the field.

Keywords: type 2 diabetes, bariatric surgery, insulin resistance, beta-cell function, glucose absorption, glucose utilization, intestinal gluconeogenesis, hepato-portal glucose sensing

INTRODUCTION

Obesity has become in the last decades the most prevalent metabolic alteration. The pathogenesis of obesity is related to multiple biological processes (genetic, neurobiological, hormonal), being frequently accompanied by psychopathological characteristics (1, 2). Good evidence from meta-analyses and nonrandomized and randomized clinical trials (RCT) has shown that obesity-metabolic surgery is the most effective treatment for patients with type 2 diabetes mellitus (T2DM) (3–12). When compared to intensive medical therapy and lifestyle intervention, metabolic surgery has shown superiority in achieving glycemic improvement, reducing number of medications and cardio-metabolic risk factors, which translates in long-term benefits on cardiovascular morbidity and mortality (3–5, 7, 9–12). Two of these RCTs, extending to 5 years follow-up, have shown that metabolic surgery induces euglycemia in 31–77% of cases (7, 10). Despite the fact that glycemic remission rates differ according to the type of surgery, duration of disease and criteria used to define remission, it has been consistently shown that over 80% of patients maintain good postoperative glycemic control despite reduced or no glucose-lowering drugs (7, 10).

There are different types of metabolic surgery which include the laparoscopic adjustable gastric band, the vertical sleeve gastrectomy (VSG), the Roux-en-Y gastric bypass (RYGB), and the biliopancreatic diversion (BPD) procedure, among other variants. The most common ones performed worldwide are the VSG, RYGB, and the gastric band. The mechanisms underlying glycemic improvement after these procedures have not yet been fully understood but involve a complex interaction among improvements in beta cell function and insulin secretion, insulin sensitivity, intestinal gluconeogenesis, and changes in glucose utilization and absorption by the gut alongside changes in the secretory pattern and morphology of adipose tissue. Therefore, the present review aims to provide a comprehensive analysis of what is known so far to better understand the mechanisms through which metabolic surgery improves glycemic control, in order to facilitate future research in the field.

BETA CELL FUNCTION AND INSULIN SECRETION

The physiological ß-cell response is characterized by a biphasic pattern, with an acute initial peak, representing the first phase insulin secretion, which typically happens within the first 30 min after meal consumption. This is followed by a gradually increasing insulin secretion which draws a smaller hump: second phase, 30–180 min after the oral glucose load (13–15). Although plasma glucose concentration is the major stimulus of insulin secretion in the fasting state, gastrointestinal tract-derived signals, mainly the gut hormones released from the endocrine cells, play an important postprandial role. This is explained by the known "incretin effect," where an enhanced insulin secretion can be observed when a glucose load is given orally as compared to intravenously. This incretin effect can contribute to as much as half of the insulin secretion after a meal (16). This gut-dependent nutrient-induced insulin secretion is mainly driven by two incretin gut hormones: glucagon-like peptide 1 (GLP-1) and glucose-dependent insulinotropic polypeptide (GIP) (16, 17).

The current understanding of T2DM is based on a concept of a gradual failure of pancreatic β-cell function in the context of increasing insulin resistance. Once the pancreas is not able to compensate for this insulin resistance, hyperglycemia ensues and the deterioration of the residual ß-cell reserve is accelerated. This β-cell dysfunction is characterized by the loss of sensitivity (i.e., the slope of the insulin secretion/plasma glucose dose-response relationship or the ability to acutely increase insulin release with increasing glycaemia) and an impaired insulin secretion (i.e., total insulin output in response to a nutrient stimulus) (18, 19).

Metabolic surgery (**Figure 1**) partly restores the dysfunction of the β-cell (19–21). The acute insulin response a surrogate of β-cell sensitivity increases after RYGB, BPD, and VSG or gastric banding (19, 22). This can be observed when using oral tests [oral glucose and mixed meal tolerance tests (OGTT, MMTT)], where an earlier and enhanced post-prandial increase in insulin concentration can be observed as compared to the pre-operative response (22). However, as there is a concomitant improvement in insulin sensitivity, less insulin is required to maintain euglycemia and, therefore, a decrease in the total area under the curve for insulin is observed after all types of procedures (23). The underlying physiological mechanisms are not yet well understood. Several contributors have been proposed in this regard, such as caloric restriction, the removal of glucose toxicity (which can enhance glucose sensing), the improvement in insulin resistance (which decreases the β-cell workload) or changes in gastrointestinal tract-derived signals (i.e., incretin hormones) (24). The enhanced GLP-1 secretion is believed by many to be an important weight loss-independent factor contributing to the postoperative improvement seen in β-cell function following VSG, RYGB, and BPD (20, 22, 23, 25–29). Indeed, antagonism with exendin-(9-39) (Ex-9) of the GLP-1 receptor results in a blunted insulin response after a meal and higher post-prandial glucose concentrations (30). However, these findings are not universal. Some studies also blocking GLP-1 by Ex-9 administration (humans) or in animal models by developing GLP-1 receptor deficient or knockout mice for instance have found different results. When Ex-9 was administered after RYGB surgery, despite observing a worsening in glycemic control, it did not recapitulate the glucose tolerance observed at baseline (31). This is in agreement with another human study comparing RYGB patients with a group undergoing an intensive lifestyle modification therapy where the glucose tolerance deterioration during Ex-9 infusion was similar in both groups (31). Moreover, in GLP-1 knockout mice following surgery the improvements observed in glycemic control, weight or eating behavior did not differ from those observed in wild-type mice (31). Despite supporting the important effect of GLP-1 on glucose-mediated insulin secretion, these findings point out at the relevance of other factors as responsible for the sustained improvement in glycemic control following metabolic surgery. Therefore, some researchers support calorie restriction as the main responsible factor for the acute improvement in the β-cell function seen after metabolic surgery, which reduces glucose levels and therefore the glucose toxicity (32–34). Undoubtedly, the combination of the GLP-1 release with caloric restriction enhances β-cell function in the early post-operative period. This is further achieved through the beneficial effects of weight loss and euglycemia on the β-cell. Nonetheless, it is worth noting that the most important predictor of the degree of postoperative improvement in β-cell dysfunction is the preoperative pancreatic reserve itself: the more "exhausted" the β-cell is before surgery, the less likely a patient is to achieve glycemic remission postoperatively (20, 21, 28, 35).

INSULIN SENSITIVITY

In physiological conditions, when glucose homeostasis is in equilibrium, hepatic glucose production, and renal glucose clearance are balanced with glucose utilization due to the insulin effect in the different tissues. After a meal, insulin release is produced in order to firstly suppress hepatic glucose production to then enhance glucose uptake into peripheral tissues. Hence

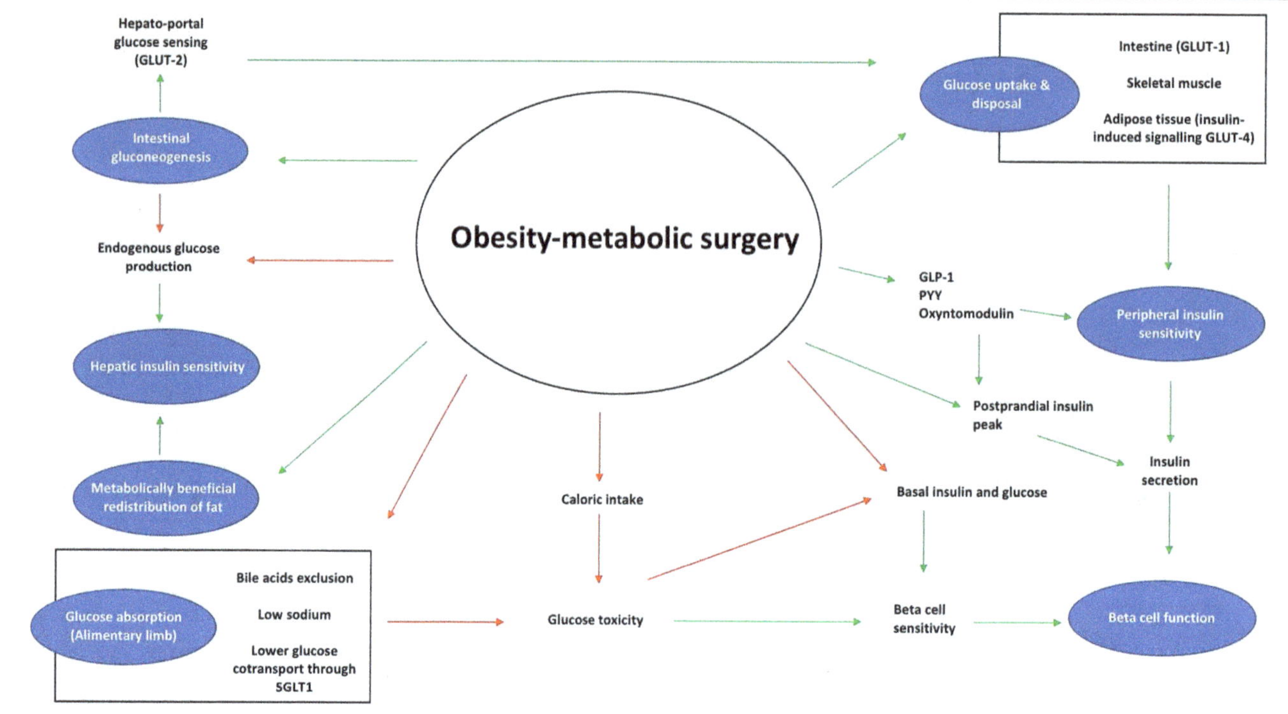

FIGURE 1 | Effects of metabolic surgery on glucose homeostasis. Diabetes remission results from improvements in β-cell function, insulin sensitivity, and changes within the adipose tissue and the gut. Red arrows, represent an inhibitory effect; Green arrows, represent a stimulating effect.

insulin sensitivity is a reflection of how a given peripheral insulin concentration accelerates glucose disappearance. Thus, in insulin resistance states, higher levels of plasma glucose are observed with higher insulin levels required to compensate for the hyperglycemia.

The mechanisms underlying the improvements seen in insulin sensitivity differ depending on the timing of assessment: early vs. late postoperative period. Within days, an improvement in glycemic control and insulin sensitivity can be observed. Most of the studies have shown that this early improvement is secondary to an increase in hepatic insulin sensitivity as indicated by a reduction in endogenous glucose production (25, 36). In contrast, peripheral insulin sensitivity, including skeletal muscle and adipose tissue, does not change during the early postoperative period, but improves gradually thereafter, exerting a close correlation with weight loss (25, 37). This is consistently seen after all metabolic surgery procedures (38). The exception is the BPD, after which an improvement in both, hepatic and peripheral insulin sensitivity since early stages and to a greater extent compared to weight-matched controls undergoing other obesity interventions can be observed (19, 39).

The increase in hepatic insulin sensitivity is due to a decrease in liver fat content secondary to an increase in lipolysis, which mobilizes fatty substrates to circulation and forces lipid oxidation (37). Interestingly, this can be also achieved with short-term caloric restriction independently of weight loss (40, 41). Therefore, the improvement in hepatic insulin sensitivity seen early after surgery could be just the result of postoperative calorie restriction. Several studies comparing different surgical procedures (VSG, RYGB) vs. a very low-calorie diet (VLCD) have shown that metabolic surgery does not reduce hepatic insulin sensitivity beyond the improvements achieved with caloric restriction (33, 34, 42, 43). However, none of these studies accounted for surgical stress. For instance, C-reactive protein, considered a marker of inflammation, infection or surgical stress quickly increases after any surgery, reaching maximum levels 2–3 days postoperatively. This also happens after metabolic surgery even after non-complicated procedures (44). So, the fact that metabolic surgery had the same improvement in insulin sensitivity as the VLCD means that metabolic surgery may be adding a small additional benefit as the observed just with calorie restriction.

In the late postoperative period, between 3 and 6 months after surgery, weight loss exerts an important role, and is the main driver of the additional improvement in insulin sensitivity. At this stage, an improvement in peripheral insulin sensitivity, which occurs after substantial weight loss takes place and that correlates with the magnitude of weight loss can be observed (19, 25, 36, 37, 39, 45). For instance, a 30% reduction in body mass index predicts a 50% increase in insulin sensitivity as seen in the European Group for the Study of Insulin Resistance (EGIR) cohort among others (19, 39, 46). As mentioned before, BPD surgery is the exception to this statement as it can rapidly improve both, hepatic and peripheral insulin sensitivity before significant weight loss occurs, although the mechanisms are not yet completely understood (47).

The long-term improvement in insulin sensitivity and body weight achieved after metabolic surgery has been mainly ascribed, in VSG, RYGB, and BPD, to the postprandial increase in anorexigenic gut hormones (i.e., GLP-1, peptide YY, and oxyntomodulin), favoring enhanced satiety to a meal which ultimately leads to reduction in calorie and food intake (48). The exception here is gastric banding, after which no increase in anorexigenic hormones takes place (49, 50). The gastric band appears to enhance satiety through neural mechanisms and the subsequent weight loss is the main mediator contributing to the increase in insulin sensitivity after it (49). The increase in gut hormones secretion has been explained through different mediators depending on the type of surgery. In the case of RYGB or BPD, the bypass of the small bowel, bile acids or changes in the gut microbiome have been postulated as possible mediators (51). It has been shown that bile acids indirectly regulate glucose through the G-protein-coupled bile acid receptor, Gpbar1 (TGR5) receptor expressed on L-cells, causing release of GLP-1 upon binding (51–53). With regards to gut microbiota changes, it is still uncertain whether it is directly related to the improvement in glycemic control following surgery. However, if a fecal transplant from healthy volunteers is performed to individuals with metabolic syndrome, an improvement in insulin sensitivity can be observed which correlates with an increased population of butyrate-producing gut microbiota (54). Moreover, some studies have shown that gut microbiota transplantation from RYGB-treated subjects to non-operated ones, results in weight loss and decreased adiposity (55, 56). Nevertheless, in none of these studies glucose nor insulin tolerance was measured (55, 56). Therefore, more studies are needed in order to elucidate to what extent and by which mechanisms the gut microbiome improves glucose metabolism after metabolic surgery. On the other hand, VSG does not have an effect on bile acids circulation. The increase in gut hormones release seem to be secondary to an increase in gastric emptying, which induces a fast transit of nutrients into the small bowel that stimulates gut hormones secretion (57), although the exact mechanism remains unknown (28).

GLUCOSE ABSORPTION

After metabolic surgery glucose metabolism changes within the gut. A lower glucose absorption has been shown to happen following RYGB and VSG, although the mechanism through which this happens differs. After RYGB, undigested nutrients reach the common channel where they meet bile acids and other digestive secretions enabling nutrient absorption. It has been shown that glucose absorption is blunted in the alimentary limb and increases in the common limb secondary to the altered bile acids traffic (58). Endoluminal glucose is absorbed through the apical sodium glucose cotransporter 1 (SGLT1), which incorporates sodium and glucose into the enterocyte from the luminal side. Therefore, the intestinal absorption of glucose requires the presence of sodium, which is originated from bile and other digestive fluids. Thus, after RYGB, there is a modification in bile acid trafficking that results in the alimentary limb not being exposed to these digestive fluids, without sodium present to be co-transported with glucose. In fact, despite SGLT1 expression or function being preserved, bile acids exclusion itself is sufficient to reduce the intestinal sodium-glucose cotransport in the alimentary limb (58). In this context, bile acids modulate the intestinal trafficking of endogenous sodium by decreasing the endoluminal content of sodium in the alimentary limb (58). This also explains why glucose uptake in the alimentary limb can be restored by giving a sodium-rich solution (59). It can be stated that SGLT-2 inhibitors are for the kidney what metabolic surgery is for SGLT-1 in the gut. In fact, some studies have already shown that in patients with T2DM, the inhibition of SGLT1 results in a reduction in postprandial glucose concentrations and an improvement in glycemic control (60, 61).

With regards to VSG, a lower glucose absorption in the small intestine has been shown (59, 62). Following VSG, a large part of the stomach is removed and therefore, there is a reduction in the leptin- and ghrelin-expressing cells. Ghrelin increases appetite, reduces gastric emptying, regulates energy expenditure and decreases glucose-induced insulin release and whole-body insulin sensitivity (63, 64). Therefore, after VSG surgery a negative correlation has been shown between ghrelin concentrations and insulin sensitivity and secretion (64). Gastric leptin is produced in the stomach and secreted into the small intestine, where it is believed to promote glucose absorption by enhancing the glucose transporter-2 (GLUT2) in the jejunum (62, 65). A recent study showed that after VSG surgery there was a decrease in glucose absorption which was enhanced with the addition of an oral gavage of leptin (62). Therefore, it has recently been postulated that after VSG, leptin depletion is one of the main factors contributing to the improvement in glucose homeostasis, rather than gut adaptation as seen after RYGB (62).

GLUCOSE UPTAKE AND UTILIZATION WITHIN THE GUT

Despite similar beneficial metabolic effects of VSG and RYGB surgeries, the changes within the gut differ. It has been shown, that after RYGB surgery there is a morphological adaptation of the alimentary limb characterized by mucosal hyperplasia and hypertrophy. These changes in the intestinal mucosa are triggered by the exposure to undigested nutrients by the alimentary limb mucosa and are not found after VSG surgery (59, 66, 67). There is emerging evidence that this hyperplasia and hypertrophy produces a reprogramming of glucose metabolism and increases the metabolic rate in order to meet the higher energetic demand, which boosts the carbohydrate consumption by the gut (59, 67–70). This higher metabolic rate and increased glucose uptake by the alimentary limb can be demonstrated through the use of [^{18}F]-fluoro-2-deoxyglucose positron emission tomography-computed tomography where the remodeled intestine exhibits the second highest glucose consumption after the brain (59, 67, 70). In fact, a positive correlation between the intestinal glucose uptake and glycemic improvement was shown, consistent with an improvement in whole-body glucose disposal (67). This process is characterized by an overexpression of the basolateral glucose transporter-1 (GLUT1), which increases the supply of glucose to the enterocyte in the same way as has been shown to do to proliferative cancer cells in response to hypoxia (59). GLUT1 plays an important role in early intestinal tissue growth and therefore is highly expressed in the fetus to then disappear progressively (71). Interestingly, this increase in the glucose utilization by the gut, secondary to the enhanced intestinal expression of GLUT1 after RYGB, is independent of weight loss or improvements in insulin secretion and sensitivity (67). It is worth noting that there is also an increase in the intestinal glucose uptake in the common limb driven by an enhancement of apical SGLT1 activity operating synergistically with the basolateral GLUT1 in order to meet the higher energy requirements (59, 67). All these findings, place the gut within the group of organs/peripheral tissues responsible for increasing glucose disposal after metabolic surgery (59, 67, 70).

INTESTINAL GLUCONEOGENESIS AND THE HEPATO-PORTAL GLUCOSE SENSING

The glucose release by the small intestine is triggered by two major gluconeogenesis enzymes: glucose-6-phosphatase (Glc6Pase) and phosphoenolpyruvate carboxykinase (PEPCK) (72, 73). When both enzymes are induced, newly synthesized glucose is released into the portal blood. This is detected by the hepato-portal glucose sensing which ultimately modulates the endogenous glucose production by the liver (74, 75). This system requires the presence of a specific glucose transporter (GLUT-2) and is potentiated by GLP-1, through which the portal sensing of glucose appearance suppresses hepatic gluconeogenesis and modulates whole-body glucose disposal, stimulating the glucose uptake by peripheral tissues (76–78). Moreover, portal sensing of intestinal gluconeogenesis induces a reduction in food intake (74, 79–81). These metabolic effects produced by the hepato-portal nervous system seem to take place through the autonomic nervous system around the portal vein which connects to central hypothalamic nuclei (72, 74, 78).

Along these lines, several studies have shown that after RYGB surgery, there is an increased expression and activity of the PEPCK and Glc6Pase enzymes in the distal jejunum and ileum as compared with gastric banding (72). This translates into an increased glucose release by the gut to the portal blood which suppresses hepatic glucose production and food intake (72). These effects where not observed in weight-matched mice after gastric banding, which suggests that at least some of the metabolic improvements seen after RYGB are independent of calorie restriction or weight loss. On the other hand, when GLUT-2 was downregulated in mice undergoing metabolic surgery, there was an impairment in the hepato-portal sensing, which affected insulin sensitivity and body weight (72). Therefore, an increase in the intestinal gluconeogenesis and the stimulation of the hepato-portal glucose sensor via a GLUT-2-dependent pathway has been postulated as one of the mechanisms through which RYGB improves insulin sensitivity and reduces food intake contributing to the resolution of hyperglycemia. However, human studies are needed to corroborate this hypothesis.

ADIPOSE TISSUE

It is well-known that adipose tissue dysfunction and an excess of body fat, specifically its central deposition in the abdominal viscera decreases insulin sensitivity and β-cell function and is an independent risk factor for T2DM and cardiovascular disease (82–85). This is due to the fact that the adipose tissue is an active endocrine and paracrine organ which releases numerous hormones, cytokines, and molecules which not only influence body weight, food intake, and energy homeostasis but also regulate glucose and lipid metabolism (86, 87). There is an increasing number of adipocyte-derived hormones which include leptin, adiponectin, resistin, acylation-stimulating protein, retinol-binding protein-4, and visfatin, among others (86, 87). Whilst the existence of as yet unidentified factors controlling body weight and metabolism should be noted (88), what we do know so far is that, except for adiponectin, circulating concentrations of these hormones are increased in obesity and insulin-resistant states, and decrease after weight-loss (51, 89). With regards to cytokines, excess adiposity is characterized by the promotion of chronic, low-grade inflammation which has been implicated in the development of T2DM (87).

As mentioned before, following metabolic surgery significant weight loss takes place. Whilst it would make sense to lose both fat mass and fat-free mass as seen after conventional dieting, it has been shown that after surgically-induced weight loss, body composition improves with a reduction in body fat percentage alongside a minimal drop in fat-free mass (90). Moreover, not only there is an overall body fat loss, but the visceral and intramuscular depot are also reduced (90, 91). This metabolically beneficial redistribution of fat further contributes to the glucose metabolism improvement seen after surgically-induced weight loss: there is an improvement in hepatic insulin sensitivity mediated by the decreased visceral and total adiposity as well as by the refrained muscle mass loss which boosts glucose uptake by the skeletal muscle (91).

But not only body composition improves, adipose tissue itself experiences several changes which include changes in the secretory profile, adipocyte, morphology, and glucose and lipid metabolism. With regards to the adipokines, there is a reduction in leptin and inflammatory cytokines such as TNF-α and several interleukins and an increase in adiponectin concentrations, which translates in a reduction in several cardio-metabolic risk factors (51, 91–95). Moreover, adiponectin concentrations have been shown to correlate with the degree of T2DM remission, being lower in those sub-optimal responders to metabolic surgery (94).

Adipose-specific glucose disposal is enhanced by insulin. The insulin receptor is a tyrosine kinase which activation causes the translocation from the intracellular storage compartment to the plasma membrane of the insulin-sensitive glucose transporter 4 (GLUT4) (96). The activity of the insulin-stimulated AMP-activated protein kinase (AMPK) and GLUT4 transporter are downregulated in patients with obesity and T2DM with the selective inactivation of its gene impairing insulin-dependent adipose glucose disposal leading to T2DM (86, 97–99). It has been shown that after weight loss the insulin-stimulated kinase activity is restored (100) and there is an improvement in insulin-induced signaling and GLUT4 activity in adipose tissue 1-year post RYGB surgery (101–103). These correlated with plasma adiponectin levels and whole-body insulin sensitivity assessed by the hyperinsulinemic euglycemic clamp (101). Several studies have also shown that adipose cell morphology also changes after metabolic surgery: there is an increase in the lipolysis pathways and adipose cell hyperplasia and a reduction in the size which improves whole-body insulin sensitivity (93, 104, 105). All these results, support the role of the adipose tissue as one of the contributors to the glycemic improvement seen after metabolic surgery.

CONCLUSION

Metabolic surgery is the most efficient treatment for inducing diabetes remission in obese patients with T2DM. Diabetes remission results from improvements in β-cell function, insulin sensitivity and changes within the gut and adipose tissue. The early improvement seen in postoperative glycemic control is due to an increase in insulin sensitivity secondary to a reduction in hepatic endogenous glucose production and caloric restriction, and an improvement in beta-cell function secondary to an enhancement in GLP-1 release. The long-term benefits in glycemic control are in part due to changes in gut hormone secretion that promote fat mass loss which improves glucose uptake by peripheral tissues (peripheral insulin sensitivity). On the other hand, the exclusion of the proximal intestinal segment after RYGB surgery, changes the gut physiology, affecting glucose absorption and utilization by the gut which contributes to the achievement of diabetes remission after metabolic surgery. Further in-depth understanding of these mechanisms could be used not only to improve the design and effectiveness of these procedures but also to accelerate the identification of targets for drug development.

AUTHOR CONTRIBUTIONS

BP-P and GF were the guarantors of this work and, as such, take full responsibility for the work as a whole and the decision to submit and publish the manuscript. JE and AM contributed to discussions and reviewed the paper, and gave their approval to the final version of the manuscript.

FUNDING

This work was supported by the Spanish Institute of Health ISCIII (Subdirección General de Evaluación and Fondos FEDER PI16/01217; Plan Estatal *I* + *D* + *I*/2013–2016). CIBER Fisiopatología de la Obesidad y Nutrición (CIBEROBN) was an initiative of the ISCIII, Spain. The funding source had no role in the writing of the manuscript or the decision to submit it for publication.

REFERENCES

1. Bray GA, Kim KK, Wilding JPH. Obesity: a chronic relapsing progressive disease process. A position statement of the World Obesity Federation. *Obes Rev.* (2017) 18:715–23. doi: 10.1111/obr.12551
2. Villarejo C, Fernandez-Aranda F, Jimenez-Murcia S, Penas-Lledo E, Granero R, Penelo E, et al. Lifetime obesity in patients with eating disorders: increasing prevalence, clinical and personality correlates. *Eur Eat Disord Rev.* (2012) 20:250–4. doi: 10.1002/erv.2166
3. Courcoulas AP, Belle SH, Neiberg RH, Pierson SK, Eagleton JK, Kalarchian MA, et al. Three-year outcomes of bariatric surgery vs lifestyle intervention for type 2 diabetes mellitus treatment: a randomized clinical trial. *JAMA Surg.* (2015) 150:931–40. doi: 10.1001/jamasurg.2015.1534
4. Cummings DE, Arterburn DE, Westbrook EO, Kuzma JN, Stewart SD, Chan CP, et al. Gastric bypass surgery vs intensive lifestyle and medical intervention for type 2 diabetes: the CROSSROADS randomised controlled trial. *Diabetologia.* (2016) 59:945–53. doi: 10.1007/s00125-016-3903-x
5. Fruhbeck G. Bariatric and metabolic surgery: a shift in eligibility and success criteria. *Nat Rev Endocrinol.* (2015) 11:465–77. doi: 10.1038/nrendo.2015.84
6. Kehagias I, Karamanakos SN, Argentou M, Kalfarentzos F. Randomized clinical trial of laparoscopic Roux-en-Y gastric bypass versus laparoscopic sleeve gastrectomy for the management of patients with BMI < 50 kg/m2. *Obes Surg.* (2011) 21:1650–6. doi: 10.1007/s11695-011-0479-x
7. Mingrone G, Panunzi S, De Gaetano A, Guidone C, Iaconelli A, Nanni G, et al. Bariatric-metabolic surgery versus conventional medical treatment in obese patients with type 2 diabetes: 5 year follow-up of an open-label, single-centre, randomised controlled trial. *Lancet.* (2015) 386:964–73. doi: 10.1016/S0140-6736(15)00075-6
8. Risstad H, Sovik TT, Engstrom M, Aasheim ET, Fagerland MW, Olsen MF, et al. Five-year outcomes after laparoscopic gastric bypass and laparoscopic duodenal switch in patients with body mass index of 50 to 60: a randomized clinical trial. *JAMA Surg.* (2015) 150:352–61. doi: 10.1001/jamasurg.2014.3579
9. Rubino F, Nathan DM, Eckel RH, Schauer PR, Alberti KG, Zimmet PZ, et al. Metabolic surgery in the treatment algorithm for type 2 diabetes: a joint statement by International Diabetes Organizations. *Obes Surg.* (2017) 27:2–21. doi: 10.1007/s11695-016-2457-9
10. Schauer PR, Bhatt DL, Kirwan JP, Wolski K, Aminian A, Brethauer SA, et al. Bariatric surgery versus intensive medical therapy for diabetes - 5-year outcomes. *N Engl J Med.* (2017) 376:641–51. doi: 10.1056/NEJMoa1600869
11. Sheng B, Truong K, Spitler H, Zhang L, Tong X, Chen L. The long-term effects of bariatric surgery on type 2 diabetes remission, microvascular and macrovascular complications, and mortality: a systematic review and meta-analysis. *Obes Surg.* (2017) 27:2724–32. doi: 10.1007/s11695-017-2866-4
12. Yan Y, Sha Y, Yao G, Wang S, Kong F, Liu H, et al. Roux-en-Y gastric bypass versus medical treatment for type 2 diabetes mellitus in obese patients: a systematic review and meta-analysis of randomized controlled trials. *Medicine.* (2016) 95:e3462. doi: 10.1097/MD.0000000000003462
13. Cersosimo E, Solis-Herrera C, Trautmann ME, Malloy J, Triplitt CL. Assessment of pancreatic β-cell function: review of methods and clinical applications. *Curr Diabetes Rev.* (2014) 10:2–42. doi: 10.2174/1573399810666140214093600
14. Mari A, Ahren B, Pacini G. Assessment of insulin secretion in relation to insulin resistance. *Curr Opin Clin Nutr Metab Care.* (2005) 8:529–33. doi: 10.1097/01.mco.0000171130.23441.59
15. Stumvoll M, Mitrakou A, Pimenta W, Jenssen T, Yki-Jarvinen H, Van Haeften T, et al. Use of the oral glucose tolerance test to assess insulin release and insulin sensitivity. *Diabetes Care.* (2000) 23:295–301. doi: 10.2337/diacare.23.3.295
16. Drucker DJ. The biology of incretin hormones. *Cell Metab.* (2006) 3:153–65. doi: 10.1016/j.cmet.2006.01.004

17. Muscelli E, Mari A, Casolaro A, Camastra S, Seghieri G, Gastaldelli A, et al. Separate impact of obesity and glucose tolerance on the incretin effect in normal subjects and type 2 diabetic patients. *Diabetes.* (2008) 57:1340–8. doi: 10.2337/db07-1315
18. Ferrannini E. The stunned beta cell: a brief history. *Cell Metab.* (2010) 11:349–52. doi: 10.1016/j.cmet.2010.04.009
19. Ferrannini E, Mingrone G. Impact of different bariatric surgical procedures on insulin action and beta-cell function in type 2 diabetes. *Diabetes Care.* (2009) 32:514–20. doi: 10.2337/dc08-1762
20. Nannipieri M, Mari A, Anselmino M, Baldi S, Barsotti E, Guarino D, et al. The role of beta-cell function and insulin sensitivity in the remission of type 2 diabetes after gastric bypass surgery. *J Clin Endocrinol Metab.* (2011) 96:E1372–9. doi: 10.1210/jc.2011-0446
21. Weiss R. Effects of Roux-en-Y gastric bypass on beta-cell function. *Diabetes.* (2014) 63:1171–3. doi: 10.2337/db13-1897
22. Kashyap SR, Daud S, Kelly KR, Gastaldelli A, Win H, Brethauer S, et al. Acute effects of gastric bypass versus gastric restrictive surgery on beta-cell function and insulinotropic hormones in severely obese patients with type 2 diabetes. *Int J Obes.* (2010) 34:462–71. doi: 10.1038/ijo.2009.254
23. Dirksen C, Jorgensen NB, Bojsen-Moller KN, Jacobsen SH, Hansen DL, Worm D, et al. Mechanisms of improved glycaemic control after Roux-en-Y gastric bypass. *Diabetologia.* (2012) 55:1890–901. doi: 10.1007/s00125-012-2556-7
24. Batterham RL, Cummings DE. Mechanisms of diabetes improvement following bariatric/metabolic surgery. *Diabetes Care.* (2016) 39:893–901. doi: 10.2337/dc16-0145
25. Jorgensen NB, Jacobsen SH, Dirksen C, Bojsen-Moller KN, Naver L, Hvolris L, et al. Acute and long-term effects of Roux-en-Y gastric bypass on glucose metabolism in subjects with Type 2 diabetes and normal glucose tolerance. *Am J Physiol Endocrinol Metab.* (2012) 303:E122–31. doi: 10.1152/ajpendo.00073.2012
26. Laferrere B, Teixeira J, McGinty J, Tran H, Egger JR, Colarusso A, et al. Effect of weight loss by gastric bypass surgery versus hypocaloric diet on glucose and incretin levels in patients with type 2 diabetes. *J Clin Endocrinol Metab.* (2008) 93:2479–85. doi: 10.1210/jc.2007-2851
27. Michaud A, Grenier-Larouche T, Caron-Dorval D, Marceau S, Biertho L, Simard S, et al. Biliopancreatic diversion with duodenal switch leads to better postprandial glucose level and beta cell function than sleeve gastrectomy in individuals with type 2 diabetes very early after surgery. *Metab Clin Exp.* (2017) 74:10–21. doi: 10.1016/j.metabol.2017.06.005
28. Nannipieri M, Baldi S, Mari A, Colligiani D, Guarino D, Camastra S, et al. Roux-en-Y gastric bypass and sleeve gastrectomy: mechanisms of diabetes remission and role of gut hormones. *J Clin Endocrinol Metab.* (2013) 98:4391–9. doi: 10.1210/jc.2013-2538
29. Rubino F, Gagner M, Gentileschi P, Kini S, Fukuyama S, Feng J, et al. The early effect of the Roux-en-Y gastric bypass on hormones involved in body weight regulation and glucose metabolism. *Ann Surg.* (2004) 240:236–42. doi: 10.1097/01.sla.0000133117.12646.48
30. Jorgensen NB, Dirksen C, Bojsen-Moller KN, Jacobsen SH, Worm D, Hansen DL, et al. Exaggerated glucagon-like peptide 1 response is important for improved beta-cell function and glucose tolerance after Roux-en-Y gastric bypass in patients with type 2 diabetes. *Diabetes.* (2013) 62:3044–52. doi: 10.2337/db13-0022
31. Vidal J, de Hollanda A, Jimenez A. GLP-1 is not the key mediator of the health benefits of metabolic surgery. *Surg Obes Relat Dis.* (2016) 12:1225–9. doi: 10.1016/j.soard.2016.02.029
32. Dutia R, Brakoniecki K, Bunker P, Paultre F, Homel P, Carpentier AC, et al. Limited recovery of beta-cell function after gastric bypass despite clinical diabetes remission. *Diabetes.* (2014) 63:1214–23. doi: 10.2337/db13-1176
33. Isbell JM, Tamboli RA, Hansen EN, Saliba J, Dunn JP, Phillips SE, et al. The importance of caloric restriction in the early improvements in insulin sensitivity after Roux-en-Y gastric bypass surgery. *Diabetes Care.* (2010) 33:1438–42. doi: 10.2337/dc09-2107
34. Steven S, Hollingsworth KG, Small PK, Woodcock SA, Pucci A, Aribasala B, et al. Calorie restriction and not glucagon-like peptide-1 explains the acute improvement in glucose control after gastric bypass in Type 2 diabetes. *Diabet Med.* (2016) 33:1723–31. doi: 10.1111/dme.13257
35. Souteiro P, Belo S, Neves JS, Magalhaes D, Silva RB, Oliveira SC, et al. Preoperative beta cell function is predictive of diabetes remission after bariatric surgery. *Obes Surg.* (2017) 27:288–94. doi: 10.1007/s11695-016-2300-3
36. Bojsen-Moller KN, Dirksen C, Jorgensen NB, Jacobsen SH, Serup AK, Albers PH, et al. Early enhancements of hepatic and later of peripheral insulin sensitivity combined with increased postprandial insulin secretion contribute to improved glycemic control after Roux-en-Y gastric bypass. *Diabetes.* (2014) 63:1725–37. doi: 10.2337/db13-1307
37. Camastra S, Gastaldelli A, Mari A, Bonuccelli S, Scartabelli G, Frascerra S, et al. Early and longer term effects of gastric bypass surgery on tissue-specific insulin sensitivity and beta cell function in morbidly obese patients with and without type 2 diabetes. *Diabetologia.* (2011) 54:2093–102. doi: 10.1007/s00125-011-2193-6
38. Gastaldelli A, Iaconelli A, Gaggini M, Magnone MC, Veneziani A, Rubino F, et al. Short-term effects of laparoscopic adjustable gastric banding versus Roux-en-Y gastric bypass. *Diabetes Care.* (2016) 39:1925–31. doi: 10.2337/dc15-2823
39. Muscelli E, Mingrone G, Camastra S, Manco M, Pereira JA, Pareja JC, et al. Differential effect of weight loss on insulin resistance in surgically treated obese patients. *Am J Med.* (2005) 118:51–7. doi: 10.1016/j.amjmed.2004.08.017
40. Henry RR, Scheaffer L, Olefsky JM. Glycemic effects of intensive caloric restriction and isocaloric refeeding in noninsulin-dependent diabetes mellitus. *J Clin Endocrinol Metab.* (1985) 61:917–25. doi: 10.1210/jcem-61-5-917
41. Kelley DE, Wing R, Buonocore C, Sturis J, Polonsky K, Fitzsimmons M. Relative effects of calorie restriction and weight loss in noninsulin-dependent diabetes mellitus. *J Clin Endocrinol Metab.* (1993) 77:1287–93. doi: 10.1210/jcem.77.5.8077323
42. Lingvay I, Guth E, Islam A, Livingston E. Rapid improvement in diabetes after gastric bypass surgery: is it the diet or surgery? *Diabetes Care.* (2013) 36:2741–7. doi: 10.2337/dc12-2316
43. Pournaras DJ, Nygren J, Hagstrom-Toft E, Arner P, le Roux CW, Thorell A. Improved glucose metabolism after gastric bypass: evolution of the paradigm. *Surg Obes Relat Dis.* (2016) 12:1457–65. doi: 10.1016/j.soard.2016.03.020
44. Csendes A, Burgos AM, Roizblatt D, Garay C, Bezama P. Inflammatory response measured by body temperature, C-reactive protein and white blood cell count 1, 3, and 5 days after laparotomic or laparoscopic gastric bypass surgery. *Obes Surg.* (2009) 19:890–3. doi: 10.1007/s11695-008-9702-9
45. Campos GM, Rabl C, Peeva S, Ciovica R, Rao M, Schwarz JM, et al. Improvement in peripheral glucose uptake after gastric bypass surgery is observed only after substantial weight loss has occurred and correlates with the magnitude of weight lost. *J Gastrointest Surg.* (2010) 14:15–23. doi: 10.1007/s11605-009-1060-y
46. Ferrannini E, Natali A, Bell P, Cavallo-Perin P, Lalic N, Mingrone G. Insulin resistance and hypersecretion in obesity. European Group for the Study of Insulin Resistance (EGIR). *J Clin Invest.* (1997) 100:1166–73. doi: 10.1172/JCI119628
47. Bradley D, Magkos F, Klein S. Effects of bariatric surgery on glucose homeostasis and type 2 diabetes. *Gastroenterology.* (2012) 143:897–912. doi: 10.1053/j.gastro.2012.07.114
48. le Roux CW, Aylwin SJ, Batterham RL, Borg CM, Coyle F, Prasad V, et al. Gut hormone profiles following bariatric surgery favor an anorectic state, facilitate weight loss, and improve metabolic parameters. *Ann Surg.* (2006) 243:108–14. doi: 10.1097/01.sla.0000183349.16877.84
49. Korner J, Inabnet W, Febres G, Conwell IM, McMahon DJ, Salas R, et al. Prospective study of gut hormone and metabolic changes after adjustable gastric banding and Roux-en-Y gastric bypass. *Int J Obes.* (2009) 33:786–95. doi: 10.1038/ijo.2009.79
50. Romero F, Nicolau J, Flores L, Casamitjana R, Ibarzabal A, Lacy A, et al. Comparable early changes in gastrointestinal hormones after sleeve gastrectomy and Roux-En-Y gastric bypass surgery for morbidly obese type 2 diabetic subjects. *Surg Endosc.* (2012) 26:2231–9. doi: 10.1007/s00464-012-2166-y

51. Madsbad S, Dirksen C, Holst JJ. Mechanisms of changes in glucose metabolism and bodyweight after bariatric surgery. *Lancet Diabet Endocrinol.* (2014) 2:152–64. doi: 10.1016/S2213-8587(13)70218-3
52. Kohli R, Bradley D, Setchell KD, Eagon JC, Abumrad N, Klein S. Weight loss induced by Roux-en-Y gastric bypass but not laparoscopic adjustable gastric banding increases circulating bile acids. *J Clin Endocrinol Metab.* (2013) 98:E708–12. doi: 10.1210/jc.2012-3736
53. Patti ME, Houten SM, Bianco AC, Bernier R, Larsen PR, Holst JJ, et al. Serum bile acids are higher in humans with prior gastric bypass: potential contribution to improved glucose and lipid metabolism. *Obesity.* (2009) 17:1671–7. doi: 10.1038/oby.2009.102
54. Vrieze A, Van Nood E, Holleman F, Salojarvi J, Kootte RS, Bartelsman JF, et al. Transfer of intestinal microbiota from lean donors increases insulin sensitivity in individuals with metabolic syndrome. *Gastroenterology.* (2012) 143:913–6.e917. doi: 10.1053/j.gastro.2012.06.031
55. Liou AP, Paziuk M, Luevano JM Jr, Machineni S, Turnbaugh PJ, Kaplan LM. Conserved shifts in the gut microbiota due to gastric bypass reduce host weight and adiposity. *Sci Transl Med.* (2013) 5:178ra141. doi: 10.1126/scitranslmed.3005687
56. Tremaroli V, Karlsson F, Werling M, Stahlman M, Kovatcheva-Datchary P, Olbers T, et al. Roux-en-Y gastric bypass and vertical banded gastroplasty induce long-term changes on the human gut microbiome contributing to fat mass regulation. *Cell Metab.* (2015) 22:228–38. doi: 10.1016/j.cmet.2015.07.009
57. Shah S, Shah P, Todkar J, Gagner M, Sonar S, Solav S. Prospective controlled study of effect of laparoscopic sleeve gastrectomy on small bowel transit time and gastric emptying half-time in morbidly obese patients with type 2 diabetes mellitus. *Surg Obes Relat Dis.* (2010) 6:152–7. doi: 10.1016/j.soard.2009.11.019
58. Baud G, Daoudi M, Hubert T, Raverdy V, Pigeyre M, Hervieux E, et al. Bile diversion in Roux-en-Y gastric bypass modulates sodium-dependent glucose intestinal uptake. *Cell Metab.* (2016) 23:547–53. doi: 10.1016/j.cmet.2016.01.018
59. Cavin J-B, Couvelard A, Lebtahi R, Ducroc R, Arapis K, Voitellier E, et al. Differences in alimentary glucose 1 absorption and intestinal disposal of blood glucose following Roux-en-Y gastric bypass vs sleeve gastrectomy. *Gastroenterology.* (2015) 150:454–64. doi: 10.1053/j.gastro.2015.10.009
60. Dobbins RL, Greenway FL, Chen L, Liu Y, Breed SL, Andrews SM, et al. Selective sodium-dependent glucose transporter 1 inhibitors block glucose absorption and impair glucose-dependent insulinotropic peptide release. *Am J Physiol Gastrointest Liver Physiol.* (2015) 308:G946–54. doi: 10.1152/ajpgi.00286.2014
61. Rosenstock J, Cefalu WT, Lapuerta P, Zambrowicz B, Ogbaa I, Banks P, et al. Greater dose-ranging effects on A1C levels than on glucosuria with LX4211, a dual inhibitor of SGLT1 and SGLT2, in patients with type 2 diabetes on metformin monotherapy. *Diabetes Care.* (2015) 38:431–8. doi: 10.2337/dc14-0890
62. Du J, Hu C, Bai J, Peng M, Wang Q, Zhao N, et al. Intestinal glucose absorption was reduced by vertical sleeve gastrectomy via decreased gastric leptin secretion. *Obes Surg.* (2018) 28:3851–61. doi: 10.1007/s11695-018-3351-4
63. Dimitriadis GK, Randeva MS, Miras AD. Potential hormone mechanisms of bariatric surgery. *Curr Obes Rep.* (2017) 6:253–65. doi: 10.1007/s13679-017-0276-5
64. Sista F, Abruzzese V, Clementi M, Carandina S, Amicucci G. Effect of resected gastric volume on ghrelin and GLP-1 plasma levels: a prospective study. *J Gastrointest Surg.* (2016) 20:1931–41. doi: 10.1007/s11605-016-3292-y
65. Ducroc R, Guilmeau S, Akasbi K, Devaud H, Buyse M, Bado A. Luminal leptin induces rapid inhibition of active intestinal absorption of glucose mediated by sodium-glucose cotransporter 1. *Diabetes.* (2005) 54:348–54. doi: 10.2337/diabetes.54.2.348
66. Mumphrey MB, Hao Z, Townsend RL, Patterson LM, Berthoud HR. Sleeve gastrectomy does not cause hypertrophy and reprogramming of intestinal glucose metabolism in rats. *Obes Surg.* (2015) 25:1468–73. doi: 10.1007/s11695-014-1547-9
67. Saeidi N, Meoli L, Nestoridi E, Gupta NK, Kvas S, Kucharczyk J, et al. Reprogramming of intestinal glucose metabolism and glycemic control in rats after gastric bypass. *Science.* (2013) 341:406–10. doi: 10.1126/science.1235103
68. Hansen CF, Bueter M, Theis N, Lutz T, Paulsen S, Dalboge LS, et al. Hypertrophy dependent doubling of L-cells in Roux-en-Y gastric bypass operated rats. *PLoS ONE.* (2013) 8:e65696. doi: 10.1371/journal.pone.0065696
69. Magkos F, Bradley D, Eagon JC, Patterson BW, Klein S. Effect of Roux-en-Y gastric bypass and laparoscopic adjustable gastric banding on gastrointestinal metabolism of ingested glucose. *Am J Clin Nutr.* (2016) 103:61–5. doi: 10.3945/ajcn.115.116111
70. Mäkinen J, Hannukainen JC, Karmi A, Immonen HM, Soinio M, Nelimarkka L, et al. Obesity-associated intestinal insulin resistance is ameliorated after bariatric surgery. *Diabetologia.* (2015) 58:1055–62. doi: 10.1007/s00125-015-3501-3
71. Pacha J. Development of intestinal transport function in mammals. *Physiol Rev.* (2000) 80:1633–67. doi: 10.1152/physrev.2000.80.4.1633
72. Troy S, Soty M, Ribeiro L, Laval L, Migrenne S, Fioramonti X, et al. Intestinal gluconeogenesis is a key factor for early metabolic changes after gastric bypass but not after gastric lap-band in mice. *Cell Metab.* (2008) 8:201–11. doi: 10.1016/j.cmet.2008.08.008
73. Yanez AJ, Nualart F, Droppelmann C, Bertinat R, Brito M, Concha II, et al. Broad expression of fructose-1,6-bisphosphatase and phosphoenolpyruvate carboxykinase provide evidence for gluconeogenesis in human tissues other than liver and kidney. *J Cell Physiol.* (2003) 197:189–97. doi: 10.1002/jcp.10337
74. Mithieux G. The new functions of the gut in the control of glucose homeostasis. *Curr Opin Clin Nutr Metab Care.* (2005) 8:445–9. doi: 10.1097/01.mco.0000172587.17385.aa
75. Sindelar DK, Chu CA, Neal DW, Cherrington AD. Interaction of equal increments in arterial and portal vein insulin on hepatic glucose production in the dog. *Am J Physiol.* (1997) 273:E972–80. doi: 10.1152/ajpendo.1997.273.5.E972
76. Burcelin R, Da Costa A, Drucker D, Thorens B. Glucose competence of the hepatoportal vein sensor requires the presence of an activated glucagon-like peptide-1 receptor. *Diabetes.* (2001) 50:1720–8. doi: 10.2337/diabetes.50.8.1720
77. Burcelin R, Dolci W, Thorens B. Glucose sensing by the hepatoportal sensor is GLUT2-dependent: *in vivo* analysis in GLUT2-null mice. *Diabetes.* (2000) 49:1643–8. doi: 10.2337/diabetes.49.10.1643
78. Thorens B, Larsen PJ. Gut-derived signaling molecules and vagal afferents in the control of glucose and energy homeostasis. *Curr Opin Clin Nutr Metab Care.* (2004) 7:471–8. doi: 10.1097/01.mco.0000134368.91900.84
79. Burcelin R, Dolci W, Thorens B. Portal glucose infusion in the mouse induces hypoglycemia: evidence that the hepatoportal glucose sensor stimulates glucose utilization. *Diabetes.* (2000) 49:1635–42. doi: 10.2337/diabetes.49.10.1635
80. Russek M. Participation of hepatic glucoreceptors in the control of intake of food. *Nature.* (1963) 197:79–80. doi: 10.1038/197079b0
81. Russek M. Demonstration of the influence of an hepatic glucosensitive mechanism on food-intake. *Physiol Behav.* (1970) 5:1207–9. doi: 10.1016/0031-9384(70)90218-0
82. Gomez-Ambrosi J, Catalan V, Rodriguez A, Andrada P, Ramirez B, Ibanez P, et al. Increased cardiometabolic risk factors and inflammation in adipose tissue in obese subjects classified as metabolically healthy. *Diabetes Care.* (2014) 37:2813–21. doi: 10.2337/dc14-0937
83. Gomez-Ambrosi J, Gonzalez-Crespo I, Catalan V, Rodriguez A, Moncada R, Valenti V, et al. Clinical usefulness of abdominal bioimpedance (ViScan) in the determination of visceral fat and its application in the diagnosis and management of obesity and its comorbidities. *Clin Nutr.* (2018) 37:580–9. doi: 10.1016/j.clnu.2017.01.010
84. Gomez-Ambrosi J, Silva C, Galofre JC, Escalada J, Santos S, Gil MJ, et al. Body adiposity and type 2 diabetes: increased risk with a high body fat percentage even having a normal BMI. *Obesity.* (2011) 19:1439–44. doi: 10.1038/oby.2011.36
85. Perez-Pevida B, Diaz-Gutierrez J, Miras AD, Silva C, Romero S, Salvador J, et al. High body adiposity drives glucose intolerance and increases

cardiovascular risk in normoglycemic subjects. *Obesity.* (2018) 26:672–82. doi: 10.1002/oby.22147
86. Fruhbeck G, Gomez-Ambrosi J. Control of body weight: a physiologic and transgenic perspective. *Diabetologia.* (2003) 46:143–72. doi: 10.1007/s00125-003-1053-4
87. Van Gaal LF, Mertens IL, De Block CE. Mechanisms linking obesity with cardiovascular disease. *Nature.* (2006) 444:875–80. doi: 10.1038/nature05487
88. Fruhbeck G, Gomez-Ambrosi J. Rationale for the existence of additional adipostatic hormones. *FASEB J.* (2001) 15:1996–2006. doi: 10.1096/fj.00-0829hyp
89. Gomez-Ambrosi J, Salvador J, Paramo JA, Orbe J, de Irala J, Diez-Caballero A, et al. Involvement of leptin in the association between percentage of body fat and cardiovascular risk factors. *Clin Biochem.* (2002) 35:315–20. doi: 10.1016/S0009-9120(02)00320-X
90. Gomez-Ambrosi J, Andrada P, Valenti V, Rotellar F, Silva C, Catalan V, et al. Dissociation of body mass index, excess weight loss and body fat percentage trajectories after 3 years of gastric bypass: relationship with metabolic outcomes. *Int J Obes.* (2017) 41:1379–87. doi: 10.1038/ijo.2017.134
91. Frikke-Schmidt H, O'Rourke RW, Lumeng CN, Sandoval DA, Seeley RJ. Does bariatric surgery improve adipose tissue function? *Obes Rev.* (2016) 17:795–809. doi: 10.1111/obr.12429
92. Faraj M, Havel PJ, Phelis S, Blank D, Sniderman AD, Cianflone K. Plasma acylation-stimulating protein, adiponectin, leptin, and ghrelin before and after weight loss induced by gastric bypass surgery in morbidly obese subjects. *J Clin Endocrinol Metab.* (2003) 88:1594–602. doi: 10.1210/jc.2002-021309
93. Hoffstedt J, Andersson DP, Eriksson Hogling D, Theorell J, Naslund E, Thorell A, et al. Long-term protective changes in adipose tissue after gastric bypass. *Diabetes Care.* (2017) 40:77–84. doi: 10.2337/dc16-1072
94. Malin SK, Bena J, Abood B, Pothier CE, Bhatt DL, Nissen S, et al. Attenuated improvements in adiponectin and fat loss characterize type 2 diabetes non-remission status after bariatric surgery. *Diabetes Obes Metab.* (2014) 16:1230–8. doi: 10.1111/dom.12376
95. Swarbrick MM, Stanhope KL, Austrheim-Smith IT, Van Loan MD, Ali MR, Wolfe BM, et al. Longitudinal changes in pancreatic and adipocyte hormones following Roux-en-Y gastric bypass surgery. *Diabetologia.* (2008) 51:1901–11. doi: 10.1007/s00125-008-1118-5
96. Kanzaki M. Insulin receptor signals regulating GLUT4 translocation and actin dynamics. *Endocr J.* (2006) 53:267–93. doi: 10.1507/endocrj.KR-65
97. Abel ED, Peroni O, Kim JK, Kim YB, Boss O, Hadro E, et al. Adipose-selective targeting of the GLUT4 gene impairs insulin action in muscle and liver. *Nature.* (2001) 409:729–33. doi: 10.1038/35055575
98. Friedman JE, Dohm GL, Leggett-Frazier N, Elton CW, Tapscott EB, Pories WP, et al. Restoration of insulin responsiveness in skeletal muscle of morbidly obese patients after weight loss. Effect on muscle glucose transport and glucose transporter GLUT4. *J Clin Invest.* (1992) 89:701–5. doi: 10.1172/JCI115638
99. Yang Q, Graham TE, Mody N, Preitner F, Peroni OD, Zabolotny JM, et al. Serum retinol binding protein 4 contributes to insulin resistance in obesity and type 2 diabetes. *Nature.* (2005) 436:356–62. doi: 10.1038/nature03711
100. Freidenberg GR, Reichart D, Olefsky JM, Henry RR. Reversibility of defective adipocyte insulin receptor kinase activity in non-insulin-dependent diabetes mellitus. Effect of weight loss. *J Clin Invest.* (1988) 82:1398–406. doi: 10.1172/JCI113744
101. Albers PH, Bojsen-Moller KN, Dirksen C, Serup AK, Kristensen DE, Frystyk J, et al. Enhanced insulin signaling in human skeletal muscle and adipose tissue following gastric bypass surgery. *Am J Physiol Regul Integr Comp Physiol.* (2015) 309:R510–24. doi: 10.1152/ajpregu.00228.2014
102. Goktas Z, Moustaid-Moussa N, Shen CL, Boylan M, Mo H, Wang S. Effects of bariatric surgery on adipokine-induced inflammation and insulin resistance. *Front Endocrinol.* (2013) 4:69. doi: 10.3389/fendo.2013.00069
103. Xu XJ, Apovian C, Hess D, Carmine B, Saha A, Ruderman N. Improved insulin sensitivity 3 months after RYGB surgery is associated with increased subcutaneous adipose tissue AMPK activity and decreased oxidative stress. *Diabetes.* (2015) 64:3155–9. doi: 10.2337/db14-1765
104. Eriksson-Hogling D, Andersson DP, Backdahl J, Hoffstedt J, Rossner S, Thorell A, et al. Adipose tissue morphology predicts improved insulin sensitivity following moderate or pronounced weight loss. *Int J Obes.* (2015) 39:893–8. doi: 10.1038/ijo.2015.18
105. Ryden M, Andersson DP, Bergstrom IB, Arner P. Adipose tissue and metabolic alterations: regional differences in fat cell size and number matter, but differently: a cross-sectional study. *J Clin Endocrinol Metab.* (2014) 99:E1870–6. doi: 10.1210/jc.2014-1526

18

Diabetic Ketoacidosis Post Bariatric Surgery

Ivania M. Rizo and Caroline M. Apovian*

Section of Endocrinology, Diabetes, Nutrition, and Weight Management, Boston University School of Medicine and Boston Medical Center, Boston, MA, United States

***Correspondence:**
Ivania M. Rizo
ivania.rizo@bmc.org

In patients with type 2 diabetes, bariatric surgery can lead to significant improvements in glycemic control and diabetes remission. We present a case of a Hispanic female with type 2 diabetes phenotype who underwent bariatric surgery and post-operatively stopped her insulin therapy due to multiple reasons, including decreased oral intake and concern for hypoglycemia. Ultimately, she developed diabetic ketoacidosis. She does not fit into the classical type 2 diabetes or type 1 diabetes definition but into the heterogeneous subgroup of diabetes called ketosis-prone diabetes.

Keywords: bariatric surgery, diabetic ketoacidosis, type 2 diabetes, Roux-en-Y gastric bypass, ketosis-prone diabetes mellitus

INTRODUCTION

Diabetes mellitus is a heterogeneous group of metabolic conditions all linked together by hyperglycemia. It primarily falls into two broad categories: type 1 and type 2. The most prevalent category, type 2 diabetes (T2D), is defined by a combination of resistance to insulin action and an inadequate compensatory insulin secretory response (1). Type 1 diabetes (T1D) results in an absolute deficiency of insulin secretion. It can be identified with certain background genetic susceptibility and serological evidence of an autoimmune T-cell mediated pathological process occurring in the pancreatic islets. Diabetic ketoacidosis (DKA) has been considered a key clinical feature of T1D although it has been reported in subjects who lack the T1D phenotype. An additional subgroup of diabetes has been emerging called ketosis-prone diabetes (KPDM). KPDM is a heterogeneous syndrome characterized by patients who present with DKA or unprovoked ketosis but do not necessarily have the phenotype of autoimmune type 1 diabetes. Most patients with KPDM are overweight or obese and usually present with a short history of hyperglycemic symptoms (2).

DKA is one of the most serious complications associated with diabetes. It is defined as a triad of uncontrolled hyperglycemia, metabolic acidosis, and increased total body ketones (3). Serum glucose is invariably elevated, barring pregnancy, or concurrent use of sodium-glucose co-transporter 2 (SGLT2) inhibitor, where glucose may be relatively normal. The metabolic abnormalities seen in DKA result from a relative deficiency in insulin combined with an increase in counter-regulatory hormones such as glucagon, catecholamines, growth hormone, and cortisol.

Bariatric surgery has emerged as a valuable tool for the treatment of diabetes and obesity. Bariatric surgery results in significant weight loss and may result in T2D remission. Mingrone et al. demonstrated a 75% remission in T2D 2 years status post RYGB or biliopancreatic diversion (4). Although it is also used in T1D and obesity with significant reduction in insulin requirements and modest improvements in hemoglobin A1c, those with T1D would not be able to stop insulin post-operatively. Prior to bariatric surgery it is essential to identify individuals with diabetes who will not be able to stop insulin despite significant weight loss or decreased oral intake.

CASE PRESENTATION

Thirty-year-old Hispanic female with past medical history of T2D, hypertension, and Roux-en-Y (RYGB) gastric bypass presented to an academic urban medical center emergency room with nausea and abdominal pain and was found to have DKA.

The patient was diagnosed with T2D at age 15, while being hospitalized for an unrelated matter. Notably, at the time of diagnosis, she had obesity with a BMI of 56.4 kilograms per square meter (kg/m^2). Insulin therapy was initiated at this time. The patient retrospectively reported being non-compliant with the insulin regimen since diagnosis and never developed DKA prior to this hospital admission. The struggle with diabetes was common in her family as her mother and two sisters are reported to have T2D.

The patient underwent laparoscopic RYGB gastric bypass 4 months prior to DKA presentation. Prior to RYGB, the patient was on Glargine 30 units per day, Lispro 15 units before meals, metformin 1,000 mg twice daily and empagliflozin 10 mg per day. Hemoglobin A1c was 9.9% 1 month prior to bariatric surgery. Patient was placed on an insulin drip intraoperatively and on post-operative day 0, insulin drip which was turned off when point of care glucose was 188 mg/dL. She was transitioned to Glargine 16 units per day and low dose insulin sliding scale that consisted of 1 unit of Lispro with meals for every 50 mg/dL glucose above 150 mg/dL. Nutritional insulin was held because the patient was on a clear liquid diet. On post-operative day 2, she was transitioned to high protein full liquid meals. The patient was discharged from the hospital on Glargine 10 units per day and metformin 1,000 mg twice a day. Empagliflozin was discontinued post operatively.

Two weeks after laparoscopic gastric bypass, the patient was seen in the bariatric clinic. She was tolerating the high protein full liquid diet without difficulty. She was taking Glargine 10 units once a day as prescribed and fasting blood glucose values were ranging from 80 to 125 mg/dL. At the time of her clinic visit, her diet was advanced to soft and moist proteins. The patient did not follow up at her scheduled 6-week post-operative appointment. Two months later, she presented to the emergency room with DKA.

At the emergency room, she reported 8 days of fevers, nausea, vomiting, poor oral intake, cough, and dizziness. She had stopped taking Glargine ~2 months prior to DKA presentation due to decreased oral intake and fear of hypoglycemia, although no hypoglycemia was recorded. She noted polyuria and polydipsia for some time. However, as her glucometer had broken, she had not obtained any blood glucose values. Otherwise, she had felt well until 8 days prior to presentation to emergency room. During that time, she reported a fever up to 105°F, and there were sick contacts in her house including small children with upper respiratory infection. The patient also noted difficulty tolerating solid foods. As a result, she was primarily eating protein shakes and liquids.

Abbreviations: DKA, diabetic ketoacidosis; RYGB, roux-en-y gastric bypass; SGLT2, SGLT 2 inhibitor; T2D, type 2 diabetes; T1D, type 1 diabetes; BMI, body mass index; KPDM, ketosis-prone diabetes mellitus; WBC, white blood cell count.

TABLE 1 | Initial laboratory values.

	Laboratory	Patient Values (Normal Ranges)
Venous blood gas	pH	7.09 (7.32–7.42)
	PCO2	24 mm Hg (35–45 mmHg)
	PO2	40 mmHg (30–50 mmHg)
	Bicarbonate	7.0 mmol/L (22–29 mmHg)
	Lactate	1.8 mmol/L (0.9–1.7 mmol/L)
Chemistry	Blood glucose	504 mg/dL (70–100 mg/dL)
	Sodium	128 mmol/L (135–145 mmol/L)
	Potassium	4.8 mmol/L (3.1–5.3 mmol/L)
	Chloride	99 mmol/L (98–110 mmol/L)
	Creatinine	1.4 mg/dL (0.5–1.1mg/dL)
	Glomerular filtration rate	44 mL/ min/1.73 m2 (>60 mL/ min/1.73m2)
	Albumin	4.6 g/dL (3.5–5.0 g/dL)
Hematology	Hemoglobin	15.7 g/dL (11.8–16.0g/dL)
	White blood cells	26.5 K/UL (4.0–11.0 K/UL)
	Platelets	352 K/UL (150–400 K/UL)

Initial labs were significant for hyperglycemia with blood glucose of 504 mg/dL, creatinine of 1.4 mg/dL, bicarbonate of 6 mmol/L, anion gap of 23 mEq/L, pH of 7.09, and urine ketones 2+ (**Table 1**). Her hemoglobin A1c was 9.2% at time of admission. Her Urinalysis and urine culture were not positive, comprehensive respiratory panel was not significant and Chest Xray at time of admission did not find any significant findings. At time of admission she had lost 17.27 kg since bariatric surgery, placing her at 78 kg and BMI of 34.84 kg/m^2. She was placed on continuous insulin infusion and fluid hydration per the DKA insulin drip protocol. After 24 hours, she was transitioned from the insulin drip to a basal- bolus insulin regimen. Ultimately, she was discharged on Glargine 20 units once a day and Lispro 6 units with meals. All KPDM patients should be discharged from initial DKA admission on insulin for safety reasons. The need for insulin can be assessed in the weeks post-discharge.

Sixteen days after discharge from the hospital, the patient was seen in the outpatient Endocrine clinic. She was doing well other than reporting a dry cough. We performed laboratory analysis which revealed concurrent blood glucose of 196 mg/dL and C-peptide of 1.36 ng/mL, glutamic acid de- carboxylase-65 antibody <5 IU/mL (anti-GAD), islet cell antibody negative, and Hemoglobin A1c of 9.3%. Zinc transporter 8 antibody was not checked.

DISCUSSION

In this case report, we describe a Hispanic female with phenotypic early onset T2D associated with class 3 obesity who had undergone RYGB gastric bypass and presented 3 months post-bariatric surgery with DKA. Our patient had overlapping features between types 1 and 2 diabetes. She had phenotypic T2D obesity, high risk ethnicity for T2D, and abdominal adiposity but developed ketoacidosis. Her subtype of diabetes does not clearly fit a type 1 or 2 diabetes definition and is most consistent with ketosis-prone diabetes mellitus (KPDM).

It was initially thought that most cases of KPDM present in African persons and in African-American individuals in the United States, but KPDM has been reported in Hispanics such as our patient (5). Several case series have reported that up to half of African-Americans and Hispanics hospitalized with DKA have a clinical presentation compatible with KPDM (6). Most patients with KPDM are overweight or obese with newly diagnosed diabetes or an acute course of hyperglycemia. As was seen in our patient, there is often a strong family history of T2D.

KPDM is a heterogeneous form of diabetes. It can be classified by the presence or absence of autoantibodies and the presence or absence of β- cell functional reserve (Aβ classification) (7). Individuals with islet cell autoantibodies are classified as A+ and those without A–. In addition, individuals with β- cell reserve, once the period of acute metabolic decompensation has resolved are labeled β+ vs. β- if there is no beta cell reserve. The largest subgroup of KPDM is the A–β+ (negative autoantibodies and positive beta cell reserve). Our patient had negative antibodies with β cell reserve. These patients resemble individuals with T2D obesity phenotype and account for 50% of all KPDM (5).

Nalini et al. further divided the A–β+ KPDM group into unprovoked vs. provoked DKA. Approximately 50% of the A–β+ subgroup present with new onset diabetes and DKA without clinically evident precipitating factors. The rest of this subgroup has a history of long-standing diabetes and develops ketoacidosis in the setting of an acute illness or non-compliance with antidiabetic treatment. In a cohort studied by Nalini et al. (8), the majority of unprovoked A–β+ KPDM were male, African American, with greater BMI, while the majority of provoked A–β+ KPDM were female and Hispanic similar to our patient (8). In addition, the unprovoked A–β+ KPDM have greater improvement in β- cell function, better glycemic control and twice the rate of insulin discontinuation 12 months after DKA event. The unprovoked group had association with a type 1 diabetes resistance allele DQB1*0602 vs. the provoked group had increased frequency of type 1 susceptibility alleles DQB1*0302 and DRB1*04. These specific immunological factors may contribute to the decline in beta function seen in the provoked KPDM group. These data suggest patients with unprovoked or provoked A–ß+ KPDM have distinct underlying mechanisms of ß cell dysfunction. Approximately 60% of all A-β+ KPDM patients are insulin dependent after 10 years (9).

There is no gold standard for the diagnosis of KPDM. However, islet antibodies and C-peptide levels should be obtained for all patients with suspected KPDM. C-peptide reflects endogenous insulin secretion by pancreatic β cells; it can be measured fasting or with a stimulation test. Islet-specific pancreatic antibodies include antibodies against glutamic acid decarboxylase (GAD 65 Ab) and antibodies against islet cells (ICA Ab). Assessment of both β- secretory reserve and β-cell autoimmunity should be performed after complete resolution of DKA to minimize the effects of glucose toxicity. Zinc transporter 8 antibody was not checked in our case. It is an additional marker of autoimmune diabetes and when combined with antibodies to insulin, GAD, or protein tyrosine kinase IA-1 it can raise the detection rate of autoimmunity to 94% in new onset cases of T1DM. Zinc transporter 8 antibody does decrease with increasing age, but may have been helpful in this case (10). In the Aβ KPDM classification, β+ is defined as a fasting C-peptide concentration >1 ng/ml and peak serum C-peptide concentration after glucagon stimulation >1.5 ng/ml (measured at 5 and 10 min after intravenous injection of 1 mg glucagon) (7).

Our patient has a random C-peptide of 1.36 ng/mL non-fasting, which does correspond to β cell secretory reserve but not as accurately as a fasting or stimulated C-peptide. The aforementioned cut offs predict β- cell function after six and 12 months and glycemic control after 1 year. A high ratio (>11) of fasting C- peptide (in nmol/L) to glucose (ml/L) predicts the potential safe discontinuation of insulin (7). Patients with long-standing diabetes and provoked DKA have a decreased chance of insulin discontinuation (7). Nalini et al. demonstrated a lesser ß cell improvement and poorer glycemic control in the provoked A-β+ KPDM group than in the unprovoked group. Our patient had a >10-year history of diabetes and presented with provoked DKA making it likely she will be insulin dependent.

DKA has been reported post bariatric surgery in type 1 and type 2 diabetes. DKA can occur post bariatric surgery in T2D but is uncommon and mild (11). Aminian et al. reported 12 patients who developed DKA after bariatric surgery at an academic center from January 2005 to December 2015. Sixty-six percent of patients who developed DKA had T1D and thirty three percent had T2D. The median interval between bariatric surgery and DKA development was 12 days (range was 0–61 days). Three out of the four patients with T2D who developed DKA were on insulin prior to surgery. Two out of the three patients had been on insulin for many years and the discontinuation of insulin post operatively was thought to be the cause of DKA. Additional precipitation factors included infection and poor oral intake (11). Arminian et al., recommend optimizing glycemic control before surgery, administering basal insulin on the morning of surgery, and using perioperative infusion protocols in the perioperative period to prevent post-operative DKA. Our patient did not have optimal glycemic control prior to surgery and also had a history of non-compliance with medications putting her at high- risk of post-operative complications. There are currently no case reports specifying KPDM and DKA post bariatric surgery.

Infection is the most common precipitating event in DKA. Our patient initially had a white blood cell count (WBC) of 26.5 U/KL concerning for infection at presentation of DKA. Repeat WBC within 24 h was 16.9 U/KL with 85% polymorphonuclear leukocytes. Although it is common to have leukocytosis with DKA, a WBC > 25.0 U/KL is more likely to be related to occult infection (3). Although there was no definitive infection found and WBC decreased and normalized by the time of discharge, a viral infection was suspected as the precipitating event in our patient in addition to the discontinuation of insulin.

In addition, the patient had a history of using empagliflozin, a sodium glucose cotransporter- 2 (SGLT2) inhibitor. SGLT2s can cause DKA and usually present as euglycemic and moderate hyperglycemic DKA (11). Our patient reported stopping SGLT2 ~3 months prior to presentation, making this precipitant less likely.

Although bariatric surgery can lead to diabetes remission, it is essential to know the type of diabetes a patient has prior to bariatric surgery. KPDM is more common in the non-Caucasian population and in particular provoked DKA is more prevalent in Hispanics. This case demonstrates caution must be used in discontinuation of insulin post bariatric surgery for non-Caucasian patients on insulin for many years despite a T2D phenotype. Patients need to be educated on potential for DKA post-operatively and signs and symptoms of DKA specially with discontinuation of insulin post operatively or other precipitants such as infection. Our patient had a classic T2D phenotype but given her presentation of provoked DKA and history of insulin use prior to bariatric surgery it is very likely she will be insulin dependent to avoid DKA even with a significant decrease in insulin requirements.

REFERENCES

1. American Diabetes Association. Diagnosis and classification of diabetes mellitus. *Diabetes Care* (2010) 33:S62–9. doi: 10.2337/dc10-S062
2. Vellanki P, Umpierrez GE. Diabetic Ketoacidosis; a common debut of diabetes among African Americans with type 2 diabetes. *Endocrine Pract.* (2017) 23:971–8. doi: 10.4158/EP161679.RA
3. Kitabchi AE, Miles JM, Umpierrez GE, Fisher JN. Hyperglycemic crises in adult patients with diabetes. *Diabetes Care* (2009) 32:1335–41. doi: 10.2337/dc09-9032
4. Mingrone G, Panunzi S, Gaetano A, Guidone C, Iaconelli A, Leccesi L, et al. Bariatric surgery versus conventional medical therapy for type 2 Diabetes. *N Engl J Med.* (2012) 366:1577–85. doi: 10.1056/NEJMoa1200111
5. Steenkamp DW, Alexanian SM, Sternthal E. Approach to the patient with atypical diabetes. *CMAJ.* (2014) 186:678–84. doi: 10.1503/cmaj.130185
6. Smiley D, Chandra P, Umpierrez GE. Update on diagnosis, pathogenesis and management of ketosis-prone Type 2 diabetes mellitus. *Diabetes Manage.* (2011) 1:589–600. doi: 10.2217/dmt.11.57
7. Balasubramanyam A, Nalini R, Hampe CS, Maldonado M. Syndromes of Ketosis-Prone diabetes mellitus. *Endocrine Rev.* (2008) 29:292–302. doi: 10.1210/er.2007-0026
8. Nalini R, Ozer K, Maldonado M, Patel S, Hampe CS, Guthikonda A, et al. Presence or absence of know DKA precipitant defines distinct syndromes of "A-β+" Ketosis- Prone Diabetes (KPD) based on long term beta cell function, HLA class II alleles, and gender predilection. *Metabolism* (2010) 59:1448–55. doi: 10.1016/j.metabol.2010.01.009
9. Mauvais-Jarvis F, Sobngwi E, Porcher R, Riveline JP, Kevorkian JP, Vaisse C, et al. Ketosis-Prone type 2 *Diabetes* in patients of sub-Saharan African origin. *Diabetes* (2004) 53:645–53. doi: 10.2337/diabetes.53.3.645
10. Lampasona V, Petrone A, Tibert C, Capizzi M, Spoletini M, di Pietro S, et al. Zinc transporter 8 antibodies complement GAD and IA-2 antibodies in the identification and characterization of adult-onset autoimmune diabetes. *Diabetes Care* (2010) 33:104–8. doi: 10.2337/dc0 8-2305
11. Aminian A, Kashyap SR, Bruguera B, Punchai S, Sharma G, Froylich D, et al. Incidence and clinical features of diabetic ketoacidosis after bariatric and metabolic surgery. *Diabetes Care* (2016) 39:e50–3. doi: 10.2337/dc15-2647

AUTHOR CONTRIBUTIONS

IR critically reviewed for important intellectual content and wrote the first draft. CA contributed to writing the manuscript. IR and CA provided approval for publication of the content, agreed to be accountable for all aspects of the work in ensuring that questions related to the accuracy or integrity of any part of the work are appropriately investigated and resolved.

19

Obesity, Male Reproductive Function and Bariatric Surgery

Angelo Di Vincenzo, Luca Busetto, Roberto Vettor and Marco Rossato*

Department of Medicine—DIMED, Center for the Study and Integrated Management of Obesity, Clinica Medica 3, University-Hospital of Padova, Padova, Italy

***Correspondence:**
Angelo Di Vincenzo
divincenzoang@gmail.com

Overweight and obesity are associated with several chronic complications, such as type 2 diabetes, arterial hypertension and atherosclerotic cardiovascular diseases, with relevant consequences for patients and public health systems. Reproductive function abnormalities, such as obesity-related secondary hypogonadism, erectile dysfunction and infertility, represent other abnormalities negatively affecting the quality of life of men suffering from obesity but, despite their high prevalence, these are often understated because of a general lack of awareness in clinical practice. Obesity and gonadal function are closely related, with obesity being associated with hypogonadism that is reversed by body weight reduction thus ameliorating reproductive and sexual health. Clinical studies specifically evaluating the impact of non-surgical weight loss on testosterone levels sometimes showed conflicting results, whereas extensive literature has demonstrated that weight loss after bariatric surgery is correlated with an increase in testosterone levels greater than that obtained with only lifestyle interventions, suggesting the role of surgery also for the treatment of hypogonadism in obese male. However, studies concerning the consequences of bariatric surgery on overall reproductive function in the male, including also sexual activity and fertility, are limited and data regarding long-term effects are lacking. Here we present a brief review summarizing the evidence regarding the interplay between obesity and reproductive abnormalities in the obese male, together with the role of bariatric surgery for the treatment of these complications, describing both the positive effects and the limitations of this procedure.

Keywords: obesity, testosterone, male hypogonadism, sexual function, erectile function, fertility, weight loss, bariatric surgery

INTRODUCTION

Appropriate management of patients with obesity needs a complete evaluation and treatment of each associated cardiovascular, metabolic and endocrine disturbance (1, 2). However, despite their high prevalence, reproductive function abnormalities are often undertreated in obese population compared to the cardio-metabolic comorbidities.

As for the other well-known complications of obesity, bariatric surgery seems to be the most effective treatment for reproductive abnormalities in obese males, frequently ensuring the complete normalization of testosterone levels, along with long-term weight maintenance, although the evidence of the effects on fertility and sexual activity is still scarce. The mechanisms linking hypothalamic-pituitary-gonadal axis, obesity and metabolic surgery are far from being completely understood, and surgical weight loss sometimes is not sufficient to ameliorate sexual function and, consequently, the quality of life. To this regard, we performed a comprehensive review of the available literature to summarize the actual evidence concerning the interplay between obesity and reproductive abnormalities and the role of bariatric surgery for the treatment of these complications, analyzing the possible underlying mechanisms but also exposing its limitations.

OBESITY AND MALE REPRODUCTIVE FUNCTION

Obesity is associated with a constellation of endocrine disturbances and, among them, reproductive function abnormalities are now recognized as relevant clinical problems in subjects with obesity. It is well-known that in women obesity is associated with menstrual irregularity, reduced fertility, higher prevalence of polycystic ovary syndrome (PCOS) (3), but also with gestational diabetes, pregnancy-related hypertension and increased risk of obesity in the offspring. In men with obesity, hypogonadism, erectile dysfunction (ED) and reduced fertility represent complications seriously affecting patient quality of life and health (4–8). Thus, their control may represent another therapeutic target in these subjects.

Sex Hormones in Obesity

Abnormal levels of sex hormones are often observed in men with obesity. Male-obesity secondary hypogonadism (MOSH) represents an endocrine dysfunction with a reported prevalence of about 45% in moderate-severe obesity (9). Furthermore, it has been reported that the prevalence of hypogonadism in obese male is higher in the presence of type 2 diabetes (T2D) (10, 11).

MOSH is characterized by different signs and symptoms, such as sexual dysfunction, depression, fatigue, decreased lean body mass and also reduced mineral bone density, which further impact on patients' health. Hormonal abnormalities characterizing MOSH are represented by decreased free and total testosterone plasma levels, together with decreased sex-hormone binding globulin (SHBG) and increased estradiol plasma levels. Usually, in this situation, gonadotropins are inappropriately low or normal, resembling a hypogonadotropic hypogonadism, but in a less percentage of patients with metabolic syndrome higher gonadotropin levels may be observed (12).

Low testosterone and high estradiol plasma levels are common features of the metabolic syndrome, and an inverse relationship between body mass index (BMI) or waist circumference and testosterone plasma levels over all age group of patients has been extensively shown (13–15). To this respect, it is largely accepted that the development of MOSH depends on adipose tissue expansion and adipocyte dysfunction. An elevated waist circumference is the expression of increased visceral adipose tissue (VAT), which can result in an enhancement of *in-situ* aromatase activity (16). This enzyme is highly expressed in adipose tissue and is thought to be responsible for the increased conversion of circulating testosterone to 17 β-estradiol in men with obesity, favoring the development of secondary hypogonadism. At the same time, this condition leads to a vicious cycle in which low testosterone contributes to maintaining high body weight and excessive abdominal fat deposition (17). In fact, testosterone may be responsible for several metabolic effects influencing also adipocyte biology by interacting with the androgen receptor that is expressed in adipose tissue, thus preventing visceral fat accumulation and improving insulin sensitivity. Furthermore, testosterone might exert a protective role from gluco-toxicity damage on pancreatic β-cells, due to an antioxidant activity on pancreatic islets preventing the β-cell apoptosis (18) or to a modulation of the renin-angiotensin-aldosterone pathway by reducing the expression of angiotensin II type 1 receptor (AGTR1), as previously reported (19). These effects may be lost with the reduction of circulating testosterone levels, and this may explain the relationship between low testosterone plasma levels and development of insulin resistance and T2D. This could be the case not only for men with MOSH, but also for age-related late-onset hypogonadism as well as in men undergoing androgen suppression for prostate cancer. Sex hormones balance has a crucial role in energy homeostasis, energy expenditure and then body mass composition. To this respect, it is interesting to note that the effects of testosterone on adipose tissue seem mediated also by skeletal muscle. In fact, *in vitro* experimental studies have shown that testosterone may interact with androgen-receptor to promote myogenic commitment of pluripotent mesenchymal cell and inhibit adipogenic differentiation via Wnt signaling (20, 21). Furthermore, increased serum levels of leptin and pro-inflammatory cytokines produced by inflamed adipose tissue (such as IL-6 and TNF-α) might have an additional suppressive effect on reproductive function. In particular, leptin has been hypothesized to negatively affect testicular steroidogenesis acting both at central and peripheral level, diminishing the pulse amplitude of luteinizing hormone releasing hormone (LHRH)/luteinizing hormone (LH) or through the activation of its receptor present on Leydig cell (22, 23).

It is also relevant to note that metabolic complications associated with obesity, T2D in particular, further affect gonadal function and testosterone levels. Different studies have reported that low testosterone levels predict the development of T2D in men and are inversely correlated with dyslipidemia and blood pressure levels (24–27). In agreement with this observation, it has been reported that higher testosterone levels are associated with a lower risk of T2D (28). Finally, androgen deprivation treatment in patients with prostate cancer is also related to an increased risk for the development of T2D (29). On the other hand, testosterone replacement therapy has been shown to be effective in weight loss and glucose homeostasis in patients with hypogonadism and metabolic syndrome.

Different mechanisms have been suggested to explain how insulin resistance, T2D and hypogonadism are interconnected in males. The effect of hyperinsulinemia on lowering testosterone concentrations has been evaluated many years ago (30, 31), showing that insulin acts both at central level, impairing the activity of gonadotropin releasing-hormone (GnRH) secreting neurons, and peripherally, where it may suppress SHBG synthesis (32), LH signaling (33), or modulate Leydig cell activity (34). The association becomes even more complex when associated complications develop. Obstructive sleep apnoea is a condition characterized by low circulating testosterone levels, but testosterone replacement in these patients has been associated with a worsening of clinical symptoms (35). Furthermore, it has been reported that the relationship between testosterone plasma levels and non-alcoholic fatty liver disease (NAFLD) shows a gender difference: low testosterone levels are independently associated with NAFLD in men and post-menopausal women (36), whereas testosterone levels are inversely associated with NAFLD in women (37), and increased levels of testosterone in PCOS patients are observed in association with NAFLD (38, 39).

Thus, the treatment of hypogonadism in patients with obesity, T2D or metabolic syndrome should consider also to the management of associated metabolic complications. To this respect testosterone replacement therapy in hypogonadal obese men has been previously suggested. Different studies have confirmed that testosterone replacement therapy in obese men leads not only to the amelioration of sexual activity, but also to the reduction of body weight, improved insulin sensitivity and reduction of other well-known cardiovascular risk factors, such as cholesterol plasma levels and inflammatory markers (40–43).

Taken together, this evidence shows a bidirectional interconnection between testosterone deficiency and metabolic diseases, a relation becoming further intriguing considering that low testosterone plasma levels have been recognized as an additional risk factor for cardiovascular disease (44, 45), and thus hypogonadism may account as another clinical complication of obesity (**Figure 1**). So, the identification of MOSH in obese subjects is strongly recommended for a complete risk stratification.

Sexual Activity, Erectile Function, and Fertility in Obesity

Obesity has a relevant negative impact not only on sex hormones levels but also on the overall sexual performance. Furthermore, according to some observations, adipose tissue expansion seems to influence also gonadal activity and spermatogenesis, leading to the reduction of fertility in obese males. BMI seems to be independently correlated with erectile function, with a high prevalence of overweight and obesity in patients suffering for ED. In comparison with normal BMI subjects, patients with a BMI higher than 28,7 Kg/m^2 show a 30% higher risk of ED (46), and it has been reported that patients with obesity waiting for bariatric surgery show a higher probability to suffer from ED with respect to those following non-surgical weight loss programs (47). In addition, in patients with ED, the presence of obesity and associated metabolic complications seems to affect further the severity of the disease, even reducing the responsiveness to phosphodiesterase 5 (PDE5) inhibitors (largely used for ED treatment) in subjects with higher BMI levels (48). Apart from the effect of MOSH and abnormal sex hormones levels, vascular and microvascular abnormalities associated with VAT expansion and chronic low-grade systemic inflammation, may represent another possible link between obesity and ED. In fact, obesity is associated with several clinical markers of subclinical atherosclerosis, such as endothelial dysfunction and impaired activity of endothelial nitric oxide, which may be at least in part responsible for the development of ED in this population. With these pathophysiological mechanisms in mind, the overlap between obesity and ED seems to represent a point of connection between adipose tissue expansion and vascular complications. Then, the presence of ED in obese subjects may account for an increased cardiovascular risk.

On the contrary, conflicting results have been observed in studies evaluating the correlation between BMI and sperm parameters, such as sperm concentration and total sperm count, although it is generally accepted that men with obesity seem to have a higher risk of azoospermia or oligozoospermia (49–51). The mechanisms by which obesity may influence fertility are complex and heterogeneous. Hyperinsulinemia and hyperleptinemia, classical features of obesity, may have a direct effect on spermatogenesis because of oxidative stress and inflammatory state, with loss of sperm DNA integrity (52, 53). Obesity might act centrally as for hypogonadism, influencing the hypothalamus-pituitary-testis axis. Furthermore, it is also possible that increased VAT may be responsible for an increased scrotal temperature which could impair testicular function.

The different treatments of obesity, such as lifestyle modification, pharmacological and surgical therapy are associated with an improvement of the different obesity-associated diseases along with weight loss, and body weight reduction appears to be effective also for MOSH. The different studies on the effects of behavioral modifications on male obese reproductive function have shown discordant results (54–56). On the contrary, a huge amount of literature has demonstrated that surgical weight loss is associated with an increase in testosterone plasma levels higher than that obtained with lifestyle modifications alone, probably reflecting the correlation between the severity of obesity and the grade of gonadal activity impairment. In fact, after surgical weight loss, an increase of testosterone plasma levels is observed in patients with MOSH, with a magnitude of androgen rise greater in those patients losing more weight (57), often leading to completely revert hypogonadism (58). However, at the moment, the effects of bariatric surgery on reproductive function in obese males remain not entirely known, and their explanation might be relevant to define future therapeutic options in obese males with MOSH and/or other reproductive abnormalities with contraindication to bariatric surgery.

ROLE OF SURGICAL WEIGHT LOSS ON REPRODUCTIVE FUNCTION IN MALE OBESITY

Considering their prevalence, obesity-associated gonadal dysfunctions may represent an important target for bariatric surgery. A recent meta-analysis has shown that, in patients undergoing bariatric surgery, PCOS was present in 36% of women whether MOSH was present in 64% of men, with a high percentage of remission after surgery (96% for PCOS, 87% for MOSH) (59). Below we present a brief description of the effects of bariatric surgery on male sex hormones plasma levels, ED and semen quality.

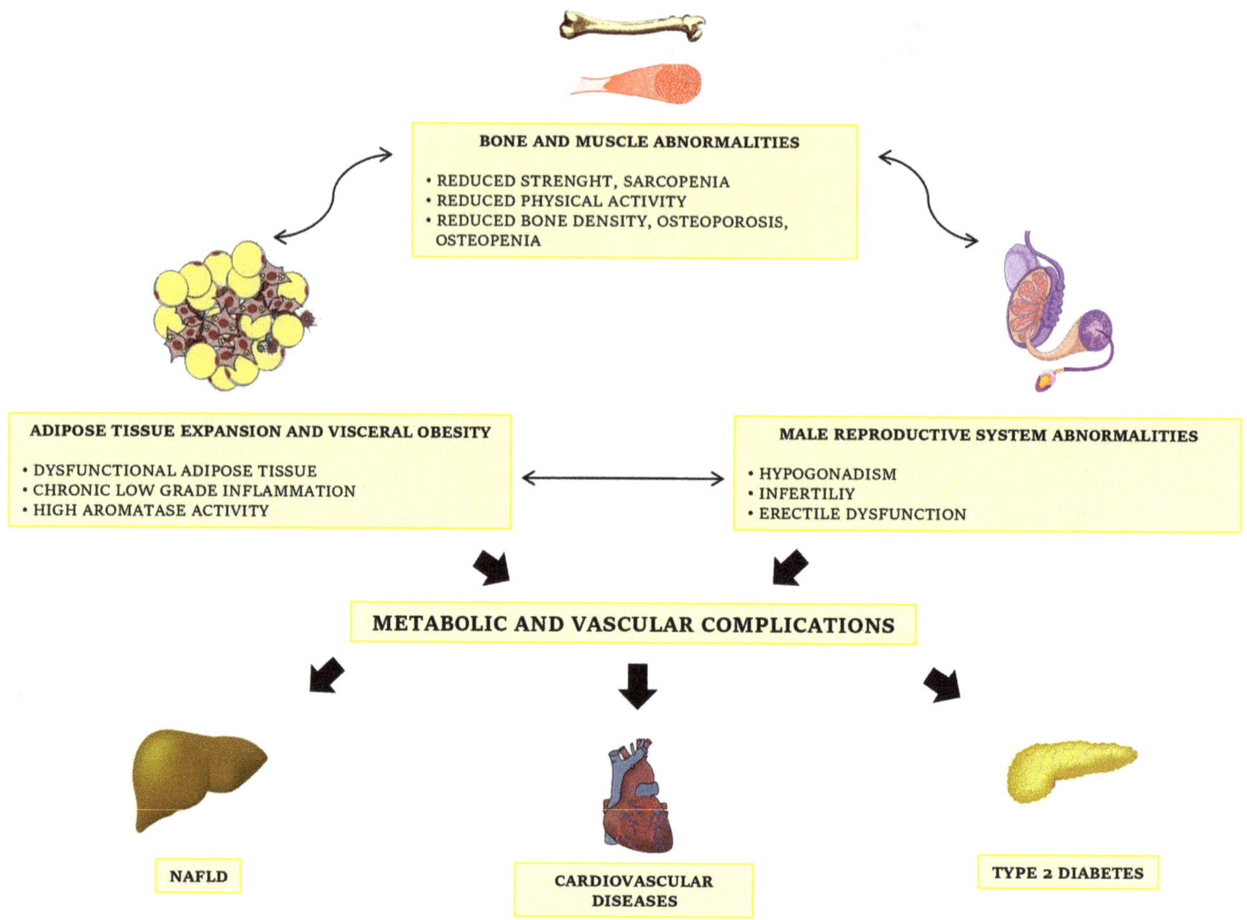

FIGURE 1 | The complex interconnections between obesity, metabolic diseases and male gonadal function.

Bariatric Surgery and Sex Hormones Plasma Levels

As previously mentioned, exogenous testosterone has been proven to be effective in hypogonadal obese men also in the amelioration of anthropometric and metabolic parameters (40–43, 60), and it could be a helpful treatment strategy in this population. However, androgen replacement therapy still has a reduced diffusion among physicians, probably because of apprehension for the possible adverse effects, such as exacerbation of OSA, worsening in lower urinary tract symptoms, and the risk of neoplastic prostate disease. In addition, exogenous testosterone may exert a negative feedback on releasing of gonadotropins which may further influence the fertility status. Weight loss has a great role in increasing testosterone levels, and a rapid weight loss obtained with lifestyle modifications has shown a beneficial effect in subjects with obesity. Niskanen et al. demonstrated that after a 9-week very-low-calorie diet there was an increase in SHBG and total testosterone plasma levels that were maintained also during weight control period (61). The results of a recent study evaluating the effects of medical treatment (dietary intervention and physical exercise) with the aim of 10% weight loss, confirmed a significant increase of total testosterone and a reduction of 17-β estradiol plasma levels after weight loss (62). Other studies evaluating the effects of calorie restriction on testosterone plasma levels reported conflicting results, while more promising results have been obtained from studies associating diet and testosterone replacement therapy (63).

On the other hand bariatric surgery is linked to greater effects on reproductive hormones abnormality in the male. Extensive literature has shown the positive effect of bariatric surgery on MOSH and this effect is irrespective of the type of surgery. Calderón et al demonstrated that significant postoperative outcomes on weight loss, HOMA index, fasting glucose, waist circumference, but also total and free testosterone plasma levels were not different between different bariatric surgery procedures such as gastric bypass, adjustable gastric banding or sleeve gastrectomy (64, 65). A limitation of these studies is represented by the heterogeneity of surgical procedures, sometimes considering the effects both of restrictive and malabsorptive surgery, which might be responsible for a relevant bias. However, after surgical weight reduction, many different studies have shown that the increase in total testosterone plasma levels is directly associated with amelioration of metabolic parameters whatever the surgical technique utilized, such as biliopancreatic diversion, vertical banded gastroplasty, and Roux-en-Y gastric by-pass (RYGB) (66–68), confirming the existence of an intricate hypothalamic-gonadal-adipocyte axis.

A positive effect of bariatric surgery on sex hormones plasma levels is commonly observed after a mid- or long-term follow up, but it can also present a rapid onset, already at 1 month from sleeve gastrectomy or RYGB (69, 70). With the maintenance of weight loss and appropriate weight control, the effects of bariatric surgery on sex hormones levels may be observed also for longer times. Pham et al recently performed an ancillary analysis from STAMPEDE trial, evaluating free and total testosterone levels 5 years after sleeve gastrectomy or RYGB in obese men with T2D. Patients who underwent bariatric surgery showed a higher increase in total and free testosterone levels with respect to medical patients in the long period (84.1 vs. 9.6%, $p = 0.008$, and 47.4 vs. −2.2%, $p = 0.013$), without significant changes in estradiol levels (71). Interestingly the increase in free testosterone observed in this study was associated with a reduction in body weight, high sensitivity-C reactive protein and leptin plasma levels, but not with an improvement in glycemic control. These results may be explained by the development of more severe abnormalities of gonadal function occurring when obesity coexists with other metabolic diseases, showing that adipose tissue dysfunction and systemic inflammation further influence gonadal activity in addition to insulin resistance and glucose metabolism alterations.

To this regard, the effects of bariatric surgery on gonadal function may be directly linked to body weight loss and, in particular, to visceral fat mass reduction. A recent study evaluating the correlation between sex hormones plasma levels and VAT (measured with magnetic resonance imaging), confirmed that visceral fat area is the main parameter associated with testosterone levels at baseline and, in addition, showed that after bariatric surgery visceral fat area is negatively associated with the increase in total testosterone plasma levels (72). VAT is well known to represent the most relevant risk factor associated with cardio-metabolic risk in patients with obesity Furthermore it probably accounts also for the development of hypogonadism in obese male, since abnormalities of adipocyte function in VAT result in negative effects on endocrine system, given that the imbalanced production of adipokines and inflammatory mediators such as leptin, IL-6, and TNF may directly influence testicular activity *in vitro* (23, 73), but evidence is lacking *in vivo*. Moreover, the reduction in VAT, that expresses higher aromatase activity with respect to the subcutaneous adipose tissue (SAT), may result in a reduced conversion of circulating testosterone leading to the reduction of estradiol and increase in testosterone plasma levels.

However, there are other clinical circumstances which may influence the amplitude of the effects of metabolic surgery on sex hormones recovery beyond weight loss *per se*. Age represents a relevant determinant for amelioration of MOSH, probably because younger subjects could have a greater response of testicular function to hypothalamic-pituitary hormones (in particular to the increase of LH levels) (74) or conversely because of an abnormal hypothalamic responsiveness to circulating sex hormones (75). To this respect, another limitation of the studies evaluating the post-surgical recovery of hypogonadism is represented by the age of studied subjects, who are usually young men when at the time of bariatric surgery.

The improvement of testosterone plasma levels may favor a condition in which the restoration of muscle strength and resistance leads to increased physical activity, amelioration of obesity-related sarcopenia and positive effects also on osteopenia and articular function, globally contributing to weight loss maintenance (76). Considering the experimental evidence regarding the influence of bone on testicular function (77), metabolic surgery may present these intriguing additional effects. To this regard, Samavat et al observed that osteocalcin, a bone hormone produced by osteoblasts, which seems to play a role on the regulation of testis function, increased after bariatric surgery, and this increase was parallel with the rising in free testosterone levels (78).

Bariatric Surgery and Erectile Function

A healthy lifestyle can preserve or restore erectile function in men, in particular in men with obesity who are at higher risk for ED because of associated metabolic and neuro-vascular abnormalities. Esposito et al showed the beneficial effects of lifestyle changes (reduced caloric intake and increased physical activity) on ED in subjects with obesity in a randomized controlled trial in which the intervention group, receiving detailed advice about how to achieve a loss of 10% or more by, obtained a significant improvement in the International Index of Erectile Function (IIEF) score (79). The beneficial effects of a moderate (10%) weight loss on sexual function have been confirmed by others (80).

As demonstrated by a recent meta-analysis, bariatric surgery leads to a significant improvement of ED as assessed by IIEF (81). ED is commonly reported by patients with severe obesity in the pre-operative period, but it may be improved by surgical induced weight loss. Dallal et al. showed that gastric bypass may revert also a severe sexual dysfunction (evaluated in this study with the Brief Male Sexual Function Inventory), with the excess of weight loss independently predicting the entity of the improvement (82). As for the increase in total testosterone plasma levels, bariatric surgery seems to guarantee an early amelioration of erectile function at six but also 1 month from surgery (83–85).

Surgical weight loss can ameliorate erectile dysfunction, as evaluated by IIEF questionnaire, probably through a modification in sex hormones plasma levels, in particular increasing follicle-stimulating hormone (FSH), total and free testosterone (86). Nonetheless it is also possible that bariatric surgery acts with a more complex mechanism. In a retrospective study conducted on Chinese obese patients with ED, Kun et al demonstrated the beneficial effects of RYGB on erectile function and showed the correlation between IIEF score and arterial integrity (both cavernosal and carotid artery, evaluated with Doppler ultrasound), irrespective of baseline BMI (87). In fact, the amplitude of the improvement of sexual function on IIEF seems to be independent of the increase of sex hormones plasma levels, confirming a more profound alteration of sexual function in obese patients which is not associated with testosterone activity alone. In a prospective observational case-series study, Mora et al observed, using a multivariate regression analysis, that variations of BMI and not hormonal and metabolic factors were independent predictors of IIEF score improvement at 1 year from bariatric surgery (88).

However, there are no univocal data about long term effects of surgical weight loss, and bariatric surgery does not always guarantee a complete normalization of erectile function. This observation is probably linked to the weight regain or to the persistence of metabolic abnormalities (89, 90), or also to psychological issues. A retrospective study by Ranasinghe et al evaluating a male obese population undergoing laparoscopic gastric banding showed an improvement of IIEF score without overall sexual function improvement: in particular, erectile index and orgasmic function worsened when adjusted for time (91). On the contrary, other studies evaluating pre- and post-surgical sexuality in male obese subjects, described positive effects of surgical weight loss, pointing also to the role of psychological issues on overall sexual activity (92, 93).

Bariatric Surgery and Semen Quality

Beyond the sex hormonal status and related clinical symptoms, bariatric surgery may potentially be associated not only with the improvement of reproductive hormones and related clinical symptoms but also with amelioration of semen parameters possibly resulting in improved fertility. Samavat et al analyzed the effects of RYGB on semen quality after 6 months from the procedure in a cohort study. They observed an increased sperm count, motility and ejaculate volume after treatment although not reaching the statistical significance. In addition, they also showed a reduction in sperm DNA fragmentation and semen IL-8, unconventional parameters of semen quality (94). Increase in total testosterone plasma levels may be partially responsible for these modifications, but these results also confirm the hypothesis regarding a deep, complex effect of obesity on reproduction, testicular activity and fertility in men, which may be reversed only partially by weight loss. Obesity may affect directly the biochemical activity of the testis, as demonstrated by lower levels of inhibin B observed in obese men, and bariatric surgery can potentially improve also this parameter (95). On the contrary, a retrospective study by Legro et al showed no amelioration in semen parameters of obese men that underwent gastric bypass (96). A previous prospective randomized study of Reis et al comparing surgical procedure and medical follow-up showed similar results: gastric by-pass obtained a significant increase in IIEF score, total and free testosterone levels in the intervention group, but did not affect sperm quality (97). In a prospective study of El Bardisi et al evaluating effects of sleeve gastrectomy on semen parameters, semen quality was not affected by surgical weight loss except for subgroups of men with pre-existing azoospermia or oligospermia (98). Some reports have also described the possibility that bariatric surgery may negatively influence sperm parameters, probably because of nutritional deficiency and induction of a systemic catabolic state with consequent accumulation of toxic metabolites (99–101). However, taken together, these data are relatively too weak to definitely clarify the situation, and more controlled studies in large populations are needed regarding this topic.

CONCLUSION

Bariatric surgery seems to be effective to improve free and total testosterone plasma levels in obese men, even if more evidence is needed about changes of other hormones such as gonadotropins and adrenal sex steroids. In addition, while testosterone plasma levels improvement is maintained for a long-term, restored erectile function seems not to be a durable effect, even if increased semen quality is not guaranteed after metabolic surgery. These conditions may be explained by the complex pathophysiology of reproductive function abnormalities occurring in men with obesity. In particular, adipose tissue expansion and consequent biochemical activity impairment (cytokines and adipokines production, increase peripheral androgens aromatization) may be responsible for reduced levels of testosterone while different and even more complex mechanisms, involving not only sex hormones levels but also neuro-vascular abnormalities and gonadal specific alterations, could be responsible for erectile dysfunction and infertility. To this regard, metabolic surgery may present some limitations; however, with respect to non-surgical weight loss, bariatric surgery remains the most effective treatment for a rapid improvement of global sexual activity and hypogonadism, so it could be considered as a relevant option for severely obese hypogonadal males.

AUTHOR CONTRIBUTIONS

DVA and RM equally wrote the article. VR and BL revised the paper.

ACKNOWLEDGMENTS

We used for our figure images from: Pixabay.com and Freepik.com-designed by Brgfx.

REFERENCES

1. Bray GA, Frühbeck G, Ryan DH, Wilding JP. Management of obesity. *Lancet* (2016) 387:1947–56. doi: 10.1016/S0140-6736(16)00271-3
2. Garvey WT, Mechanick JI, Brett EM, Garber AJ, Hurley DL, Jastreboff AM, et al. American association of clinical endocrinologists and american college of endocrinology comprehensive clinical practice guidelines for medical care of patients with obesity. *Endocr Pract.* (2016) 22:842–84. doi: 10.4158/EP161356.ESGL
3. Lim SS, Davies MJ, Norman RJ, Moran LJ. Overweight, obesity and central obesity in women with polycystic ovary syndrome: a systematic review and meta-analysis. *Hum Reprod Update* (2012) 18:618–37. doi: 10.1093/humupd/dms030
4. Hafner RJ, Watts JM, Rogers J. Quality of life after gastric bypass for morbid obesity. *Int J Obes.* (1991) 15:555–60.

5. Moore RH, Sarwer DB, Lavenberg JA, Lane IB, Evans JL, Volger S, et al. Relationship between sexual function and quality of life in obese persons seeking weight reduction. *Obesity* (2013) 21:1966–74. doi: 10.1002/oby.20398
6. Poggiogalle E, Di Lazzaro L, Pinto A, Migliaccio S, Lenzi A, Donini LM. Health-related quality of life and quality of sexual life in obese subjects. *Int J Endocrinol.* (2014) 2014:847871. doi: 10.1155/2014/847871
7. Dong JY, Zhang YH, Qin LQ. Erectile dysfunction and risk of cardiovascular disease: meta-analysis of prospective cohort studies. *J Am Coll Cardiol.* (2011) 58:1378–85. doi: 10.1016/j.jacc.2011.06.024
8. Eisenberg ML, Li S, Behr B, Cullen MR, Galusha D, Lamb DJ, et al. Semen quality, infertility and mortality in the USA. *Hum Reprod.* (2014) 29:1567–74. doi: 10.1093/humrep/deu106
9. Calderón B, Gómez-Martín JM, Vega-Piñero B, Martín-Hidalgo A, Galindo J, Luque-Ramírez M, et al. Prevalence of male secondary hypogonadism in moderate to severe obesity and its relationship with insulin resistance and excess body weight. *Andrology* (2016) 4:62–7. doi: 10.1111/andr.12135
10. Dandona P, Dhindsa S. Update: hypogonadotropic hypogonadism in type 2 diabetes and obesity. *J Clin Endocrinol Metab.* (2011) 96:2643–51. doi: 10.1210/jc.2010-2724
11. Chughtai B, Lee RK, Te AE, Kaplan SA. Metabolic syndrome and sexual dysfunction. *Curr Opin Urol.* (2011) 21:514–8. doi: 10.1097/MOU.0b013e32834b8681
12. Dhindsa S, Furlanetto R, Vora M, Ghanim H, Chaudhuri A, Dandona P. Low estradiol concentrations in men with subnormal testosterone concentrations and type 2 diabetes. *Diabetes Care* (2011) 34:1854–9. doi: 10.2337/dc11-0208
13. Stanworth RD, Jones TH. Testosterone in obesity, metabolic syndrome and type 2 diabetes. *Front Horm Res.* (2009) 37:74–90. doi: 10.1159/000176046
14. Makhsida N, Shah J, Yan G, Fisch H, Shabsigh R. Hypogonadism and metabolic syndrome: implications for testosterone therapy. *J Urol.* (2005) 174:827–34. doi: 10.1097/01.ju.0000169490.78443.59
15. Svartberg J. Epidemiology: testosterone and the metabolic syndrome. *Int J Impot Res.* (2007) 19:124–8. doi: 10.1038/sj.ijir.3901499
16. Wake DJ, Strand M, Rask E, Westerbacka J, Livingstone DE, Soderberg S, et al. Intra-adipose sex steroid metabolism and body fat distribution in idiopathic human obesity. *Clin Endocrinol.* (2007) 66:440–6. doi: 10.1111/j.1365-2265.2007.02755.x
17. Cohen PG. Aromatase, adiposity, aging and disease. The hypogonadal-metabolic-atherogenic-disease and aging connection. *Med Hypotheses* (2001) 56:702–8. doi: 10.1054/mehy.2000.1169
18. Hanchang W, Semprasert N, Limjindaporn T, Yenchitsomanus PT, Kooptiwut S. Testosterone protects against glucotoxicity-induced apoptosis of pancreatic β-cells. (INS-1) and male mouse pancreatic islets. *Endocrinology* (2013) 154:4058–67. doi: 10.1210/en.2013-1351
19. Kooptiwut S, Hanchang W, Semprasert N, Junking M, Limjindaporn T, Yenchitsomanus PT. Testosterone reduces AGTR1 expression to prevent β-cell and islet apoptosis from glucotoxicity. *J Endocrinol.* (2015) 224:215–24. doi: 10.1530/JOE-14-0397
20. Singh R, Artaza JN, Taylor WE, Gonzalez-Cadavid NF, Bhasin S. Androgens stimulate myogenic differentiation and inhibit adipogenesis in C3H 10T1/2 pluripotent cells through an androgen receptor-mediated pathway. *Endocrinology* (2003) 144:5081–8. doi: 10.1210/en.2003-0741
21. Singh R, Artaza JN, Taylor WE, Braga M, Yuan X, Gonzalez-Cadavid NF, et al. Testosterone inhibits adipogenic differentiation in 3T3-L1 cells: nuclear translocation of androgen receptor complex with beta-catenin and T-cell factor 4 may bypass canonical Wnt signaling to down-regulate adipogenic transcription factors. *Endocrinology* (2006) 147:141–54. doi: 10.1210/en.2004-1649
22. Martin LJ. Implications of adiponectin in linking metabolism to testicular function. *Endocrine* (2014) 46:16–28. doi: 10.1007/s12020-013-0102-0
23. Isidori AM, Caprio M, Strollo F, Moretti C, Frajese G, Isidori A, et al. Leptin and androgens in male obesity: evidence for leptin contribution to reduced androgen levels. *J Clin Endocrinol Metab.* (1999) 84:3673–80. doi: 10.1210/jc.84.10.3673
24. Svartberg J, von Mühlen D, Schirmer H, Barrett-Connor E, Sundfjord J, Jorde R. Association of endogenous testosterone with blood pressure and left ventricular mass in men. The Tromsø Study. *Eur J Endocrinol.* (2004) 150:65–71. doi: 10.1530/eje.0.1500065
25. Traish AM, Feeley RJ, Guay A. Mechanisms of obesity and related pathologies: androgen deficiency and endothelial dysfunction may be the link between obesity and erectile dysfunction. *FEBS J.* (2009) 276:5755–67. doi: 10.1111/j.1742-4658.2009.07305.x
26. Stellato RK, Feldman HA, Hamdy O, Horton ES, McKinlay JB. Testosterone, sex hormone-binding globulin, and the development of type 2 diabetes in middle-aged men: prospective results from the Massachusetts male aging study. *Diabetes Care* (2000) 23:490–4. doi: 10.2337/diacare.23.4.490
27. Haffner SM, Shaten J, Stern MP, Smith GD, Kuller L. Low levels of sex hormone-binding globulin and testosterone predict the development of non-insulin-dependent diabetes mellitus in men. MRFIT research group multiple risk factor intervention trial. *Am J Epidemiol.* (1996) 143:889–97. doi: 10.1093/oxfordjournals.aje.a008832
28. Ding EL, Song Y, Malik VS, Liu S. Sex differences of endogenous sex hormones and risk of type 2 diabetes: a systematic review and meta-analysis. *JAMA* (2006) 295:1288–99. doi: 10.1001/jama.295.11.1288
29. Keating NL, O'Malley AJ, Freedland SJ, Smith MR. Diabetes and cardiovascular disease during androgen deprivation therapy: observational study of veterans with prostate cancer. *J Natl Cancer Inst.* (2010) 102:39–46. doi: 10.1093/jnci/djp404
30. Pasquali R, Macor C, Vicennati V, Novo F, De lasio R, Mesini P, et al. Effects of acute hyperinsulinemia on testosterone serum concentrations in adult obese and normal-weight men. *Metabolism* (1997) 46:526–9. doi: 10.1016/S0026-0495(97)90189-X
31. Pasquali R, Casimirri F, De lasio R, Mesini P, Boschi S, Chierici R, et al. Insulin regulates testosterone and sex hormone-binding globulin concentrations in adult normal weight and obese men. *J Clin Endocrinol Metab.* (1995) 80:654–658.
32. Tsai EC, Matsumoto AM, Fujimoto WY, Boyko EJ. Association of bioavailable, free, and total testosterone with insulin resistance: influence of sex hormone-binding globulin and body fat. *Diabetes Care* (2004) 27:861–8. doi: 10.2337/diacare.27.4.861
33. Benitez A, Perez Diaz J. Effect of streptozotocin-diabetes and insulin treatment on regulation of Leydig cell function in the rat. *Horm Metab Res.* (1985) 17:5–7. doi: 10.1055/s-2007-1013433
34. Pitteloud N, Hardin M, Dwyer AA, Valassi E, Yialamas M, Elahi D, et al. Increasing insulin resistance is associated with a decrease in Leydig cell testosterone secretion in men. *J Clin Endocrinol Metab.* (2005) 90:2636–41. doi: 10.1210/jc.2004-2190
35. Cole AP, Hanske J, Jiang W, Kwon NK, Lipsitz SR, Kathrins M, et al. Impact of testosterone replacement therapy on thromboembolism, heart disease and obstructive sleep apnoea in men. *BJU Int.* (2018) 121:811–8. doi: 10.1111/bju.14149
36. Yim JY, Kim J, Kim D, Ahmed A. Serum testosterone and non-alcoholic fatty liver disease in men and women in the US. *Liver Int.* (2018) 38:2051–59. doi: 10.1111/liv.13735
37. Jaruvongvanich V, Sanguankeo A, Riangwiwat T, Upala S. Testosterone, sex hormone-binding globulin and nonalcoholic fatty liver disease: a systematic review and meta-analysis. *Ann Hepatol.* (2017) 16:382–94. doi: 10.5604/01.3001.0009.8593
38. Rocha ALL, Faria LC, Guimarães TCM, Moreira GV, Cândido AL, Couto CA, et al. Non-alcoholic fatty liver disease in women with polycystic ovary syndrome: systematic review and meta-analysis. *J Endocrinol Invest.* (2017) 40:1279–88. doi: 10.1007/s40618-017-0708-9
39. Kumarendran B, O'Reilly MW, Manolopoulos KN, Toulis KA, Gokhale KM, Sitch AJ, et al. Polycystic ovary syndrome, androgen excess, and the risk of nonalcoholic fatty liver disease in women: a longitudinal study based on a United Kingdom primary care database. *PLoS Med.* (2018) 15:e1002542. doi: 10.1371/journal.pmed.1002542
40. Saad F, Haider A, Doros G, Traish A. Long-term treatment of hypogonadal men with testosterone produces substantial and sustained weight loss. *Obesity* (2013) 21:1975–81. doi: 10.1002/oby.20407
41. Haider A, Yassin A, Doros G, Saad F. Effects of long-term testosterone therapy on patients with 'diabesity': results of observational studies of pooled analyses in obese hypogonadal men with type 2 diabetes. *Int J Endocrinol.* (2014) 2014:683515. doi: 10.1155/2014/683515

42. Haider A, Yassin A, Doros G, Traish AM, Saad F. Reductions of weight and waist size in 362 hypogonadal men with obesity grades I to III under long-term treatment with testosterone undecanoate. (TU): observational data from two registry studies. In: *Abstract (SAT-0940) Presented at the Endocrine Society's 96th Annual Meeting* (2014).
43. Yassin A, Doros G. Testosterone therapy in hypogonadal men results in sustained and clinically meaningful weight loss. *Clin Obes.* (2013) 3:73–83. doi: 10.1111/cob.12022
44. Vikan T, Schirmer H, Njølstad I, Svartberg J. Endogenous sex hormones and the prospective associations with cardiovascular disease and mortality in men. The Tromso Study. *Eur J Endocrinol.* (2009) 161:435–42.doi: 10.1530/EJE-09–0284.
45. Yeap BB, Hyde Z, Almeida OP, Norman PE, Chubb SA, Jamrozik K, et al. Lower testosterone levels predict incident stroke and transient ischemic attacks in older men. *J Clin Endocrinol Metab.* (2009) 94:2353–9. doi: 10.1210/jc.2008-2416
46. Bacon CG, Mittleman MA, Kawachi I, Giovannucci E, Glasser DB, Rimm EB. Sexual function in men older than 50 years of age: results from the health professionals follow-up study. *Ann Intern Med.* (2003) 139:161–8. doi: 10.7326/0003-4819-139-3-200308050-00005
47. Sarwer DB, Spitzer JC, Wadden TA, Rosen RC, Mitchell JE, Lancaster K, et al. Sexual functioning and sex hormones in persons with extreme obesity and seeking surgical and nonsurgical weight loss. *Surg Obes Relat Dis.* (2013) 9:997–1007. doi: 10.1016/j.soard.2013.07.003
48. Demir O, Akgul K, Akar Z, Cakmak O, Ozdemir I, Bolukbasi A, et al. Association between severity of lower urinary tract symptoms, erectile dysfunction and metabolic syndrome. *Aging Male.* (2009) 12:29–34. doi: 10.1080/13685530902777425
49. Andersen JM, Herning H, Aschim EL, Hjelmesæth J, Mala T, Hanevik HI, et al. Body mass index is associated with impaired semen characteristics and reduced levels of anti-müllerian hormone across a wide weight range. *PLoS ONE* (2015) 10:e0130210. doi: 10.1371/journal.pone.0130210
50. MacDonald AA, Herbison GP, Showell M, Farquhar CM. The impact of body mass index on semen parameters and reproductive hormones in human males: a systematic review with meta-analysis. *Hum Reprod Update* (2010) 16:293–311. doi: 10.1093/humupd/dmp047
51. Sermondade N, Faure C, Fezeu L, Shayeb AG, Bonde JP, Jensen TK, et al. BMI in relation to sperm count: an updated systematic review and collaborative meta-analysis. *Hum Reprod Update* (2013) 19:221–31. doi: 10.1093/humupd/dms050
52. Leisegang K, Bouic PJ, Menkveld R, Henkel RR. Obesity is associated with increased seminal insulin and leptin alongside reduced fertility parameters in a controlled male cohort. *Reprod Biol Endocrinol.* (2014) 12:34. doi: 10.1186/1477-7827-12-34
53. Agarwal A, Virk G, Ong C, du Plessis SS. Effect of oxidative stress on male reproduction. *World J Mens Health* (2014) 32:1–17. doi: 10.5534/wjmh.2014.32.1.1
54. Armamento-Villareal R, Aguirre LE, Qualls C, Villareal DT. Effect of lifestyle intervention on the hormonal profile of frail, obese older men. *J Nutr Health Aging* (2016) 20:334–40. doi: 10.1007/s12603-016-0698-x
55. Kaukua J, Pekkarinen T, Sane T, Mustajoki P. Sex hormones and sexual function in obese men losing weight. *Obes Res.* (2003) 11:689–94. doi: 10.1038/oby.2003.98
56. Leenen R, van der Kooy K, Seidell JC, Deurenberg P, Koppeschaar HP. Visceral fat accumulation in relation to sex hormones in obese men and women undergoing weight loss therapy. *J Clin Endocrinol Metab.* (1994) 78:1515–20.
57. Pellitero S, Olaizola I, Alastrue A, Martínez E, Granada ML, Balibrea JM, et al. Hypogonadotropic hypogonadism in morbidly obese males is reversed after bariatric surgery. *Obes Surg.* (2012) 22:1835–42. doi: 10.1007/s11695-012-0734-9
58. Samavat J, Facchiano E, Lucchese M, Forti G, Mannucci E, Maggi M, et al. Hypogonadism as an additional indication for bariatric surgery in male morbid obesity? *Eur J Endocrinol.* (2014) 171:555–60. doi: 10.1530/EJE-14-0596
59. Escobar-Morreale HF, Santacruz E, Luque-Ramírez M, Botella Carretero JI. Prevalence of 'obesity-associated gonadal dysfunction' in severely obese men and women and its resolution after bariatric surgery: a systematic review and meta-analysis. *Hum Reprod Update* (2017) 23:390–408. doi: 10.1093/humupd/dmx012
60. Saad F, Yassin A, Doros G, Haider A. Effects of long-term treatment with testosterone on weight and waist size in 411 hypogonadal men with obesity classes I-III: observational data from two registry studies. *Int J Obes.* (2016) 40:162–70. doi: 10.1038/ijo.2015.139
61. Niskanen L, Laaksonen DE, Punnonen K, Mustajoki P, Kaukua J, Rissanen A. Changes in sex hormone-binding globulin and testosterone during weight loss and weight maintenance in abdominally obese men with the metabolic syndrome. *Diabetes Obes Metab.* (2004) 6:208–15. doi: 10.1111/j.1462-8902.2004.00335.x
62. De Lorenzo A, Noce A, Moriconi E, Rampello T, Marrone G, Di Daniele N, et al. MOSH Syndrome. (Male Obesity Secondary Hypogonadism): clinical assessment and possible therapeutic approaches. *Nutrients* (2018) 10: E474. doi: 10.3390/nu10040474
63. Heufelder AE, Saad F, Bunck MC, Gooren L. Fifty-two-week treatment with diet and exercise plus transdermal testosterone reverses the metabolic syndrome and improves glycemic control in men with newly diagnosed type 2 diabetes and subnormal plasma testosterone. *J Androl.* (2009) 30:726–33. doi: 10.2164/jandrol.108.007005
64. Calderón B, Galdón A, Calañas A, Peromingo R, Galindo J, García-Moreno F, et al. Effects of bariatric surgery on male obesity-associated secondary hypogonadism: comparison of laparoscopic gastric bypass with restrictive procedures. *Obes Surg.* (2014) 24:1686–92. doi: 10.1007/s11695-014-1233-y
65. Botella-Carretero JI, Balsa JA, Gómez-Martin JM, Peromingo R, Huerta L, Carrasco M, et al. Circulating free testosterone in obese men after bariatric surgery increases in parallel with insulin sensitivity. *J Endocrinol Invest.* (2013) 36:227–32. doi: 10.3275/8469
66. Alagna S, Cossu ML, Gallo P, Tilocca PL, Pileri P, Alagna G, et al. Biliopancreatic diversion: long-term effects on gonadal function in severely obese men. *Surg Obes Relat Dis.* (2006) 2:82–6. doi: 10.1016/j.soard.2006.01.005
67. Bastounis EA, Karayiannakis AJ, Syrigos K, Zbar A, Makri GG, Alexiou D. Sex hormone changes in morbidly obese patients after vertical banded gastroplasty. *Eur Surg Res.* (1998) 30:43–7. doi: 10.1159/000008556
68. Hammoud A, Gibson M, Hunt SC, Adams TD, Carrell DT, Kolotkin RL, et al. Effect of Roux-en-Y gastric bypass surgery on the sex steroids and quality of life in obese men. *J Clin Endocrinol Metab.* (2009) 94:1329–32. doi: 10.1210/jc.2008-1598
69. Boonchaya-Anant P, Laichuthai N, Suwannasrisuk P, Houngngam N, Udomsawaengsup S, Snabboon T. Changes in testosterone levels and sex hormone-binding globulin levels in extremely obese men after bariatric surgery. *Int J Endocrinol.* (2016) 2016:1416503. doi: 10.1155/2016/1416503
70. Di Vincenzo A, Silvestrin V, Bertoli E, Foletto M, Pagano C, Fabris R, et al. Short-term effects of surgical weight loss after sleeve gastrectomy on sex steroids plasma levels and PSA concentration in men with severe obesity. *Aging Male* (2018). doi: 10.1080/13685538.2018.1528445. [Epub ahead of print].
71. Pham NH, Bena J, Bhatt DL, Kennedy L, Schauer PR, Kashyap SR. Increased free testosterone levels in men with uncontrolled type 2 diabetes five years after randomization to bariatric surgery. *Obes Surg* (2018) 28:277–80. doi: 10.1007/s11695-017-2881-5
72. Liu F, Tu Y, Zhang P, Bao Y, Han J, Jia W. Decreased visceral fat area correlates with improved total testosterone levels after Roux-en-Y gastric bypass in obese Chinese males with type 2 diabetes: a 12-month follow-up. *Surg Obes Relat Dis.* (2018) 14:462–8. doi: 10.1016/j.soard.2017.11.009
73. Tena-Sempere M, Pinilla L, González LC, Diéguez C, Casanueva FF, Aguilar E. Leptin inhibits testosterone secretion from adult rat testis *in vitro*. *J Endocrinol.* (1999) 161:211–8. doi: 10.1677/joe.0.1610211
74. Facchiano E, Scaringi S, Veltri M, Samavat J, Maggi M, Forti G, et al. Age as a predictive factor of testosterone improvement in male patients after bariatric surgery: preliminary results of a monocentric prospective study. *Obes Surg.* (2013) 23:167–72. doi: 10.1007/s11695-012-0753-6
75. Luconi M, Samavat J, Seghieri G, Iannuzzi G, Lucchese M, Rotella C, et al. Determinants of testosterone recovery after bariatric surgery: is it only a matter of reduction of body mass index? *Fertil Steril.* (2013) 99:1872–9.e1. doi: 10.1016/j.fertnstert.2013.02.039

76. Neunhaeuserer D, Gasperetti A, Savalla F, Gobbo S, Bullo V, Bergamin M, et al. Functional evaluation in obese patients before and after sleeve gastrectomy. *Obes Surg.* (2017) 27:3230–9. doi: 10.1007/s11695-017-2763-x
77. Liao M, Guo X, Yu X, Pang G, Zhang S, Li J, et al. (2013). Role of metabolic factors in the association between osteocalcin and testosterone in Chinese men. *J Clin Endocrinol Metab.* 98:3463–9. 10.1210/jc.2013–1805.
78. Samavat J, Facchiano E, Cantini G, Di Franco A, Alpigiano G, Poli G, et al. Osteocalcin increase after bariatric surgery predicts androgen recovery in hypogonadal obese males. *Int J Obes* (2014) 38:357–63. doi: 10.1038/ijo.2013.228
79. Esposito K, Giugliano F, Di Palo C, Giugliano G, Marfella R, D'Andrea F, et al. Effect of lifestyle changes on erectile dysfunction in obese men: a randomized controlled trial. *JAMA* (2004) 291:2978–2984. doi: 10.1001/jama.291.24.2978
80. Khoo J, Piantadosi C, Worthley S, Wittert GA. Effects of a low-energy diet on sexual function and lower urinary tract symptoms in obese men. *Int J Obes.* (2010) 34:1396–403 doi: 10.1038/ijo.2010.76
81. Glina FPA, de Freitas Barboza JW, Nunes VM, Glina S, Bernardo WM. What is the impact of bariatric surgery on erectile function? A systematic review and meta-analysis. *Sex Med Rev.* (2017) 5:393–402. doi: 10.1016/j.sxmr.2017.03.008
82. Dallal RM, Chernoff A, O'Leary MP, Smith JA, Braverman JD, Quebbemann BB. Sexual dysfunction is common in the morbidly obese male and improves after gastric bypass surgery. *J Am Coll Surg.* (2008) 207:859–64. doi: 10.1016/j.jamcollsurg.2008.08.006
83. Aleid M, Muneer A, Renshaw S, George J, Jenkinson AD, Adamo M, et al. Early effect of bariatric surgery on urogenital function in morbidly obese men. *J Sex Med.* (2017) 14:205–14. doi: 10.1016/j.jsxm.2016.12.004
84. Groutz A, Gordon D, Schachter P, Amir H, Shimonov M. Effects of bariatric surgery on male lower urinary tract symptoms and sexual function. *Neurourol Urodyn.* (2017) 36:636–9. doi: 10.1002/nau.22980
85. Efthymiou V, Hyphantis T, Karaivazoglou K, Gourzis P, Alexandrides TK, Kalfarentzos F, et al. The effect of bariatric surgery on patient HRQOL and sexual health during a 1-year postoperative period. *Obes Surg.* (2015) 25:310–8. doi: 10.1007/s11695-014-1384-x
86. Reis LO, Favaro WJ, Barreiro GC, de Oliveira LC, Chaim EA, Fregonesi A, et al. Erectile dysfunction and hormonal imbalance in morbidly obese male is reversed after gastric bypass surgery: a prospective randomized controlled trial. *Int J Androl.* (2010) 33:736–44. doi: 10.1111/j.1365-2605.2009.01017.x
87. Kun L, Pin Z, Jianzhong D, Xiaodong H, Haoyong Y, Yuqian B, et al. Significant improvement of erectile function after Roux-en-Y gastric bypass surgery in obese Chinese men with erectile dysfunction. *Obes Surg.* (2015) 25:838–44. doi: 10.1007/s11695-014-1465-x
88. Mora M, Aranda GB, de Hollanda A, Flores L, Puig-Domingo M, Vidal J. Weight loss is a major contributor to improved sexual function after bariatric surgery. *Surg Endosc.* (2013) 27:3197–204. doi: 10.1007/s00464-013-2890-y
89. Rosenblatt A, Faintuch J, Cecconello I. Sexual hormones and erectile function more than 6 years after bariatric surgery. *Surg Obes Relat Dis.* (2013) 9:636–40. doi: 10.1016/j.soard.2012.06.010
90. Sarwer DB, Spitzer JC, Wadden TA, Rosen RC, Mitchell JE, Lancaster K, et al. Sexual functioning and sex hormones in men who underwent bariatric surgery. *Surg Obes Relat Dis.* (2015) 11:643–51. doi: 10.1016/j.soard.2014.12.014
91. Ranasinghe WK, Wright T, Attia J, McElduff P, Doyle T, Bartholomew M, et al. Effects of bariatric surgery on urinary and sexual function. *BJU Int.* (2011) 107:88–94. doi: 10.1111/j.1464-410X.2010.09509.x
92. Kinzl JF, Trefalt E, Fiala M, Hotter A, Biebl W, Aigner F. Partnership, sexuality, and sexual disorders in morbidly obese women: consequences of weight loss after gastric banding. *Obes Surg.* (2001) 11:455–8. doi: 10.1381/096089201321209323
93. Camps MA, Zervos E, Goode S, Rosemurgy AS. Impact of bariatric surgery on body image perception and sexuality in morbidly obese patients and their partners. *Obes Surg.* (1996) 6:356–60. doi: 10.1381/096089296765556700
94. Samavat J, Cantini G, Lotti F, Di Franco A, Tamburrino L, Degl'Innocenti S, et al. (2018). Massive weight loss obtained by bariatric surgery affects semen quality in morbid male obesity: a preliminary prospective double-armed study. *Obes Surg.* 28:69–76. doi: 10.1007/s11695-017-2802-7
95. Globerman H, Shen-Orr Z, Karnieli E, Aloni Y, Charuzi I. Inhibin B in men with severe obesity and after weight reduction following gastroplasty. *Endocr Res.* (2005) 31:17–26. doi: 10.1080/07435800500228971
96. Legro RS, Kunselman AR, Meadows JW, Kesner JS, Krieg EF, Rogers AM, et al. Time-related increase in urinary testosterone levels and stable semen analysis parameters after bariatric surgery in men. *Reprod Biomed Online* (2015) 30:150–6. doi: 10.1016/j.rbmo.2014.10.014
97. Reis LO, Zani EL, Saad RD, Chaim EA, de Oliveira LC, Fregonesi A. Bariatric surgery does not interfere with sperm quality–a preliminary long-term study. *Reprod Sci.* (2012) 19:1057–62. doi: 10.1177/1933719112440747
98. El Bardisi H, Majzoub A, Arafa M, AlMalki A, Al Said S, Khalafalla K, et al. Effect of bariatric surgery on semen parameters and sex hormone concentrations: a prospective study. *Reprod Biomed Online* (2016) 33:606–11. doi: 10.1016/j.rbmo.2016.08.008
99. Lazaros L, Hatzi E, Markoula S, Takenaka A, Sofikitis N, Zikopoulos K, et al. Dramatic reduction in sperm parameters following bariatric surgery: report of two cases. *Andrologia* (2012) 44:428–32. doi: 10.1111/j.1439-0272.2012.01300.x
100. Sermondade N, Massin N, Boitrelle F, Pfeffer J, Eustache F, Sifer C, et al. Sperm parameters and male fertility after bariatric surgery: three case series. *Reprod Biomed Online* (2012) 24:206–10. doi: 10.1016/j.rbmo.2011.10.014
101. di Frega AS, Dale B, Di Matteo L, Wilding M. Secondary male factor infertility after Roux-en-Y gastric bypass for morbid obesity: case report. *Hum Reprod.* (2005) 20:997–8. doi: 10.1093/humrep/deh707

20

Short-Term Changes in Mental, Physical, and Social Factors after Metabolic Bariatric Surgery in Adolescents

Ariela Goldenshluger[1†], Tamar Maor[1†], Renana Via-Kagan[2], Orly Zelekha[2] and Yftach Gepner[1]*

[1] Department of Epidemiology and Preventive Medicine, Sackler Faculty of Medicine, School of Public Health, Sylvan Adams Sports Institute, Tel-Aviv University, Tel-Aviv, Israel, [2] Israel Center for Disease Control, Ministry of Health, Jerusalem, Israel

Correspondence:
Yftach Gepner
gepner@tauex.tau.ac.il

[†] These authors have contributed equally to this work

Background: Metabolic bariatric surgery (MBS) is an effective treatment for adolescents with severe obesity. However, changes in mental, physical, and social factors, as well as their association with the extent of excess weight loss (%EWL) after MBS, remain controversial.

Methods: We followed 97 adolescents (64% females, aged 17 $\pm$ 0.9 years, BMI 46.1 $\pm$ 5.9 kg/m^2) before and 9 months following MBS in a multi-center, prospective cohort study. Changes in mental, physical, and social factors were assessed by self-reported questionnaires, and associations with %EWL were evaluated after adjustment for potential confounders.

Results: The body mass index (BMI) decreased by 30%, and all physical parameters significantly improved ($p \leq 0.001$). Energy level increased by 24%, mood level by 14%, and mental health by 9.5% ($p \leq 0.002$). Social parameters were also improved, with a significant decrease in social rejection ($p = 0.02$), and an increase in participation in after-school social activities ($p = 0.008$). Mental health improvement was associated with baseline social rejection ($r = 0.514$, $p < 0.001$). The improvement in all factors was not related to the extent of %EWL.

Conclusion: Metabolic bariatric surgery MBS in adolescents led to a meaningful decrease in BMI and to an improvement in short-term physical, mental, and social factors that were not related to %EWL. Patients experiencing social rejection may improve their mental health following BS.

Keywords: bariatric surgery, physical status, adolescents, obesity, mental health, social rejection

INTRODUCTION

The prevalence of severe obesity [BMI of $\geq$35 or >120% of the 95th percentile] has increased in the last decades among adults and adolescents (1–3) and remains a worldwide public health concern (4). Although lifestyle modification is a beneficial strategy to decrease some extent of body weight (5–7), metabolic bariatric surgery (MBS) has been found as a beneficial intervention for severe obesity and its related comorbidities in the long term for adolescents (7–9). A systematic review of 49 studies ($n = 3{,}007$) of adolescents undergoing MBS and long-term, multicenter, and prospective trials reported a 26–31% reduction in BMI, and significant remission of diabetes (86–100%), dyslipidemia (64–83%), and hypertension (68–92%) (7, 10–12). Despite the evidence for metabolic health benefits from MBS among adolescents, these candidates are a high-risk group. Since, adolescents with obesity are more likely to endorse lower self-esteem, depression, reduced quality of life, and anhedonia (13, 14), and even it has been shown that mental factors could affect the chances to perform MBS and complete the preoperative program (14). Nationally, it is recommended an optimal multidisciplinary follow-up including visits to the bariatric surgeon, dietitian, and pediatrician for all patients, and a mental health professional follow-up according to personal need (15). Following surgery, the quality of life (QoL) in adolescents has been associated with long-term weight loss maintenance (16). Previous studies have reported an improvement in QoL in adolescents from 1 to 5 years after MBS (10, 11, 17, 18). However, 5 years following MBS, the improvement in QoL was mainly physical, not mental (19). The association between changes in mental, mental, and physical factors and weight loss and changes after MBS in adolescents remains unclear. Therefore, the objectives of this study were to evaluate the mental, physical, and social factor changes from baseline and to assess the association between those changes and EWL%, using a nationwide prospective cohort of adolescents after MBS.

METHODS

This prospective cohort study was conducted among adolescents who underwent MBS at 21 different medical institutions in Israel, between October 2017 and December 2019, using data from the Israeli National Registry of Adolescents Bariatric Surgery, a mandatory registry created by the Ministry of Health, in which all bariatric surgeries performed in adolescents in Israel, are registered. The registry includes data collected at a baseline visit in the bariatric Clinic before the surgery and the follow-up, performed by self-reported telephonic questionnaires. All patients and their families were provided informed consent for the study. The study was approved by the Institutional Review Board number of the Tel HaShomer Medical Center (6199-19-SMC) and by the Tel Aviv University's Helsinki committee (0001814-1).

Mental, Physical, and Social Factors

All study participants were requested to complete a baseline questionnaire before surgery regarding physical and social functioning and mental health factors. The questionnaire (**Supplementary Material 1**) is mandatory at baseline as part of the National Bariatric Registry, which gathers information about every adolescent undergoing bariatric surgery in the country. National guidelines for MBS in patients under the age of 18 years, are part of the Ministry of Health's medical director notice 27/2017 (August 2017) (15) and encourage follow-up of adolescents undergoing bariatric surgeries in Israel. The questionnaire included sets of questions on health status (e.g., obesity-related co-morbidities, chronic pain related to weight, smoking habits, and substance use), physical (energy level, and hygiene-related difficulties), mental (sadness, hopeless feeling, low self-esteem, and history of self-hurt attempt) and social factors (social rejection, after-school activities participation), as well as sets of questions on dietary patterns (vomiting, overeating episodes, loss of control eating, and eating at night, dietitian visits). Parents and adolescents (in the presence of a parent and with given permission) completed the questionnaire during the preoperative visit to the bariatric clinic. Preoperative presence of comorbidities was contributed by a physician at the bariatric medical center and based on medical records. The follow-up telephonic questionnaire was completed by Israeli National Registry of Adolescents Bariatric Surgery research assistants and the research team interviewers, at a mean of 8.8 ± 3.4 months post-surgery.

Questions regarding "Energy level" and "Mood level" have five-point Likert scale answers and were converted to a 0–100 scale. Dichotomous questions (yes/no) regarding physical state (e.g., snoring, pain affected by weight, physical activity habits), social factors (after-school social activities and social rejection), and mental health factors (sadness, low self-esteem, hopelessness, suicidal thoughts, and self-hurt attempts history) were performed.

The mental health questions were grouped as a mental health score with a higher score on a 0–100 scale meaning a better status (Cronbach's Alpha of 0.67).

%EWL Calculations

The %EWL was calculated by using the formula:

$$\%EWL = \frac{[(initial\ weight) - (post\ operativeweight)]}{[(initial\ weight) - (ideal\ body\ weight)]} \times 100$$

The ideal body weight was defined by the weight corresponding to a BMI of 25 kg/m^2, according to the American Society for Metabolic and Bariatric Surgery outcome reporting standards (20). The initial weight and height were taken from the measurement by the medical center during the preoperative visit, and the post-operative weight was self-reported at the interview.

Statistical Analysis

Baseline characteristics of those who agreed to be interviewed after surgery and those who refused were compared by a t-test or Chi-square test for continuous and categorical variables, respectively. Changes in mental, physical, and social factors were examined by a paired t-test for numeric variables and by a McNemar test for dichotomous variables. The association between factor changes and %EWL was assessed using the Pearson correlation for numerical variables. In addition, we divided the participants into below and above median %EWL [(%EWL < 67% ($n = 48$), and %EWL ≥ 67% ($n = 46$)] and compared the change in mental, physical, and social factors between weight loss categories by t-test for numerical variables and by a Chi-squared test for dichotomous variables. A univariate linear regression model was used to evaluate the association between dependent

TABLE 1 | Baseline characteristics of the participants before metabolic bariatric surgery.

		Male ($n = 35$)	Female ($n = 62$)	Total ($n = 97$)	*P*
Demographic characteristics					
Age, years		17.1 ± 0.9	17.0 ± 0.9	17.0 ± 0.9	0.58
Ethnic group, *n* (%)	Jewish	31 (88.6%)	51 (83.6%)[a]	82 (85.4%)[a]	0.51
	Arabic	4 (11.4%)	10 (16.4%)[a]	14 (14.6%)[a]	
Clinical characteristics					
Surgery procedure, *n* (%)	Sleeve gastrectomy	31 (88.6%)	53 (85.5%)	84 (86.6%)	0.76*
	Roux-en Y gastric bypass	0	2 (3.2%)	2 (2.1%)	
	Single anastomosis gastric bypass	3 (8.6%)	7 (11.3%)	10 (10.3%)	
	Gastric band	1 (2.9%)	0	1 (1%)	
BMI, kg/m^2		45.4 ± 5.5	46.5 ± 6.1	46.1 ± 5.9	0.39
Comorbidities:					
Diabetes, *n* (%)		2 (5.7%)	8 (12.9%)	10 (10.3%)	0.32**
Hypertension, *n* (%)		12 (34.3%)	3 (4.8%)	15 (15.5%)	<0.001
Dyslipidemia, *n* (%)		12 (34.3%)	17 (27.4%)	29 (29.9%)	0.48
Fatty liver, *n* (%)		26 (76.5%)[a]	39 (62.9%)	65 (67.7%)[a]	0.17
Obstructive sleep apnea, *n* (%)		7 (20.0%)	18 (29.0%)	25 (25.8%)	0.33
Urinary incontinence, *n* (%)		0[e]	3 (5.2%)[d]	3 (3.4%)[f]	-
Orthopedic ¥, *n* (%)		8 (22.9%)	14 (22.6%)	22 (22.7%)	0.97
Reflux, *n* (%)		6 (17.1%)	4 (6.5%)	10 (10.3%)	-
Anxiety, *n* (%)		0[c]	4 (6.6%)[a]	4 (4.3%)[d]	–
Depression, *n* (%)		1 (3.0%)[b]	4 (6.6%)[a]	5 (5.3%)[c]	–
ADHD, *n* (%)		4 (12.1%)[b]	24 (40.7%)[c]	28 (30.4%)[e]	0.004
Smoking, *n* (%)		5 (14.7%)[a]	6 (10.0%)[b]	11 (11.7%)[c]	0.52**
SBP, mmHg		133 ± 16	123 ± 13[a]	127 ± 14[a]	0.003
DBP, mmHg		72.8 ± 10	72.7 ± 11[a]	72.8 ± 11[a]	0.96
Irregular periods, *n* (%)		–	21 (33.9%)[a]	–	–
PCOS, *n* (%)	-	–	7 (11.3%)	–	

Data in the table are presented as mean ± SD for numerical variables and n (%) for dichotomous variables. t- test was used to evaluate differences for numerical variables and Chi-square test for nominal variables. All statistical analyses were two sided with a significance of < 0.05. Irregular periods and PCOS were examined only for females.
**calculated as sleeve gastrectomy vs. other procedures by Fisher's exact test.*
***calculated by Fisher's exact test, [a]1 participant is missing, [b]2 are missing, [c]3 are missing, [d]4 are missing, [e]5 are missing, [f]9 are missing.*
ADHD, attention deficit and hyperactivity disorders; BMI, body mass index; SBP, systolic blood pressure; DBP, diastolic blood pressure; kg, kilograms; m, meters; mmHg, millimeters of mercury; PCOS, polycystic ovary syndrome. ¥ Orthopedic pain related to body weight.

variables of mental, physical, and social factors changes (for numerical parameters) and potential independent variables: age, gender, baseline BMI, ethnic group, dietitian meetings number, and number of comorbidities. A multivariate linear regression model assessed associations between significant variables in the univariate analysis and was adjusted for possible confounders: age, gender, and baseline BMI or gender, baseline BMI, and time from surgery. Additionally, a sensitivity analysis of the self-reported weight, before surgery compared to documented weight at hospitalization, was performed. All statistical analyses were two-sided with a significance of $p < 0.05$.

RESULTS

In total, 107 out of 123 adolescents who underwent MBS from 10/2017-to 12/2019 were contacted and 16 refused to participate. We excluded five participants, who were less or beyond the follow-up time frame, and five participants who underwent additional surgery after the MBS. In total, 97 adolescents were interviewed at 8.8 ± 3.4 months post-surgery. Baseline characteristics are summarized in **Table 1** by gender (62 females and 35 males, aged 17 ± 0.9 years, with a BMI of 46.1 ± 5.9). Sleeve gastrectomy was the most common surgical procedure (86.6%). The dietary patterns report showed a sense of loss of control while eating ($n = 38$, 40.4%), night eating ($n = 48$, 51.1%), excess eating ($n = 47$, 50%), and vomiting ($n = 3$, 3.2%). Females had lower systolic blood pressure, lower rates of hypertension diagnosis, and higher rates of Attention-Deficit Hyperactivity Disorder (ADHD) ($p = 0.003$, $p < 0.001$, and $p = 0.004$, respectively). Except for gender, there were no other significant differences in baseline characteristics between participants and those who refused to be interviewed (**Supplementary Material 2**).

TABLE 2 | Changes in body weight and physical, social and mental parameters 9 months after metabolic bariatric surgery in adolescents.

	Pre-surgery	Post-surgery	improvement in those with pre-condition	*N*	P
Weight parameters					
Weight (kg)	127.7 ± 17.9	89.1 ± 15.1	–	94	<0.001
BMI (kg/m²)	45.9 ± 5.9	32.2 ± 5.6	–	94	<0.001
Physical and social parameters					
Snoring*, *n* (%)	43 (56.6%)	6 (7.9%)	38 (88.3%)	76	<0.001
Pain*, *n* (%)	39 (46.4%)	16 (19.0%)	33 (84.6%)	84	0.001
Physical activity*, *n* (%)	35 (42.2%)	72 (86.7%)	40 (83.3%)¥	83	<0.001
After-school social activities*, *n* (%)	35 (47.3%)	52 (70.3%)	27 (69.2%)	74	0.008
Social rejection*, *n* (%)	13 (17.1%)	4 (5.4%)	11 (84.6%)	76	0.02
Energy level** (0–100 scale)	61.0 ± 29.1	80.1 ± 21.2	–	84	<0.001
Mood level** (0–100 scale)	80.5 ± 21.5	91.5 ± 17.7	–	82	<0.001
Mental health score* (0–100 scale)**	88.8 ± 21.8	97.2 ± 8.1	–	50	0.002
Sadness, n (%)*	11 (13.9%)	3 (3.8%)	10 (90.9%)	79	0.039
Low self-esteem, n (%)*	8 (15.4%)	4 (7.7%)	6 (75%)	52	0.289
Hopelessness, n (%)*	14 (17.9%)	5 (6.4%)	13 (92.8%)	78	0.049
Suicidal thoughts, n (%)*	3 (5.6%)	0	3 (100%)	54	–
Self-hurt attempts, n (%)*	2 (3.6%)	1 (1.8%)	1 (50%)	55	1
Smoking	11 (12.9%)	19 (22.3%)	10 (13.3)¥¥	85	0.039

Data in the table are presented as mean ± SD for numerical variables n (%) for dichotomous variables. Paired t- test was used to evaluate differences for numerical variables and McNemar test for nominal variables. All statistical analyses were two sided with a significance of < 0.05. Pre-τsurgery weight and height were measured at the medical center on hospitalization. Post-surgery weight is based on self-reported data, post-surgery height was taken from the measurement of the medical center pre-surgery.
**Dichotomous questions (yes/no). **Ordinal scale question (0–100 scale, higher score means better status). ***Sum of all the dichotomous questions below (0–100 scale, higher score means better mental health). ¥ From those who did not performed any physical activity prior to surgery; ¥¥ from those who did not smoke prior to surgery.*
BMI, body mass index; kg, kilograms; m, meters.

Mental, Physical, and Social Factors and Weight Changes After Surgery

Mean weight loss was 38.6 ± 11.2 kg, %EWL was 68.5 ± 19.9%, percent of total body weight loss (TWL%) was 30.1 ± 7.4%, and the BMI had decreased by 13.8 ± 3.7 kg/m² ($p < 0.001$). Seventy-one (82.6%) participants took multivitamins every week, 81 (91%) were at a dietitian follow-up and 41 (46.6%) were under mental follow-up by a social worker o psychologist. Fifteen participants (29.4%, $n = 51$ respondents) reported having improved a personal hygiene problems after surgery. In addition, physical factors (snoring, pain affected by weight, and physical activity) had improved significantly ($p \leq 0.001$). However, 10 (22.2%) participants, who did not suffer from pain before surgery, reported onset of chronic pain by the follow-uptime. The energy level increased by 24% from 61 ± 29.1 to 80.1 ± 21.2 post-surgery ($p < 0.001$), while the mood level had increased by 14% from 80.5 ± 21.5 to 91.5 ± 17.7 ($p < 0.001$). Social parameters also improved, with a decrease in social rejection from 13 (17.1%) pre-surgery to 4 (5.4%) post-surgery ($p = 0.02$), and an increase in participation in after-school social activities. The mental health score increased by 9.5% from 88.8 ± 21.8 pre-surgery to 97.2 ± 8.1 post-surgery ($p = 0.002$), although not all the individual components showed a significant improvement when calculated separately (**Table 2**).

Among the participants that underwent an additional surgery ($n = 5$), their EWL% was 73.5 ± 14.7% after a mean follow-up of 11 months (vs. 68.5 ± 19.9% after a mean of 9 months in the study group), and they visited 4.8 ± 2.2 times the ER, and were 3.3 ± 1/5 times hospitalized. Similar improvements in mental, physical, and social factors were found between those who underwent additional bariatric surgery and those with one metabolic bariatric surgery.

When comparing between sexes, males had a higher %EWL than females (75.7 ± 18.2% vs. 64.3 ± 19.7% respectively, $p = 0.006$). Social rejection improved significantly in females ($n = 10$, 83% of those presenting social rejection at baseline, $p = 0.012$), but not in males. Both females and males improved physical symptoms comparing to baseline, such as snoring ($n = 23$, 88%, $p < 0.001$ in those with snoring prior to the surgery for females and $n = 15$, 88%, $p = 0.001$ for males) and weight-related pain ($n = 20$, 83.3%, $p = 0.019$ for females and $n = 13$, 86.6%, $p = 0.21$ for males). Other parameters were comparable between males and females.

Association Between %EWL and Baseline Parameters

We divided our sample into two categories, based on median %EWL: %EWL < 67 ($n = 48$, mean of 53%), and %EWL ≥ 67 ($n = 46$, mean of 82%; **Table 3**). Three participants were excluded from the analysis (did not report weight after surgery). As expected, a long time from surgery to interview was associated with a higher %EWL ($p = 0.010$). More females achieved a lower %EWL than males (79.1% in the lower EWL% group compared to 45.6% in the higher EWL% group, $p = 0.001$), and those with a

TABLE 3 | Baseline characteristics and quality of life changes post-surgery across percent excess weight loss categories.

	EWL<67 % n = 48	EWL≥67 % n = 46	p
Baseline characteristics			
Female gender	38 (79.1%)	21 (45.6%)	0.001
Baseline BMI, kg/m^2	48.2 ± 6.4	43.6 ± 4.2	<0.001
Age, years	16.8 ± 1.0	17.3 ± 0.6	0.002
Time from surgery to interview, months	8.0 ± 3.0	9.8 ± 3.7	0.010
Physical, social and mental health changes			
Snoring (remission*)	19 (90.4%) n = 21	19 (86.3%) n = 22	–
Pain (remission*)	16 (84.2%) n = 19	17 (85.0%) n = 20	–
Physical activity (improvement**)	18 (81.8%) n = 22	22 (88.0%) n = 25	–
After-school social activities (improvement**)	12 (66.6%) n = 18	14 (70.0%) n = 20	–
Social rejection (remission*)	7 (77.9%) n = 9	4 (100%) n = 4	–
Δ Energy (0–100 scale)	19.5 ± 31.3 n = 41	19.0 ± 43.4 n = 42	0.956
Δ Mood level (0–100 scale)	10.0 ± 23.8 n = 40	10.9 ± 25.0 n = 41	0.858
Δ Mental health score (0–100 scale)	8.4 ± 18.0 n = 26	8.3 ± 18.5 n = 24	0.980

Group division is based on EWL% median = 67%. Data in the table are presented as mean ± SD for numerical variables and n (%) for dichotomous variables. T-test was used to evaluate differences for numerical variables and Chi square test for nominal variables. P is missing if one or more cells have an expected count <5. All statistical analyses were two sided with significance of < 0.05. %EWL was calculated from measured height and weight at baseline, and from the post-surgery self-reported weight. Total N is 94, as three participants do not have post-surgery weight self-report. N is listed for a parameter when not all the group was relevant / data was missing. Energy level, mood level and mental health score are 0–100 scales; higher score means a better status.

**From those who answered "yes" at baseline. **from those who answered "no" at baseline. %EWL, Percent excess weight loss; BMI, Body mass index; Δ, (post-surgery score) – (pre-surgery score).*

higher baseline BMI achieved a lower EWL compared to those with lower baseline BMI ($p < 0.001$). In addition, there were no associations detected between %EWL and changes in mental, physical, and social parameters.

Association Between Changes in Mental Health Parameters and Baseline Parameters

Associations between changes in energy and mood levels, mental health score, physical and social factors, and independent variables, such as age, gender, ethnic group, and baseline BMI were examined by a univariate linear regression model.

The change in mental health score was significantly associated to baseline social rejection ($r = 0.514$, $p < 0.001$), meaning that the mental health score of participants, who reported social rejection at baseline, improved more than those who did not report experiencing this condition. This association remained significant after adjusting for age, gender, and baseline BMI. The results were similar after the sensitivity analysis and baseline weights values (reported vs. measured) were highly correlated ($r = 0.82, p < 0.001$).

DISCUSSION

In this short-term nationwide prospective cohort study, we found that MBS in adolescents led to a 30% reduction in BMI and an increase in physical, mental, and social parameters. However, the improvement in those QoL factors was not associated with %EWL.

All physical parameters in our study, including snoring, pain related to weight, physical activity, and energy level, improved postoperatively following MBS, by previous literature's physical subscales (19, 21–23). A study that evaluated the quality of life using SF-36 on adolescents showed that reflux, nausea, and diarrhea after surgery worsened physical status over time, but remained higher than baseline and showed that the highest improvement after surgery was related to physical functioning, physical role functioning and general health (19). Mental health has shown to be similar in adolescents after MBS compared to adolescents with obesity taking part in a non-surgical lifestyle modification program (23). Up to 5 years after surgery, mental health status has remained similar (19) and has improved mainly concerning mental functioning scores (22) or partially concerning two of four mental health domains ($n = 81$) (8). Similarly, our findings showed an improvement in mental health scores, mainly in 2 domains, in addition to all physical and social factors. Similar to previous studies, the rate of weight loss was not associated with social, physical, and mental parameter changes in our study. A previous review of 10 studies ($n = 322$) (24) and studies evaluating adolescents' mental health (25) and psychopathology (26) 2 years following surgery showed that changes in BMI did not necessarily correlate with improvement in quality of life. However, another study reported that a greater percentage of weight loss was associated with better weight and physical quality of life 2 years post-surgery (23). Another large study of 242 adolescents reported 6% lower odds of having musculoskeletal pain and 10% lower odds of having lower extremity pain per 10% reduction of BMI postoperatively (21). In our study, the significance of this association was difficult to determine (including snoring, pain, and physical activity) probably due to the sample size and change in pain is mainly relevant for those who reported the condition at baseline. Since most physical functioning questions in our study are dichotomous and considering previous literature findings, the association between %EWL and physical patterns, especially pain, might exist. Additionally, our study showed an increase in smoking percentage in accordance with an American cohort that showed a rise in smoking habits in teens who underwent bariatric surgery and those who did not (27).

We detected a meaningful correlation between improvement in mental health scores and baseline social rejection. This finding emphasizes the importance of peer relationships in youth (28) and their meaningful contribution to mental health improvement among teenagers undergoing MBS. It also reflects the potential impact of obesity stigma on teens seeking MBS and the opportunity for health status improvement for those who experience stigmatization. The impact of weight-related stigma was mentioned elsewhere (29, 30) and was unrelated to BMI and associated with poorer weight-related quality of life.

There are several limitations in the design of this study. The questionnaire was written for parents and for adolescents, who mainly answer it together and there is no record of whether the responder is a parent or an adolescent. The pre-surgery questionnaire was self-completed by the adolescents with their parents without the mediation of an interviewer, and the post-surgery questionnaire was completed by phone interview. Despite that the questionnaire was not fully validated, the sensitivity analysis for the weight report suggested that the reported weights were reliable. In addition, the information regarding the reason for the additional bariatric surgery of five participants was missing. Although these limitations are meaningful, the main results on physical and mental factors are consistent with literature reports, assuming that the questions add valuable data. In addition, the time from surgery to interview varied with a range of 4–16 months, while a higher %EWL was associated with a longer time from surgery to interview. This finding provides a logical directionality for the weight changes. This short-term represents mainly the weight loss phase, and as shown previously in the AMOS study, a longer follow-up of 2 years may show a slow-down in weight loss (8, 11) and weight regain in some patients. To reduce the effect of time from surgery was inserted into the multivariate regressions model to adjust this possible confounder. Another limitation of the study is the finding that more males refused to be interviewed than females, which could lead to a possible selection bias, although baseline characteristics were mainly similar, and the analyses were adjusted for gender. This higher proportion of females reflect the bariatric population. It is important to point out that these results reflect physical, social factors, and mental health of the ongoing weight loss phase. Further studies should examine this scope in a longer-term after the surgery.

CONCLUSION

The MBS in adolescents, during the weight loss phase, leads to a meaningful decrease in BMI and improvement in physical, mental, and social factors. Although the correlation to EWL% was not found, patients experiencing social rejection may benefit from MBS, especially in short-term mental health. Further studies should investigate mental, physical, and social parameters in a longer-term post-surgery.

ETHICS STATEMENT

The studies involving human participants were reviewed and approved by the Institutional Review Board of the Tel HaShomer Medical Center (SMC-6199-19). Written informed consent to participate in this study was provided by the participants' legal guardian/next of kin.

AUTHOR CONTRIBUTIONS

TM, RV-K, OZ, and YG conceived and carried out the study. TM, AG, YG, and OZ analyzed the data and wrote the manuscript. All authors approved the final version of the manuscript.

REFERENCES

1. Michalsky M, Kramer RE, Fullmer MA, Polfuss M, Porter R, Ward-Begnoche W, et al. Developing criteria for pediatric/adolescent bariatric surgery programs. *Pediatrics.* (2011) 128:S65–70. doi: 10.1542/peds.2011-0480F
2. Geva N, Pinhas-Hamiel O, Reichman B, Derazne E, Vivante A, Barak Y, et al. The association between obesity and secular trend of stature: a nationwide study of 2. 8 million adolescents over five decades. *Int J Obes.* (2019) 43:1932–9. doi: 10.1038/s41366-019-0371-7
3. Bentham J, Di Cesare M, Bilano V, Bixby H, Zhou B, Stevens GA, et al. Worldwide trends in body-mass index, underweight, overweight, and obesity from 1975 to 2016: a pooled analysis of 2416 population-based measurement studies in 128·9 million children, adolescents, and adults. *Lancet.* (2017) 390:2627–42. doi: 10.1016/S0140-6736(17)32129-3
4. Grover SA, Kaouache M, Rempel P, Joseph L, Dawes M, Lau DCW, et al. Years of life lost and healthy life-years lost from diabetes and cardiovascular disease in overweight and obese people: a modelling study. *Lancet Diabetes Endocrinol.* (2015) 3:114–22. doi: 10.1016/S2213-8587(14)70229-3
5. Gepner Y, Shelef I, Schwarzfuchs D, Zelicha H, Tene L, Yaskolka Meir A, et al. Effect of distinct lifestyle interventions on mobilization of fat storage pools. *Circulation.* (2017) 137:1143–57. doi: 10.1161/CIRCULATIONAHA.117.030501
6. Sigal RJ, Alberga AS, Goldfield GS, Prud'homme D, Hadjiyannakis S, Gougeon R, et al. Effects of aerobic training, resistance training, or both on percentage body fat and cardiometabolic risk markers in obese adolescents: the healthy eating aerobic and resistance training in youth randomized clinical trial. *JAMA Pediatr.* (2014) 168:1006–14. doi: 10.1001/jamapediatrics.2014.1392
7. Inge TH, Courcoulas AP, Jenkins TM, Michalsky MP, Mary L. Five-year outcomes of gastric bypass in adolescents as compared with adults. *N Engl J Med.* (2019) 381:e17. doi: 10.1056/NEJMc1908751
8. Olbers T, Gronowitz E, Werling M, Mårlid S, Flodmark CE, Peltonen M, et al. Two-year outcome of laparoscopic Roux-en-Y gastric bypass in adolescents with severe obesity: results from a Swedish Nationwide Study (AMOS). *Int J Obes.* (2012) 36:1388–95. doi: 10.1038/ijo.2012.160
9. Sarno LA, Lipshultz SE, Harmon C, De La Cruz-Munoz NF, Balakrishnan PL. Short- and long-term safety and efficacy of bariatric surgery for

severely obese adolescents: a narrative review. *Pediatr Res.* (2020) 87:202–9. doi: 10.1038/s41390-019-0532-3
10. Qi L, Guo Y, Liu CQ, Huang ZP, Sheng Y, Zou DJ. Effects of bariatric surgery on glycemic and lipid metabolism, surgical complication and quality of life in adolescents with obesity: a systematic review and meta-analysis. *Surg Obes Relat Dis.* (2017) 13:2037–55. doi: 10.1016/j.soard.2017.09.516
11. Olbers T, Beamish AJ, Gronowitz E, Flodmark CE, Dahlgren J, Bruze G, et al. Laparoscopic Roux-en-Y gastric bypass in adolescents with severe obesity (AMOS): a prospective, 5-year, Swedish nationwide study. *Lancet Diabetes Endocrinol.* (2017) 5:174–83. doi: 10.1016/S2213-8587(16)30424-7
12. Inge TH, Jenkins TM, Xanthakos SA, Dixon JB, Daniels SR, Zeller MH, et al. Long-term outcomes of bariatric surgery in adolescents with severe obesity (FABS-5+): a prospective follow-up analysis. *Lancet Diabetes Endocrinol.* (2017) 5:165–73. doi: 10.1016/S2213-8587(16)30315-1
13. Herget S, Rudolph A, Hilbert A, Blüher S. Psychosocial status and mental health in adolescents before and after bariatric surgery. A systematic literature review. *Obes Facts.* (2014) 7:233–45. doi: 10.1159/000365793
14. Franklin EV, Klement J, Mulpuri N, Qureshi FG. Mental health factors associated with progression to adolescent metabolic and bariatric surgery. *Surg Obes Relat Dis.* (2021) 17:1855–63. doi: 10.1016/j.soard.2021.06.014
15. Ministry of Health. *Bariatric Surgery Criteria for Adolescents of the Ministry of Health.* (2017). Available online at: https://www.health.gov.il/hozer/mr27_2017.pdf (accessed April 16, 2022).
16. Ryder JR, Gross AC, Fox CK, Kaizer AM, Rudster K. Factors associated with long-term weight loss maitenance following bariatric surgery in adolescents with severe obesity. *Int J Obes.* (2018) 42:102–7. doi: 10.1038/ijo.2017.193
17. O'Brien PE, Sawyer SM, Laurie C, Brown WA, Skinner S, Veit F, et al. Laparoscopic adjustable gastric banding in severely obese adolescents. *JAMA.* (2010) 303:113–7. doi: 10.1001/jama.2010.81
18. Inge TH, Courcoulas AP, Jenkins TM, Michalsky MP, Helmrath MA, Brandt ML, et al. Weight loss and health status 3 years after bariatric surgery in adolescents. *N Engl J Med.* (2015) 374:113–23. doi: 10.1056/NEJMoa1506699
19. Dewberry L, Khoury J, Schmiege S, Jenkins T, Boles R, Inge T. Gastrointestinal symptoms in relation to quality of life after metabolic surgery in adolescents. *Surg Obes Relat Dis.* (2020) 16:554–61. doi: 10.1016/j.soard.2019.12.025
20. Brethauer SA, Kim J, Chaar M, Papasavas P, Eisenberg D, Rogers A, et al. Standardized outcomes reporting in metabolic and bariatric surgery. *Surg Obes Relat Dis.* (2015) 11:489–506. doi: 10.1016/j.soard.2015.02.003
21. Bout-Tabaku S, Gupta R, Jenkins TM, Ryder JR, Baughcum AE, Jackson RD, et al. Musculoskeletal pain, physical function, and quality of life after bariatric surgery. *Pediatrics.* (2019) 144:e20191399. doi: 10.1542/peds.2019-1399
22. Sysko R, Devlin MJ, Hildebrandt TB, Brewer SK, Zitsman JL, Walsh BT. Psychological outcomes and predictors of initial weight loss outcomes among severely obese adolescents receiving laparoscopic adjustable gastric banding. *J Clin Psychiatry.* (2012) 73:1351–7. doi: 10.4088/JCP.12m07690
23. Reiter-Purtill J, Ley S, Kidwell KM, Mikhail C, Austin H, Chaves E, et al. Change, predictors and correlates of weight- and health-related quality of life in adolescents 2-years following bariatric surgery. *Int J Obes.* (2020) 44:1467–78. doi: 10.1038/s41366-019-0394-0
24. Hillstrom KA, Graves JK. A review of depression and quality of life outcomes in adolescents post bariatric surgery. *J Child Adolesc Psychiatr Nurs.* (2015) 28:50–9. doi: 10.1111/jcap.12104
25. Järvholm K, Karlsson J, Olbers T, Peltonen M, Marcus C, Dahlgren J, et al. Two-year trends in psychological outcomes after gastric bypass in adolescents with severe obesity. *Obesity.* (2015) 23:1966–72. doi: 10.1002/oby.21188
26. Hunsaker SL, Garland BH, Rofey D, Reiter-Purtill J, Mitchell J, Courcoulas A, et al. A multisite 2-year follow up of psychopathology prevalence, predictors, and correlates among adolescents who did or did not undergo weight loss surgery. *J Adolesc Heal.* (2018) 63:142–50. doi: 10.1016/j.jadohealth.2017.12.021
27. Zeller MH, Kidwell KM, Reiter-Purtill J, Jenkins TM, Michalsky MP, Mitchell JE, et al. Cigarette use and adolescent metabolic and bariatric surgery. *Obesity.* (2021) 29:579–86. doi: 10.1002/oby.23084
28. Somerville LH, Somerville L, Dir C, Sci P. Special issue on the teenage brain: Sensitivity to social evaluation NIH public access author manuscript. *Curr Dir Psychol Sci.* (2013) 22:121–7. doi: 10.1177/0963721413476512
29. Sarwer DB, Fabricatore AN, Eisenberg MH, Sywulak LA, Wadden TA. Self-reported stigmatization among candidates for bariatric surgery. *Obesity.* (2008) 16(Suppl. 2):S75–9. doi: 10.1038/oby.2008.450
30. Sarwer DB, Fabricatore AN, Eisenberg MH, Sywulak LA, Wadden TA. Correction to: self-reported stigmatization among candidates for bariatric surgery. *Obesity.* (2010) 18:652. doi: 10.1038/oby.2009.484

21

Altered Glucose Metabolism and Glucose Transporters in Systemic Organs after Bariatric Surgery

Ju Hun Oh[1,2], *Chan Woo Kang*[2], *Eun Kyung Wang*[2], *Jung Ho Nam*[1,2], *Soohyun Lee*[2], *Kyeong Hye Park*[4], *Eun Jig Lee*[2], *Arthur Cho*[3*] *and Cheol Ryong Ku*[2*]

[1] *Brain Korea 21 PLUS Project for Medical Science, Yonsei University, College of Medicine, Seoul, South Korea,* [2] *Department of Internal Medicine, Endocrinology, Institute of Endocrine Research, Yonsei University College of Medicine, Seoul, South Korea,* [3] *Department of Nuclear Medicine, Yonsei University College of Medicine, Seoul, South Korea,* [4] *Division of Endocrinology and Metabolism, Department of Internal Medicine, National Health Insurance Service Ilsan Hospital, Goyang, South Korea*

Correspondence:
Cheol Ryong Ku
cr079@yuhs.ac
Arthur Cho
artycho@yuhs.ac

The Roux-en-Y gastric bypass (RYGB) is highly effective in the remission of obesity and associated diabetes. The mechanisms underlying obesity and type 2 diabetes mellitus remission after RYGB remain unclear. This study aimed to evaluate the changes in continuous dynamic FDG uptake patterns after RYGB and examine the correlation between glucose metabolism and its transporters in variable endocrine organs using ^{18}F-fluoro-2-deoxyglucose positron emission tomography images. Increased glucose metabolism in specific organs, such as the small intestine and various fat tissues, is closely associated with improved glycemic control after RYGB. In Otsuka Long-Evans Tokushima Fatty rats fed with high-fat diets, RYGB operation increases intestine glucose transporter expression and various fat tissues' glucose transporters, which are not affected by insulin. The fasting glucose decrement was significantly associated with RYGB, sustained weight loss, post-RYGB oral glucose tolerance test (OGTT) area under the curve (AUC), glucose transporter, or glycolytic enzymes in the small bowel and various fat tissues. High intestinal glucose metabolism and white adipose tissue-dependent glucose metabolism correlated with metabolic benefit after RYGB. These findings suggest that the newly developed glucose biodistribution accompanied by increased glucose transporters is a mechanism associated with the systemic effect of RYGB.

Keywords: bariatric surgery, diabetes mellitus, glucose metabolism, glucose transporter, obesity

INTRODUCTION

Bariatric surgery provides a long-term solution for patients with severe obesity. Bariatric surgeries are effective for both substantial weight loss and improved glucose metabolism, resulting in the remission of type 2 diabetes mellitus (DM) (1–7), especially in patients with a history of diabetes for less than 5 years (4, 5, 8), and the effects are superior to conventional non-surgical diabetes therapy (4, 5). Among bariatric surgeries, Roux-en Y gastric bypass (RYGB) has the most powerful therapeutic effect on the resolution of DM and obesity. In most patients undergoing RYGB, improved glycemic control occurs initially within days before sustained weight loss, implicating the possibility of a weight-independent mechanism of bariatric surgery (9). In addition, several studies indicated that bariatric surgeries enhance the systemic hormone levels or signaling peptides, including GLP-1, GLP-2, CCK, 5-HT, PYY, and IGFBP-2 (10–16), causing alterations in bile acids and related pathways (17–19). However, to date, most studies mainly focused on the intestine after bariatric surgery (20–24), which cannot fully explain clinical improvement (16, 17, 25). Meanwhile, few studies focus on systemic metabolism change.

^{18}F-fluoro-2-deoxyglucose (FDG) positron emission tomography (PET)/computed tomography (CT) is used in the diagnosis of cancer malignancies by capturing the high FDG uptake of cancer cells. Also, the FDG uptake pattern shows the biodistribution of physiological glucose disposal. We previously reported that after bariatric surgery, intestinal glycolysis and glucose excretion through the intestine were substantially increased, which contributed to the rapid and lasting beneficial effect on glycemic control that is predominantly weight loss independent (21, 24). Moreover, in this study, we observed the change of systemic glucose metabolism not only in robust intestinal FDG uptake but also in various organs. Although systemic increment of glucose metabolism was observed, whether this newly developed glucose metabolism is correlated with metabolic improvement after RYGB remains unclear.

This study aimed to evaluate the changes in continuous dynamic FDG uptake patterns after RYGB and examine the correlation between glucose metabolism and its transporters in variable endocrine organs.

METHODS

Animals

All animal experiments were carried out under an Institutional Animal Care and Use Committee-approved protocol and institutional guidelines for the proper and humane use of animals. Four-week-old male Otsuka Long-Evans Tokushima Fatty (OLETF) rats were provided by the Tokushima Research Institute (Otsuka Pharmaceutical). OLETF rats were fed a high-fat diet (D12492, Research Diets, USA) for 16 weeks and were assigned to two types of surgery (RYGB: n=10 and sham surgery: n=4). The rats were housed at 22 ± 1°C under a 12-12 h light-dark cycle, with *ad libitum* access to water and food. Positron emission tomography (PET) was performed after an overnight fast before the surgery and 2, 4, and 8 weeks post-surgery and was processed as described below.

Roux-En Y Gastric Bypass

RYGB was performed under anesthesia as described in a previous study (21). The length of the entire small intestine was measured from the Treitz ligament. The jejunum was cut 18 cm downstream from the Treitz ligament. In a jejuno-gastric anastomosis, an end-to-side gastrojejunostomy was performed, and the other end of the cut jejunum was anastomosed to the small intestine 20 cm distal to the gastrojejunostomy resulting in a long common limb.

Sham Operation

The Sham group was used as a control. The sham surgery was performed as described in a previous study (21). Briefly, sham surgery consisted of laparotomy, a 1-cm enterotomy on the jejunum, and re-anastomosis without transection of jejunum and stomach.

Micro-Positron Emission Tomography and Radiotracer Counting

μPET imaging was performed according to a previously published paper protocol (21, 24). After an overnight fast, approximately 1 mCi of 18F-fluoro-2-deoxyglucose (FDG) was injected *via* tail vein injection. One hour after FDG injection, a 10 min μPET scan was conducted using Inveon PET (Siemens Medical Solutions, Knoxville, KY, USA). The maximum standardized uptake value (SUVmax), averaged uptake value (SUVmean), SUVmax normalized to rodents' weight (maxSUV), and SUVmean normalized to rodents' weight (meanSUV) were measured with the volume of interest (VOI) drawn on multiple tissues on PET images using the pMOD software (version 4.3, Switzerland). The SUVmax of the VOI was measured using the following formula: (decay-corrected activity [kBq] per tissue volume [mL])/(injected 18F-FDG activity [kBq] per body mass [g]). Immediately after μPET scan, the rats were euthanized in a CO_2 chamber, and tissues were excised, weighted, and subjected to gamma counting (Wallac Wizard 3" 1480 Gamma Counter; PerkinElmer, Akron, OH, USA). FDG tissue biodistribution data were decay-corrected according to the time of FDG injection and normalized to both the tissue weight (g) and radioactivity level. In counting FDG activity in the various tissues, the counts per minute were normalized to the dose of radioactivity injected.

Quantitative real-Time Polymerase Chain Reaction

Total RNA from tissues was isolated using the RNeasy Mini Kit (Qiagen, Germantown, MD, USA) according to the manufacturer's protocol. cDNA was synthesized using the ReverTra Ace (Toyobo, Osaka, Japan). qRT-PCR was performed using the ABI StepOne Plus Real-Time PCR machine (Applied Biosystems, Foster City, CA, USA). The primers used in this study are listed in **Table S1**. The relative transcriptional expression of target genes was evaluated by Eq. $2^{-\Delta Ct}$ (ΔCt = Ct of target gene minus Ct of reference gene of each organ tissue).

Statistical Analysis

All data were expressed as means ± SEM. Statistical analyses were performed using the Prism software version 4.0.0 (GraphPad, La Jolla, CA, USA). Each experiment was performed at least three times. All data were analyzed for statistical significance using the student's t test. In addition, Spearman correlation analyses were performed for comparing post-op OGTT AUC, post-op fasting glucose, post-op weight, post-op FDG radioactivity, post-op glucose transporter and glucose metabolism enzyme mRNA level. Also, in the RYGB column, sham group was set as 0 and RYGB group was set as 1, and correlation analysis was performed to analyze the correlation between operation type and glucose biodistribution.

Statistical significance was set at $p < 0.05$, and differences are indicated using asterisks (*$p < 0.05$, **$p < 0.01$, ***$p < 0.001$).

RESULT

FDG PET/CT Scanning Cases of Changes in Systemic Glucose Biodistribution After Gastrectomy in Human and RYGB in Rodents

Previous our study showed that increased intestinal glycolysis significantly correlated with reduction in HbA1c levels (21, 24). To further characterize the systemic glucose metabolism, we focused not only on small bowel but also the whole-body organs. We performed baseline and post-surgical FDG µPET in RYGB-operated rats. Pre-operated OLETF rats showed that low FDG uptake in the intestine and fat layer (**Figures 1A-C**). After RYGB surgery, it was confirmed that robust FDG uptake was observed in the intestine and subcutaneous layer (**Figures 1D-F**). We gained similar observations in patients who underwent FDG-PET/CT 1 year after Roux-en-Y gastroesophagectomy for gastric cancer. FDG-PET/CT showed elevated FDG uptake not only in small bowel but also in the subcutaneous fat layer (**Figures 1 G-J**), which is similar to observations from RYGB-operated rats (**Figures 1D-F**). Thus, these results indicated that newly developed glucose metabolism occurred in surgical groups after bariatric surgery.

Altered Glucose Distribution After RYGB

When comparing PET images of patients who underwent bariatric surgery with PET images after RYGB with OLETF rats examined in this experiment, it was confirmed that, similar to humans, changes in systemic glucose metabolism and small intestine occurred in OLETF rats after RYGB (**Figure 1**).

To confirm our previous finding of the occurrence of a newly FDG uptake pattern and unexpected glucose retention and secretion in the intestine (21, 24), OLETF rats were fed a 60% high-fat diet for 16 weeks and were subjected to RYGB. All sham-operated rats gained or maintained weight, whereas those that were subjected to RYGB lost weight robustly and sustainably for 8 weeks (**Figure 2A**). We conducted OGTT and measured fasting glucose at 8 weeks post-surgery. As expected, compared to sham operation, RYGB resulted in improved glucose control (**Figures 2B, C**). Absolute body weight (702.1 ± 10.67 vs. 590.23 ± 6.25 g, $p<0.01$), fasting glucose levels (10.439 ± 0.212 vs. 7.849 ± 0.169 mmol/L, $p<0.01$), and body weight changes (%reduction compared with preoperative weight, +4.06% vs. –

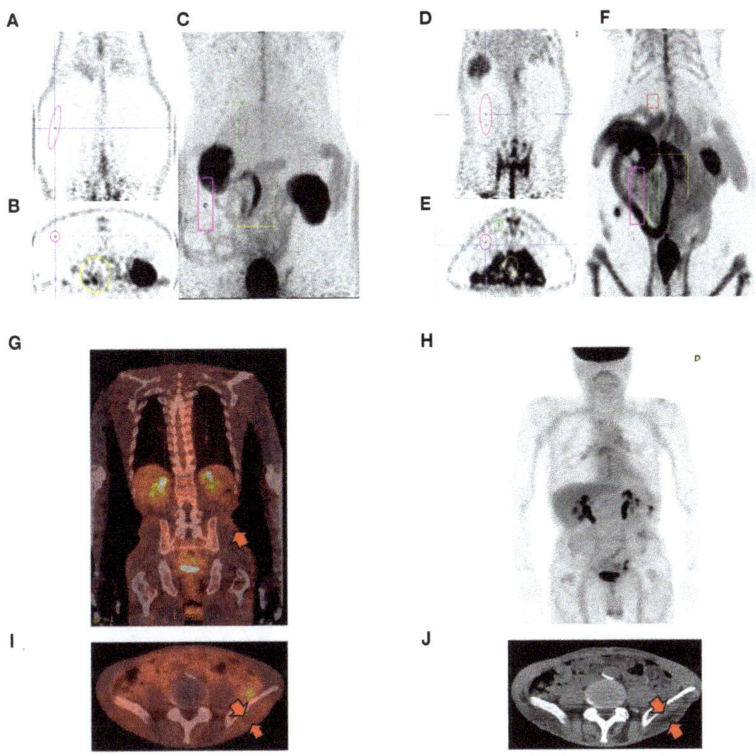

FIGURE 1 | Representative PET cases of altered systemic glucose distribution. **(A-C)** pre-operative OLETFrat showing low FDG uptake in the subcutaneous fat layer. Note low FDG uptake in the bowel in MIP images. **(D-F)** post-operative OLETFrat showing increased FDG uptake in the subcutaneous layer 2 months after surgery. (**A**, **D** coronal PET, **B**, **E** axial PET, **C, F** maximum intensity projection (MIP) **(G-J)** Representative case of changes in biodistribution after gastrectomy. A 49-year-old male patient underwent Roux-en-Y gastroesophagectomy due to stomach cancer. FDG PET/CT was performed one year after surgery for surveillance. Fusion coronal **(G)** and axial fusion **(I)** images shows elevated FDG uptake in the corresponding subcutaneous fat layer (arrows, **J**).

25.2%, respectively), fasting glucose changes (%reduction compared with preoperative glucose, +15.9% vs. -42.6%, respectively) were significantly lower in RYGB-operated rats (**Figures 2A-C**).

To evaluate whether RYGB enhanced systemic glucose uptake, we performed baseline and post-RYGB dynamic FDG μPET. List-mode-time-of-flight data acquisition started immediately after the intravenous FDG administration and lasted for 1 h. Dynamic PET images were reconstructed, and six spherical regions of interest (ROI), each with 20 mm diameter, were placed on the six segments of each organ, avoiding any blood vessels. The averaged FDG activity in all six ROIs was extracted from the dynamic images to form a global Time Activity Curves (TAC) (**Figures 2D-G**). ^{18}FDG distribution was characterized by rapid liver uptake, followed by clearance through the other organ, including the kidney and bladder (**Figures 1B, 2D**). Rapid liver uptake of FDG was increased in RYGB rats but preceded a washout of FDG radioactivity over 60 min, and the difference between the two groups disappeared (**Figure 2D**). This phenomenon also occurred in muscles (**Figure 2F**). In contrast, compared to sham surgery rats, fat-specific radioactivity was still retained at 60 min in RYGB-operated rats (**Figure 2G**). Also, a previous study (21) showed that although FDG did not accumulate in the intestine of sham-surgery rats, the intestine of RYGB-treated rats showed a high accumulation of the FDG (**Figure 2E**).

To evaluate systemic changes in glucose metabolism after RYGB operation, multiple tissues were excised and subjected to

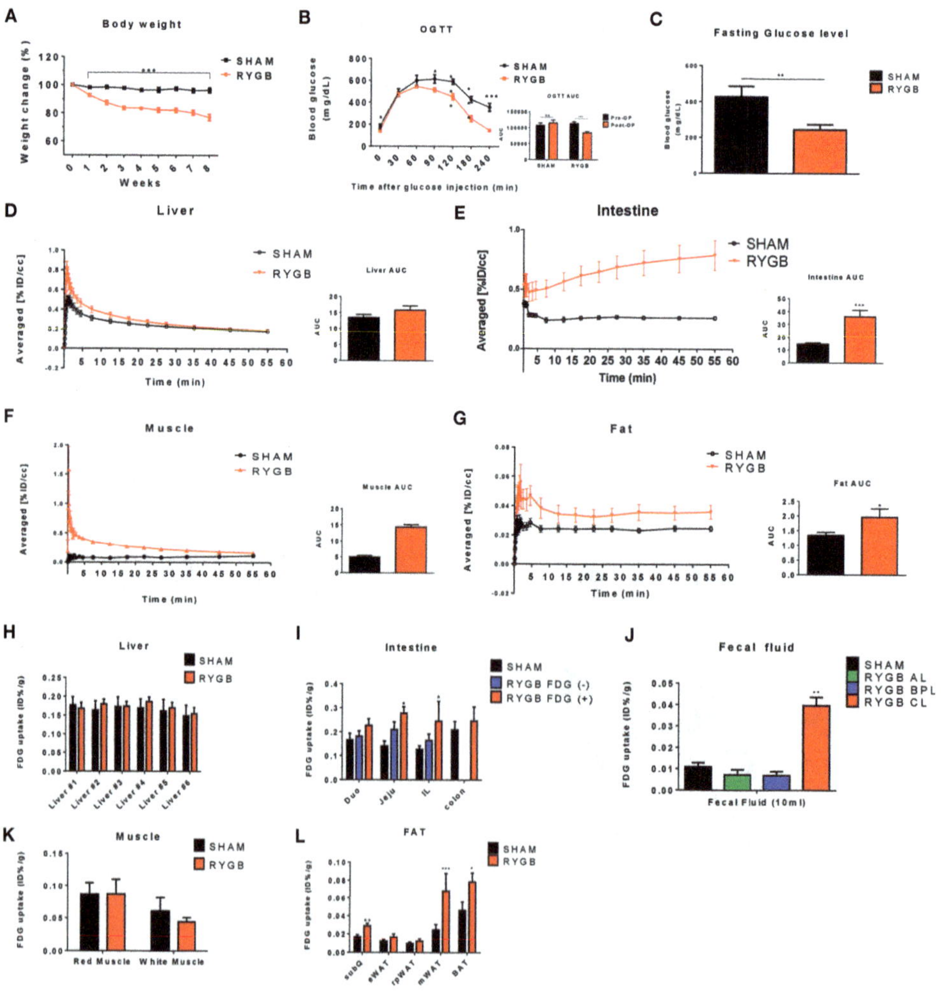

FIGURE 2 | Altered glucose distribution after RYGB. Metabolic parameters in adult male Otsuka Ling-Evans Tokushima fatty (OLETF) rats showing weekly body weight change **(A)** measured every week over 8 weeks, oral glucose tolerance test (OGTT) data **(B)**, and fasting glucose level **(C)** in sham-operated and RYGB-operated rats. Representative 2-Deoxy-2-[18F]-fluoro-D-glucose (FDG)-PET image analysis in OLETF rats. OLETF rats Time Activity Curves (TAC) obtained from 60-min dynamic PET imaging and AUC graph of liver **(D)**, intestine **(E)**, muscle **(F)**, and mesenteric fat **(G)**. Liver #1~#6 denote Right Median Lobe (#1), Right Superior Lobe (#2), Right Median Lobe (#3), Left Median Lobe (#4), Left Lateral Lobe (#5), Caudate Lobe (#6), respectively **(H)**. FDG biodistribution analysis (gamma counting) in RYGB-operated and sham-operated rats in various organs, including the liver **(H)**, intestine **(I)**, intestinal lumen phosphate buffered saline (PBS) washing analysis **(J)**, muscle **(K)**, and various fat tissues **(L)**. Number of mice in all panels **(A–C)** (males; RYGB, 10; sham, 4). All data are presented as mean ± SEM, *p<0.05, **p<0.01, ***p<0.001 vs. sham.

gamma counting of FDG radioactivity immediately after μPET. FDG tissue biodistribution analysis showed that FDG uptake in the intestine and fat was higher in RYGB-operated rats compared with that in sham-operated rats, whereas no difference in the FDG uptake in the liver and muscle was observed (**Figures 2H, K**). Furthermore, excreted FDG into common limbs (CL) of the intestine lumen was increased in RYGB-operated CL compared to that of RYGB-operated alimentary limbs (AL), biliopancreatic limbs (BPL), and sham-operated rats (**Figure 2J**). Taken together, these data indicated that RYGB induced a newly glucose biodistribution through the intestine and fat tissue and that RYGB-induced improved glycemic control might be correlated with this newly glucose biodistribution.

Expression of Glucose Transporters in Various Organs

Because systemic glucose uptake was observed in various tissues after RYGB, we evaluated which glucose uptake and glucose metabolism genes could influence this glucose homeostasis. Glucose transporter (GLUT) and enzyme genes were observed in tissues based on reverse transcription PCR (RT-PCR) analysis (**Figure 3**). In the intestine, we selected regions of each limb of the intestine with higher levels of FDG uptake (FDG +) or basal levels (FDG -) using gamma counting. Corresponding sections of sham-operated rats were used as controls. Consistent with previous study (21), in the AL of the intestine, GLUT1 and Hexokinase (HK) genes showed a sequential increase corresponding to FDG uptake increase patterns (sham jejunum, AL FDG (-), AL FDG (+)) (**Figure 3A**). Other GLUT genes were unchanged or decreased in sham and RYGB. Similarly, in CL, GLUT1 and HK genes were upregulated in FDG (+) AL (**Figure 3B**). However, no genes in the BPL of the intestine were differently regulated in RYGB rats (**Figure 3C**). We removed various fat tissues, including the inguinal white adipose tissue (iWAT), epididymal WAT (eWAT), brown adipose tissue (BAT), retroperitoneal WAT (rpWAT), and mesentery WAT (mWAT), to identify which fats contribute to the improvement of glucose homeostasis of RYGB-operated rats. In all fats, except for eWAT, GLUT1 expression was increased in RYGB-operated rats than that in sham rats (**Figures 3D-H**). In the rpWAT of RYGB-operated rats, GLUT1-5 expressions were significantly increased (**Figure 3D**). In the liver, GLUT1 and GLUT2 showed a significantly increased in RYGB-operation rats (**Figure 3I**). In accordance with above dynamic PET data, no genes were significantly altered in the muscle (**Figures 3J, K**). These results indicated that GLUT and HK are robustly associated with systemic and newly glucose biodistribution by RYGB.

Correlation Analysis Between Glucose Distribution and Glucose Transporters

To document the relationships between glucose uptake and metabolism related genes and system metabolic changes, we conducted correlation analysis. Operation type, post-op OGTT AUC, post-op fating glucose level, post-op weight, FDG radioactivity, and GLUT1-5 genes were used as multiple parameters for Pearson or Spearman correlation analysis. Since FDG uptake was increased in the AL of the intestine, CL of the intestine, and various adipose tissues among various organs, we conducted a correlation analysis with intestine and WAT (**Figure 4**). Correlation analysis showed that: (1) operation type, post-op AUC, post-op fasting glucose, and post-op weight were positively correlated (**Figures 4A-E**); (2) in the AL of intestine, RYGB surgery correlated with FDG radioactivity and GLUT1 expression, whereas post-op AUC, fasting glucose level, and weight were negatively associated with FDG uptake and GLUT1 expression (**Figure 4A**); (3) in the CL of intestine, RYGB surgery correlated with CL FDG radioactivity and CL GLUT1 expression, whereas post-op AUC, fasting glucose level, and weight were negatively associated with CL FDG uptake, CL GLUT1 expression, and SGLT1 expression (**Figure 4B**); (4) in iWAT, RYGB surgery correlated with iWAT FDG radioactivity, iWAT GLUT1 expression, and GLUT5 expression, whereas post-op AUC, fasting glucose level, and weight were negatively associated with iWAT FDG uptake and GLUT1 expression, while post-FDG uptake was positively associated with GLUT2, GLUT3, and SGLT1 expression (**Figure 4C**); (5) in mWAT, post-op AUC negatively associated with mWAT GLUT1, GLUT2, and SLGT2 expression, whereas post-op fasting glucose level and weight were negatively associated with mWAT FDG uptake (**Figure 4D**); (6) in rpWAT, RYGB surgery correlated with rpWAT FDG radioactivity, rpWAT GLUT1 expression, and GLUT5 expression (**Figure 4E**), whereas post-op AUC, fasting glucose level, and weight were negatively associated with iWAT FDG uptake and GLUT1 expression. These data are consistent with systemic glucose metabolism changes in RYGB-operated patients and rats. These results indicated that systemic glucose metabolism changes are robustly associated with upregulation of GLUT1, and related transporter genes underwent RYGB.

DISCUSSION

The biological mechanism of improved hyperglycemia and weight loss by bariatric remains unelucidated. Previous studies focused on the anatomical changes of the intestine or gut oriented hormones, such as glucagon-like peptide 1. Here, we demonstrate that the potential image-based semi-quantitative FDG activity of systemic glycolytic activity correlated with improved glycemic control and robust weight loss brought by RYGB in a rodent model. We analyzed the correlation between increased systemic glucose metabolism and RYGB-induced improvement in metabolic changes. We have shown that (1) the increased glucose metabolism not only in AL and CL of the intestine but also in mWAT, rpWAT, and iWAT; (2) the increased expression of glucose transporter subtypes in organs showed improved glucose metabolism after RYGB; and (3) the correlation between increased organ-specific glucose metabolism and improved hyperglycemia in rats after RYGB.

Insulin-induced glucose disposal occurs in muscle, fat, and various organs in normal physiology (26). After bariatric surgery

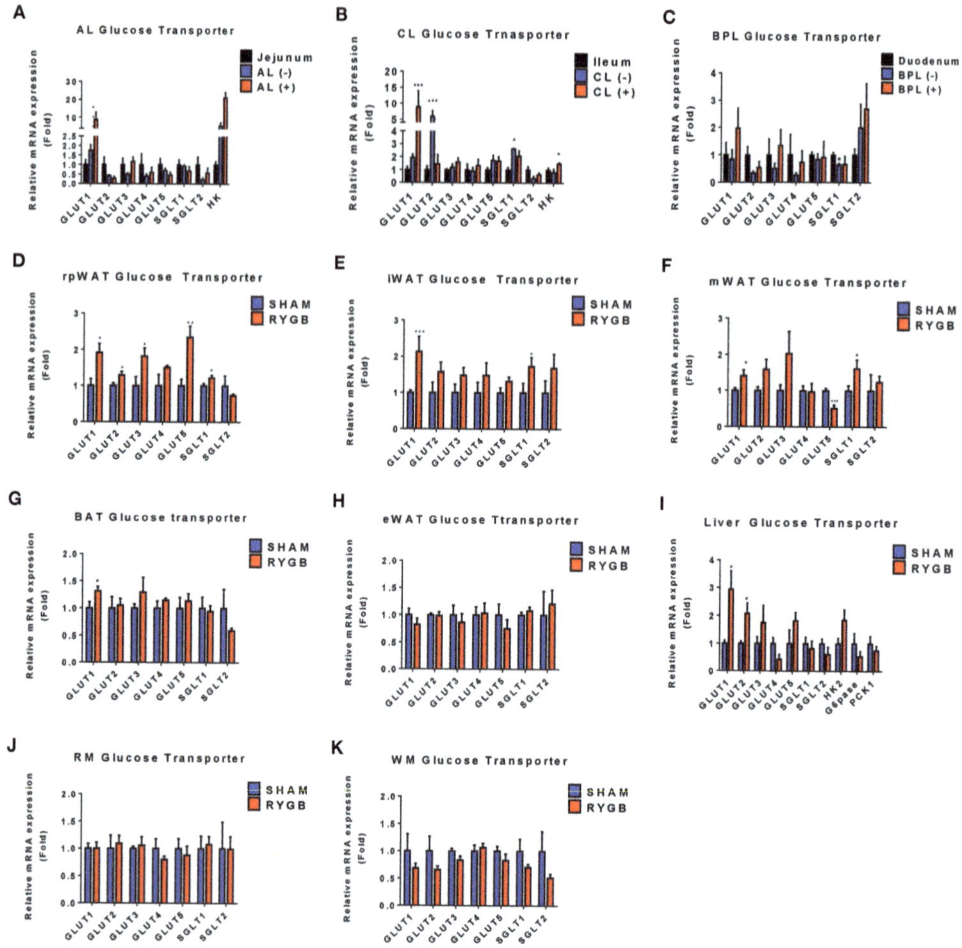

FIGURE 3 | Expression of Glucose transporters in various organs. Subtypes of glucose transporters are altered in RYGB-operated OLETF rats. The expression of glucose transporter subtype in alimentary limbs (AL), common limb (CL), and biliopancreatic limb (BPL) of RYGB-operated rats and the corresponding limbs of sham-operated rats **(A-C)**. The fold change was calculated based on the corresponding sham-operated bowel (jejunum for the CL, duodenum for the biliopancreatic limbs (BPL), and ileum for the CL). (–) or (+) denotes FDG negativity or positivity of individual rats, respectively. The expression of glucose transporter subtype in retroperitoneal white adipose tissue (rpWAT) **(D)**, inguinal WAT (iWAT) **(E)**, mesentery WAT (mWAT) **(F)**, brown adipose tissue (BAT) **(G)**, epididymal WAT (eWAT) **(H)**, liver **(I)**, red muscle (RM) **(J)**, and white muscle (WM) **(K)**. The fold change was calculated based on the corresponding sham-operated rats' organs. All data are presented as mean ± SEM, *$p<0.05$, **$p<0.01$, ***$p<0.001$ vs. sham.

in obese patients with T2D, micro-PET analysis revealed a possible increase in systemic glucose uptake (**Figures 1, 2**). FDG uptake was not changed in the muscle, a representative glucose disposed organ, but newly increased in the intestine and various fat tissues. According to the TAC graph, FDG was trapped for over 60 min in both the intestine and fat, unlike in muscles and liver (**Figure 2**). Some studies showed that bariatric surgery leads to a significant improvement in hepatic insulin sensitivity, which is accompanied by increased hepatic glucose uptake and reduced endogenous glucose production in human T2D or non-T2D patients (27). However, our results showed that hepatic glucose uptake was comparable. Several studies demonstrated that FDG uptake in the liver was lower or comparable in RYGB-operated groups (20, 21), which may be caused by a glucose analogue in which FDG cannot be metabolized. It is postulated that Glucose-6-phophatase (G6pase) is expressed in liver and this enzyme may affect the retention of FDG in liver. Also, in the muscle, an earlier FDG uptake surge was observed but preceded a slow washout of FDG radioactivity over the remaining 60 min and showed that insulin-induced glucose disposal does not change. Previous studies showed that bariatric surgery induced improvement in glycemic control independently with insulin secretion or sensitivity (20, 21, 28, 29). Unlike in liver or muscle, FDG retention is maintained in various fat tissues, including mWAT, iWAT, and rpWAT, which are the organ where glucose is uptaken by insulin-induced GLUT4 activity (30). However, our data showed that although GLUT4 expression is comparable, the expression of GLUT1 was increased. This result indicated that the high expression of GLUT1, whose activity is independent of insulin, contributes to increased glucose uptake after RYGB surgery. Similar to reprogrammed intestinal glucose

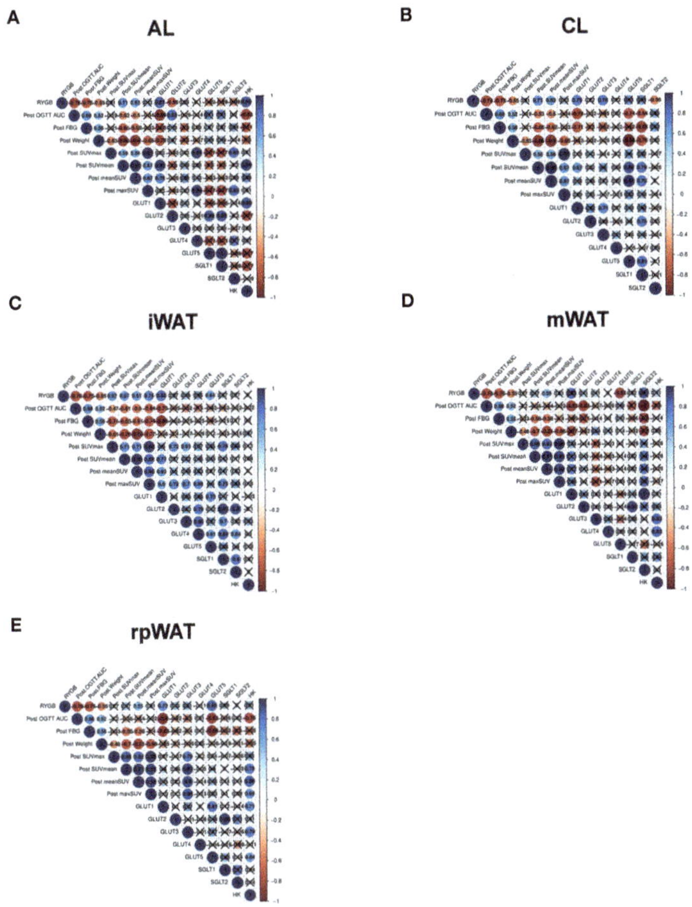

FIGURE 4 | Correlation analysis between glucose distribution and glucose transporters Spearman's correlation among post-operated OGTT AUC, post-operated weight, postoperated fasting glucose, operation type, the maximum standardized FDG uptake value (SUVmax), the averaged standardized FDG value, and each normalized to weight (maxSUV, meanSUV), and the expression levels of glucose transporters in **(A)** AL, **(B)** CL, **(C)** iWAT, **(D)** mWAT, and **(E)** rpWAT, representing significant FDG uptake in TAC images in RYGB-operated OLETF rats. Nonsignificant correlations (p-value > 0.05) are indicated by crosses.

metabolism after RYGB is mediated by GLUT1, GLUT1 contributes to glucose absorption in various fat tissues. Accordingly, systemic reprogrammed glucose absorption patterns were mediated independently of insulin-mediated effects.

Our results indicate that compared with sham-operated rats, GLUT1 is upregulated in organs with increased FDG uptake of RYGB-operated animals. GLUT1 and glycolysis genes are increased in the intestine after bariatric surgery (20, 21, 23, 28, 31). Consistent with previous studies (23, 32), intestinal glucose transporter GLUT2 and SGLT1 expression were downregulated in the AL and CL of RYGB-operated rats. In organs with a high FDG uptake, GLUT1 expression was increased. mWAT, iWAT, and rpWAT showed the increased expression of GLUT1 after RYGB surgery. Conversely, GLUT1 expression was comparable in the organ with no change in FDG uptake after RYGB. It can be inferred that the insulin-independent higher FDG uptake in fat is due to the increase in GLUT1. GLUT1 is rarely expressed in mature intestine and white adipose tissue (33). Intestinal hypertrophy and increasing villus length are caused by intestinal glucose uptake through GLUT1 after RYGB (20, 21, 34, 35). In our previous study, Amphiregulin (AREG)/Epidermal growth factor receptor (EGFR) signaling is upregulated in RYGB rats and human intestine, and AREG increases glucose uptake and secretion through EGFR-mediated GLUT1 expression and trafficking (21). Also, oxygen is insufficient due to numerous build-up processes occurring in the small intestine, which leads to the overexpression of GLUT1 by HIF1-a (36). We speculate that soluble factors such as AREG not only affect the intestine, but also affect the various organs through circulating through the blood. AREG may regulate GLUT1 expression in various fats throughout the body. In fact, it was reported that overexpression of AREG in white adipose tissue of db/db mice reduced mouse weight and fat weight and beta-oxidation signaling and TCA cycle would be increased in white adipose tissue (37). Furthermore, the T Helper cell modulates intestinal stem cell renewal and intestinal morphology (38). Previous studies showed that AREG, which originated from T helper 2 cells, results in the upregulation of the GLUT1 expression (21). Therefore, the intestinal derived signal may affect the glucose disposal of fat tissues independent of insulin action or intestine-derived T helper 2 cells systemically similar to other immune cells (39).

The current study has several limitations. First, we only used ^{18}F-fluoro-2-deoxyglucose (FDG). However, glucose is trapped in the cell in the form of glucose-6-phosphate (G6P). G6P is a late limiting step in glucose metabolism. FDG in the intestine and fat tissues was retained for over 60 min; therefore, if glucose had been used instead of FDG, it would have been metabolized. Also, previous study showed that ^{14}C-Glucose disposal and excretion was similar to those of FDG. Second, we only showed correlation and not causation through experiments. However, to our knowledge, this study is the first to demonstrate the quantitative measurements of post-RYGB FDG uptake in various organs and show dynamic glucose retention. This study supports the RYGB-induced new systemic glucose distribution. Further studies are needed to identify the signaling pathways inducing GLUT1-mediated systemic glucose disposal, which may be new drug targets to mimic the RYGB-induced improvement in metabolic changes.

In conclusion, the induction of GLUT1 levels by RYGB is robust and is correlated with improved metabolic changes. This novel finding may support the unknown mechanism effect of RYGB.

ETHICS STATEMENT

The studies involving human participants were reviewed and approved by Approved by Severance Hospital's institutional review board. The ethics committee waived the requirement of written informed consent for participation. The animal study was reviewed and approved by Institutional Animal Care and Use Committee (IACUC) at the Yonsei University Health System. Written informed consent was not obtained from the individual(s) for the publication of any potentially identifiable images or data included in this article.

AUTHOR CONTRIBUTIONS

Conceptualization: CKu and AC. Data curation and formal analysis: CKu, JO, KP, and AC. Funding acquisition: CKu. Investigation and methodology: CKu, JO, CKa, EW, JN, SL, and AC. Supervision and validation: CKu, JO and AC. Visualization: CKu, JO, and AC. Writing original draft: CKu, JO, and AC. Writing review and editing: CKu, JO, EL, KP, and AC. All authors contributed to the article and approved the submitted version.

ACKNOWLEDGMENTS

We would like to thank Byung Gon Kim and Jung-Hyun Ji, members of the laboratory animal research Centre of ABMRC at Yonsei University College of Medicine, for their technical support with animal experiments.

REFERENCES

1. Rubino F. Bariatric Surgery: Effects on Glucose Homeostasis. *Curr Opin Clin Nutr Metab Care* (2006) 9(4):497–507. doi: 10.1097/01.mco.0000232914.14978.c5
2. Buchwald H, Avidor Y, Braunwald E, Jensen MD, Pories W, Fahrbach K, et al. Bariatric Surgery: A Systematic Review and Meta-Analysis. *Jama* (2004) 292 (14):1724–37. doi: 10.1001/jama.292.14.1724
3. Mingrone G, Panunzi S, De Gaetano A, Guidone C, Iaconelli A, Leccesi L, et al. Bariatric Surgery Versus Conventional Medical Therapy for Type 2 Diabetes. *N Engl J Med* (2012) 366(17):1577–85. doi: 10.1056/NEJMoa1200111
4. Schauer PR, Bhatt DL, Kirwan JP, Wolski K, Aminian A, Brethauer SA, et al. Bariatric Surgery Versus Intensive Medical Therapy for Diabetes - 5-Year Outcomes. *N Engl J Med* (2017) 376(7):641–51. doi: 10.1056/NEJMoa1600869
5. Mingrone G, Panunzi S, De Gaetano A, Guidone C, Iaconelli A, Nanni G, et al. Bariatric-Metabolic Surgery Versus Conventional Medical Treatment in Obese Patients With Type 2 Diabetes: 5 Year Follow-Up of an Open-Label, Single-Centre, Randomised Controlled Trial. *Lancet* (2015) 386(9997):964–73. doi: 10.1016/S0140-6736(15)00075-6
6. Chambers AP, Jessen L, Ryan KK, Sisley S, Wilson-Pérez HE, Stefater MA, et al. Weight-Independent Changes in Blood Glucose Homeostasis After Gastric Bypass or Vertical Sleeve Gastrectomy in Rats. *Gastroenterology* (2011) 141(3):950–8. doi: 10.1053/j.gastro.2011.05.050
7. Lingvay I, Guth E, Islam A, Livingston E. Rapid Improvement in Diabetes After Gastric Bypass Surgery: Is it the Diet or Surgery? *Diabetes Care* (2013) 36(9):2741–7. doi: 10.2337/dc12-2316
8. Abarca-Gómez L., Abdeen Z.A., Hamid Z.A.., Abu-Rmeileh N.M., Acosta-Cazares B., Acuin C., et al. Worldwide Trends in Body-Mass Index, Underweight, Overweight, and Obesity From 1975 to 2016: A Pooled Analysis of 2416 Population-Based Measurement Studies in 128·9 Million Children, Adolescents, and Adults. *Lancet* (2017) 390(10113):2627–42. doi: 10.1016/S0140-6736(17)32129-3
9. Jørgensen NB, Jacobsen SH, Dirksen C, Bojsen-Møller KN, Naver L, Hvolris L, et al. Acute and Long-Term Effects of Roux-En-Y Gastric Bypass on Glucose Metabolism in Subjects With Type 2 Diabetes and Normal Glucose Tolerance. *Am J Physiol Endocrinol Metab* (2012) 303(1):E122–31. doi: 10.1152/ajpendo.00073.2012
10. Stefater MA, Wilson-Pérez HE, Chambers AP, Sandoval DA, Seeley RJ. All Bariatric Surgeries Are Not Created Equal: Insights From Mechanistic Comparisons. *Endocr Rev* (2012) 33(4):595–622. doi: 10.1210/er.2011-1044
11. Laferrère B. Do We Really Know Why Diabetes Remits After Gastric Bypass Surgery? *Endocrine* (2011) 40(2):162–7. doi: 10.1007/s12020-011-9514-x
12. Falkén Y, Hellström PM, Holst JJ, Näslund E. Changes in Glucose Homeostasis After Roux-En-Y Gastric Bypass Surgery for Obesity at Day Three, Two Months, and One Year After Surgery: Role of Gut Peptides. *J Clin Endocrinol Metab* (2011) 96(7):2227–35. doi: 10.1210/jc.2010-2876

13. Mumphrey MB, Patterson LM, Zheng H, Berthoud HR. Roux-En-Y Gastric Bypass Surgery Increases Number But Not Density of CCK-, GLP-1-, 5-HT-, and Neurotensin-Expressing Enteroendocrine Cells in Rats. *Neurogastroenterol Motil* (2013) 25(1):e70–9. doi: 10.1111/nmo.12034
14. Holst JJ. Enteroendocrine Secretion of Gut Hormones in Diabetes, Obesity and After Bariatric Surgery. *Curr Opin Pharmacol* (2013) 13(6):983–8. doi: 10.1016/j.coph.2013.09.014
15. Ramracheya RD, McCulloch LJ, Clark A, Wiggins D, Johannessen H, Olsen MK, et al. PYY-Dependent Restoration of Impaired Insulin and Glucagon Secretion in Type 2 Diabetes Following Roux-En-Y Gastric Bypass Surgery. *Cell Rep* (2016) 15(5):944–50. doi: 10.1016/j.celrep.2016.03.091
16. Faramia J, Hao Z, Mumphrey MB, Townsend RL, Miard S, Carreau A-M, et al. IGFBP-2 Partly Mediates the Early Metabolic Improvements Caused by Bariatric Surgery. *Cell Rep Med* (2021) 2(4):100248. doi: 10.1016/j.xcrm.2021.100248
17. Ryan KK, Tremaroli V, Clemmensen C, Kovatcheva-Datchary P, Myronovych A, Karns R, et al. FXR Is a Molecular Target for the Effects of Vertical Sleeve Gastrectomy. *Nature* (2014) 509(7499):183–8. doi: 10.1038/nature13135
18. Flynn CR, Albaugh VL, Cai S, Cheung-Flynn J, Williams PE, Brucker RM, et al. Bile Diversion to the Distal Small Intestine has Comparable Metabolic Benefits to Bariatric Surgery. *Nat Commun* (2015) 6(1):7715. doi: 10.1038/ncomms8715
19. DePaoli AM, Zhou M, Kaplan DD, Hunt SC, Adams TD, Learned RM, et al. FGF19 Analog as a Surgical Factor Mimetic That Contributes to Metabolic Effects Beyond Glucose Homeostasis. *Diabetes* (2019) 68(6):1315–28. doi: 10.2337/db18-1305
20. Saeidi N, Meoli L, Nestoridi E, Gupta NK, Kvas S, Kucharczyk J, et al. Reprogramming of Intestinal Glucose Metabolism and Glycemic Control in Rats After Gastric Bypass. *Science* (2013) 341(6144):406–10. doi: 10.1126/science.1235103
21. Kwon IG, Kang CW, Park JP, Oh JH, Wang EK, Kim TY, et al. Serum Glucose Excretion After Roux-En-Y Gastric Bypass: A Potential Target for Diabetes Treatment. *Gut* (2021) 70(10):1847–56. doi: 10.1136/gutjnl-2020-321402
22. Ribeiro-Parenti L, Jarry A-C, Cavin J-B, Willemetz A, Le Beyec J, Sannier A, et al. Bariatric Surgery Induces a New Gastric Mucosa Phenotype With Increased Functional Glucagon-Like Peptide-1 Expressing Cells. *Nat Commun* (2021) 12(1):110. doi: 10.1038/s41467-020-20301-1
23. Cavin JB, Couvelard A, Lebtahi R, Ducroc R, Arapis K, Voitellier E, et al. Differences in Alimentary Glucose Absorption and Intestinal Disposal of Blood Glucose After Roux-En-Y Gastric Bypass vs Sleeve Gastrectomy. *Gastroenterology* (2016) 150(2):454–64.e9. doi: 10.1053/j.gastro.2015.10.009
24. Ku CR, Lee N, Hong JW, Kwon IG, Hyung WJ, Noh SH, et al. Intestinal Glycolysis Visualized by FDG PET/CT Correlates With Glucose Decrement After Gastrectomy. *Diabetes* (2017) 66(2):385–91. doi: 10.2337/db16-1000
25. Aron-Wisnewsky J, Prifti E, Belda E, Ichou F, Kayser BD, Dao MC, et al. Major Microbiota Dysbiosis in Severe Obesity: Fate After Bariatric Surgery. *Gut* (2019) 68(1):70–82. doi: 10.1136/gutjnl-2018-316103
26. Dimitriadis G, Mitrou P, Lambadiari V, Maratou E, Raptis SA. Insulin Effects in Muscle and Adipose Tissue. *Diabetes Res Clin Pract* (2011) 93:S52–S9. doi: 10.1016/S0168-8227(11)70014-6
27. Immonen H, Hannukainen JC, Iozzo P, Soinio M, Salminen P, Saunavaara V, et al. Effect of Bariatric Surgery on Liver Glucose Metabolism in Morbidly Obese Diabetic and Non-Diabetic Patients. *J Hepatol* (2014) 60(2):377–83. doi: 10.1016/j.jhep.2013.09.012
28. Kim M, Son YG, Kang YN, Ha TK, Ha E. Changes in Glucose Transporters, Gluconeogenesis, and Circadian Clock After Duodenal-Jejunal Bypass Surgery. *Obes Surg* (2015) 25(4):635–41. doi: 10.1007/s11695-014-1434-4
29. Isbell JM, Tamboli RA, Hansen EN, Saliba J, Dunn JP, Phillips SE, et al. The Importance of Caloric Restriction in the Early Improvements in Insulin Sensitivity After Roux-En-Y Gastric Bypass Surgery. *Diabetes Care* (2010) 33(7):1438–42. doi: 10.2337/dc09-2107
30. Leto D, Saltiel AR. Regulation of Glucose Transport by Insulin: Traffic Control of GLUT4. *Nat Rev Mol Cell Biol* (2012) 13(6):383–96. doi: 10.1038/nrm3351
31. Deal RA, Tang Y, Fletcher R, Torquati A, Omotosho P. Understanding Intestinal Glucose Transporter Expression in Obese Compared to Non-Obese Subjects. *Surg Endosc* (2018) 32(4):1755–61. doi: 10.1007/s00464-017-5858-5
32. Stearns AT, Balakrishnan A, Tavakkolizadeh A. Impact of Roux-En-Y Gastric Bypass Surgery on Rat Intestinal Glucose Transport. *Am J Physiol Gastrointest Liver Physiol* (2009) 297(5):G950–7. doi: 10.1152/ajpgi.00253.2009
33. Thorens B. Glucose Transporters in the Regulation of Intestinal, Renal, and Liver Glucose Fluxes. *Am J Physiol* (1996) 270(4 Pt 1):G541–53. doi: 10.1152/ajpgi.1996.270.4.G541
34. Bueter M, Löwenstein C, Olbers T, Wang M, Cluny NL, Bloom SR, et al. Gastric Bypass Increases Energy Expenditure in Rats. *Gastroenterology* (2010) 138(5):1845–53. doi: 10.1053/j.gastro.2009.11.012
35. Hansen CF, Bueter M, Theis N, Lutz T, Paulsen S, Dalbøge LS, et al. Hypertrophy Dependent Doubling of L-Cells in Roux-En-Y Gastric Bypass Operated Rats. *PloS One* (2013) 8(6):e65696. doi: 10.1371/journal.pone.0065696
36. Chen C, Pore N, Behrooz A, Ismail-Beigi F, Maity A. Regulation of Glut1 mRNA by Hypoxia-Inducible Factor-1. Interaction Between H-Ras and Hypoxia. *J Biol Chem* (2001) 276(12):9519–25. doi: 10.1074/jbc.M010144200
37. Yang B, Kumoto T, Arima T, Nakamura M, Sanada Y, Kumrungsee T, et al. Transgenic Mice Specifically Expressing Amphiregulin in White Adipose Tissue Showed Less Adipose Tissue Mass. *Genes Cells* (2018) 23(3):136–45. doi: 10.1111/gtc.12558
38. Biton M, Haber AL, Rogel N, Burgin G, Beyaz S, Schnell A, et al. T Helper Cell Cytokines Modulate Intestinal Stem Cell Renewal and Differentiation. *Cell* (2018) 175(5):1307–20.e22. doi: 10.1016/j.cell.2018.10.008
39. Rojas OL, Pröbstel AK, Porfilio EA, Wang AA, Charabati M, Sun T, et al. Recirculating Intestinal IgA-Producing Cells Regulate Neuroinflammation *via* IL-10. *Cell* (2019) 176(3):610–24.e18. doi: 10.1016/j.cell.2018.11.035

22

Metabolite Changes after Metabolic Surgery – Associations to Parameters Reflecting Glucose Homeostasis and Lipid Levels

Sofie Ahlin[1,2], Consuelo Cefalo[2], Isabel Bondia-Pons[3], Kajetan Trošt[3], Esmeralda Capristo[2], Luca Marini[2], Montserrat Romero[4,5,6], Antonio Zorzano[4,5,6], Amalia Gastaldelli[7], Geltrude Mingrone[2,8†] and John J. Nolan[3,9†]*

[1] Department of Molecular and Clinical Medicine, Institute of Medicine, The Sahlgrenska Academy at the University of Gothenburg, Gothenburg, Sweden, [2] Department of Medical and Surgery Sciences, Fondazione Policlinico Universitario A. Gemelli Istituto di Ricovero e Cura a Carattere Scientifico (IRCCS), Rome, Italy, [3] Research Department, Steno Diabetes Center, Gentofte, Denmark, [4] Departament de Bioquímica i Biomedicina Molecular, Facultat de Biologia, Universitat de Barcelona, Barcelona, Spain, [5] Institute for Research in Biomedicine (IRB Barcelona), Barcelona Institute of Science and Technology (BIST), Barcelona, Spain, [6] CIBERDEM, Centro de Investigación Biomédica en Red (CIBER) de Diabetes y Enfermedades Metabólicas Asociadas, Barcelona, Instituto de Salud Carlos III, Barcelona, Spain, [7] Cardiometabolic Risk Laboratory, Institute of Clinical Physiology, Consiglio Nazionale delle Ricerche (CNR), Pisa, Italy, [8] Department of Diabetes & Nutritional Sciences, Faculty of Life Sciences & Medicine, King's College, London, United Kingdom, [9] Department of Clinical Medicine, Trinity College, Dublin, Ireland

Correspondence:
Sofie Ahlin
sofie.ahlin@gu.se

[†]These authors share senior authorship

Aims: To test the hypothesis that adipose tissue gene expression patterns would be affected by metabolic surgery and we aimed to identify genes and metabolic pathways as well as metabolites correlating with metabolic changes following metabolic surgery.

Materials and Methods: This observational study was conducted at the Obesity Unit at the Catholic University Hospital of the Sacred Heart in Rome, Italy. Fifteen patients, of which six patients underwent Roux-en-Y gastric bypass and nine patients underwent biliopancreatic diversion, were included. The participants underwent an oral glucose tolerance test and a hyperinsulinemic euglycemic clamp. Small polar metabolites were analyzed with a two-dimensional gas chromatography coupled to time-of-flight mass spectrometry (GC×GC-TOFMS). Gene expression analysis of genes related to metabolism of amino acids and fatty acids were analyzed in subcutaneous adipose tissue. All procedures were performed at study start and at follow-up (after 185.3 ± 72.9 days).

Results: Twelve metabolites were significantly changed after metabolic surgery. Six metabolites were identified as 3-indoleacetic acid, 2-hydroxybutyric acid, valine, glutamic acid, 4-hydroxybenzeneacetic acid and alpha-tocopherol. The branched chain amino acids displayed a significant decrease together with a decrease in BCAT1 adipose tissue mRNA levels. Changes in the identified metabolites were associated to changes in lipid, insulin and glucose levels.

Conclusions: Our study has identified metabolites and metabolic pathways that are altered by metabolic surgery and may be used as biomarkers for metabolic improvement.

Keywords: metabolic surgery, metabolomics, branched chain amino acids (BCAA), adipose tissue, metabolic pathway

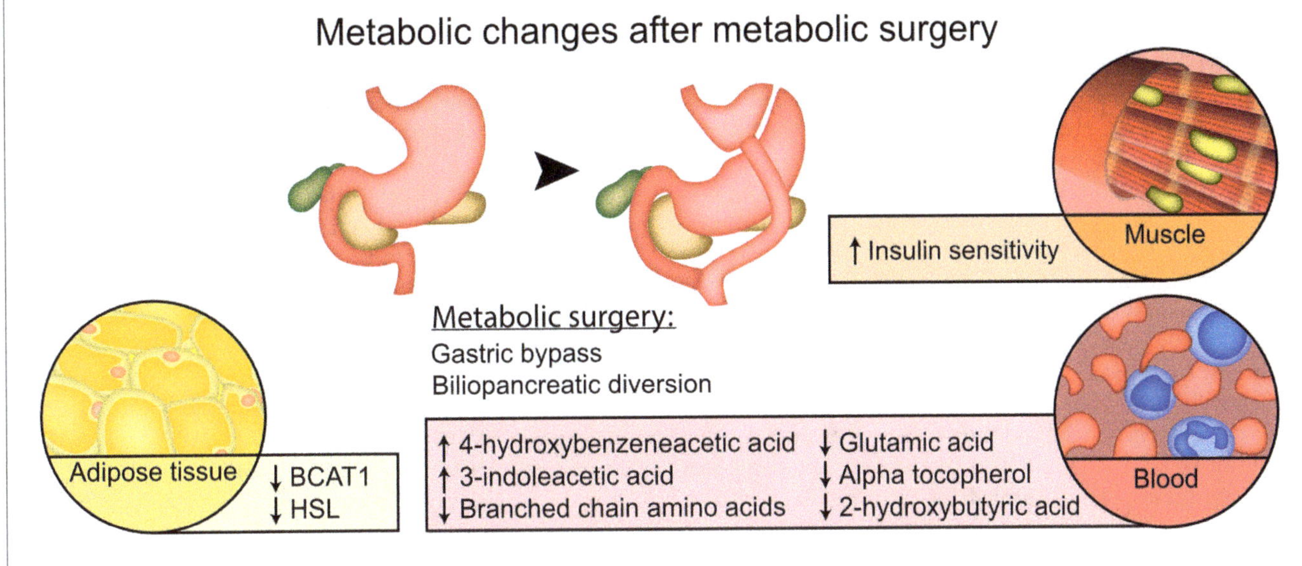

GRAPHICAL ABSTRACT |

INTRODUCTION

Treatment with metabolic surgery usually results in a long-term weigh loss (1) but is also associated with remission of type 2 diabetes, improvement of insulin resistance and prevention of cardiovascular disease (2–4). For some metabolic surgery procedures, where a part of the small intestine is bypassed, the improvement in glucose metabolism exceeds what is predicted and these benefits occur before the patients have started to lose weight (5, 6). This raises the possibility that there are additional mediators of the metabolic improvement after metabolic surgery other than weight loss.

Metabolites are the product of the activity of the genome, transcriptome and proteome and are thought to be the closest link to an organism's phenotype (7, 8). Hence, metabolomics analysis is considered a very suitable method to investigate complex conditions such as type 2 diabetes and insulin resistance (9). However, how metabolites are regulated by different metabolic surgery procedures and how they are related to the metabolic improvement is less well understood.

Using an integrative approach to analyze adipose tissue gene expression in parallel with metabolite profiling, we aimed to identify metabolic pathways and metabolites related to the metabolic improvement after metabolic surgery.

MATERIALS AND METHODS

Ethics Statement

The ethics committee at the Catholic University Hospital of the Sacred Heart, Rome, Italy, approved all study protocols. Participants gave informed consent to participate.

Study Participants

Recruitment of participants was performed at the Catholic University Hospital of the Sacred Heart in Rome, Italy. In total 15 patients were recruited of which six patients underwent Roux-en-Y gastric bypass (RYGBP) and nine patients underwent biliopancreatic diversion (BPD) as treatment for obesity. The surgeon decided the surgical procedure for each participant. Usually BPD is used for patients with higher BMI (>45 kg/m^2) (10). Inclusion criteria were a body mass index of 40 kg/m^2 or more, no previous diagnosis of type 2 diabetes with a HbA1c ≤ 7% and willingness to participate in the study. Major endocrine disease, malignancies and liver cirrhosis were established as exclusion criteria. Follow-up visits were performed after 185.3 ± 72.9 days.

Blood samples from participants in a fasting state were collected together with anthropometry both at study start and at follow-up. All participants also underwent an oral glucose tolerance test. Blood chemistry was performed at the central laboratory of the Catholic University Hospital of the Sacred Heart in Rome, Italy.

Hyperinsulinemic-Euglycemic Clamp

Peripheral insulin sensitivity was assessed by a hyperinsulinemic-euglycemic clamp in participants that had fasted overnight (11), which has previously been described in detail (12). At the start of the test, two venous accesses were established, one in the antecubital vein for infusions and another was inserted into a hand vein. The hand was heated in a heated air box set at 60°C to obtain arterialized blood samples. A primed constant insulin infusion at the rate of 6 pmol/min/kg was given to the participant together with a variable glucose infusion that was adjusted every 5 minutes on the basis on blood glucose measurements so that blood glucose concentration was stable at the fasting value for 2 h. The last 40 minutes of the test was used to calculate whole body glucose uptake (M, mg/kg/min). All samples were stored at – 80°C before further analysis.

Other Measurements of Insulin Sensitivity and Insulin Secretion

Homeostatic model assessment of insulin resistance (HOMA-IR) (13) and oral glucose insulin sensitivity (OGIS) (14) were calculated. Insulin secretion was estimated with C-peptide deconvolution (15, 16).

Adipose Tissue Gene Expression

Subcutaneous adipose tissue biopsies were obtained from participants before at study start and at follow-up. The biopsies were taken from the umbilical area, snap frozen in liquid nitrogen and stored in -80°C until further analysis. Analysis of mRNA levels of genes related to the metabolism of branched chain amino acids, fatty acid metabolism and amino acid metabolism were performed. mRNA isolation was performed using magnetic beads. Subcutaneous white adipose tissue was sorted into lysis buffer. Directly after tissue sorting, the plate containing lysis buffer and lysed tissue was incubated for 15 minutes at 65°C. Subsequently, RNA was purified using RNA Clean XP bead suspension (Agencourt Bioscience). RNA was quantified using the Quant-iT RNA Assay kit (Life Technologies), and after that cDNA synthesis was performed by Pico Profiling. mRNA isolation and cDNA synthesis was carried out at Functional Genomics Platform of IRB Barcelona (17).

Quantitative real-time PCR was performed using the ABI Prism 7900 HT real-time PCR machine (Applied Biosystems) and the SYBR Green PCR Master Mix (Applied Biosystems), using Peptidylprolyl Isomerase A (PPIA) as internal controls for normalization. The following genes involved in branched chain amino acid metabolism were analyzed: branched chain amino acid transaminase 1 (BCAT1), branched chain amino acid transaminase 2 (BCAT2), Branched chain ketoacid dehydrogenase α (BCKDHα) and branched chain ketoacid dehydrogenase β (BCKDHβ). Additional gene expression analysis of genes related to amino acid metabolism were also performed for the following genes: glutamate dehydrogenase (GDH), asparagine synthetase (AS), glycine amidinotransferase (AT); and for the following genes related to fatty acid metabolism: acetyl-CoA carboxylase α (ACCα), patatin like phospholipase domain containing 2 (ATGL), Fatty acid synthase (FASN), Hormone sensitive lipase (HSL), diacylglycerol O-acyltransferase 1 (DGAT1), perilipin 1 (PLIN1), perilipin 2 (PLIN2). For primer sequences, please, see **Supplemental Table S1**.

Small Polar Metabolites by Two-Dimensional Gas Chromatography Coupled to Time-of-Flight Mass Spectrometry (GC×GC-TOFMS)

Small polar metabolites were analyzed with two-dimensional gas chromatography coupled to time-of-flight mass spectrometry (GC×GC-TOFMS). Proteins from 30 µl plasma were precipitated using 400 µl methanol. Then 10 µl of group specific internal standards (heptadecanoic acid-d33 (175.36 mg/l), valine-d8 (35.72 mg/l), succinic acid-d4 (58.54 mg/l) and glutamic acid-d5 (110.43 mg/l)) were added and the samples were vortexed and left to precipitate on ice for 30 min. Half of the supernatant was evaporated to dryness after centrifugation for 3 min at 10000 rpm. An MPS autosampler (Gerstel, Mülheim an der Ruhr, Germany) was used to derivatize evaporated samples. The two step- derivatization started by adding 25 µl of methoxyamine hydrochloride (98%) and the samples were incubated for 1 hour at 45°C. Then, 25 µl of N-methyl-N-trimethylsilyltrifluoroacetamide was added as a second step in the derivatization and the samples were again incubated for 1 hour at 45°C. Retention index standards (n-alkanes, 25 µl, 8 mg/l) and an injection standard (4,4′-dibromooctafluorobiphenyl in hexane, 50 µl, 9.8 mg/l) were added and 1 µl of the derivatized sample was injected into the system (Pegasus 4D from Leco, St. Joseph, MI, USA).

A system of 3 columns were used for chromatographic separation. The first column was a 1.7 m deactivated retention gap column (0.53 mm ID, FS deactivated, Agilent technologies, USA) followed by a 10 m × 0.18 mm I.D. Rxi-5 ms (Restek Corp., Bellefonte, PA, USA) primary column and a 1.5 m × 0.1 mm I.D. BPX-50 (SGE Analytical Science, Austin, TX, USA) secondary column. The temperature program included the following steps: 50°C for 2 minutes followed by a gradually increasing temperature by steps of 7°C/minute up to 240°C and finally 25°C/minute to 300°C where it was held for 3 min. The secondary column had a slightly different temperature program that was maintained 20°C higher than in the primary column.

Raw data were processed with ChromaTOF version 4.32 (LECO Corporation, St. Joseph, MI). Signal to noise values higher than 100 was used as an inclusion criterion. The area of selected ions was used for target compounds and the total ion chromatogram area was used for untargeted compounds. External calibration curves with at least 6 concentration points were used to quantify selected compounds. Results were then exported as text files for further processing with Guineu software (18).

The samples were aligned and normalized with internal standards. Compounds belonging to chemical background or outside of the linear range were excluded. Small polar metabolites were identified using an in-house library, the NIST14 mass spectral library, and the Golm metabolome database (19). Metabolites verified with the in-house library were assigned as class 1, metabolites reaching similarity higher than 850 and a retention index difference lower than 30 were assigned to class 2. Other metabolites which did not meet the previous requirement were assigned as class 3 and were characterized by their spectra and Golm group annotation.

The coefficient of variation of compounds quantified by external calibration curve and measured on quality control plasma was on average 11% (n=8). The coefficient of variation of spiked compounds across the sample set also reached on average 11% (n=36). Metabolites that were present in more than 80% of the samples were included into further statistical analysis.

Statistical Analysis

Baseline characteristics are presented as means ± standard deviations (SD) or numbers and percent. Paired t-tests were used to analyze differences at study start and at follow-up. Student's t-tests were used to analyze differences between the two surgery groups at study start and at follow-up. Fisher's exact test was used for comparisons between the surgery groups of categorical data. Data on anthropometry and metabolic parameters were log2-transformed to achieve normal distribution. Metabolomics data were normalized by using log2-transformed values and scaled into zero mean and unit variance (autoscaling) (20) to obtain metabolite profiles comparable to each other. P-value < 0.05 was considered statistically significant. For the metabolomics data a false discovery rate of q-value < 0.05 was for correction of multiple comparisons. Spearman correlation analysis was performed on fold changes of relative concentrations (after versus before metabolic surgery) of metabolomic data and metabolic parameters to select variables for linear regression analysis. The fold changes were then log2-transformed (log2(post/pre)) to achieve linear relationships before linear regression analysis. For statistical analysis of gene expression, gene expression was normalized to mean value at study start and differences at study start and at follow-up were calculated with paired T-test. All statistical analyses were performed by using the R Project for Statistical Computing version 3.x. and IBM SPSS statistics software 21.0 (IBM Corp. NY. USA).

RESULTS

Participants' Characteristics at Study Start and Follow-Up

Participants' characteristics at study start and at follow-up are presented in **Table 1**. The participants treated with biliopancreatic diversion (BPD) were different from the participants treated with Roux-en Y gastric bypass (RYGB) in some aspects at study start. All patients treated with RYGB were men (n = 6, 100%) compared to four men of nine included patients in the BPD group (44.4%, p-value 0.044). The patients in the RYGB group also had significantly lower BMI compared to the BPD group (45.3 kg/m^2 ± 5.7 vs 55.9 kg/m^2 ± 9.7, p-value 0.034.

Indices for adiposity (weight, BMI) and parameters reflecting glucose homeostasis (fasting glucose, HbA1c and whole-body glucose uptake) were significantly improved after metabolic surgery for both the RYGB and BPD group (**Table 1**). Total serum cholesterol and S-LDL-cholesterol were significantly reduced after intervention in the BPD group, but this was not observed in the RYGB group (**Table 1**).

Small Polar Metabolites

In total, 378 small polar metabolites were observed in the GC×GC-TOF-MS database after normalization and filtering. Out of them, 73 metabolites were identified, mainly as amino acids, organic acids and fatty acids.

Twelve metabolites were significantly (p-value < 0.05; q-value < 0.05) altered at follow-up compared with the study start (pre vs post) in the whole study population (**Table 2**). Six of these 12 metabolites could be identified as 3-indoleacetic acid, 2-hydroxybutyric acid, valine, glutamic acid, 4-hydroxybenzeneacetic acid and alpha-tocopherol. 3-indoleacetic acid and 4-hydroxybenzeneacetic acid displayed an increase at follow-up

TABLE 1 | Participants' characteristics at study start and at follow-up visit.

	ALL		BPD		RYGB		% differences		
	At study start	At follow-up	At study start	At follow-up	At study start	At follow-up	ALL	BPD	RYGB
Number	15	15	9	9	6	6	15	9	6
Days until follow-up		185.3 ± 72.9		183.7 ± 61.8		187.8 ± 93.6			
Men, n (%)	10 (66.7)	–	4 (44.4) *	–	6 (100) *	–	–	–	–
Age, years	44.3 ± 8.3	–	44.7 ± 8.1	–	43.7 ± 9.4	–	–	–	–
Weight, kg	151.0 ± 24.8 ###	110.4 ± 22.2 ###	156.3 ± 28.7 ###	109.4 ± 26.8 ###	143.0 ± 16.7 ##	112.0 ± 15.1 ##	-26.5 ± 10.8	-29.8 ± 12.0	21.6 ± 7.0
% Excess weight loss	–	53.3 ± 19.9	–	55.5 ± 20.9	–	50.0 ± 19.7	–	–	–
BMI, kg/m^2	51.7 ± 9.7 ###	37.7 ± 7.7 ###	55.9 ± 9.7 * ###	39.1 ± 8.9 ###	45.3 ± 5.7 * ##	35.5 ± 5.5 ##	-26.1 ± 11.4	-29.2 ± 13.0	-21.6 ± 7.0
Change in BMI	–	-14.0 ± 7.2	–	-16.9 ± 7.9 *	–	-9.7 ± 3.1 *	–	–	–
Glucose, mg/dl	97.5 ± 17.0 ###	76.8 ± 11.1 ###	101.7 ± 20.7 #	76.7 ± 13.8 #	91.3 ± 6.3 ##	77.0 ± 6.3 ##	-19.8 ± 13.9	-22.6 ± 17.1	-15.6 ± 6.3
Total cholesterol, mg/dl	189.6 ± 28.2 ###	138.1 ± 28.6 ###	197.0 ± 31.3 ###	124.7 ± 17.3 * ###	178.5 ± 20.2	158.2 ± 31.2 *	-25.0 ± 22.1	-35.2 ± 13.7 *	-9.8 ± 24.7 *
HDL-cholesterol, mg/dl	47.1 ± 9.5	41.7 ± 12.3	47.9 ± 7.9	38.9 ± 13.2	46.0 ± 12.4	45.5 ± 11.0	-8.0 ± 38.5	-14.0 ± 42.1	0.5 ± 35.5
LDL-cholesterol, mg/dl	119.5 ± 22.1 ##	74.9 ± 27.5 ##	127.9 ± 16.3 ##	61.6 ± 14.2 * ##	107.8 ± 25.6	92.7 ± 32.0 *	-37.8 ± 23.9	-50.0 ± 15.2 *	-20.8 ± 24.4 *
Triglycerides, mg/dl	134.9 ± 58.5	109.6 ± 49.3	141.4 ± 52.7	116.2 ± 61.1	126.3 ± 69.7	99.7 ± 25.2	-8.7 ± 46.2	-16.4 ± 19.6	1.7 ± 69.2
Type 2 diabetes	2	0	1	0	1	0	–	–	–
HbA1c, mmol/mol	41.4 ± 3.7 ###	36.5 ± 2.6 ###	42.1 ± 4.0 #	37.3 ± 2.5 #	40.3 ± 3.3 ##	35.3 ± 2.3 ##	-11.3 ± 8.1	-10.7 ± 9.8	-12.2 ± 5.3
Whole body glucose uptake, M, mg/kg/min	2.7 ± 1.4 ###	6.0 ± 2.2 ###	2.3 ± 1.2 ###	6.1 ± 2.3 ###	3.3 ± 1.7 #	5.7 ± 2.3 #	151.0 ± 116.5	188.2 ± 119.4	95.2 ± 94.6
HOMA-IR	3.3 ± 2.2 ##	1.1 ± 0.6 ##	3.0 ± 2.2	1.3 ± 0.6	3.6 ± 2.3 #	0.9 ± 0.5 #	-42.7 ± 62.4	-25.4 ± 74.7	-68.6 ± 25.5
Insulin secretion, pmol/min/m^2	223.4 ± 100.7	196.6 ± 140.0	226.2 ± 89.9	173.9 ± 98.0	219.2 ± 124.2	230.6 ± 192.9	-14.3 ± 37.1	-20.4 ± 37.6	-5.1 ± 37.8

*Data are presented as mean values ± standard deviation or numbers and percent. * = p-values < 0.05 in comparisons between the BPD group and the RYGB group at study start and follow-up. # = p-values < 0.05, ## = p-values < 0.01 and ### = p-values < 0.001 in comparisons at study start and at follow-up in each study group. BMI, Body Mass Index; HDL-cholesterol, high density lipoprotein cholesterol; LDL-cholesterol, low density lipoprotein cholesterol; HbA1c, glycated hemoglobin; HOMA-IR, Homeostatic Model Assessment for Insulin Resistance.*

TABLE 2 | Small polar metabolites with signficant change between study start and follow-up in the total surgery group (n = 15).

Metabolite (relative concentration)	At study start	At follow-up	p-value	q-value
ID no. 400	6.45 ± 1.56	39.89 ± 37.04	0.00012	0.026
3-indoleacetic acid	57.34 ± 53.48	309.37 ± 362.84	0.00016	0.018
ID no. 493	9.31 ± 4.88	17.71 ± 5.79	0.00018	0.013
ID no. 361	7.21 ± 3.63	37.23 ± 35.10	0.00022	0.012
ID no. 294	565.07 ± 194.45	349.27 ± 194.06	0.00030	0.013
2-hydroxybutyric acid	399.49 ± 209.60	164.03 ± 85.83	0.00039	0.014
Valine	574.80 ± 131.67	395.01 ± 109.86	0.00075	0.023
ID no. 296	182.64 ± 66.16	343.78 ± 144.47	0.0012	0.033
ID no. 580	13.90 ± 9.77	32.91 ± 17.23	0.0016	0.039
Glutamic acid	244.25 ± 85.84	141.77 ± 80.66	0.0017	0.037
4 hydroxybenzeneacetic acid	22.83 ± 31.43	152.01 ± 164.83	0.0017	0.034
Alpha tocopherol	28.75 ± 9.11	19.62 ± 8.40	0.0019	0.036

The data are presented as mean relative concentration ± standard deviation. Paired T-test on log2-transformed values was used to analyse differences in metabolite levels at study start and follow-up. False discovery rate was used to adjust for multiple testing.

whereas the other identified metabolites were decreased. None of the small polar metabolites displayed a significant difference between the BPD and RYGBP group at study start or at follow-up.

Changes in GSG Index, Branched Chain Amino Acids, Aromatic Amino Acids and Saturated Fatty Acids After Metabolic Surgery

We also analyzed changes in groups of metabolites known to be associated to metabolic diseases (21) such as branched chain amino acids (BCAA = leucine, valine, isoleucine), aromatic amino acids (AAA = phenylalanine + tyrosine + tryptophan), GSG index [calculated from amino acids involved in oxidative stress and the synthesis of glutathione, Glutamate/(Serine+ Glycine)], a marker of liver fibrosis in non-alcoholic fatty liver disease (NAFLD) (22) and saturated fatty acids (Palmitic acid + Stearic acid) at study start and at follow-up.

GSG index and BCAA displayed a significant decrease after metabolic surgery (p-value 0.0004 and p-value 0.004, respectively, **Table 3**). No differences in GSG-index, BCAA, AAA or saturated fatty acids were observed between the BPD group and RYGB group at study start but at follow-up the RYGB group displayed a significantly lower levels of AAA (p-value 0.006) compared with the BPD group (p-value 0.006, **Table 3**).

Associations Between the Changes of Small Polar Metabolites and Changes in Metabolic Parameters

Several correlations between parameters reflecting glucose homeostasis and the metabolites regulated by metabolic surgery were observed in Spearman correlation analyses (**Figure 1**). The change in 3-indoleacetic acid and the change in 4-hydroxybenzeneacetic acid were negatively correlated to the change in glucose. The changes in alpha-tocopherol was positively correlated to both changes in s-insulin and changes in HOMA-IR. 2-hydroxyburyric acid was correlated to OGIS. In linear regression analysis the change in 3-indoleacetic acid and the change in 4-hydroxybenzeneacetic acid could predict the change in glucose ($R^2 = 0.745$; p-value<0.001 and $R^2 = 0.709$; p-value 0.003; **Supplemental Figures S1A, B**). In addition, alpha tocopherol could significantly predict the change in s-insulin ($R^2 = 0.263$; p-value 0.050; **Supplemental Figure S1C**) but could not predict the change in HOMA-IR ($R^2 = 0.253$; p-value 0.056) and 2-hydroxybutyric acid could not predict the change in OGIS in a linear regression analysis ($R^2 = 0.235$; p-value 0.067). No changes in metabolites were correlated to changes in insulin sensitivity estimated with whole body glucose uptake.

Correlations were also observed between changes in serum lipid levels and metabolites regulated by metabolic surgery (**Figure 1**). The change in valine, alpha-tocopherol and branched chain amino acids were all negatively correlated to changes in s-cholesterol. Changes in 2-hydroxybutyric acid, glutamic acid and GSG-index were negatively correlated to changes in HDL-cholesterol. In addition, the change in valine and branched chain amino acids also displayed negative correlations to the change in LDL-cholesterol. A linear

TABLE 3 | Changes in GSG index, branched chain amino acids, aromatic amino acids and saturated fatty acids after metabolic surgery.

	ALL		BPD		RYGB	
	At study start	At follow-up	At study start	At follow-up	At study start	At follow-up
GSG-index	0.69 ± 0.26 ###	0.31 ± 0.20 ###	0.66 ± 0.25 #	0.34 ± 0.23 #	0.73 ± 0.29 #	0.28 ± 0.14 #
Branched chain amino acids	1243.65 ± 341.90 ##	888.37 ± 283.09 ##	1129.64 ± 199.39	981.62 ± 285.96	1414.67 ± 453.01 ###	748.50 ± 233.30 ###
Aromatic amino acids	415.81 ± 98.78	345.50 ± 117.68	397.24 ± 107.24	405.40 ± 80.22 **	443.67 ± 85.85 #	255.65 ± 111.07 ** #
Saturated fatty acids	5007.40 ± 866.23	4501.13 ± 1374.79	5282.23 ± 752.38	4882.31 ± 1359.03	4595.15 ± 924.87	3929.37 ± 1297.38

** = p-values < 0.01 in comparisons between the BPD group and the RYGB group at study start and follow-up. # = p-values < 0.05, ## = p-values < 0.01 and ### = p-values < 0.001 in comparisons study start vs follow-up in each study group.

regression model further established that the change in valine (R^2 0.0609; p-value 0.001), alpha-tocopherol (R^2 0.374; p-value 0.015) and branched chain amino acid (R^2 0.594; p-value 0.001) could predict the change in s-cholesterol (**Supplemental Figure S2** panel A–C) and that changes in 2-hydroxybutyric acid (R^2 0.672; p-value 0.001), glutamic acid (R^2 0.668; p-value 0.001) and GSG-index (R^2 0.534; p-value 0.007) could predict the change in HDL-cholesterol (**Supplemental Figure S2**, panel D–F). Furthermore, changes in valine (R^2 0.712; p-value 0.001) and branched chain amino acids (R^2 0.688; p-value 0.001) could predict the change in LDL-cholesterol (**Supplemental Figure S2** panel G, H).

Adipose Tissue Gene Expression Analysis

Among the genes involved in branched chain amino acid metabolism BCAT1 displayed a significant reduction in mRNA levels in adipose tissue after surgery (p-value 0.003, **Figure 2A**). The changes in BCAT1 gene expression (log2(post/pre)) was not correlated to the changes in BCAA concentrations (log2(post/pre) (correlation coefficient -0.282; p-value 0.309). The gene expression of HSL (Hormone sensitive lipase), was also reduced in adipose tissue after metabolic surgery (p-value 0.017, **Figure 2B**). No significant changes in gene expression of genes related to amino acid metabolism (GDH, AS and AT) were observed (**Figure 2C**).

DISCUSSION

In this study we have investigated metabolic pathways and metabolites that are altered after metabolic surgery and related to the metabolic improvement by using an integrative approach analyzing adipose tissue gene expression in parallel with plasma metabolite profiling.

In our study branched chain amino acids, as well as glutamic acid, were down regulated after metabolic surgery, in line with previous studies (23–25). Serum levels of both BCAA as well as glutamic acid have previously been associated with insulin resistance (26–28). However, the changes in valine and BCAA or glutamic acid were not able to predict the changes in parameters reflecting glucose homeostasis in our study. Instead, changes in valine, BCAA and glutamic acid could predict changes in serum cholesterol levels. Interestingly, BCAAs have been shown to influence hepatic lipid metabolism both *in vitro* and *in vivo* (29), which may explain our observed association.

The previous reported links between circulating BCAA and metabolic function (26–28) have highlighted the importance of well-functioning BCAA metabolism. It has been suggested that elevated levels of branched chain amino acid associated with obesity could be a consequence of alterations of the BCAA catabolizing enzymes in adipose tissue (30). A recent report showed that BCAA catabolizing enzymes in visceral adipose tissue are decreased in women with obesity (31), which might account for the increased circulating levels of BCAA observed in the obese state. However, our results do not support this hypothesis. Instead we observed a decrease in adipose tissue

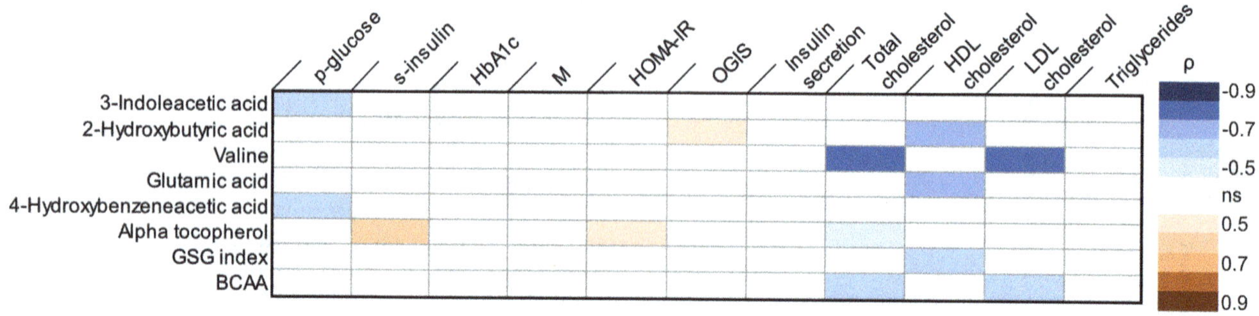

FIGURE 1 | Correlations between changes in metabolic parameters [log2 (post/pre)] and changes in metabolites [log2 (post/pre)] in Spearman correlation analyses. Blue color indicates a significant negative correlation coefficient and red color a significant positive correlation coefficient. HbA1c, glycated hemoglobin; M, whole body glucose uptake; OGIS, oral glucose insulin sensitivity; HDL-cholesterol, High density lipoprotein cholesterol; LDL, low density lipoprotein cholesterol; BCAA, branched chain amino acids. ns, not significant.

BCAT1 gene expression in adipose tissue after metabolic surgery, which are in line with a study reporting that a decrease of mRNA *BCAT1* in the adipose tissue is a marker for weight loss maintenance after a low calorie diet (32).

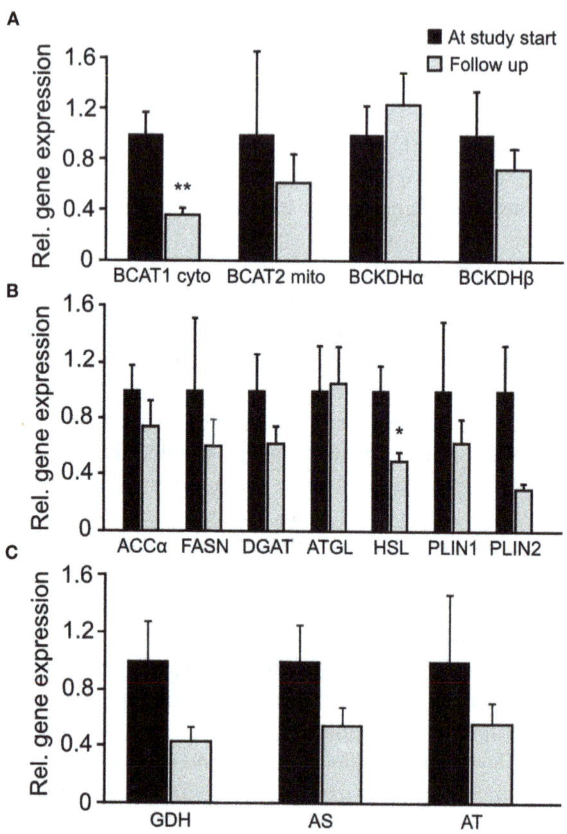

FIGURE 2 | Changes in the entire cohort in relative gene expression of adipose tissue genes involved in **(A)** branched chain amino acid metabolism **(B)** fatty acid metabolism **(C)** amino acid metabolism. *p-value < 0.05. **p-value < 0.01.

Branched chain amino acids can downregulate the synthesis of the 3-indoleacetic acid in bacteria (33) present in in the gut (34). Thus, it is possible that the decreased levels of branched chain amino acids after metabolic surgery could result in the increased levels of 3-indoleacetic observed in our study. 3-indoleacetic acid is produced by tryptophan and a recent study has suggested that changes in indole tryptophan metabolites from gut bacteria can be responsible for the beneficial metabolic effects of metabolic surgery (35). This is an interesting hypothesis as the change in 3-indoleacetic acid could predict the change in circulating glucose levels in our study.

Additional three individual metabolites were regulated by metabolic surgery in our study: 2-hydroxybutyric acid, a derivate from alpha-ketobutyrate that is produced in the liver by the catabolism of threonine and methionine and glutathione synthesis, and alpha-tocopherol that both were decreased after metabolic surgery and 4-hydroxybeneacetic acid, produced from tyrosine in bacteria in the gut (34), which was increased. The decrease of 2-hydroxybutyric acid after metabolic surgery was correlated to HOMA-IR in a previous study (36). However, in our study the change of 2-hydroxybutyric acid was not associated with any of the parameters reflecting glucose homeostasis. A more interesting finding was the association of 4-hydroxybenzeneacetic acid to changes in glucose levels and the association between alpha tocopherol and fasting insulin levels. Furthermore, regulation of 4-hydroxybenzeneacetic acid after metabolic surgery has, to the best of our knowledge, not been reported before. Hence, both alpha tocopherol and 4-hydroxybezeneacetic acid may be interesting targets for future studies on glucose homeostasis after metabolic surgery.

A decrease in hormone sensitive lipase (HSL) was also observed after metabolic surgery in our study. A decrease of adipose tissue HSL mRNA levels after weight loss has been reported in women with obesity (37) whereas others report a reduction of HSL adipose tissue mRNA levels in obesity (38). The mechanism behind the reduction in HSL mRNA levels in adipose tissue in our study is unclear, but the promoter region of the HSL gene contains a glucose responsive region (39) and the improved insulin sensitivity and reduction in glucose levels after metabolic surgery may have an impact on HSL gene expression levels.

Our study has limitations. The study contains a relatively small number of patients, and it is reasonable to believe that there are other metabolite changes after metabolic surgery that we are not able to demonstrate here due to limited statistical power. In addition, no major differences in metabolites between the two surgery types were observed. This is probably due to a small number of patients in each group so the study did not have power enough to detect such differences. However, the two surgical procedures studied here, RYGB and BPD are different in some aspects such as differences in fat malabsorption and the weight loss achieved (40). Hence, it is reasonable to believe that some differences in metabolites might be detected but our study did not have power to detect such differences.

We here show that plasma concentrations of branched chain amino acids and adipose tissue mRNA levels of BCAT1 were down-regulated after metabolic surgery. In addition, results from this study have identified some new candidates, such as 4-hydroxybenzeneacetic acid, 2-hydroxybutyric acid and alpha tocopherol that may be used as biomarkers for the early metabolic improvement after metabolic surgery, which include short-term metabolic changes related to caloric restriction and improved hepatic insulin resistance as well as enteroendocrine changes (41). Future studies are needed to further validate our results in other study cohorts and with longer follow-up.

ETHICS STATEMENT

The studies involving human participants were reviewed and approved by the ethics committee at the Catholic University Hospital of the Sacred Heart, Rome, Italy. The patients/participants provided their written informed consent to participate in this study.

AUTHOR CONTRIBUTIONS

CC, EC, and LM collected data. AZ and MR. coordinated and performed the gene expression analysis. IB-P and KT coordinated and performed the metabolomics lab analysis. SA, AG, GM, JN, and AZ data interpretation. SA and GM wrote the manuscript. GM, JN, and AZ are responsible for study design. All authors contributed to discussion and reviewed/edited the manuscript. All authors contributed to the article and approved the submitted version.

FUNDING

This study was funded by The Catholic university hospital of the Sacred heart, the Health & Medical Care Committee of the Region Västra Götaland (grant no. VGFOUREG-931560), the Swedish research council (grant no. 2016-00522), and the Magnus Bergvall Foundation (grant no 2019-03489). IB-P is grateful to the Novo Nordisk Foundation for her Clinical Research Fellow grant.

ACKNOWLEDGMENTS

We are thankful to Jonas Carlsten for helping us designing the visual abstract.

REFERENCES

1. Carlsson LM, Peltonen M, Ahlin S, Anveden A, Bouchard C, Carlsson B, et al. Bariatric Surgery and Prevention of Type 2 Diabetes in Swedish Obese Subjects. *N Engl J Med* (2012) 367(8):695–704. doi: 10.1056/NEJMoa1112082
2. Mingrone G, Panunzi S, De Gaetano A, Guidone C, Iaconelli A, Nanni G, et al. Bariatric-Metabolic Surgery Versus Conventional Medical Treatment in Obese Patients With Type 2 Diabetes: 5 Year Follow-Up of an Open-Label, Single-Centre, Randomised Controlled Trial. *Lancet* (2015) 386(9997):964–73. doi: 10.1016/S0140-6736(15)00075-6
3. Sjostrom L, Peltonen M, Jacobson P, Ahlin S, Andersson-Assarsson J, Anveden A, et al. Association of Bariatric Surgery With Long-Term Remission of Type 2 Diabetes and With Microvascular and Macrovascular Complications. *JAMA* (2014) 311(22):2297–304. doi: 10.1001/jama.2014.5988
4. Sjostrom L. Review of the Key Results From the Swedish Obese Subjects (SOS) Trial - A Prospective Controlled Intervention Study of Bariatric Surgery. *J Intern Med* (2013) 273(3):219–34. doi: 10.1111/joim.12012
5. Gastaldelli A, Iaconelli A, Gaggini M, Magnone MC, Veneziani A, Rubino F, et al. Short-Term Effects of Laparoscopic Adjustable Gastric Banding Versus Roux-En-Y Gastric Bypass. *Diabetes Care* (2016) 39(11):1925–31. doi: 10.2337/dc15-2823
6. Guidone C, Manco M, Valera-Mora E, Iaconelli A, Gniuli D, Mari A, et al. Mechanisms of Recovery From Type 2 Diabetes After Malabsorptive Bariatric Surgery. *Diabetes* (2006) 55(7):2025–31. doi: 10.2337/db06-0068
7. Patti GJ, Yanes O, Siuzdak G. Innovation: Metabolomics: The Apogee of the Omics Trilogy. *Nat Rev Mol Cell Biol* (2012) 13(4):263–9. doi: 10.1038/nrm3314
8. Zamboni N, Saghatelian A, Patti GJ. Defining the Metabolome: Size, Flux, and Regulation. *Mol Cell* (2015) 58(4):699–706. doi: 10.1016/j.molcel.2015.04.021
9. Newgard CB. Metabolomics and Metabolic Diseases: Where Do We Stand? *Cell Metab* (2017) 25(1):43–56. doi: 10.1016/j.cmet.2016.09.018
10. Skogar ML, Sundbom M. Duodenal Switch Is Superior to Gastric Bypass in Patients With Super Obesity When Evaluated With the Bariatric Analysis and Reporting Outcome System (BAROS). *Obes Surg* (2017) 27(9):2308–16. doi: 10.1007/s11695-017-2680-z
11. DeFronzo RA, Tobin JD, Andres R. Glucose Clamp Technique: A Method for Quantifying Insulin Secretion and Resistance. *Am J Physiol* (1979) 237(3): E214–23. doi: 10.1152/ajpendo.1979.237.3.E214
12. Ahlin S, Cefalo C, Bondia-Pons I, Capristo E, Marini L, Gastaldelli A, et al. Bile Acid Changes After Metabolic Surgery Are Linked to Improvement in Insulin Sensitivity. *Br J Surg* (2019) 106(9):1178–86. doi: 10.1002/bjs.11208
13. Matthews DR, Hosker JP, Rudenski AS, Naylor BA, Treacher DF, Turner RC. Homeostasis Model Assessment: Insulin Resistance and Beta-Cell Function From Fasting Plasma Glucose and Insulin Concentrations in Man. *Diabetologia* (1985) 28(7):412–9. doi: 10.1007/BF00280883
14. Mari A, Pacini G, Murphy E, Ludvik B, Nolan JJ. A Model-Based Method for Assessing Insulin Sensitivity From the Oral Glucose Tolerance Test. *Diabetes Care* (2001) 24(3):539 48. doi: 10.2337/diacare.24.3.539

15. Hovorka R, Jones RH. How to Measure Insulin Secretion. *Diabetes Metab Rev* (1994) 10(2):91–117. doi: 10.1002/dmr.5610100204
16. Van Cauter E, Mestrez F, Sturis J, Polonsky KS. Estimation of Insulin Secretion Rates From C-Peptide Levels. Comparison of Individual and Standard Kinetic Parameters for C-Peptide Clearance. *Diabetes* (1992) 41 (3):368–77. doi: 10.2337/diab.41.3.368
17. Gonzalez-Roca E, Garcia-Albeniz X, Rodriguez-Mulero S, Gomis RR, Kornacker K, Auer H. Accurate Expression Profiling of Very Small Cell Populations. *PLoS One* (2010) 5(12):e14418. doi: 10.1371/journal.pone.0014418
18. Castillo S, Mattila I, Miettinen J, Oresic M, Hyotylainen T. Data Analysis Tool for Comprehensive Two-Dimensional Gas Chromatography/Time-of-Flight Mass Spectrometry. *Anal Chem* (2011) 83(8):3058–67. doi: 10.1021/ac103308x
19. Kopka J, Schauer N, Krueger S, Birkemeyer C, Usadel B, Bergmuller E, et al. GMD@CSB.DB: The Golm Metabolome Database. *Bioinformatics* (2005) 21 (8):1635–8. doi: 10.1093/bioinformatics/bti236
20. van den Berg RA, Hoefsloot HC, Westerhuis JA, Smilde AK, van der Werf MJ. Centering, Scaling, and Transformations: Improving the Biological Information Content of Metabolomics Data. *BMC Genomics* (2006) 7:142. doi: 10.1186/1471-2164-7-142
21. Masoodi M, Gastaldelli A, Hyotylainen T, Arretxe E, Alonso C, Gaggini M, et al. Metabolomics and Lipidomics in NAFLD: Biomarkers and Non-Invasive Diagnostic Tests. *Nat Rev Gastroenterol Hepatol* (2021) 18:835–56. doi: 10.1038/s41575-021-00502-9
22. Gaggini M, Carli F, Rosso C, Buzzigoli E, Marietti M, Della Latta V, et al. Altered Amino Acid Concentrations in NAFLD: Impact of Obesity and Insulin Resistance. *Hepatology* (2018) 67(1):145–58. doi: 10.1002/hep.29465
23. Lopes TI, Geloneze B, Pareja JC, Calixto AR, Ferreira MM, Marsaioli AJ. Blood Metabolome Changes Before and After Bariatric Surgery: A (1)H NMR-Based Clinical Investigation. *Omics* (2015) 19(5):318–27. doi: 10.1089/omi.2015.0009
24. Magkos F, Bradley D, Schweitzer GG, Finck BN, Eagon JC, Ilkayeva O, et al. Effect of Roux-En-Y Gastric Bypass and Laparoscopic Adjustable Gastric Banding on Branched-Chain Amino Acid Metabolism. *Diabetes* (2013) 62 (8):2757–61. doi: 10.2337/db13-0185
25. Aasheim ET, Elshorbagy AK, Diep LM, Sovik TT, Mala T, Valdivia-Garcia M, et al. Effect of Bariatric Surgery on Sulphur Amino Acids and Glutamate. *Br J Nutr* (2011) 106(3):432–40. doi: 10.1017/S0007114511000201
26. Lynch CJ, Adams SH. Branched-Chain Amino Acids in Metabolic Signalling and Insulin Resistance. *Nat Rev Endocrinol* (2014) 10(12):723–36. doi: 10.1038/nrendo.2014.171
27. Newgard CB, An J, Bain JR, Muehlbauer MJ, Stevens RD, Lien LF, et al. A Branched-Chain Amino Acid-Related Metabolic Signature That Differentiates Obese and Lean Humans and Contributes to Insulin Resistance. *Cell Metab* (2009) 9(4):311–26. doi: 10.1016/j.cmet.2009.02.002
28. Seibert R, Abbasi F, Hantash FM, Caulfield MP, Reaven G, Kim SH. Relationship Between Insulin Resistance and Amino Acids in Women and Men. *Physiol Rep* (2015) 3(5). doi: 10.14814/phy2.12392
29. Bishop CA, Schulze MB, Klaus S, Weitkunat K. The Branched-Chain Amino Acids Valine and Leucine Have Differential Effects on Hepatic Lipid Metabolism. *FASEB J* (2020) 34(7):9727–39. doi: 10.1096/fj.202000195R
30. Herman MA, She P, Peroni OD, Lynch CJ, Kahn BB. Adipose Tissue Branched Chain Amino Acid (BCAA) Metabolism Modulates Circulating BCAA Levels. *J Biol Chem* (2010) 285(15):11348–56. doi: 10.1074/jbc.M109.075184
31. Boulet MM, Chevrier G, Grenier-Larouche T, Pelletier M, Nadeau M, Scarpa J, et al. Alterations of Plasma Metabolite Profiles Related to Adipose Tissue Distribution and Cardiometabolic Risk. *Am J Physiol Endocrinol Metab* (2015) 309(8):E736–46. doi: 10.1152/ajpendo.00231.2015
32. Viguerie N, Montastier E, Maoret JJ, Roussel B, Combes M, Valle C, et al. Determinants of Human Adipose Tissue Gene Expression: Impact of Diet, Sex, Metabolic Status, and Cis Genetic Regulation. *PLoS Genet* (2012) 8(9): e1002959. doi: 10.1371/journal.pgen.1002959
33. Parsons CV, Harris DM, Patten CL. Regulation of Indole-3-Acetic Acid Biosynthesis by Branched-Chain Amino Acids in Enterobacter Cloacae UW5. *FEMS Microbiol Lett* (2015) 362(18):fnv153. doi: 10.1093/femsle/fnv153
34. Keller R, Pedroso MZ, Ritchmann R, Silva RM. Occurrence of Virulence-Associated Properties in Enterobacter Cloacae. *Infect Immun* (1998) 66 (2):645–9. doi: 10.1128/IAI.66.2.645-649.1998
35. Galligan JJ. Beneficial Actions of Microbiota-Derived Tryptophan Metabolites. *Neurogastroenterol Motil* (2018) 30(2):e13283. doi: 10.1111/nmo.13283
36. Shantavasinkul PC, Muehlbauer MJ, Bain JR, Ilkayeva OR, Craig DM, Newgard CB, et al. Improvement in Insulin Resistance After Gastric Bypass Surgery Is Correlated With a Decline in Plasma 2-Hydroxybutyric Acid. *Surg Obes Relat Dis* (2018) 14(8):1126–32. doi: 10.1016/j.soard.2018.03.033
37. Kolehmainen M, Vidal H, Ohisalo JJ, Pirinen E, Alhava E, Uusitupa MI. Hormone Sensitive Lipase Expression and Adipose Tissue Metabolism Show Gender Difference in Obese Subjects After Weight Loss. *Int J Obes Relat Metab Disord* (2002) 26(1):6–16. doi: 10.1038/sj.ijo.0801858
38. Large V, Reynisdottir S, Langin D, Fredby K, Klannemark M, Holm C, et al. Decreased Expression and Function of Adipocyte Hormone-Sensitive Lipase in Subcutaneous Fat Cells of Obese Subjects. *J Lipid Res* (1999) 40(11):2059–66. doi: 10.1016/S0022-2275(20)32429-9
39. Smih F, Rouet P, Lucas S, Mairal A, Sengenes C, Lafontan M, et al. Transcriptional Regulation of Adipocyte Hormone-Sensitive Lipase by Glucose. *Diabetes* (2002) 51(2):293–300. doi: 10.2337/diabetes.51.2.293
40. Carswell KA, Vincent RP, Belgaumkar AP, Sherwood RA, Amiel SA, Patel AG, et al. The Effect of Bariatric Surgery on Intestinal Absorption and Transit Time. *Obes Surg* (2014) 24(5):796–805. doi: 10.1007/s11695-013-1166-x
41. Knop FK, Taylor R. Mechanism of Metabolic Advantages After Bariatric Surgery: It's All Gastrointestinal Factors Versus It's All Food Restriction. *Diabetes Care* (2013) 36(Suppl 2):S287–91. doi: 10.2337/dcS13-2032

23

Metabolic Surgery on Patients with Polycystic Ovary Syndrome

Wenwen Yue[1†], Xin Huang[2†], Wenjing Zhang[1], Shumin Li[3,4], Xu Liu[1], Yian Zhao[5], Jiaxin Shu[5], Teng Liu[2], Weihua Li[6] and Shaozhuang Liu[2*]*

[1] School of Nursing and Rehabilitation, Cheeloo College of Medicine, Shandong University, Jinan, China, [2] Division of Bariatric and Metabolic Surgery, Department of General Surgery, Qilu Hospital of Shandong University, Jinan, China, [3] Center for Reproductive Medicine, Cheeloo College of Medicine, Shandong University, Jinan, China, [4] Key Laboratory of Reproductive Endocrinology of Ministry of Education, Shandong University, Jinan, China, [5] Cheeloo College of Medicine, Shandong University, Jinan, China, [6] Operating Theater, Qilu Hospital of Shandong University, Jinan, China

***Correspondence:**
Shaozhuang Liu
liushaozhuang@sdu.edu.cn
Weihua Li
swan05311@163.com

[†]These authors have contributed equally to this work

Polycystic ovary syndrome (PCOS) is a complicated reproductive endocrine disease that is closely related to obesity. Metabolic surgery ameliorates a series of clinical manifestations and related comorbidities of PCOS. However, the overall efficacy of metabolic surgery on PCOS remains uncertain. This systematic review and meta-analysis aimed to evaluate the therapeutic effects of metabolic surgery on obese patients with PCOS. A systematic literature search for relevant studies was conducted on PubMed, Embase, Web of Science, and the Cochrane Library from inception to June 2021. Data extraction and quality evaluation were performed by three researchers, and RevMan 5.4 software was used to conduct the meta-analysis. A total of 14 studies involving 501 obese patients with PCOS were included. Incidence of PCOS in obese women ranged from 5.5% to 63.5% among the included studies. The results showed the incidence of abnormal menstruation decreased from 81% to 15% (OR=0.03, 95% confidence interval (CI): 0.01–0.08), while the incidence of hirsutism dropped from 71% to 38% (OR=0.21, 95% CI: 0.06–0.74). Serum total testosterone and free testosterone levels decreased by 25.92 ng/dL (MD = -25.92, 95% CI: -28.90– -22.93) and 2.28 ng/dL (SMD = -2.28, 95% CI: -3.67– -0.89), respectively. Sex hormone-binding globulin (SHBG) levels increased by 26.46 nmol/L (MD = 26.46, 95% CI: 12.97–39.95). Serum anti-Mullerian hormone (AMH) levels decreased by 1.29 ng/mL (MD = -1.29, 95% CI: -1.92– -0.66). Small sample size studies revealed that pregnancy rates ranged from 95.2% to 100% postoperatively. Metabolic surgery contributed to marked improvement of abnormal menstruation, hirsutism, and levels of free testosterone, total testosterone, SHBG, and AMH in patients with PCOS. Our findings indicate that patients with PCOS are expected to benefit from metabolic surgery, and could help potentially improve their reproductive outcomes. Metabolic surgery could thus be a new viable option for the clinical treatment of PCOS.

Keywords: polycystic ovary syndrome, metabolic surgery, bariatric surgery, obesity, meta-analysis, systematic review

1 INTRODUCTION

Polycystic ovary syndrome (PCOS) is the most common endocrinopathy affecting women of reproductive age and is characterized by ovulation dysfunction, hyperandrogenism, and polycystic ovarian morphology (PCOM). The prevalence of PCOS ranges from 8% to 13% depending on the diagnostic criteria and study population (1, 2). Women with PCOS exhibit menstrual irregularities, hirsutism, and infertility. In addition, this syndrome can lead to long-term comorbidities, including obesity, type 2 diabetes mellitus, cardiometabolic diseases, endometrial carcinoma, and psychological disorders (3–5).

The pathogenesis of PCOS is multifactorial and remains unclear. However, a close relationship between obesity and the development of PCOS has been reported, with >50% of patients with PCOS as obese or overweight (6). In addition, hyperandrogenism, chronic inflammation, and family history of diabetes contributed to insulin resistance as the main pathogenetic mechanism of PCOS, with 50-70% of patients with PCOS exhibiting insulin resistance and compensatory hyperinsulinism (7, 8). Insulin resistance is considered an intrinsic feature of the syndrome, independent of body weight. However, obesity, a frequent feature among PCOS patients (60-70%), has a major contribution to the aggravation of insulin resistance (9). Studies have suggested that weight loss improves reproductive and metabolic dysfunction and reduces the risk of diabetes and cardiovascular disease (10, 11). Currently, lifestyle management targeting weight reduction is the first-line treatment for PCOS (12).

Metabolic surgery is the most effective and sustainable treatment for morbid obesity. Its therapeutic effects include resolution of type 2 diabetes, hypertension, hyperlipidemia, cardiovascular disease, and obstructive sleep apnea (13, 14). In addition, a few small-scale studies have indicated the positive effects of metabolic surgery on PCOS, including improvement of abnormal menstruation, hirsutism, fertility, and associated metabolic problems (10, 15). These findings suggested that metabolic surgery could be a potential treatment for PCOS; therefore, it has been recommended as an experimental therapy (2). However, there is no consensus on the use of metabolic surgery for the treatment of PCOS due to insufficient evidence. In the present study, we conducted a systematic review and meta-analysis to evaluate the therapeutic effects of metabolic surgery on PCOS.

2 METHODS

This systematic review and meta-analysis was conducted and reported according to the Systematic Reviews and Meta-analyses guidelines (16, 17) (a checklist of the guidelines is provided in the **Supplementary Material**). A prespecified study protocol was developed and registered on PROSPERO (registration number: CRD42021251524).

2.1 Data Sources and Search Strategy

A comprehensive literature search was conducted on PubMed, Embase, Web of Science, and the Cochrane Library from their inception to June 2021. The search was focused on trials of metabolic surgery for treating PCOS and included the following search terms: (bariatric OR "metabolic surgery" OR "gastric bypass" OR "sleeve gastrectomy" OR "gastric banding") AND ("polycystic ovary syndrome" OR "polycystic ovarian" OR "PCOS"). An email was forwarded to the corresponding author when there was no access to the full text. **Supplementary Table 1** lists the detailed search term.

Eligibility Criteria

The inclusion criteria were as follows: (1) studies were randomized controlled trials (RCTs) or observational trials of metabolic surgery on patients with PCOS; (2) participants were diagnosed with obesity and PCOS and had undergone metabolic surgery; (3) participants were premenopausal women, with no restrictions for race or country; (4) studies should include at least ten patients, and study design had at least 6-month follow-up; (5) studies were published in English; and (6) studies reported at least one of the listed outcomes of interest–abnormal menstruation, hirsutism, and levels of total testosterone, free testosterone, anti-Mullerian hormone (AMH), and sex hormone-binding globulin (SHBG).

The exclusion criteria were as follows: (1) studies were in the form of abstracts, case reports, letters, comments, reviews, meta-analyses, and animal studies; (2) studies included no surgical intervention, lacked data on the outcome of interest; and (3) studies had unreliable designs or obvious statistical errors.

2.3 Study Selection and Data Extraction

Three independent reviewers (WY, WZ and XH) screened the titles and abstracts, conducted preliminary screening according to inclusion and exclusion criteria, further reviewed, screened, and cross-checked the full texts. Disagreement was settled by consensus.

The same reviewers extracted data independently into electronic data extraction forms, and discrepancies were resolved by consensus. Extracted data included information on study characteristics (author, publication date, country, study design, surgical procedure, duration of follow-up, sample size,

TABLE 1 | Baseline characteristics of included studies and participants.

Study	Country	Study design	Follow-up (mo)	Type of surgery	Total patients (n)	PCOS (n)	Age (yr)	Preop BMI (kg/m²)	Postop BMI (kg/m²)	EWL%	Outcomes extracted
Benito et al. (18)	Spain	Prospective	48	RYGB, SG, AGB	216	53	32.1 ± 5.3	44.6± 4.7	28.5 ± 4.1	–	②③⑥⑦
Bhandari et al. (19)	India	Prospective	6	SG	75	43	27.77 ± 4.50	42.52 ± 5.71	30.76± 2.93	58.37± 11.41	①⑤⑦
Casal et al. (10)	Spain	Retrospective	10.1 ± 1.5	LSG, LRYGB	217	43	33.19 ± 4.91	45.59 ± 4.97	27.73 ± 4.34		①
Chiofalo et al. (20)	Italy	Retrospective	12	SG, RYGB	55	29	30 ± 6	44 ± 7	–	65 ± 19	⑤⑦
Christ and Falcone, (21)	USA	Retrospective	22.8 ± 3.6	–	930	44	36.1 ± 2.3	44.2 ± 2.1	35.4 ± 1.5	–	②③⑦
Christinajoice et al. (22)	India	Retrospective	36	LSG, RYGB, LAGB	45	29	24.7 ± 10.2	41.5 ± 6.8		66.9 ± 24	④
Dilday et al. (23)	USA	Retrospective	12	SG	1385	119	31.5 ± 1.08	41.9 ± 5.2	29.55 ± 5.7	65.83 ± 21.8	⑦
Eid et al. (24)	USA	Retrospective	27.5 ± 16	LRYGB	24	24	34 ± 9.7	50 ± 7.5	30 ± 4.5	56.7	①④⑦
Eid et al. (25)	USA	Retrospective	12	LRYGB	14	14	36.3 ± 8.4	44.8 ± 1.6	29.2 ± 5.9	66.5	①②③④⑦
Escobar-Morreale et al. (26)	Spain	Prospective	12 ± 5	BPD, RYGB	36	17	29.8 ± 5.3	50.7 ± 7.1	41 ± 9	–	①②③⑦
Jamal et al. (27)	USA	Retrospective	46.7 ± 35.3	LRYGB	566	31	32 ± 5.8	52.8 ± 9.08	34.3 ± 5.7	64	④⑦
Singh et al. (28)	India	Prospective	12	LSG, LGB	50	18	29.7 ± 5.9	44.9 ± 7.5	–	63 ± 7.91	②④
Turkmen et al. (29)	Sweden	Prospective	6	RYGB	13	13	29.92 ± 7.12	47.15 ± 7.57	35.46 ± 7.04	–	①②⑥⑦
Wang et al. (30)	China	Prospective	12	LSG	48	24	25.5(22-35)	35.2(29-45.7)	31.7 ± 2.8	54 ± 24	①②⑦

BMI, body mass index; EWL%, excess weight loss percentage; SG, sleeve gastrectomy; RYGB, Roux-en-Y gastric bypass; AGB, adjustable gastric banding; LAGB, laparoscopic adjustable gastric banding; BPD, biliopancreatic diversion; LSG, laparoscopic sleeve gastrectomy; LRYGB, laparoscopic Roux-en-Y gastric bypass; LGB, laparoscopic gastric bypass; PCOS, polycystic ovary syndrome; ①, abnormal menstruation; ②, total testosterone; ③, free testosterone; ④, hirsutism; ⑤, AMH; ⑥, SHBG; ⑦, BMI.

PCOS cases), participant characteristics (age, body mass index [BMI]), and the outcomes mentioned above.

2.4 Quality Assessment and Risk of Bias

The methodological quality of RCTs was assessed using the Cochrane risk of bias tool (31). The quality of non-randomized studies was assessed using the MINORS scale (32). A higher score indicated a higher quality study. Disagreement among the reviewers was resolved by discussion. Funnel plots were examined to assess the publication bias.

2.5 Statistical Analysis

Statistical analyses were performed using Review Manager 5.4 (from the Cochrane Collaboration, http://www.cochrane.org). Odds ratios (OR) with 95% confidence intervals were calculated for dichotomous data. Mean difference (MD) or standardized mean difference (SMD) with 95% confidence intervals was calculated for continuous data. Heterogeneity was evaluated using Cochran's Q test, and the degree of inconsistency (I^2). I^2 values <30%, 30% to 50%, and >50% were interpreted as low, moderate, and considerable heterogeneity, respectively. We performed the meta-analysis using a fixed-effect model if there was no significant heterogeneity among studies; otherwise, a random-effect model was applied, and sensitivity analysis was performed to confirm the validity of the analysis results. In this meta-analysis, the test level was set to α=0.05. Publication bias was evaluated using funnel plots.

3 RESULTS

3.1 Search Results and Quality of Studies

The study selection process is summarized (**Figure 1**). From a total of 879 records, 192 were excluded due to duplication, 629 were excluded by title and abstract screening, and 44 were excluded after a further detailed review. A total of 14 studies conducted on 501 obese patients with PCOS were eligible and were in the meta-analysis (10, 18–30). After the quality assessment, no study was excluded because of lack of reliability (**Supplementary Table 2**).

3.2 Characteristics of Studies and Participants

The characteristics of the included studies are summarized **in Table 1**. These articles were published between 2005 and 2021. Overall, 3674 participants and 501 obese patients with PCOS were included in our analyses. Among the included studies, incidence of PCOS in obese women ranged from 5.5% to 63.5%.

3.3 Meta-Analysis Results

3.3.1 Abnormal Menstruation

Ten studies reported at least 6-month follow-up outcomes of abnormal menstruation (10, 19, 21, 24–30). Heterogeneity was considerable among studies (I^2 = 66%, P=0.002); thus, the random-effects model was used for analysis. Meta-analysis results showed that metabolic surgery could reduce the incidence of

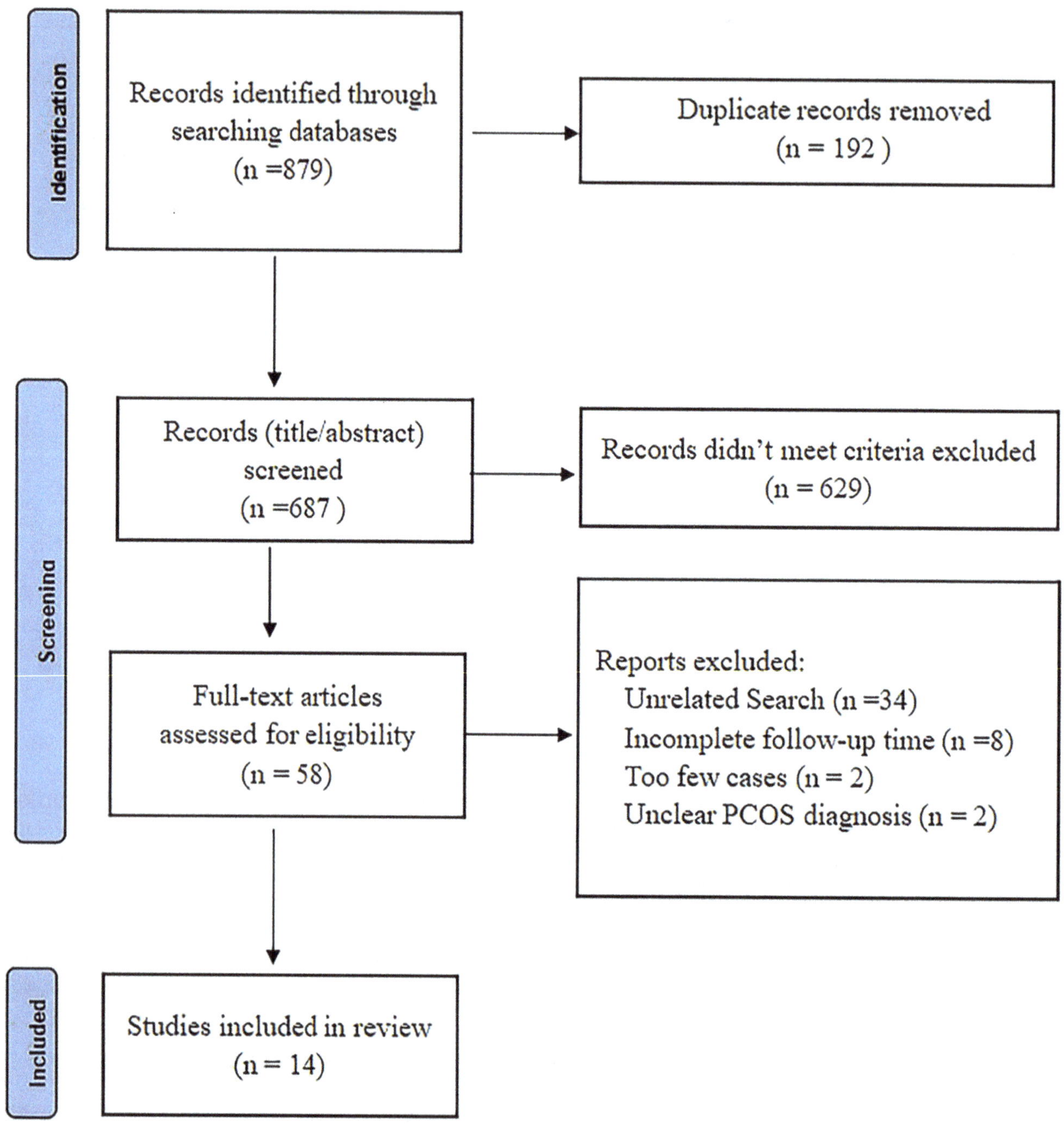

FIGURE 1 | PRISMA diagram of the systematic review.

menstrual abnormalities from 82% to 15% in women with PCOS [OR=0.03, 95%CI (0.01, 0.08), P<0.001] (**Figure 2A**).

3.3.2 Hirsutism

Changes in hirsutism were reported in five studies with 105 patients (21, 24, 25, 27, 28). Due to the high heterogeneity (I^2 = 69%, P<0.1), the random-effects model was employed. Data from the analysis revealed that metabolic surgery reduced the incidence of hirsutism from 71% to 38% [OR=0.21, 95%CI (0.06, 0.74), P=0.01] (**Figure 2B**).

3.3.3 Total Testosterone

Seven articles reported changes in total testosterone levels (18, 21, 25, 26, 28–30). The fixed-effects model was used for analysis because the heterogeneity was low (I^2 = 0%, P>0.1). The results showed a decrease of 25.92 ng/dL in total testosterone in patients

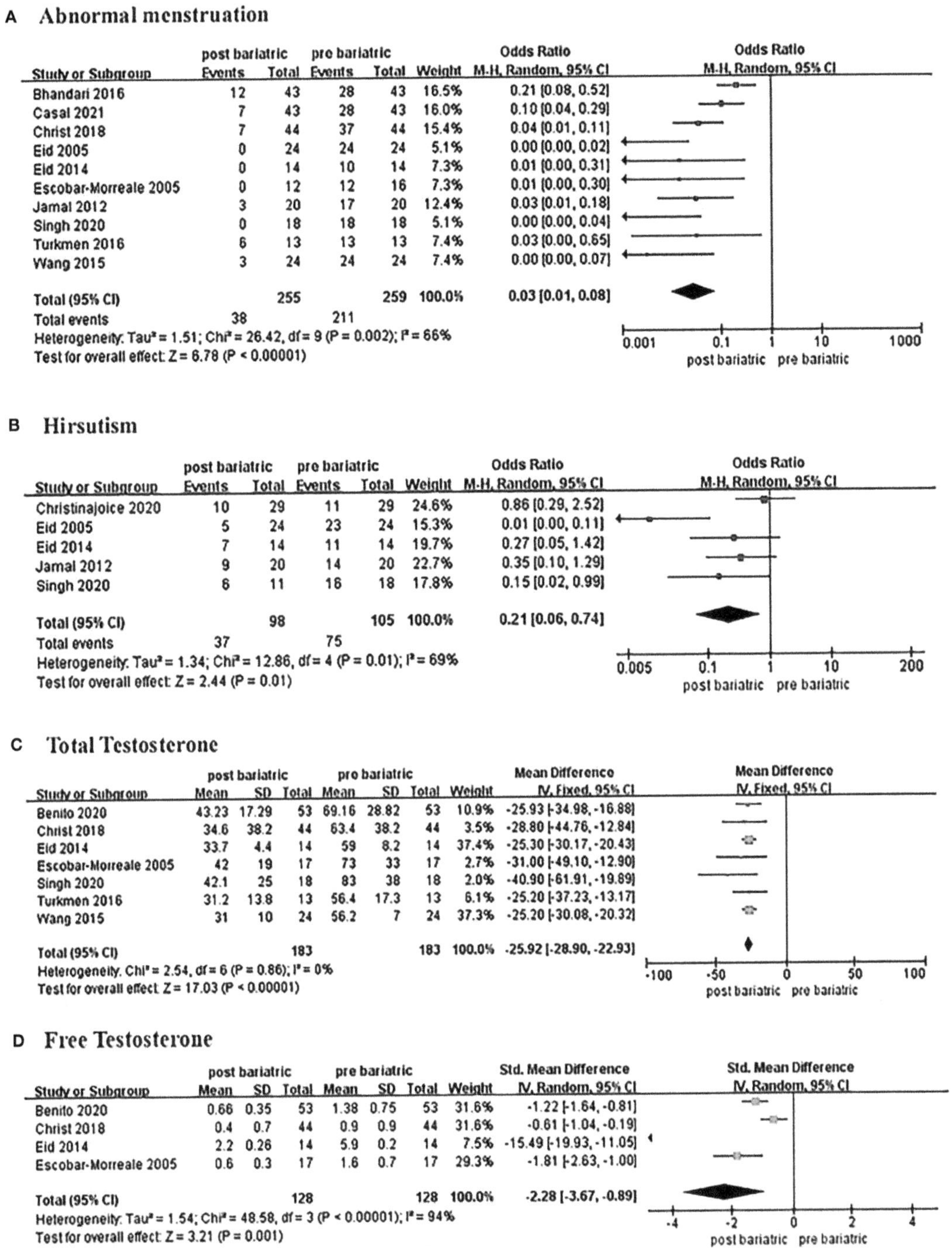

FIGURE 2 | Forrest plots showing changes of abnormal menstruation **(A)**, hirsutism **(B)**, total testosterone **(C)**, and free testosterone **(D)** in women with PCOS after metabolic surgery.

with PCOS after surgery [MD = -25.92, 95%CI (-28.90, -22.93), P< 0.00001] **(Figure 2C)**.

3.3.4 Free Testosterone

Four studies contributed to the meta-analysis in terms of free testosterone levels (18, 21, 25, 26) in 128 women with PCOS. Heterogeneity was considerable (I^2 = 94%, P<0.1) with regard to the measurement methods; hence, we adopted the standard mean difference (SMD) to summarize the data. The results of the meta-analysis showed that free testosterone in women with PCOS decreased by approximately 2.28 ng/dL after metabolic surgery [SMD = -2.28, 95%CI (-3.67, -0.89), P=0.001] **(Figure 2D)**.

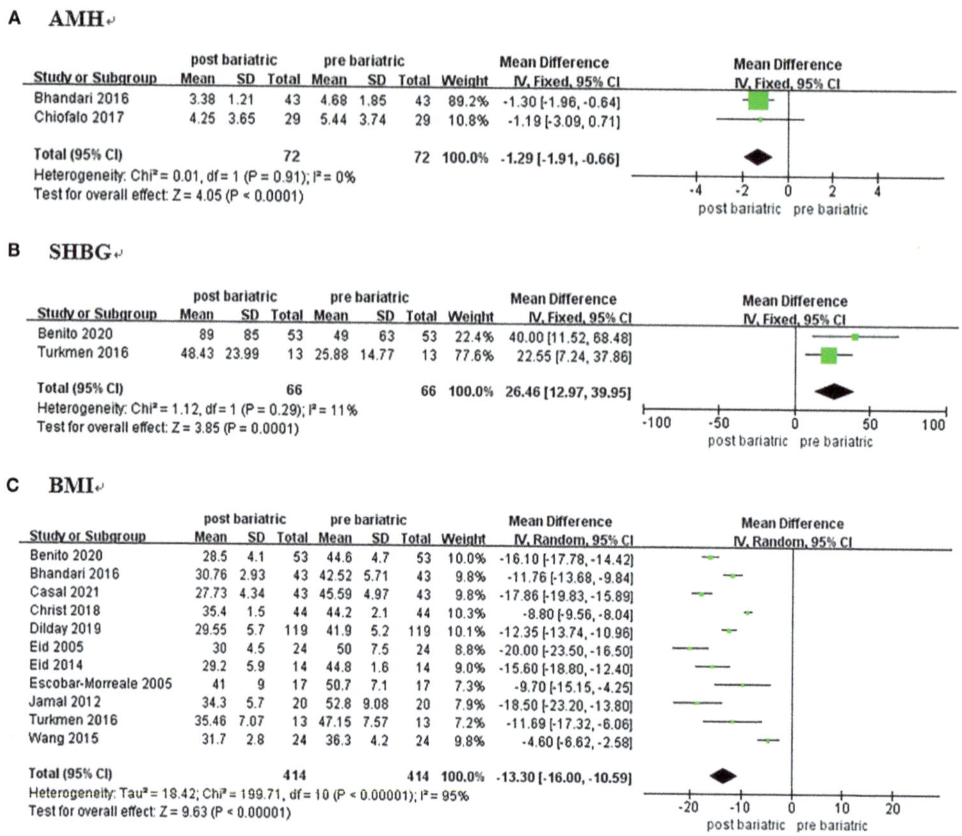

FIGURE 3 | Forrest plots showing changes of AMH **(A)**, SHBG **(B)**, and BMI **(C)** in women with PCOS after metabolic surgery.

3.3.5 AMH

Two studies compared the pre and postoperative differences in AMH (19, 20); a total of 72 women with PCOS were included. As there was low heterogeneity (I^2 = 0%, P>0.1), the estimate was assessed with fixed-effects model. There was a significant difference between groups [MD = -1.29, 95%CI (-1.92, -0.66), P<0.00001)] **(Figure 3A)**, and the results showed that AMH decreased by approximately 1.29 ng/mL after surgery.

3.3.6 SHBG

Two studies on 66 patients reporting pre and postoperative SHBG data were included (18, 29). The analysis was performed using a fixed-effects model because of low heterogeneity (I^2 = 11%, P=0.29). The results showed that SHBG in women with PCOS increased by approximately 26.46 nmol/L after metabolic surgery [MD = 26.46, 95%CI (12.97, 39.95), P = 0.001] **(Figure 3B; Table 2)**.

3.3.7 Body Mass Index

Eleven studies reported BMI among 414 patients (10, 18, 19, 21, 23–27, 29, 30). There was considerable heterogeneity detected (I^2 = 95%, P<0.00001), and the meta-analysis was performed with the random-effects model. BMI of the patients decreased by approximately 13.30 kg/m^2 after surgery [MD = -13.30, 95%CI (-16.00, -10.59), P< 0.00001] **(Figure 3C)**.

3.3.8 Fertility and Pregnancy Outcomes

Three studies reported the reproductive outcomes of women after surgery and revealed that 31/32 patients with PCOS with a desire to conceive became pregnant after surgery (18, 24, 27). Jamal et al. (27) found that no pregnancy or postpartum complications were reported after surgery. The study by Benito et al. (18) showed that the live birth rates were 81.0% after surgery.

3.4 Publication Bias

Publication bias was assessed using funnel plots for two outcomes (abnormal menstruation and BMI) as the number of included studies was more than 10. The results suggested the presence of publication bias in these studies (**Figure 4**).

4 DISCUSSION

This study is an updated systematic review and meta-analysis of the effects of metabolic surgery on PCOS. Fourteen high-quality studies including 501 patients were analyzed. The primary outcomes included changes in abnormal menstruation, hirsutism, and total and free testosterone levels. In addition, data on AMH and SHBG levels were integrated to gain a more comprehensive understanding of the beneficial effects of metabolic surgery. BMI and reproductive outcomes were also discussed. The principal findings of this study were as follows: (1) the incidence of abnormal menstruation decreased from 81% to 15% after metabolic surgery; (2) the incidence of hirsutism decreased from 71% to 38%; and (3) serum free testosterone, total testosterone, and AMH levels decreased, while SHBG levels increased postoperatively.

IR has been implicated in the pathogenesis of anovulation and infertility in PCOS, and abnormalities in insulin action have been observed in a variety of reproductive tissues in PCOS women (33). Obese women are more likely to have ovulatory dysfunction due to compensatory hyperinsulinism, hyperandrogenism and dysregulation of the hypothalamic-pituitary-ovarian axis, which manifests as sparse ovulation and menstrual abnormalities (34). Escobar-Morreale et al. (26) reported that weight reduction induced by Roux-en-Y gastric bypass (RYGB)/biliopancreatic diversion (BPD) contributed to the restoration of menstruation. In this study, the BMI decreased by 13.30 kg/m^2, and the incidence of abnormal menstruation decreased from 81% to 15%. Two similar meta-analyses conducted previously revealed that the remission rates of abnormal menstruation were 49% and 77%, respectively (15, 35). Although metabolic surgery improved abnormal menstruation, a few patients still experienced menstrual irregularities after surgery. Therefore, predictors of improvement in abnormal menstruation after surgery need to be clarified.

Furthermore, hyperandrogenemia is considered a core pathophysiological feature of PCOS. It impairs follicular growth and maturation and causes abnormal menstruation, sparse ovulation, and hirsutism (36, 37). As previously suggested, obese patients are more prone to IR, and both obesity and IR represent the fundamental features of PCOS, which contribute to its pathogenesis and reinforce hyperandrogenemia (38). SHBG binds testosterone and reduces free testosterone levels in the blood (39). Women with PCOS and lower serum SHBG levels have a higher risk of developing hyperandrogenism, obesity, type 2 diabetes, metabolic syndrome, and cardiovascular disease (39, 40). Our study showed that SHBG levels increased by 26.46 nmol/L postoperatively, while free testosterone and total testosterone levels decreased by 2.28 ng/dL and 25.92 ng/dL, respectively. In addition, the incidence of hirsutism decreased from 71% to 38%. We considered that metabolic surgery was superior to medication for improving hyperandrogenemia. In a previous meta-analysis, SHBG levels increased by 7.8 nmol/L and free testosterone levels decreased by 1.77 ng/dL after metformin + GLP-1 receptor agonist treatment (41).

AMH is a glycoprotein produced by granulosa cells when follicle growth is initiated (42). Excessive production of AMH in the ovaries, which inhibits normal follicle growth, is considered an important feature of PCOS (43, 44). Elevated serum AMH levels lead to PCOM and oligomenorrhea among women with PCOS (45). The present study initially integrated data on AMH levels in patients after metabolic surgery, and the findings indicated a decrease of 1.29 ng/mL. Changes in PCOM were not analyzed due to the lack of data; only one study reported a decrease from 50% to 44% (21). Weight loss helps regulate serum AMH levels, improve PCOM, and restore menstruation (46). Therefore, further studies are required to determine the effects of metabolic surgery on AMH and PCOM in patients with PCOS.

The reproductive outcomes of patients in three studies were reviewed, and a significant improvement in pregnancy and fertility outcomes was noted postoperatively. In a review of six studies, Butterworth et al. (6) reported that pregnancy rates ranged from 33% to 100% after metabolic surgery in patients with PCOS. However, the sample size was very small (2–11), and the follow-up time was short. Hence, Further studies are needed to outline the advantages and disadvantages of metabolic surgery in terms of reproductive outcomes. According to a previous study, metabolic surgery reduced the risk of gestational diabetes, excessive fetal growth, and shorter gestation; however, it also increased the risk of small-for-gestational-age infants and stillbirth or neonatal death (47). Based on consensus recommendations,

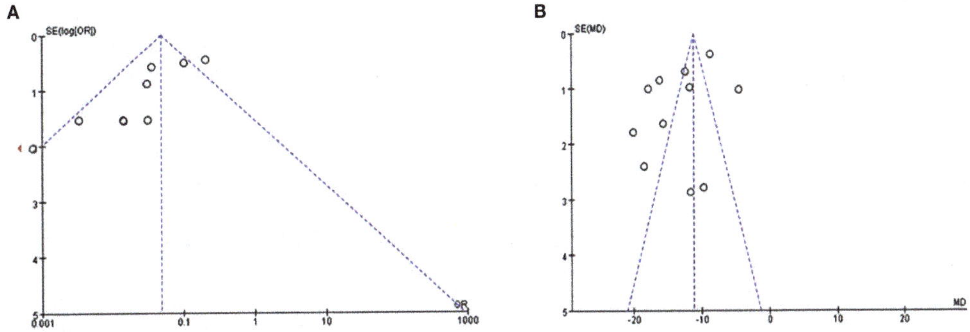

FIGURE 4 | Evaluate of publication bias by funnel plots of studies reporting on abnormal menstruation **(A)** and BMI **(B)**.

TABLE 2 | Summary for outcomes.

Outcomes	Number of studies	Number of cases	Heterogeneity test		Effect model	Meta-analysis results	
			I2(%)	P		Effect size (95%CI)	P
Abnormal menstruation	10	259	66	<.00001	REM	OR=0.03 [0.01, 0.08]	<.00001
Hirsutism	5	105	69	0.01	REM	OR=0.21 [0.06, 0.74]	0.004
Total testosterone	7	183	0	0.86	FEM	MD=-25.92 [-28.90,-22.93]	<.00001
Free testosterone	4	128	94	<.00001	REM	SMD=-2.28 [-3.67, -0.89]	0.001
AMH	2	72	0	0.91	FEM	MD=-1.29 [-1.91, -0.66]	<.00001
SHBG	2	59	0	0.46	FEM	MD=33.52 [10.87, 56.17]	0.004

CI, confidence interval; FEM, fixed effects model; MD, mean difference; OR, odds ratio; REM, random effects model; SMD, standardized mean difference.

pregnancy should be postponed to 1 year after sleeve gastrectomy/RYGB, when a stable weight is achieved (48). For obese patients with PCOS who aim for fertility and are thus seeking metabolic surgery, the appropriate time to conceive needs further discussion.

Few studies have discussed the mechanisms that improve PCOS symptoms after metabolic surgery (49–51). In obese women, IR and hyperinsulinemia promote androgen secretion leading to hyperandrogenemia. Furthermore, serum SHBG and growth hormone levels decrease, while leptin and luteinizing hormone levels increase. Thus, neuroregulation of the hypothalamic-pituitary-ovarian axis is severely disturbed, and these factors affect the occurrence and progression of PCOS at multiple levels (52, 53). Although PCOS is known to improve with weight loss and that weight loss is effective in restoring IR, hyperandrogenism, and the hypothalamic-pituitary-ovarian axis (54–56), there is a possible weight-loss-independent mechanism for PCOS improvement after metabolic surgery. Eid et al. (25) reported that menstruation recovery occurred within a few weeks after surgery, while there was no significant weight loss, which is consistent with the clinical experience of our center. And improvements in PCOS were not correlated with the degree of weight loss. There is a weight-loss-independent mechanism of diabetes mellitus control after metabolic surgery that involves changes in gut hormones, bile acids, and gut microbiota (57). These factors are also associated with the pathogenesis of PCOS (49). Therefore, we believe that changes in gut hormones, bile acids, and gut microbiota contribute to the improvement of PCOS after metabolic surgery. Nonetheless, further studies are needed to elucidate the underlying mechanism.

There has been existing reviews and meta-analyses with the same topic (15, 35, 56). However, it did not impair the innovation or value of the present study. The major strength of this study is as follows: firstly, five extra newly published articles were included (10, 18, 20, 22, 23), the latest ones of which were published in 2020 (18, 22) and 2021 (10). Secondly, AMH and SHBG, two indicators closely related to PCOS, but never evaluated in any of the existing reviews and meta-analyses mentioned above, were assessed and discussed in the present study for the first time. Thirdly, we reviewed the pregnancy rates and fertility outcomes of patients with PCOS after metabolic surgery through three articles included in this meta-analysis (18, 24, 27). We also discussed the advantages and disadvantages of metabolic surgery on reproductive outcomes in patients with PCOS, as well as the optimal timing to conceive after surgery. Furthermore, all the articles included in the present study are with a follow-up time of >6 months and the number of PCOS cases>10, thus providing more credible and convincing evidence.

It should be noted that the present study had a few limitations. The heterogeneity was considerable in a part of outcomes which may resulted due to the differences in population characteristics, duration of follow-up, and diagnostic criteria for PCOS used among studies included. Moreover, potential publication bias was observed in the current study due to unpublished articles with negative results.

5 CONCLUSION

This study demonstrated that metabolic surgery significantly improved abnormal menstruation, hirsutism, and hyperandrogenism in women with PCOS. Serum AMH levels increased, and SHBG levels decreased postoperatively. Metabolic surgery may be a new viable treatment option for obese patients with PCOS. Further studies are required to confirm these beneficial effects and elucidate the underlying mechanisms.

AUTHOR CONTRIBUTIONS

WY, XH and WZ were major contributors in writing the Manuscript. WY, XH, and WZ contributed to literature search, screening, and data extraction. SLi, XL and YZ contributed to statistical analyses. JS and TL contributed to data validation. WL and SLiu. are responsible for review and modification of the manuscript. All authors read and approved the final manuscript.

ACKNOWLEDGMENTS

All the authors of included original studies should be appreciated sincerely. We thank Elsevier Language Editing Services for English language editing.

REFERENCES

1. Lizneva D, Suturina L, Walker W, Brakta S, Gavrilova-Jordan L, Azziz R. Criteria, Prevalence, and Phenotypes of Polycystic Ovary Syndrome. *Fertil Steril* (2016) 106(1):6–15. doi: 10.1016/j.fertnstert.2016.05.003
2. Teede H, Deeks A, Moran L. Polycystic Ovary Syndrome: A Complex Condition With Psychological, Reproductive and Metabolic Manifestations That Impacts on Health Across the Lifespan. *BMC Med* (2010) 8:41. doi: 10.1186/1741-7015-8-41
3. Sedighi S, Amir Ali Akbari S, Afrakhteh M, Esteki T, Alavi Majd H, Mahmoodi Z. Comparison of Lifestyle in Women With Polycystic Ovary Syndrome and Healthy Women. *Global J Health Sci* (2014) 7(1):228–34. doi: 10.5539/gjhs.v7n1p228
4. Sirmans SM, Pate KA. Epidemiology, Diagnosis, and Management of Polycystic Ovary Syndrome. *Clin Epidemiol* (2013) 6:1–13. doi: 10.2147/CLEP.S37559
5. Williams T, Mortada R, Porter S. Diagnosis and Treatment of Polycystic Ovary Syndrome. *Am Family Physician* (2016) 94(2):106–13.
6. Butterworth J, Deguara J, Borg CM. Bariatric Surgery, Polycystic Ovary Syndrome, and Infertility. *J Obes* (2016) 2016:1871594. doi: 10.1155/2016/1871594
7. Li L, Zhang J, Deng Q, Li J, Li Z, Xiao Y, et al. Proteomic Profiling for Identification of Novel Biomarkers Differentially Expressed in Human Ovaries From Polycystic Ovary Syndrome Patients. *PloS One* (2016) 11(11): e0164538-e. doi: 10.1371/journal.pone.0164538
8. Luque-Ramírez M, Alpañés M, Escobar-Morreale H. The Determinants of Insulin Sensitivity, β-Cell Function, and Glucose Tolerance Are Different in Patients With Polycystic Ovary Syndrome Than in Women Who do Not Have Hyperandrogenism. *Fertil Steril* (2010) 94(6):2214–21. doi: 10.1016/j.fertnstert.2009.11.049
9. Fica S, Albu A, Constantin M, Dobri GA. Insulin Resistance and Fertility in Polycystic Ovary Syndrome. *J Med Life* (2008) 1(4):415–22.
10. Casals G, Andreu A, Barral Y, Ventosa S, Redondo M, Torres F, et al. Bariatric Surgery on Reproductive Outcomes: The Impact According to the Diagnosis of Polycystic Ovarian Syndrome and Surgical Procedures. *Obes Surg* (2021) 31 (6):2590–8. doi: 10.1007/s11695-021-05297-x
11. Wing RR, Lang W, Wadden TA, Safford M, Knowler WC, Bertoni AG, et al. Benefits of Modest Weight Loss in Improving Cardiovascular Risk Factors in Overweight and Obese Individuals With Type 2 Diabetes. *Diabetes Care* (2011) 34(7):1481–6. doi: 10.2337/dc10-2415
12. Legro RS, Arslanian SA, Ehrmann DA, Hoeger KM, Murad MH, Pasquali R, et al. Diagnosis and Treatment of Polycystic Ovary Syndrome: An Endocrine Society Clinical Practice Guideline. *J Clin Endocrinol Metab* (2013) 98 (12):4565–92. doi: 10.1210/jc.2013-2350
13. Cummings S, Pratt J. Metabolic and Bariatric Surgery: Nutrition and Dental Considerations. *J Am Dental Assoc (1939)* (2015) 146(10):767–72. doi: 10.1016/j.adaj.2015.06.004
14. Garvey WT, Mechanick JI, Brett EM, Garber AJ, Hurley DL, Jastreboff AM, et al. American Association of Clinical Endocrinologists and American College of Endocrinology Comprehensive Clinical Practice Guidelines for Medical Care of Patients With Obesity. *Endocr Pract* (2016) 22(Suppl 3):1–203. doi: 10.4158/EP161365.GL
15. Li YJ, Han Y, He B. Effects of Bariatric Surgery on Obese Polycystic Ovary Syndrome: A Systematic Review and Meta-Analysis. *Surg Obes Relat Dis* (2019) 15(6):942–50. doi: 10.1016/j.soard.2019.03.032
16. Liberati A, Altman DG, Tetzlaff J, Mulrow C, Gotzsche PC, Ioannidis JP, et al. The PRISMA Statement for Reporting Systematic Reviews and Meta-Analyses of Studies That Evaluate Healthcare Interventions: Explanation and Elaboration. *BMJ* (2009) 339:b2700. doi: 10.1136/bmj.b2700
17. Stroup DF, Berlin JA, Morton SC, Olkin I, Williamson GD, Rennie D, et al. Meta-Analysis of Observational Studies in Epidemiology: A Proposal for Reporting. Meta-Analysis Of Observational Studies in Epidemiology (MOOSE) Group. *Jama* (2000) 283(15):2008–12. doi: 10.1001/jama.283.15.2008
18. Benito E, Gomez-Martin JM, Vega-Pinero B, Priego P, Galindo J, Escobar-Morreale HF, et al. Fertility and Pregnancy Outcomes in Women With Polycystic Ovary Syndrome Following Bariatric Surgery. *J Clin Endocrinol Metab* (2020) 105(9):e3384–91. doi: 10.1210/clinem/dgaa439
19. Bhandari S, Ganguly I, Bhandari M, Agarwal P, Singh A, Gupta N, et al. Effect of Sleeve Gastrectomy Bariatric Surgery-Induced Weight Loss on Serum AMH Levels in Reproductive Aged Women. *Gynecol Endocrinol* (2016) 32 (10):799–802. doi: 10.3109/09513590.2016.1169267
20. Chiofalo F, Ciuoli C, Formichi C, Selmi F, Forleo R, Neri O, et al. Bariatric Surgery Reduces Serum Anti-Mullerian Hormone Levels in Obese Women With and Without Polycystic Ovarian Syndrome. *Obes Surg* (2017) 27 (7):1750–4. doi: 10.1007/s11695-016-2528-y
21. Christ JP, Falcone T. Bariatric Surgery Improves Hyperandrogenism, Menstrual Irregularities, and Metabolic Dysfunction Among Women With Polycystic Ovary Syndrome (PCOS). *Obes Surg* (2018) 28(8):2171–7. doi: 10.1007/s11695-018-3155-6
22. Christinajoice S, Misra S, Bhattacharya S, Kumar SS, Nandhini BD, Palanivelu C, et al. Impact of Bariatric Surgery on Female Reproductive Health and Maternal Outcomes. *Obes Surg* (2020) 30(2):383–90. doi: 10.1007/s11695-019-04245-0
23. Dilday J, Derickson M, Kuckelman J, Reitz C, Ahnfeldt E, Martin M, et al. Sleeve Gastrectomy for Obesity in Polycystic Ovarian Syndrome: A Pilot Study Evaluating Weight Loss and Fertility Outcomes. *Obes Surg* (2019) 29 (1):93–8. doi: 10.1007/s11695-018-3473-8
24. Eid GM, Cottam DR, Velcu LM, Mattar SG, Korytkowski MT, Gosman G, et al. Effective Treatment of Polycystic Ovarian Syndrome With Roux-En-Y Gastric Bypass. *Surg Obes Relat Dis* (2005) 1(2):77–80. doi: 10.1016/j.soard.2005.02.008
25. Eid GM, McCloskey C, Titchner R, Korytkowski M, Gross D, Grabowski C, et al. Changes in Hormones and Biomarkers in Polycystic Ovarian Syndrome Treated With Gastric Bypass. *Surg Obes Relat Dis* (2014) 10(5):787–91. doi: 10.1016/j.soard.2014.02.046
26. Escobar-Morreale HF, Botella-Carretero JI, Alvarez-Blasco F, Sancho J, San Millan JL. The Polycystic Ovary Syndrome Associated With Morbid Obesity may Resolve After Weight Loss Induced by Bariatric Surgery. *J Clin Endocrinol Metab* (2005) 90(12):6364–9. doi: 10.1210/jc.2005-1490
27. Jamal M, Gunay Y, Capper A, Eid A, Heitshusen D, Samuel I. Roux-En-Y Gastric Bypass Ameliorates Polycystic Ovary Syndrome and Dramatically Improves Conception Rates: A 9-Year Analysis. *Surg Obes Relat Dis* (2012) 8 (4):440–4. doi: 10.1016/j.soard.2011.09.022
28. Singh D, Arumalla K, Aggarwal S, Singla V, Ganie A, Malhotra N. Impact of Bariatric Surgery on Clinical, Biochemical, and Hormonal Parameters in Women With Polycystic Ovary Syndrome (PCOS). *Obes Surg* (2020) 30 (6):2294–300. doi: 10.1007/s11695-020-04487-3
29. Turkmen S, Ahangari A, Backstrom T. Roux-En-Y Gastric Bypass Surgery in Patients With Polycystic Ovary Syndrome and Metabolic Syndrome. *Obes Surg* (2016) 26(1):111–8. doi: 10.1007/s11695-015-1729-0
30. Wang K, Jiang Q, Zhi Y, Zhu Z, Zhou Z, Xie Y, et al. Contrasting Sleeve Gastrectomy With Lifestyle Modification Therapy in the Treatment of Polycystic Ovary Syndrome. *J Laparoendosc Adv Surg Tech* (2015) 25 (6):493–8. doi: 10.1089/lap.2014.0511

31. Furlan AD, Malmivaara A, Chou R, Maher CG, Deyo RA, Schoene M, et al. Updated Method Guideline for Systematic Reviews in the Cochrane Back and Neck Group. *Spine (Phila Pa 1976)* (2015) 40(21):1660–73. doi: 10.1097/BRS.0000000000001061
32. Slim K, Nini E, Forestier D, Kwiatkowski F, Panis Y, Chipponi J. Methodological Index for Non-Randomized Studies (Minors): Development and Validation of a New Instrument. *ANZ J Surg* (2003) 73(9):712–6. doi: 10.1046/j.1445-2197.2003.02748.x
33. Wang Y, Fu X, Xu J, Wang Q, Kuang H. Systems Pharmacology to Investigate the Interaction of Berberine and Other Drugs in Treating Polycystic Ovary Syndrome. *Sci Rep* (2016) 6:28089-. doi: 10.1038/srep28089
34. Broughton DE, Moley KH. Obesity and Female Infertility: Potential Mediators of Obesity's Impact. *Fertil Steril* (2017) 107(4):840–7. doi: 10.1016/j.fertnstert.2017.01.017
35. Skubleny D, Switzer NJ, Gill RS, Dykstra M, Shi X, Sagle MA, et al. The Impact of Bariatric Surgery on Polycystic Ovary Syndrome: A Systematic Review and Meta-Analysis. *Obes Surg* (2016) 26(1):169–76. doi: 10.1007/s11695-015-1902-5
36. Zeng X, Xie YJ, Liu YT, Long SL, Mo ZC. Polycystic Ovarian Syndrome: Correlation Between Hyperandrogenism, Insulin Resistance and Obesity. *Clin Chim Acta* (2020) 502:214–21. doi: 10.1016/j.cca.2019.11.003
37. Zhao X, Zhong J, Mo Y, Chen X, Chen Y, Yang D. Association of Biochemical Hyperandrogenism With Type 2 Diabetes and Obesity in Chinese Women With Polycystic Ovary Syndrome. *Int J Gynaecol Obstet* (2010) 108(2):148–51. doi: 10.1016/j.ijgo.2009.09.021
38. Regidor PA, Mueller A, Sailer M, Gonzalez Santos F, Rizo JM, Egea FM. Chronic Inflammation in PCOS: The Potential Benefits of Specialized Pro-Resolving Lipid Mediators (SPMs) in the Improvement of the Resolutive Response. *Int J Mol Sci* (2020) 22(1):384. doi: 10.3390/ijms22010384
39. Deswal R, Yadav A, Dang AS. Sex Hormone Binding Globulin - an Important Biomarker for Predicting PCOS Risk: A Systematic Review and Meta-Analysis. *Syst Biol Reprod Med* (2018) 64(1):12–24. doi: 10.1080/19396368.2017.1410591
40. Veldhuis JD, Dyer RB, Trushin SA, Bondar OP, Singh RJ, Klee GG. Immunologic and Mass-Spectrometric Estimates of SHBG Concentrations in Healthy Women. *Metabol: Clin Exp* (2014) 63(6):783–92. doi: 10.1016/j.metabol.2014.03.010
41. Xing C, Li C, He B. Insulin Sensitizers for Improving the Endocrine and Metabolic Profile in Overweight Women With PCOS. *J Clin Endocrinol Metab* (2020) 105(9):2950–63. doi: 10.1210/clinem/dgaa337
42. Iliodromiti S, Kelsey TW, Anderson RA, Nelson SM. Can Anti-Mullerian Hormone Predict the Diagnosis of Polycystic Ovary Syndrome? A Systematic Review and Meta-Analysis of Extracted Data. *J Clin Endocrinol Metab* (2013) 98(8):3332–40. doi: 10.1210/jc.2013-1393
43. Bednarska-Czerwińska A, Olszak-Wąsik K, Olejek A, Czerwiński M, Tukiendorf AA. Vitamin D and Anti-Müllerian Hormone Levels in Infertility Treatment: The Change-Point Problem. *Nutrients* (2019) 11 (5):1053. doi: 10.3390/nu11051053
44. Dumont A, Robin G, Catteau-Jonard S, Dewailly D. Role of Anti-Müllerian Hormone in Pathophysiology, Diagnosis and Treatment of Polycystic Ovary Syndrome: A Review. *Reprod Biol Endocrinol: RB&E* (2015) 13:137. doi: 10.1186/s12958-015-0134-9
45. Song DK, Oh JY, Lee H, Sung YA. Differentiation Between Polycystic Ovary Syndrome and Polycystic Ovarian Morphology by Means of an Anti-Müllerian Hormone Cutoff Value. *Korean J Internal Med* (2017) 32(4):690–8. doi: 10.3904/kjim.2016.038
46. Nybacka Å, Carlström K, Fabri F, Hellström PM, Hirschberg AL. Serum Antimüllerian Hormone in Response to Dietary Management and/or Physical Exercise in Overweight/Obese Women With Polycystic Ovary Syndrome: Secondary Analysis of a Randomized Controlled Trial. *Fertil Steril* (2013) 100 (4):1096–102. doi: 10.1016/j.fertnstert.2013.06.030
47. Johansson K, Cnattingius S, Näslund I, Roos N, Trolle Lagerros Y, Granath F, et al. Outcomes of Pregnancy After Bariatric Surgery. *N Engl J Med* (2015) 372 (9):814–24. doi: 10.1056/NEJMoa1405789
48. Shawe J, Ceulemans D, Akhter Z, Neff K, Hart K, Heslehurst N, et al. Pregnancy After Bariatric Surgery: Consensus Recommendations for Periconception, Antenatal and Postnatal Care. *Obes Rev* (2019) 20 (11):1507–22. doi: 10.1111/obr.12927
49. Giampaolino P, Foreste V, Di Filippo C, Gallo A, Mercorio A, Serafino P, et al. Microbiome and PCOS: State-Of-Art and Future Aspects. *Int J Mol Sci* (2021) 22(4):2048. doi: 10.3390/ijms22042048
50. Lin W, Wen L, Wen J, Xiang G. Effects of Sleeve Gastrectomy on Fecal Gut Microbiota and Short-Chain Fatty Acid Content in a Rat Model of Polycystic Ovary Syndrome. *Front Endocrinol* (2021) 12:747888. doi: 10.3389/fendo.2021.747888
51. Wen L, Lin W, Li Q, Chen G, Wen J. Effect of Sleeve Gastrectomy on Kisspeptin Expression in the Hypothalamus of Rats With Polycystic Ovary Syndrome. *Obes (Silver Spring)* (2020) 28(6):1117–28. doi: 10.1002/oby.22795
52. Silvestris E, de Pergola G, Rosania R, Loverro G. Obesity as Disruptor of the Female Fertility. *Reprod Biol Endocrinol: RB&E* (2018) 16(1):22. doi: 10.1186/s12958-018-0336-z
53. Wang F, Dai W, Yang XH, Guo YH, Sun YP. Analyses of Optimal Body Mass Index for Infertile Patients With Either Polycystic or Non-Polycystic Ovary Syndrome During Assisted Reproductive Treatment in China. *Sci Rep* (2016) 6:34538. doi: 10.1038/srep34538
54. Li L, Feng Q, Ye M, He Y, Yao A, Shi K. Metabolic Effect of Obesity on Polycystic Ovary Syndrome in Adolescents: A Meta-Analysis. *J Obstet Gynaecol* (2017) 37(8):1036–47. doi: 10.1080/01443615.2017.1318840
55. Terra X, Auguet T, Guiu-Jurado E, Berlanga A, Orellana-Gavaldà JM, Hernández M, et al. Long-Term Changes in Leptin, Chemerin and Ghrelin Levels Following Different Bariatric Surgery Procedures: Roux-En-Y Gastric Bypass and Sleeve Gastrectomy. *Obes Surg* (2013) 23(11):1790–8. doi: 10.1007/s11695-013-1033-9
56. Lee R, Joy Mathew C, Jose MT, Elshaikh AO, Shah L. Cancarevic I. A Review of the Impact of Bariatric Surgery in Women With Polycystic Ovary Syndrome. *Cureus* (2020) 12(10):e10811. doi: 10.7759/cureus.10811
57. Liu H, Hu C, Zhang X, Jia W. Role of Gut Microbiota, Bile Acids and Their Cross-Talk in the Effects of Bariatric Surgery on Obesity and Type 2 Diabetes. *J Diabetes Invest* (2018) 9(1):13–20. doi: 10.1111/jdi.12687

Permissions

All chapters in this book were first published by Frontiers; hereby published with permission under the Creative Commons Attribution License or equivalent. Every chapter published in this book has been scrutinized by our experts. Their significance has been extensively debated. The topics covered herein carry significant findings which will fuel the growth of the discipline. They may even be implemented as practical applications or may be referred to as a beginning point for another development.

The contributors of this book come from diverse backgrounds, making this book a truly international effort. This book will bring forth new frontiers with its revolutionizing research information and detailed analysis of the nascent developments around the world.

We would like to thank all the contributing authors for lending their expertise to make the book truly unique. They have played a crucial role in the development of this book. Without their invaluable contributions this book wouldn't have been possible. They have made vital efforts to compile up to date information on the varied aspects of this subject to make this book a valuable addition to the collection of many professionals and students.

This book was conceptualized with the vision of imparting up-to-date information and advanced data in this field. To ensure the same, a matchless editorial board was set up. Every individual on the board went through rigorous rounds of assessment to prove their worth. After which they invested a large part of their time researching and compiling the most relevant data for our readers.

The editorial board has been involved in producing this book since its inception. They have spent rigorous hours researching and exploring the diverse topics which have resulted in the successful publishing of this book. They have passed on their knowledge of decades through this book. To expedite this challenging task, the publisher supported the team at every step. A small team of assistant editors was also appointed to further simplify the editing procedure and attain best results for the readers.

Apart from the editorial board, the designing team has also invested a significant amount of their time in understanding the subject and creating the most relevant covers. They scrutinized every image to scout for the most suitable representation of the subject and create an appropriate cover for the book.

The publishing team has been an ardent support to the editorial, designing and production team. Their endless efforts to recruit the best for this project, has resulted in the accomplishment of this book. They are a veteran in the field of academics and their pool of knowledge is as vast as their experience in printing. Their expertise and guidance has proved useful at every step. Their uncompromising quality standards have made this book an exceptional effort. Their encouragement from time to time has been an inspiration for everyone.

The publisher and the editorial board hope that this book will prove to be a valuable piece of knowledge for researchers, students, practitioners and scholars across the globe.

List of Contributors

Mohammed K. Hankir
Department of Experimental Surgery, University Hospital Wuerzburg, Wuerzburg, Germany

Florian Seyfried
Department of General, Visceral, Vascular and Pediatric Surgery, University Hospital Wuerzburg, Wuerzburg, Germany

Lidia Castagneto-Gissey, James Casella-Mariolo and Giovanni Casella
Department of Surgical Sciences, Sapienza University of Rome, Rome, Italy

Geltrude Mingrone
Division of Diabetes & Nutritional Sciences, Fondazione Policlinico Universitario A. Gemelli IRCCS, Rome, Italy
Division of Diabetes & Nutritional Sciences, Università Cattolica del Sacro Cuore Rome, Rome, Italy
Division of Diabetes & Nutritional Sciences, Faculty of Life Sciences & Medicine, King's College London, London, United Kingdom

William P. Martin, James White and Neil G. Docherty
Diabetes Complications Research Centre, School of Medicine, Conway Institute of Biomolecular and Biomedical Research, University College Dublin, Dublin, Ireland

Francisco J. López-Hernández
Instituto de Estudios de Ciencias de la Salud de Castilla y León-Instituto de Investigación Biomédica de Salamanca (IECSCYL-IBSAL), Hospital Virgen Vega, Salamanca, Spain

Carel W. le Roux
Diabetes Complications Research Centre, School of Medicine, Conway Institute of Biomolecular and Biomedical Research, University College Dublin, Dublin, Ireland
Division of Investigative Science, Imperial College London, London, United Kingdom

Elina Akalestou and Guy A. Rutter
Section of Cell Biology and Functional Genomics, Division of Diabetes, Endocrinology and Metabolism, Department of Metabolism, Digestion and Reproduction, Imperial Centre for Translational and Experimental Medicine, Imperial College London, London, United Kingdom

Laurent Genser
Section of Cell Biology and Functional Genomics, Division of Diabetes, Endocrinology and Metabolism, Department of Metabolism, Digestion and Reproduction, Imperial Centre for Translational and Experimental Medicine, Imperial College London, London, United Kingdom
Department of Digestive and Hepato-Pancreato-Biliary Surgery, Liver Transplantation, Assistance Publique-Hôpitaux de Paris, Pitié-Salpêtrière University Hospital, Institut Hospitalo-Universitaire ICAN, Sorbonne Université, Paris, France

Chrysi Koliaki, Evangelia Tzeravini, Eleftheria Papachristoforou, Ioanna Severi, Nicholas Tentolouris and Alexander Kokkinos
First Department of Propaedeutic Internal Medicine and Diabetes Center, Medical School, National and Kapodistrian University of Athens, Laiko General Hospital, Athens, Greece

Elina El Deik, Melina Karaolia, Marina Noutsou and Anastasia Thanopoulou
Diabetes Center, Second Department of Internal Medicine, Medical School, Hippokratio General Hospital, National and Kapodistrian University of Athens, Athens, Greece

Aikaterini Kountouri, Konstantinos Balampanis and Vaia Lambadiari
Second Department of Internal Medicine and Research Institute, Medical School, National and Kapodistrian University of Athens, Attikon General Hospital, Athens, Greece

Giuseppe Daniele, Simone Codini, Annamaria Ciccarone, Laura Giusti and Stefano Del Prato
Department of Clinical and Experimental Medicine, University of Pisa, Pisa, Italy

Beatrice Campi and Ele Ferrannini
C.N.R. Institute of Clinical Physiology, Pisa, Italy

Alessandro Saba
Department of Surgical, Medical and Molecular Pathology and Critical Care Medicine, University of Pisa, Pisa, Italy
Laboratory of Clinical Pathology, St. Chiara University Hospital, Pisa, Italy

Russel L. Esterline
AstraZeneca Pharmaceutical, Gaithersburg, MD, United States

Jayanthi Raman and Dean Spirou
Discipline of Clinical Psychology, Graduate School of Health, University of Technology Sydney, Sydney, NSW, Australia

Lisbeth Jahren
Library Section for Medicine and Health Sciences, NTNU University Library, NTNU-Norwegian University of Science and Technology, Trondheim, Norway

Trine Tetlie Eik-Nes
Department of Neuromedicine and Movement Science, Faculty of Medicine and Health Sciences, NTNU-Norwegian University of Science and Technology, Trondheim, Norway

Emmanouil Korakas, Aikaterini Kountouri and Athanasios Raptis
Second Department of Internal Medicine, Medical School, Attikon University Hospital, National and Kapodistrian University of Athens, Athens, Greece

Alexander Kokkinos
First Department of Propaedeutic Medicine, Medical School, Laiko General Hospital, National and Kapodistrian University of Athens, Athens, Greece

Sana Sultan, Benjamin Whitelaw, Bianca M. Leca, Simon J. B. Aywlin and Georgios K. Dimitriadis
Department of Endocrinology and Metabolic Medicine, King's College Hospital NHS Foundation Trust, London, United Kingdom

Ameet G. Patel and Francesco Rubino
Department of Minimal Access Surgery, King's College Hospital NHS Foundation Trust, London, United Kingdom

Shamsi El-Hassani
Minimal Access and Bariatric Unit, Princess Royal University Hospital, King's College Hospital NHS Foundation Trust, Orpington, United Kingdom

Royce P. Vincent
Department of Clinical Biochemistry, King's College Hospital NHS Foundation Trust, London, United Kingdom

Jorunn Sandvik
Clinic of Medicine and Rehabilitation, Møre and Romsdal Hospital Trust, Alesund, Norway
Department of Surgery, Center for Obesity, St. Olav Hospital, Trondheim University Hospital, Trondheim, Norway
Obesity Research Group, Department of Clinical and Molecular Medicine, Norwegian University of Science and Technology, Trondheim, Norway

Torstein Hole
Clinic of Medicine and Rehabilitation, Møre and Romsdal Hospital Trust, Alesund, Norway
Faculty of Medicine and Health Sciences, Norwegian University of Science and Technology, Trondheim, Norway

Christian Klöckner
Department of Surgery, Center for Obesity, St. Olav Hospital, Trondheim University Hospital, Trondheim, Norway
Department of Psychology, NTNU - Norwegian University of Science and Technology, Trondheim, Norway

Bård Kulseng
Department of Surgery, Center for Obesity, St. Olav Hospital, Trondheim University Hospital, Trondheim, Norway
Obesity Research Group, Department of Clinical and Molecular Medicine, Norwegian University of Science and Technology, Trondheim, Norway

Arne Wibe
Department of Clinical and Molecular Medicine, Norwegian University of Science and Technology, Trondheim, Norway
Department of Surgery, St. Olav Hospital, Trondheim University Hospital, Trondheim, Norway

Fatima Cody Stanford and Vibha Singhal
Neuroendocrine Unit, Massachusetts General Hospital and Harvard Medical School, Boston, MA, United States
Pediatric Endocrinology, Massachusetts General Hospital and Harvard Medical School, Boston, MA, United States
MGH Weight Center, Massachusetts General Hospital, Boston, MA, United States

Tasnim Mushannen
Neuroendocrine Unit, Massachusetts General Hospital and Harvard Medical School, Boston, MA, United States
Weill Cornell Medicine, Education City, Al Rayyan, Qatar

Priscilla Cortez
Neuroendocrine Unit, Massachusetts General Hospital and Harvard Medical School, Boston, MA, United States
Department of Biology, College of Science, University of Arizona, Tucson, AZ, United States

Karen J. Campoverde Reyes
Neuroendocrine Unit, Massachusetts General Hospital and Harvard Medical School, Boston, MA, United States
Liver Research Center, Beth Israel Deaconess Medical Center, Boston, MA, United States

Hang Lee
Departments of Biostatistics and Harvard Medical School, Boston, MA, United States

Denise W. Gee
MGH Weight Center, Massachusetts General Hospital, Boston, MA, United States

Janey S. Pratt
Department of Surgery and Pediatric Surgery and Stanford University School of Medicine, Stanford, CA, United States

Paul A. Boepple
Pediatric Endocrinology, Massachusetts General Hospital and Harvard Medical School, Boston, MA, United States
MGH Weight Center, Massachusetts General Hospital, Boston, MA, United States

Miriam A. Bredella
Department of Radiology, Massachusetts General Hospital and Harvard Medical School, Boston, MA, United States

Madhusmita Misra
Neuroendocrine Unit, Massachusetts General Hospital and Harvard Medical School, Boston, MA, United States
Pediatric Endocrinology, Massachusetts General Hospital and Harvard Medical School, Boston, MA, United States

Karl J. Neff
Diabetes Complications Research Centre, Conway Institute, University College Dublin, Dublin, Ireland,

Abdullah Alkandari
Department of Surgery and Cancer, Imperial College London, London, United Kingdom
Dasman Diabetes Institute, Kuwait City, Kuwait

Hutan Ashrafian and Ara Darzi
Department of Surgery and Cancer, Imperial College London, London, United Kingdom
Institute of Global Health Innovation, Imperial College London, London, United Kingdom

Thozhukat Sathyapalan
Department of Academic Endocrinology, Diabetes, and Metabolism, Hull York Medical School, Kingston upon Hull, United Kingdom

Elaine Holmes, Thanos Athanasiou and Nigel J. Gooderham
Department of Surgery and Cancer, Imperial College London, London, United Kingdom

Stephen L. Atkin
Weill Cornell Medical College Qatar, Qatar Foundation, Doha, Qatar

Isabel Cornejo-Pareja, Mercedes Clemente-Postigo and Francisco J. Tinahones
Unidad de Gestión Clínica Endocrinología y Nutrición, Instituto de Investigación Biomédica de Málaga—IBIMA, Hospital Universitario Virgen de la Victoria, Universidad de Málaga, Málaga, Spain
Centro de Investigación Biomédica en Red (CIBER) Fisiopatología de la Obesidad y Nutrición (CIBEROBN), Instituto de Salud Carlos III (ISCIII), Málaga, Spain

Andrea G. Izquierdo and Ana B. Crujeiras
Epigenomics in Endocrinology and Nutrition Group, Instituto de Investigacion Sanitaria (IDIS), Complejo Hospitalario Universitario de Santiago (CHUS/SERGAS), Santiago de Compostela, Spain
CIBER Fisiopatologia de la Obesidad y Nutricion (CIBERobn), Madrid, Spain

Pedro R. Pereira, Tiago Morais, Sofia S. Pereira and Mariana P. Monteiro
Endocrine, Cardiovascular and Metabolic Research, Unit for Multidisciplinary Research in Biomedicine, University of Porto, Porto, Portugal
Department of Anatomy, Abel Salazar Institute of Biomedical Sciences, University of Porto, Porto, Portugal

Marta Guimarães
Endocrine, Cardiovascular and Metabolic Research, Unit for Multidisciplinary Research in Biomedicine, University of Porto, Porto, Portugal
Department of Anatomy, Abel Salazar Institute of Biomedical Sciences, University of Porto, Porto, Portugal
Department of General Surgery, Centro Hospitalar de Entre o Douro e Vouga, Santa Maria da Feira, Portugal

Mário Nora
Department of Anatomy, Abel Salazar Institute of Biomedical Sciences, University of Porto, Porto, Portugal
Department of General Surgery, Centro Hospitalar de Entre o Douro e Vouga, Santa Maria da Feira, Portugal

Belén Pérez-Pevida
Section of Investigative Medicine, Division of Diabetes, Endocrinology and Metabolism, Imperial College London, Hammersmith Campus, London, United Kingdom
Department of Endocrinology and Nutrition, Clínica Universidad de Navarra, Pamplona, Spain

Javier Escalada and Gema Frühbeck
Department of Endocrinology and Nutrition, Clínica Universidad de Navarra, Pamplona, Spain
Biomedical Research Networking Center for Physiopathology of Obesity and Nutrition (CIBEROBN), ISCIII, Pamplona, Spain
Obesity and Adipobiology Group, Instituto de Investigación Sanitaria de Navarra (IdiSNA), Pamplona, Spain

Alexander D. Miras
Section of Investigative Medicine, Division of Diabetes, Endocrinology and Metabolism, Imperial College London, Hammersmith Campus, London, United Kingdom

Ivania M. Rizo and Caroline M. Apovian
Section of Endocrinology, Diabetes, Nutrition, and Weight Management, Boston University School of Medicine and Boston Medical Center, Boston, MA, United States

Ariela Goldenshluger, Tamar Maor and Yftach Gepner
Department of Epidemiology and Preventive Medicine, Sackler Faculty of Medicine, School of Public Health, Sylvan Adams Sports Institute, Tel-Aviv University, Tel-Aviv, Israel

Renana Via-Kagan and Orly Zelekha
Israel Center for Disease Control, Ministry of Health, Jerusalem, Israel

Ju Hun Oh and Jung Ho Nam
Brain Korea 21 PLUS Project for Medical Science, Yonsei University, College of Medicine, Seoul, South Korea
Department of Internal Medicine, Endocrinology, Institute of Endocrine Research, Yonsei University College of Medicine, Seoul, South Korea

Chan Woo Kang, Eun Kyung Wang, Soohyun Lee, Eun Jig Lee and Cheol Ryong Ku
Department of Internal Medicine, Endocrinology, Institute of Endocrine Research, Yonsei University College of Medicine, Seoul, South Korea

Kyeong Hye Park
Division of Endocrinology and Metabolism, Department of Internal Medicine, National Health Insurance Service Ilsan Hospital, Goyang, South Korea

Arthur Cho
Department of Nuclear Medicine, Yonsei University College of Medicine, Seoul, South Korea

Sofie Ahlin
Department of Molecular and Clinical Medicine, Institute of Medicine, The Sahlgrenska Academy at the University of Gothenburg, Gothenburg, Sweden
Department of Medical and Surgery Sciences, Fondazione Policlinico Universitario A. Gemelli Istituto di Ricovero e Cura a Carattere Scientifico (IRCCS), Rome, Italy

Consuelo Cefalo, Esmeralda Capristo and Luca Marini
Department of Medical and Surgery Sciences, Fondazione Policlinico Universitario A. Gemelli Istituto di Ricovero e Cura a Carattere Scientifico (IRCCS), Rome, Italy

Isabel Bondia-Pons and Kajetan Trošt
Research Department, Steno Diabetes Center, Gentofte, Denmark

Montserrat Romero and Antonio Zorzano
Departament de Bioquímica i Biomedicina Molecular, Facultat de Biologia, Universitat de Barcelona, Barcelona, Spain
Institute for Research in Biomedicine (IRB Barcelona), Barcelona Institute of Science and Technology (BIST), Barcelona, Spain
CIBERDEM, Centro de Investigación Biomédica en Red (CIBER) de Diabetes y Enfermedades Metabólicas Asociadas, Barcelona, Instituto de Salud Carlos III, Barcelona, Spain

Amalia Gastaldelli
Cardiometabolic Risk Laboratory, Institute of Clinical Physiology, Consiglio Nazionale delle Ricerche (CNR), Pisa, Italy

John J Nolan
Research Department, Steno Diabetes Center, Gentofte, Denmark
Department of Clinical Medicine, Trinity College, Dublin, Ireland

Wenwen Yue, Wenjing Zhang and Xu Liu
School of Nursing and Rehabilitation, Cheeloo College of Medicine, Shandong University, Jinan, China

Xin Huang, Teng Liu and Shaozhuang Liu
Division of Bariatric and Metabolic Surgery, Department of General Surgery, Qilu Hospital of Shandong University, Jinan, China

Shumin Li
Center for Reproductive Medicine, Cheeloo College of Medicine, Shandong University, Jinan, China
Key Laboratory of Reproductive Endocrinology of Ministry of Education, Shandong University, Jinan, China

Yian Zhao and Jiaxin Shu
Cheeloo College of Medicine, Shandong University, Jinan, China

Weihua Li
Operating Theater, Qilu Hospital of Shandong University, Jinan, China

Index

A

Adiponectin, 5, 10, 26, 35, 42, 51, 87, 91, 106, 139, 141, 150, 152, 155, 160, 168, 186-187, 190, 201

Adipose Tissue, 1-2, 4, 6-11, 13-15, 17, 22, 26, 34-35, 44, 48-55, 71, 77, 86-87, 91, 93, 96, 102-103, 107-108, 139, 148-151, 155, 160, 165-168, 170-173, 182-184, 186-187, 190, 196-197, 199-200, 211, 215-217, 219-222, 225-228

Adiposity, 17, 21, 25, 27, 34, 42, 44, 49, 51-52, 55, 61-62, 78, 88, 91, 146, 148-150, 159, 166, 172, 185-186, 189, 192, 201, 223

B

Bariatric Surgery, 6-8, 10-12, 18, 21-23, 28, 33, 42-47, 51-52, 55, 57-60, 62-64, 66, 72-92, 96-103, 105-111, 116-118, 120, 124-138, 140, 142, 145, 153-157, 159-163, 167-170, 172-175, 177-182, 187-195, 197-200, 202-207, 209-213, 215-219, 227-228, 230, 237-238

Berberine, 238

Bioactivity, 146, 157

Bioavailability, 18, 20

Bioinformatics, 228

C

Caloric Restriction, 4, 50, 90, 95, 139, 147, 150, 158, 183-184, 188, 219, 227

Calorie Restriction, 85, 183-184, 186, 188, 198

Cancer, 12-23, 43, 57, 127-128, 132-133, 135-137, 162, 167, 171-172, 181, 186, 196, 201, 212-213

D

Dexamethasone, 50, 54-55, 143, 147, 158

Diabetes, 4, 6-12, 17-18, 21-22, 24-33, 35-36, 38-49, 51-62, 64-66, 68-71, 77, 80-94, 99-100, 103-104, 110-111, 113, 115-130, 132-137, 140, 148, 153-163, 169-176, 178-182, 184, 187-196, 201-202, 205-206, 209-211, 218-221, 223, 227-228, 230, 235-238

Diabetes Mellitus, 17-18, 22, 24, 31, 38, 42, 46, 53, 56-60, 62, 69-70, 80-82, 84-85, 88-90, 93, 99, 103-104, 110-111, 113, 125, 135, 137, 140, 153-155, 163, 182, 187-192, 194, 201, 211, 230, 236

Diagnostics, 170

Diastolic Blood Pressure, 83, 206

Dissection, 141, 156

Dna Binding, 48

Dna Damage, 95

Doppler Ultrasound, 199

Drug Absorption, 117

Duodenum, 10, 27, 37, 71, 84, 87, 128, 139-140, 151, 154, 169, 175, 216

Dyslipidemia, 14, 58-59, 80, 83-84, 88, 93, 110-111, 113, 115, 137, 175-176, 196, 205-206

Dysregulation, 13-14, 19, 25, 47, 53, 72-75, 78, 146-147, 165, 167, 235

E

Ejection Fraction, 45

Electron Microscopy, 32

Electronic Health Records, 77

Embryogenesis, 95

Endometrial Cancer, 17-18, 22

Endoplasmic Reticulum Stress, 90

Endothelial Cells, 77

Endothelial Dysfunction, 25, 94, 98-99, 197, 201

Endotoxemia, 156

Endotoxin, 94, 99, 156

Enterocytes, 67, 87

Epidemiology, 22, 25, 41, 46, 61-62, 181, 201, 204, 237

Epigenetic Alterations, 95, 165, 171

G

Gestation, 52, 235

Glucose Tolerance, 5, 48, 51, 64-66, 70, 81, 86-87, 90, 125, 139, 155, 183, 187-188, 211, 214, 221, 227, 237

Glutamic Acid, 70, 87-88, 192-193, 222-225

Glutathione, 224

H

Hepatitis, 18

Hormone Levels, 141, 150, 157, 212, 236-238

Hyperlipidemia, 1, 43, 53, 62, 104, 117, 230

Hyperparathyroidism, 85, 151-152, 160-161

Hyperplasia, 18, 87, 90, 147, 185, 187

I

Immunohistochemistry, 3-5, 7

Immunosuppression, 46

L

Lesions, 12, 18, 23, 25, 36

Leucocyte, 39

Leukemia, 171

Lipid Profile, 83-84, 103, 138, 163, 178

M

Magnetic Resonance Imaging, 199

Minimally Invasive Surgery, 22

Mononuclear Cells, 165

P

Parathyroid, 89, 151, 160-161

Pathogenesis, 12, 26, 42, 44, 48, 53, 85, 124, 149, 165, 167, 182, 194, 230, 235-236

Positron Emission Tomography, 185, 211-212

Post-operative Period, 83-84, 86, 113, 121, 139, 183

Postoperative Complications, 20, 153

Precision Medicine, 167, 172

Pro-inflammatory Cytokines, 17, 93-94, 149

Prognosis, 16-19, 21, 131, 169-170, 173

Prostate Cancer, 196, 201

Proteomics, 171

Proximal Femur, 160

Q

Quality Of Life, 36, 45, 57, 77, 96, 100, 102-103, 115, 137-138, 158-159, 195-196, 200-202, 205, 208-210

R

Radiofrequency, 95

S

Stem Cell, 42, 219

Streptomycin, 129

Stress Response, 158

Surgery, 1-2, 5-13, 18-24, 26-47, 51-52, 55-60, 62-64, 66, 68, 72-92, 96-163, 167-170, 172-200, 202-238

Surgical Intervention, 22, 88, 96, 100, 116, 118, 140, 153, 169-170, 175

T

Triglycerides, 34-35, 83-84, 97, 111, 113, 176, 179-180

Tryptophan, 224, 226

Tumor Microenvironment, 22

Tumor Necrosis Factor, 93

Tumor Suppressor Genes, 17

Tumorigenesis, 19

U

Ulceration, 19, 123

Ulcers, 23, 84

Ultrasound, 34, 199

Ultrasound Imaging, 34

Univariate Analysis, 206

V

Visceral Adipose Tissue, 13, 17, 22, 34, 77, 93, 96, 165

Visceral Fat, 34, 44, 54, 87, 97, 100, 146, 148, 150, 159, 189, 196, 199, 202

W

Western Blot, 5, 7

Western Diet, 50

Wnt Signaling, 196, 201

Printed in the USA
CPSIA information can be obtained
at www.ICGtesting.com
LVHW080039211023
761596LV00010BA/1834